Advanced Tuberculosis Infection Prevention and Control Practices

Jacob Angara Sheehama
https://orcid.org/0000-0001-5085-6606
University of Namibia, Namibia

IGI Global
Scientific Publishing
Publishing Tomorrow's Research Today

Vice President of Editorial	Melissa Wagner
Director of Acquisitions	Mikaela Felty
Director of Book Development	Jocelynn Hessler
Production Manager	Mike Brehm
Cover Design	Jose Rosado

Published in the United States of America by
IGI Global Scientific Publishing
701 East Chocolate Avenue
Hershey, PA, 17033, USA
Tel: 717-533-8845 | Fax: 717-533-7115
Website: https://www.igi-global.com E-mail: cust@igi-global.com

Library of Congress Cataloging-in-Publication Data

LCCN: 2025022519 (CIP Data Pending)
ISBN13: 9798337334462
Isbn13Softcover: 9798337334479
EISBN13: 9798337334486
British Cataloguing in Publication Data
A Cataloguing in Publication record for this book is available from the British Library.

Table of Contents

Detailed Table of Contents

Despite the availability of effective diagnostic tools and curative therapies, tuberculosis continues to impose a disproportionate burden on marginalized populations across both low- and high-income countries. This chapter presents a comparative analysis of TB treatment practices and infection prevention strategies in rural, resource-constrained regions and in high-income, urban settings. It explores how structural limitations—such as weak healthcare infrastructure, poor access to diagnostics, and socioeconomic disparities—shape the delivery and effectiveness of TB care in rural areas. At the same time, it shows how the developed countries, more resourceful, continue to struggle with TB among the marginalized, control of drug-resistant strains, and long-term adherence. Based on case studies from Uganda, Canada, India, and Norway, the chapter demonstrates how various healthcare models adapt to the local epidemiological pressures.

Tuberculosis (TB) in prisons remains a critical public health challenge, with infection rates significantly higher than in the general population. Overcrowding, poor ventilation, malnutrition, and substance use increase the risk of TB transmission among inmates. Correctional facilities must implement effective screening, diagnosis, treatment adherence, and follow-up mechanisms to control the disease. This study examines the impact of prison conditions on TB transmission and evaluates existing interventions, using secondary data from sources like NCRB, WHO, and CDC.

The risk of healthcare workers (HCWs) contracting tuberculosis (TB) occupationally has been significantly elevated, with prevalence rates significantly higher than those of the general population. The most hazardous factors include poor ventilation, irregular use of personal protective equipment (PPE), underlying disease histories, working with multidrug-resistant TB, and long exposure to patients with an infectious disease. High-risk groups, such as laboratory technicians, nurses, and physicians, report prevalence rates of 2,006-6,468 per 100,000 individuals. This chapter goes into detail about how well infection-control measures, regular check-ups, tuberculosis preventive treatment (TPT), and self-care practices help reduce tuberculosis among healthcare workers. The chapter also discusses the administration functions, engineering measures, screening processes, and monitoring strategies for controlling tuberculosis among healthcare workers. The chapter provides practical solutions to the challenges of protecting healthcare workers and reducing the occupational tuberculosis burden.

Healthcare workers (HCWs) are at a heightened risk of tuberculosis (TB) infection due to frequent and prolonged exposure to infected individuals in clinical settings. This study investigates the occupational risk factors contributing to TB infection among HCWs by analyzing data collected from both healthcare and non-healthcare professionals across various workplace environments. The dataset included individuals from departments such as internal medicine, infection wards, intensive care units, and administrative offices, while also considering non-healthcare sectors like education and the service industry. Preprocessing ensured clean and structured data, followed by feature selection using Particle Swarm Optimization (PSO) to isolate the most influential variables. A Bi-Stacked Artificial Neural Network (ANN) model was employed to classify TB infection risk, demonstrating strong predictive performance by capturing nonlinear relationships between occupational exposure and infection status.

Tuberculosis (TB) continues to be one of the top 10 causes of death worldwide, despite being a preventable and curable disease. According to the World Health Organization (WHO), approximately 10.6 million people fell ill with TB in 2022, and 1.3 million died, highlighting a persistent global health burden. The ongoing challenges in TB control are compounded by the emergence of multidrug-resistant TB (MDR-TB), delayed diagnosis, insufficient infection control infrastructure, and the impact of social determinants of health. In healthcare and community settings alike, TB transmission remains a major concern, especially in high-burden countries. This chapter, titled "Innovative Strategies for Tuberculosis Infection Prevention and Control," aims to explore cutting-edge approaches, novel frameworks, and integrated interventions that are reshaping the landscape of TB prevention and containment. The proposal presents a comprehensive roadmap of how innovation, driven by science, technology, policy, and community engagement, can elevate the global response to TB infection control.

Tuberculosis (TB) remains a significant public health challenge, particularly among vulnerable populations such as migrants, slum dwellers, immunocompromised individuals, and those with limited access to formal healthcare. In India, a substantial proportion of individuals with TB-like symptoms first seek care at private pharmacies, which are often overlooked in national TB control efforts. This study aims to enhance TB diagnosis and screening among such populations by leveraging a public-private mix (PPM) model and advanced machine learning techniques. A comprehensive dataset was collected from pharmacy-linked patient interactions and preprocessed for quality and consistency. Feature selection was conducted using Ant Colony Optimization (ACO) to identify key predictors. A Bi-Stacked Long Short-Term Memory (LSTM) model was then applied to capture sequential patterns in patient data and improve diagnostic accuracy.

This chapter explores the prevalence and burden of tuberculosis (TB) within prisons and correctional facilities, emphasizing the disproportionate rates of infection compared to the general population. It analyzes contributing factors such as overcrowding, poor ventilation, limited healthcare access, and co-existing vulnerabilities like HIV and substance abuse. The chapter further discusses the transmission dynamics of TB in these confined environments and the implications for public health beyond prison walls. Strategies for TB prevention, diagnosis, treatment, and continuity of care are examined, highlighting global best practices and policy recommendations. Special attention is given to the challenges posed by multidrug-resistant TB (MDR-TB) and the integration of prison health services into national TB control programs. Through data-driven insights and case examples, this chapter underscores the urgent need for comprehensive interventions to mitigate TB's impact on incarcerated populations and the broader community.

Tuberculosis (TB) remains a significant public health challenge across both rural and developed regions, though the nature and effectiveness of treatment practices vary widely. In rural settings, TB treatment is often hindered by limited access to healthcare services, diagnostic delays, poor adherence due to socioeconomic factors, and lack of health literacy. Conversely, developed countries exhibit structured treatment protocols, rapid diagnostics, and advanced monitoring systems, yet continue to face challenges such as drug-resistant TB strains and treatment among vulnerable populations like immigrants and the homeless. This study explores the disparities and commonalities in TB treatment practices using advanced data-driven methods. A dataset of global survey data was compiled and preprocessed to identify key variables influencing treatment success. Feature selection was performed using the REORA optimization algorithm, followed by analysis through a Bi-stacked LSTM model to capture deep, bidirectional patterns in treatment behaviors.

The emergence of drug-resistant tuberculosis and limitations of existing treatment regimens have underscored the urgent need for new therapeutic strategies. This chapter explores recent advancements in TB treatment, focusing on novel and repurposed drugs such as bedaquiline, delamanid, and pretomanid, along with the development of shorter, all-oral regimens. It reviews key clinical trials that have shaped current treatment guidelines and examines innovative drug delivery systems, including nanotechnology and inhaled therapies. The role of host-directed therapies, and supportive diagnostic innovations are also discussed. Challenges such as drug resistance and equitable access to new treatments are critically analysed. By highlighting ongoing research and global initiatives, the chapter emphasizes the potential of a multifaceted approach to transform TB care and contribute to global TB elimination efforts.

This chapter explores advancements in tuberculosis (TB) control, focusing on novel drugs, innovative clinical trial designs, and biotechnological breakthroughs. It highlights the transformative BPaL regimen, which shortens treatment for drug-resistant TB to six months with 90% success, alongside emerging drugs like TBAJ-876. Adaptive trial designs and real-world evidence enhance efficiency, while genomics, AI, and host-directed therapies (e.g., metformin, vitamin D) offer new therapeutic avenues. Challenges like resistance, access barriers, and ethical concerns are addressed, emphasizing equitable strategies. Public-private partnerships, such as the TB Alliance, drive progress, but diverse trial populations and rapid diagnostics are critical for global impact.

Pulmonary rehabilitation (PR) is a vital intervention for managing long-term respiratory complications that persist after tuberculosis (TB) treatment. Individuals recovering from TB often suffer from chronic dyspnea, reduced exercise tolerance, fatigue, and psychological issues, all of which contribute to a decreased quality of life. A multidisciplinary PR approach—including exercise training, inspiratory muscle strengthening, airway clearance techniques, nutritional support, and psychological counseling—has demonstrated significant benefits in improving functional capacity and alleviating symptoms. Randomized controlled trials and meta-analyses highlight the physiological and psychosocial improvements associated with PR in post-TB populations. Additionally, alternative delivery models such as community-based programs and telerehabilitation have shown promise, especially in resource-limited settings. Evidence supports the integration of PR into routine post-TB care to optimize recovery and enhance long-term health outcomes.

Preface

INTRODUCTION

As the editor of *Advanced Tuberculosis Infection Prevention and Control Practices*, I am honored to present this comprehensive resource, crafted to address one of the most persistent global health challenges: tuberculosis (TB). Despite significant strides in recent decades to combat TB, it remains endemic in many regions, with misdiagnosed, untreated or inadequately treated infectious cases driving ongoing transmission. Fundamental gaps in TB prevention and control, particularly in resource-constrained and high-burden settings, continue to undermine global efforts to end this disease. A critical barrier is the failure to systematically consider TB when individuals seek healthcare, leading to delayed or missed diagnoses and insufficient implementation of effective infection prevention and control (IPC) measures, including early and effective treatment.

This book is designed to complement the existing TB IPC practices and regulations established by Health Ministries and specialized institutions, such as correctional facilities and care homes for older adults. Its primary aim is to provide a robust scientific framework for TB infection prevention and control (TB-IPC) across diverse settings—health facilities, congregate environments, public spaces, and communities where the risk of TB transmission is elevated. The chapters within offer both technical and operational guidance, emphasizing the managerial activities and administrative controls necessary to strengthen TB-IPC at all levels of the health system.

Our goal is to equip a wide audience with the knowledge and tools to implement effective TB-IPC strategies at all times. This book is intended for frontline healthcare workers, health system officials overseeing TB, HIV/AIDS, and IPC programs, and managers of hospital services in both public and private sectors. It also serves officials in prison, police, and military services, as well as managers in private and state-owned enterprises responsible for the health and safety of their workforce. In essence, this resource is for everyone committed to reducing the burden of TB and safeguarding communities from its spread.

The development of this book has been a collaborative effort, drawing on the expertise of leading researchers, clinicians, and policymakers in the field of TB prevention and control. I extend my deepest gratitude to the contributors whose rigorous scholarship and practical insights have shaped this volume. It is my hope that *Advanced Tuberculosis Infection Prevention and Control Practices* will serve as a vital tool in the global fight against TB, fostering informed action and sustainable progress toward a world free of this disease.

ORGANIZATION OF THE BOOK

Chapter 1: TB Treatment Practice in Rural and Developed Countries

As the editor of this volume, I am pleased to introduce Chapter 1, which offers a comparative lens on tuberculosis (TB) treatment practices across rural, resource-constrained settings and high-income, urban environments. This chapter delves into the structural and socioeconomic barriers that shape TB care, such as limited diagnostic access and weak healthcare infrastructure in rural areas, contrasted with the challenges of managing drug-resistant TB and ensuring adherence among marginalized populations in developed countries. Drawing on case studies from Uganda, Canada, India, and Norway, the authors illustrate how diverse healthcare models adapt to local epidemiological pressures. This analysis underscores the critical need for tailored TB infection prevention and control (TB-IPC) strategies that address disparities while leveraging local strengths, providing actionable insights for health system planners and practitioners aiming to reduce TB transmission globally.

Chapter 2: Impact of Overcrowding on Tuberculosis Prevalence and Healthcare Accessibility in Prisons

In Chapter 2, we confront the alarming burden of TB in correctional facilities, where overcrowding, poor ventilation, and limited healthcare access create a perfect storm for disease transmission. This chapter examines how these conditions, compounded by malnutrition and substance use, drive TB prevalence rates far higher than in the general population. Using secondary data from authoritative sources like the National Crime Records Bureau (NCRB), World Health Organization (WHO), and Centers for Disease Control and Prevention (CDC), the authors identify critical gaps in screening, treatment continuity, and healthcare infrastructure, particularly during inmate transfers. The chapter proposes evidence-based policies and enhanced collaboration between prison authorities and public health agencies to strengthen TB-IPC. Its recommendations for strategic interventions offer practical solutions for mitigating TB risks in prisons, protecting both inmates and the broader community.

Chapter 3: Diagnosis and Screening of Tuberculosis in Vulnerable Populations and the Elderly

Chapter 3 focuses on the unique challenges of diagnosing and screening TB among vulnerable populations, including the elderly, incarcerated individuals, migrants, and those with HIV. These groups face heightened risks due to biological, social, and structural factors that complicate timely case detection. The authors highlight the limitations of current diagnostic approaches, despite advancements in molecular technologies, and advocate for context-specific screening protocols that address atypical presentations in elderly patients and systemic barriers in marginalized communities. By proposing integrated, community-based interventions and advanced diagnostics, this chapter aligns with the book's mission to enhance TB-IPC through equitable and accessible strategies. Its insights are vital for health workers and policymakers aiming to reduce TB transmission in high-risk settings.

Chapter 4: Battling Tuberculosis on the Frontlines: Protecting Healthcare Workers from Occupational TB

Chapter 4 shines a spotlight on the occupational risks faced by healthcare workers (HCWs), who are disproportionately affected by TB due to prolonged exposure in clinical settings. With prevalence rates among HCWs ranging from 2,006 to 6,468 per 100,000, this chapter details the hazards posed by poor ventilation, inconsistent use of personal protective equipment (PPE), and exposure to multidrug-resistant TB. It explores practical TB-IPC measures, including infection control protocols, regular screenings, TB preventive treatment (TPT), and self-care practices, to safeguard HCWs. The authors also address administrative and engineering controls, offering a comprehensive framework for reducing occupational TB burden. This chapter is essential for hospital managers and health officials seeking to protect frontline workers, a critical component of robust TB-IPC systems.

Chapter 5: A Data-Driven Framework to Assess TB Vulnerability in Healthcare Workforces

In Chapter 5, we explore a data-driven approach to understanding TB vulnerability among healthcare workers (HCWs), a key focus for effective TB-IPC. By analyzing data from diverse workplace environments, including healthcare and non-healthcare sectors, this study employs advanced computational methods—Particle Swarm Optimization (PSO) for feature selection and a Bi-Stacked Artificial Neural Network (ANN) model—to predict TB infection risk. The findings reveal critical occupational risk factors and demonstrate the power of predictive modeling in identifying high-risk groups. This chapter offers a forward-thinking framework for health system administrators to enhance TB-IPC by prioritizing targeted interventions for HCWs, ensuring safer clinical environments and reducing transmission risks.

Chapter 6: Innovative Strategies for Tuberculosis Infection Prevention and Control

Chapter 6 presents a compelling exploration of innovative strategies to combat TB, a disease that claimed 1.3 million lives in 2022 despite being preventable and curable. The authors address persistent challenges, including MDR-TB, delayed diagnoses, and inadequate infection control infrastructure, particularly in high-burden countries. This chapter introduces cutting-edge approaches—spanning scientific, technological, and policy-driven innovations—that strengthen TB-IPC in healthcare and community settings. By integrating novel frameworks and community engagement strategies, it provides a comprehensive roadmap for elevating global TB prevention efforts. This chapter is a must-read for practitioners and policymakers seeking transformative solutions to reduce TB transmission and achieve global control targets.

Chapter 7: Early TB Case Identification Using Sequential Deep Learning Models

Chapter 7 introduces an innovative approach to early TB case detection among vulnerable populations, such as migrants and slum dwellers, who often seek care at private pharmacies in high-burden settings like India. By leveraging a public-private mix (PPM) model and advanced machine learning—specifically, a Bi-Stacked Long Short-Term Memory (LSTM) model with Ant Colony Optimization (ACO) for feature selection—this study enhances diagnostic accuracy through sequential pattern analysis. This chapter underscores the importance of integrating technology into community-based TB-IPC strategies to improve early detection and reduce transmission. Its insights are particularly relevant for health officials and researchers aiming to bridge diagnostic gaps in informal healthcare settings.

Chapter 8: TB Diagnosis and Screening Among Vulnerable Populations: Bridging TB Detection Gaps Through Equity and Technology

Chapter 8 tackles the critical issue of TB diagnosis and screening in vulnerable groups, including refugees, prisoners, children, and people with HIV, where detection gaps exacerbate transmission risks. The authors review traditional and advanced diagnostic tools—such as GeneXpert, Truenat, and AI-assisted imaging—while emphasizing community-based and digital health solutions. Through case studies from high-burden countries, this chapter advocates for equitable, accessible diagnostics and intersectoral collaboration to support global TB elimination goals. Its focus on technology-driven, equity-focused TB-IPC strategies makes it an essential resource for health system planners and community health practitioners.

Chapter 9: Leveraging Media and Communication Strategies to Enhance Tuberculosis Prevention and Control Efforts

Chapter 9 explores the transformative potential of media and communication strategies in strengthening TB-IPC efforts. By examining the role of traditional and digital platforms in disseminating accurate information, reducing stigma, and promoting health-seeking behaviors, this chapter highlights the importance of culturally sensitive messaging. Through case studies and current literature, the authors evaluate the effectiveness of targeted campaigns across diverse contexts, offering best practices for integrating communication into TB control programs. This chapter is a vital guide for public health communicators and program managers aiming to enhance community engagement and reduce TB transmission through informed, inclusive strategies.

Chapter 10: Prevalence and Burden of Tuberculosis in Prisons and Correctional Facilities: Tuberculosis Infection Prevention and Practices

Chapter 10 delves into the heightened TB burden in prisons, where overcrowding, poor ventilation, and limited healthcare access drive infection rates far above those in the general population. The authors analyze transmission dynamics, compounded by vulnerabilities like HIV and substance abuse, and their implications for public health beyond prison walls. This chapter reviews global best practices for TB-IPC, including screening, diagnosis, treatment, and continuity of care, with a focus on addressing multidrug-resistant TB (MDR-TB). By offering data-driven insights and policy recommendations, it provides a blueprint for prison administrators and health officials to mitigate TB's impact in correctional settings and protect broader communities.

Chapter 11: AI-Driven Comparative Framework for TB Treatment Optimization in Diverse Settings

Chapter 11 presents a groundbreaking AI-driven framework to optimize TB treatment across rural and developed settings, addressing disparities in care delivery critical to TB-IPC. Using global survey data and advanced methods like the REORA optimization algorithm and Bi-stacked LSTM modeling, this study identifies key variables influencing treatment success. The authors highlight challenges in rural areas—such as diagnostic delays and poor adherence—while noting persistent issues in developed settings, including drug-resistant TB and treatment among vulnerable groups. This chapter offers health system planners and clinicians a data-driven approach to tailoring TB-IPC interventions, enhancing treatment outcomes, and reducing transmission in diverse contexts.

Chapter 12: New Drugs, Clinical Trials, and Innovations in Tuberculosis Treatment

Chapter 12 explores the evolving landscape of TB treatment, a critical component of TB-IPC, by focusing on novel and repurposed drugs like bedaquiline, delamanid, and pretomanid, alongside shorter, all-oral regimens. The authors review pivotal clinical trials, innovative drug delivery systems (e.g., nanotechnology, inhaled therapies), and host-directed therapies, while addressing challenges like drug resistance and equitable access. By highlighting global research initiatives, this chapter underscores the potential of multifaceted approaches to transform TB care and reduce transmission. It is an invaluable resource for clinicians, researchers, and policymakers driving TB elimination efforts.

Chapter 13: Pioneering TB Solutions: New Drugs, Clinical Trials, and the Power of Biotechnology

Chapter 13 showcases pioneering advancements in TB control, emphasizing novel drugs like the BPaL regimen and emerging agents such as TBAJ-876, which promise shorter, more effective treatments for drug-resistant TB. The authors explore innovative clinical trial designs, genomics, AI, and host-directed therapies (e.g., metformin, vitamin D), while addressing challenges like resistance and access disparities. Public-private partnerships, such as the TB Alliance, are highlighted as drivers of progress. This chapter offers a forward-looking perspective on integrating biotechnology into TB-IPC, making it essential for researchers and health officials aiming to reduce TB transmission through cutting-edge solutions.

Chapter 14: The Role of Pulmonary Rehabilitation in the Restoration of Respiratory Function After Tuberculosis

Chapter 14 highlights the critical role of pulmonary rehabilitation (PR) in addressing post-TB respiratory complications, an often-overlooked aspect of TB-IPC that supports long-term health outcomes. The authors detail how chronic dyspnea, reduced exercise capacity, and psychological issues impact quality of life in TB survivors, and how multidisciplinary PR—encompassing exercise, inspiratory muscle training, and psychosocial support—improves functional recovery. Evidence from randomized trials and meta-analyses supports PR's integration into routine post-TB care, with alternative delivery models like telerehabilitation showing promise in resource-limited settings. This chapter is essential for clinicians and rehabilitation specialists aiming to enhance post-TB recovery and reduce the broader burden of TB.

CONCLUSION

As the editor of *Advanced Tuberculosis Infection Prevention and Control Practices*, I am profoundly encouraged by the collective expertise and innovative solutions presented in this volume, which together form a robust blueprint for tackling one of the world's most enduring public health challenges: tuberculosis (TB). The chapters within this book illuminate the multifaceted nature of TB prevention and control, addressing critical gaps in diagnosis, treatment, and infection control across diverse settings—from rural communities and high-income urban centers to prisons and healthcare facilities. By exploring cutting-edge diagnostic technologies, novel treatment regimens, data-driven frameworks, and community-based interventions, this work underscores the importance of tailored, equitable, and evidence-based strategies to curb TB transmission. The contributions also highlight the urgent need to protect vulnerable populations, including healthcare workers, incarcerated individuals, migrants, and the elderly, while emphasizing the transformative potential of biotechnology, media campaigns, and pulmonary rehabilitation in strengthening TB infection prevention and control (TB-IPC).

This volume is more than a compendium of research; it is a call to action for all stakeholders—frontline health workers, policymakers, prison administrators, private sector managers, and community advocates—to unite in a shared mission to end the TB epidemic. By integrating the scientific, operational, and policy insights offered here, we can bridge systemic gaps, overcome resource constraints, and address social determinants that perpetuate TB's spread. My hope is that this book will serve as a vital resource, inspiring and equipping readers to implement effective TB-IPC measures that safeguard communities and move us closer to the World Health Organization's goal of a TB-free world by 2030. I extend my heartfelt gratitude to the contributors whose dedication and scholarship have made this work possible, and to you, the reader, for joining us in this critical endeavor.

Chapter 1
TB Treatment Practice in Rural and Developed Countries

S. Ida Evangeline
https://orcid.org/0000-0003-2997-7897
Government College of Engineering, Tirunelveli, India

ABSTRACT

Despite the availability of effective diagnostic tools and curative therapies, tuberculosis continues to impose a disproportionate burden on marginalized populations across both low- and high-income countries. This chapter presents a comparative analysis of TB treatment practices and infection prevention strategies in rural, resource-constrained regions and in high-income, urban settings. It explores how structural limitations—such as weak healthcare infrastructure, poor access to diagnostics, and socioeconomic disparities—shape the delivery and effectiveness of TB care in rural areas. At the same time, it shows how the developed countries, more resourceful, continue to struggle with TB among the marginalized, control of drug-resistant strains, and long-term adherence. Based on case studies from Uganda, Canada, India, and Norway, the chapter demonstrates how various healthcare models adapt to the local epidemiological pressures.

INTRODUCTION

Tuberculosis remains one of the most enduring and lethal infectious diseases of modern times, despite the availability of effective diagnostics, treatment, and prevention tools. In 2023 alone, TB was responsible for an estimated 1.3 million deaths and over 10 million new cases worldwide. It is a disease deeply intertwined

DOI: 10.4018/979-8-3373-3446-2.ch001

with poverty, structural inequality, and health system weaknesses. The World Health Organization (WHO) has always been aware of this and with the help of the End TB Strategy, promotes a global vision for the reduction of TB deaths by 95% and cases by 90% by 2035 in comparison with 2015. Although global efforts and biomedical advances have taken significant steps towards these aims, the burden of TB is not evenly spread – between and within countries (Vasiliu et al. 2024).

A particularly striking contrast exists between TB treatment practices and outcomes in rural, low-resource areas of low- and middle-income countries and the urbanized, technologically advanced settings of high-income nations. In the rural areas barriers like poor health infrastructure, geographic isolation, lack of healthcare workers and poor drug supply chains hinder the TB programs greatly. These challenges are usually exacerbated by deep-seated social determinants – malnutrition, stigma, illiteracy, and poverty – that slow down diagnosis and erode treatment adherence (Meintjes & Maartens, 2024).

Meanwhile, developed countries, while benefiting from advanced healthcare systems and strong policy frameworks, are not immune to TB challenges. In such settings, TB tends to be sustained among the marginalized populations like migrants, the homeless, incarcerated populations, and those with substance use disorders. These groups are socially excluded, they have less access to care, and they are at a higher risk of drug-resistant TB – issues that require special, often multi-sectoral treatment and infection control measures (Coussens et al. 2024).

This chapter sets out to compare and critically examine TB treatment practices across these two broad settings—rural regions and developed countries—with a special focus on how systemic, clinical, and societal factors influence TB control efforts. It will explore how infection prevention and control (IPC) measures are designed and implemented in divergent resource settings, and how creative models like digital adherence tools, community-based care, and integrated health services can improve treatment outcomes.

Drawing on real-world case studies, WHO technical guidance, peer-reviewed research, and lessons from global health programs, the chapter aims to present a nuanced and actionable framework for TB control. At the core of this analysis is the claim that even though the principles of TB care – early diagnosis, effective treatment, patient support, and prevention of transmission – are universal, their implementation requires local adaptation. The chapter argues for equity-oriented, adaptable TB treatment practices that are sensitive to the socio-economic and infrastructural realities of the people they serve.

Ultimately, the goal of this chapter is to inform policymakers, practitioners, and public health stakeholders about the importance of contextualizing TB treatment and IPC efforts, thereby contributing to more inclusive, effective, and sustainable strategies to end TB globally.

TB EPIDEMIOLOGY ACROSS CONTEXTS

Tuberculosis remains a leading cause of illness and death from a single infectious agent, exceedingly even HIV/AIDS in global mortality. Yet, the distribution of TB is far from uniform. Its epidemiology is a coming together of biological susceptibility, performance of health system, and socio-economic inequality. Such an understanding of this distribution is very important in creating responsive treatment and prevention strategies.

Global Trends and Burden

According to the World Health Organization's Global TB Report (2023), over 85% of TB cases occur in low- and middle-income countries (LMICs), with the highest burdens concentrated in countries like India, Indonesia, China, the Philippines, Pakistan, Nigeria, Bangladesh, and the Democratic Republic of Congo. These countries are not only responsible for most of the cases in the world but also characterize sharp disparities within- especially between urban and rural areas. In rural settings, where there is a poor infrastructure for primary care, poor disease surveillance, and use of traditional healers or informal providers, underdiagnosis and undertreatment often occur, and the disease spreads silently (Yerezhepov et al. 2024).

Delayed diagnosis is a hallmark of TB in rural settings. In rural districts of Sub-Saharan Africa or South Asia, it is not uncommon for the patients to wait weeks or months for a confirmed diagnosis because of the lack of diagnostic labs or workers with TB symptom recognition skills. This delay not only makes the severe disease progression and death more likely but also allows for the community-level transmission, especially in households with poor ventilation or crowded living conditions (Naidoo et al. 2024).

TB in High-Income Countries

In contrast, most high-income countries have successfully reduced overall TB incidence through decades of investment in housing, nutrition, public health, and universal health coverage. In countries like the United States, Canada, and Western Europe, the TB is currently a condition of particular high-risk groups. Epidemiological data show that an unfair proportion of TB cases from these countries are among immigrants from high-burden countries, indigenous population, HIV-positive individuals, and homeless or incarcerated persons (Guerrieri et al. 2024).

Urban centers in high-income countries often serve as focal points for TB outbreaks, especially in congregate settings like shelters, prisons, or poorly ventilated multi-family housing. For instance, transmission clusters among people with unstable housing in London and New York have led to outbreaks, where it is hard to follow the treatment and regular screening (Eisenhut et al. 2025).

The Challenge of Drug-Resistant TB

The emergence of drug-resistant TB (DR-TB) has added further complexity to the global epidemiological landscape. With a global threat to TB control, MDR-TB, which is resistant to both isoniazid and rifampicin, the most powerful first-line drugs, is a problem. Extensively drug-resistant TB (XDR-TB), which includes resistance to fluoroquinolones and second-line injectable drugs, is an even more difficult challenge because of scarce treatment regimens and poor outcomes (Farhat et al. 2024).

In rural areas of LMICs, DR-TB is often underdiagnosed because of the absence of advanced laboratory diagnostics such as GeneXpert or line probe assays. This results in empirical treatment on symptoms instead of resistance profiles, which does not only cure, but also spreads resistance. On the other hand, high-income countries have the capacity to detect and treat DR-TB, but they struggle with logistical and ethical issues of dealing with imported cases, long-term follow-up in mobile populations, and adherence to treatment in socially vulnerable groups (Schwab et al. 2024).

Implications for Control Strategies

The epidemiological divergence between rural LMICs and high-income countries necessitates differentiated approaches to TB control. Although rural environments lack increased diagnostic ability, community-based screening, and decentralization of care, high-income nations call for focused outreach for at-risk populations and latent TB infection management. In both settings, the social determinants of TB – poverty, stigma, housing insecurity, and malnutrition – continue to be pivotal in reducing the spread and successful treatment of TB.

This epidemiological perspective offers the initial perspective for discussing health system responses, innovations, and policy strategies of the following chapters.

HEALTHCARE INFRASTRUCTURE AND ACCESS

The ability to diagnose, treat, and prevent tuberculosis hinges critically on the strength and accessibility of a country's healthcare infrastructure. There is, however, an enormous difference between rural health systems of low-resources countries and urban healthcare networks of high-income countries. These imbalances are reflected in trained personnel, physical infrastructure, necessary medicines and referral systems – which ultimately determines the course of TB care and control.

Rural Settings in Low-Resource Environments

In many low- and middle-income countries, rural health systems remain underfunded, fragmented, and geographically dispersed. Basic facilities such as electricity, running water, or refrigeration are usually absent from the primary healthcare facilities in remote villages – making it even hard to provide the most basic health services. These clinics are likely to be staffed by a single nurse or community health worker (CHW) who has to cover a vast array of conditions, usually without any specific training in TB diagnosis and treatment (Olawade et al. 2024).

Referral systems are weak or non-existent, making it difficult to escalate suspected TB cases to district or regional hospitals where diagnostic tools like GeneXpert or chest X-ray might be available. Patients often have to travel long distances and pay out-of-pocket transport costs, leading to diagnostic delay and non-attendance. These barriers do not only impact individual outcomes, but they also contribute to community-level transmission because of untreated or insufficiently treated cases (Rahmatullah et al. 2025).

Inconsistent drug supply chains further weaken TB treatment in rural areas. Stockouts of the first-line anti-TB medications are not a rare event, and once drug regimens are interrupted, the risk of treatment failure and drug resistance skyrockets. Also, the absence of standardized recordkeeping makes it hard to follow up patient's outcomes or continuity of care during referral.

Urban and Developed Health Systems

In contrast, healthcare systems in high-income countries are characterized by integrated networks of specialized hospitals, diagnostic laboratories, electronic medical record systems, and a robust health workforce. Such systems allow for quick identification of the TB cases, tracing the contacts, and adherence promotion. Multidisciplinary TB teams, such as pulmonologists, infectious disease specialists, social workers, and case managers, are able to develop individualized care plans, especially for patients with complex social or medical needs (Chilala et al. 2024).

However, despite these structural advantages, access gaps still exist. Immigrants and refugees often face linguistic, legal, or cultural barriers when navigating unfamiliar healthcare systems. Homeless, or those who use drugs, may distrust medical institutions or have unstable contact information, which causes the breaks in the treatment. These access problems are frequently exacerbated by bureaucratic barriers, such as requirements for residence documents or insurance qualification, that slow down or discourage care (MacPherson et al. 2024).

Decentralization and Task-Shifting Strategies

To improve access in rural and underserved regions, many countries have adopted decentralization strategies that aim to bring TB services closer to the community. This involves empowering CHWs to perform TB screening, provide medications, and monitor adherence to treatment with supervisory frameworks. Task-shifting with adequate resource and regulation can significantly increase access in regions with limited trained clinicians (Okoroafor & Christmals, 2024).

In cities of developed nations, mobile TB units and outreach clinics have been employed to target high-risk populations, including the homeless or imprisoned. These services usually work hand in hand with shelters, community organizations and public health departments to provide follow up and continuity of care (Das et al. 2025).

Leveraging Technology and Integration

Telemedicine, digital adherence tools, and electronic health records offer promising avenues to overcome infrastructure limitations. In the rural settings, mobile phone-based tools can link patients to distant clinicians and allow supervision via video DOT. In urban settings, electronic warning systems can inform public health officials about the missed appointments or the emerging case clusters (Gilmour & Alene, 2024).

Finally, the integration of TB care into broader primary health services—including maternal-child health, HIV care, and chronic disease management—has emerged as a best practice. This integration does not only strengthen overall health systems, but it also reduces stigma through normalizing TB care in routine health interaction.

DIAGNOSTIC AND TREATMENT CAPABILITIES

Reliable diagnosis and effective treatment form the backbone of tuberculosis control. But the abilities to diagnose and treat TB are incomparably different in rural, low-resource settings and the health systems of developed countries. These variations affect not only the rate and accuracy of diagnosis but also the quality of treatment, monitoring, and results.

Diagnostic Gaps in Rural Settings

In rural areas of low- and middle-income countries, access to high-quality TB diagnostics remains limited. The majority of health centers continue using the sputum smear microscopy, a method that was developed more than a century ago. As much as it is cheap, it is not sensitive especially in patients with HIV co-infection, children and extrapulmonary TB. In addition, smear microscopy does not identify drug resistance.

Advanced diagnostic tools such as GeneXpert MTB/RIF—endorsed by the WHO for rapid detection of TB and rifampicin resistance—are increasingly available but still concentrated in urban centers or district-level facilities. Their application in rural clinics is limited by the necessity to have stable electricity, temperature control, maintenance, and trained personnel. Consequently, most rural patients have to travel long distances or wait for a long time before they receive their test results which in turn delays or lead to loss to follow-up (Ye et al. 2024).

Comprehensive Diagnostic Systems in High-Income Countries

Developed countries typically benefit from well-resourced diagnostic infrastructure. Suspected TB patients are quickly assessed with a mix of chest radiography, GeneXpert, liquid culture, and molecular drug susceptibility testing. Laboratories can identify the drug-sensitive and drug-resistant strains in a matter of days. Such advanced techniques as line probe assays, whole-genome sequencing, and interferon gamma release assays (IGRAs) are not only diagnostic tools but tools for epidemiological surveillance and outbreak investigations.

These countries also benefit from quality control systems, centralized electronic surveillance platforms, and effective sample transport networks – facilities that are hardly found in rural LMICs. However, even in such settings, missed opportunities can be observed because of the inexperience of providers, low suspicion in non-endemic regions, or lack of awareness among the at-risk populations (Assefa et al. 2024).

Treatment Regimens and Drug Access

Globally, the standard regimen for drug-sensitive TB includes a six-month course of isoniazid, rifampicin, pyrazinamide, and ethambutol. Although these drugs are commonly prescribed, availability and constant supply of these drugs is a challenge in most rural set ups. Repeated drug stockouts, absence of fixed-dose combination pills, and poor storage of the drugs undermines the quality of treatment. Furthermore, when patients are not treated following confirmatory testing, inappropriate regimens may be used and the risk of resistance will be enhanced.

For drug-resistant TB (DR-TB), treatment is far more complex. Second-line drugs like bedaquiline, delamanid, linezolid and clofazimine need to be monitored closely for side effects and patterns of resistance. Rural facilities are generally unable to provide such care safely and to perform the required baseline and follow-up lab investigations. In addition, the newer, shorter all-oral regimens have not been integrated into national protocols by many countries hence continued use of poisonous injectable drugs.

In contrast, developed countries can provide individualized DR-TB regimens supported by laboratory diagnostics, regular blood work, and therapeutic drug monitoring. The patients are supported through case managers, social workers, and financial subsidies. However, high costs of treatment and social determinants (e.g., homelessness, immigration status) may still interfere with care continuity, even in resource-abundant settings (Bausch et al. 2024).

Innovations in Diagnosis and Treatment Delivery

Promising developments are emerging to bridge diagnostic and treatment gaps. Portable, battery-operated diagnostic systems such as Truenat and mobile X-ray vans have proved successful among the hard-to-reach populations. Digital adherence tools such as SMS reminders, smart pill boxes, and video-supported DOT (vDOT) are flexible and minimize the load of both patients and health workers.

In both settings, simplified treatment regimens, such as the 4-month rifapentine-based regimen or the 6-month bedaquiline-based MDR-TB regimen, represent major breakthroughs. These shorter, less toxic regimens enhance adherence and decrease costs, and their implementation requires the investment in training, drug procurement systems, and regulatory changes (Goletti et al. 2024).

SOCIAL DETERMINANTS AND ADHERENCE CHALLENGES

The trajectory of tuberculosis is shaped not only by clinical care and biomedical interventions but also by the social environments in which people live, work, and seek treatment. The social determinants of health such as poverty, education, housing, stigma, and access to social services influence the TB infection risk and success of treatment deeply. These determinants play different in rural and developed contexts, but both are characterised by substantial barriers to sustained adherence and optimal outcomes.

Poverty and Structural Vulnerability

In rural areas of low- and middle-income countries, poverty is a persistent backdrop that exacerbates every stage of the TB care cascade. Malnutrition related to poor immunity increases susceptibility to TB and deteriorates clinical outcomes. Insufficient housing – particularly in multi generation homes – facilitates airborne transmission. Many patients are daily wage earners who cannot afford to miss work for clinic visits and out of pocket costs for transport, diagnostics, and supportive care, often go unrecorded but act as major barriers to adherence.

Even when TB services are offered free of charge, indirect costs remain a major barrier. Research has demonstrated that more than half of the TB-affected households in LMIC's experience catastrophic health expenditure, which is defined as expenditure that is beyond 20% of the annual household income. Lack of financial protection means that patients could delay seeking care, break treatment, or turn to uncontrolled private providers (Cintron et al. 2025).

Stigma and Psychological Barriers

TB-related stigma—rooted in fears of contagion, misconceptions about the disease, or its association with poverty and HIV—continues to obstruct care-seeking and adherence. In the rural areas, people may refuse diagnosis because of the fear of social isolation or discrimination by members of the community. TB may stigmatize women in a disproportionate manner, often affecting their marriage prospects or their reputation as a moral failing.

In developed countries, stigma often intersects with marginalization. Homeless, drug users, or HIV-positive people might internalize shame or stay away from healthcare facilities because of their past experiences of neglect or discrimination. For the undocumented immigrants, the fear of deportation may also postpone or disrupt TB care (Nasir et al. 2024).

Health Literacy and Patient Engagement

Low levels of health literacy can affect patients' understanding of TB as a curable disease and the importance of completing long treatment courses. In a number of contexts, patients can feel better within a few weeks and stop taking medicines without knowing about the risk of relapse or resistance. The complicated instructions, language barriers, or lack of trust in health workers can aggravate these issues.

In urban, high-income countries, patients may disengage due to complex health systems, poor communication, or lack of culturally competent services. It is important to make treatment plans patient-friendly and linguistically appropriate and complemented with sufficient counseling for adherence (Chauhan et al. 2024).

Adherence Support: From DOT to Digital Tools

Directly Observed Therapy, where a healthcare worker watches patients take their medication, has been a cornerstone of TB programs since the 1990s. Although it is able to enhance adherence, DOT is laborious, generally inconvenient, and can be seen as coercive. In rural areas, daily traveling to a clinic might not be possible; in the cities, it could conflict with working hours or be stigmatizing.

In response, digital adherence technologies (DATs) have been developing. These include:

- 99DOTS: A cheap system in which patients confirm taking medication by dialing toll free numbers.
- Video DOT (vDOT): Patients record or livestream themselves taking medication with mobile apps.
- Electronic pillboxes: Devices that record when pills are taken and send the information to providers.

Such tools provide more autonomy and decrease the pressure on health workers, while at the same time allowing remote monitoring and timely interventions when doses are missed. However, access to mobile devices, network coverage, and digital literacy has to be taken into consideration in implementation (Chen et al. 2024).

Community and Psychosocial Interventions

Community oriented models (treatment supporters, peer educators, TB clubs) have been found effective in rural and urban areas. These models develop trust, eliminate isolation and establish accountability. Nutritional support, mental health counseling, and housing assistance are other enablers of adherence, particularly for the vulnerable patients in high-income countries.

The inclusion of TB services within larger social protection efforts, like conditional cash transfer, food rations, or job training, can address the underlying reasons for non-adherence and improve long-term recoveries (Fuady et al. 2024).

INFECTION PREVENTION AND CONTROL PRACTICES

Infection prevention and control is a critical yet often under-implemented pillar in the management of tuberculosis, particularly in healthcare and congregate settings where transmission risk is heightened. Good IPC does not only ensure the safety of patients and caregivers but also helps achieve wider public health objectives by breaking the chain of transmission. With such clear international guidance available – such as the WHO's TB IPC policy – implementation is uneven across health systems, with vast differences between rural health centres in low-income countries to tertiary care facilities in high-income settings.

In rural and under-resourced environments, IPC faces fundamental challenges rooted in infrastructural and systemic limitations. Many rural health clinics lack even the most basic conditions conducive to infection control. Clinics are often overcrowded, poorly ventilated, and structurally incapable of supporting patient isolation. The lack of designated triage areas makes it hard to isolate the coughing or symptomatic patients from the rest. In addition, there is usually a shortage of personal protective gears like masks and respirators and even where the resources are available, they will be ineffective due to lack of training among healthcare workers. This shortcoming is made worse by the poor awareness of the IPC protocols, lack of adequate staff supervision, and the poor administrative control. Routine surveillance and effective occupational health measures are lacking in such settings, exposing the healthcare workers to TB frequently, with high rates of latent TB infection and occupational transmission as a result (Marme et al. 2024).

In contrast, health systems in high-income countries are typically equipped with a full range of IPC measures. Modern hospitals have purpose-built isolation rooms with negative-pressure ventilation systems, centralized air filtration with HEPA technology, and systems in place to identify and isolate suspected TB patients rapidly. Such facilities typically incorporate TB risk assessments into standard hospital triage and always have the same PPE requirements including N95 respirator use with annual fit testing. In addition, there is usually a robust institutional support for occupational health services such as regular screening for TB and post-exposure protocols for healthcare workers. However, IPC implementation is not equally strong in all settings. Congregate settings like shelters, prisons, and long-term care facilities tend to be behind when it comes to the use of TB-specific IPC, and low disease awareness in these non-specialist settings may lead to delayed identification and response to outbreaks.

The COVID-19 pandemic inadvertently accelerated the adoption of airborne infection control practices globally. Measures such as universal masking, improved hand hygiene, triage algorithms, and enhanced ventilation—once considered challenging to implement in low-resource settings—became more commonplace. These developments offer an opportunity to develop cross disease IPC strategies that are beneficial to TB control. For example, clinics that adopted natural ventilation or open-air triage tents for COVID-19 are now better prepared to use similar measures for TB. Additionally, mass PPE use and IPC training during the pandemic has enhanced the baseline level of awareness among health workers, and made the situation more conducive for adopting TB-specific IPC. Although there is progress, sustainable implementation of IPC takes conscious efforts and policy commitment and contextual adaptation. Examples of innovations that can be adapted to resource-limited settings include low-cost ultraviolet germicidal irradiation systems, cough-monitoring protocols, and redesign of facilities for better airflow. Capacity-building programs that involve on-site mentorship, simplified IPC checklists, and mobile supervision have worked well to enhance compliance and accountability. Notably, IPC should not be considered as an independent intervention that should be incorporated into national TB programs, aligned with the wider health system's objectives, and financed and trained through the dedicated pipelines (van der Westhuizen et al. 2024).

Overall, the technical knowledge for TB IPC is available, but the challenge is filling the gap between the implementation in diverse settings. Customizing IPC interventions to local realities of health systems – be they in terms of infrastructure improvements for rural clinics or targeted interventions in urban shelters – can deliver substantial improvements in controlling TB transmission and safeguarding vulnerable populations.

CASE STUDIES

To illustrate the real-world implications of TB treatment disparities and infection prevention efforts, this section presents case studies from both rural and developed contexts. These exemplify ways in which local challenges and adaptive strategies determine TB care outcomes.

Rural Uganda: Community-Based DOT and Health Worker Shortages

In Uganda's rural districts, community-based directly observed therapy (CB-DOT) has been deployed to increase treatment access. Community health workers (CHWs) are trained and they make visits to patients at home to administer daily medication and counseling. Although CB-DOT has enhanced the adherence and completion rates, the program suffers from chronic problems like disrupted supply of drugs, high attrition levels of CHWs because of low incentives, and lack of accurate diagnostic tools. Lack of good IPC measures in local clinics leads to high rates of TB transmission among patients and staff (Kakande et al. 2024).

Urban Canada: TB Control in Homeless Populations

In cities like Toronto, TB outbreaks have occurred within homeless shelters, prompting a public health response involving mobile chest X-ray units, rapid diagnostics, and enhanced contact tracing. Integration of social services with the TB care (such as providing housing support and substance use treatment) has been central in enhancing adherence. Nevertheless, stigma, transient populations, and mental health comorbidities still make it difficult to provide sustained care delivery even when advanced healthcare infrastructure is available (Ge et al. 2024).

India: Private Sector Engagement in Rural TB Control

In parts of rural India, the private healthcare sector plays a dominant role in TB diagnosis and treatment. Programs such as Public-Private Interface Agency (PPIA) model have integrated the informal providers with the national TB program. Through provision of free diagnostic tests and drug kits, and the incorporation of private practitioners in standardized protocols, treatment outcomes have been bettered. However, IPC is still a weak link and there are many small clinics that do not have ventilation or training on infection control (Jhaveri et al. 2024).

Norway: DR-TB Management in a High-Income Setting

Norway, with its low TB incidence, faces challenges managing imported multidrug-resistant TB (MDR-TB) cases. These cases are usually managed in special hospitals that have access to sophisticated diagnostics and second line drugs. Although cure rates are high, adherence support such as housing, translation services, and legal support is vital for positive outcomes, particularly for asylum seekers and migrant workers.

These case studies show how the resource constraints and the social complexities affect the TB control irrespective of the national income level. Solutions that are effective need to be locally tailored models that integrate clinical care with social and structural interventions (Storvig et al. 2024).

INNOVATIONS AND INTEGRATED MODELS

Amid the persistent challenges of TB treatment and infection control, both rural and developed settings have seen the emergence of innovative and integrated care models designed to improve access, adherence, and outcomes. These models utilize technology, community resources, and health system integration to provide more patient-centered, efficient, and context-sensitive solutions.

Digital Adherence Technologies

Technologies such as 99DOTS (a low-cost phone-based adherence system) and video DOT (vDOT) have gained traction as scalable alternatives to traditional DOT, especially during the COVID-19 pandemic. These tools enable remote monitoring of the intake of medication, which minimizes patient burden and increases convenience. Rural pilots in such countries as India and Ethiopia have demonstrated promising results in enhancing adherence, but a lack of digital literacy and infrastructure are obstacles (Chilala et al. 2025).

Mobile and Decentralized Diagnostic Services

To overcome geographic barriers in rural areas, mobile diagnostic units equipped with digital chest X-rays and GeneXpert machines have been deployed in regions like South Africa and Bangladesh. These services take early detection to the underserved communities, thus allowing for prompt treatment initiation and community transmission prevention (Zulu et al. 2024).

Public-Private Mix Models

Recognizing the role of informal and private providers in TB care, especially in rural and urban LMICs, public-private mix approaches have been formalized. These models encourage private providers to report cases and follow the national guidelines and send patients to public health programs for free diagnoses and drugs, increasing quality and continuity of care (Vidyasagaran et al. 2024).

Integrated TB-HIV and Primary Healthcare Services

In settings with high co-infection rates, such as sub-Saharan Africa, integrated TB-HIV services have streamlined care pathways and reduced mortality. Partnership with maternal and child health services, non-communicable disease (NCD) programs, and community-based care platforms has also enhanced case identification and minimized loss to follow-ups (Maseko et al. 2025).

Patient-Centered and Community-Based Care

Models that prioritize patient needs—such as home-based care, flexible treatment schedules, nutritional and psychosocial support—have shown better treatment adherence and satisfaction. Drugs in Peru and Nepal have managed to mobilize cured TB patients as peer supporters, thus creating community trust and curbing stigma.

Taken together, these innovations are a paradigm shift from vertical, facility-oriented TB control programs to horizontal, integrated and patient-responsive care models. However, their effectiveness relies on sustainable funding, local ownership, and integration with the wider health system goals (Martín et al. 2024).

POLICY IMPLICATIONS AND RECOMMENDATIONS

The complex interplay of social, structural, and clinical factors influencing TB treatment outcomes demands policy responses that are both adaptive and equity driven. Lessons from different environments – rural and developed – point to the need for policies that strike a balance between global standards and local realities.

Aligning with the WHO End TB Strategy

While the WHO End TB Strategy outlines universal goals—early diagnosis, effective treatment, patient support, and transmission prevention—its implementation must be tailored to context. In rural areas, it translates into increasing the capacity of primary healthcare, making decentralized diagnostic tools, and promoting community-based care. In high-income settings, it takes continuous focus on vulnerable populations and intersectoral collaboration to address social determinants (Junqueira-Kipnis et al. 2024).

Investing in Health System Resilience

Governments and partners must invest in strengthening health systems, especially in under-resourced rural regions. This entails ensuring there are infrastructure improvements, reliable drug supply chains, development of human resources and integrated service delivery platforms that bring together TB care with maternal health, HIV and chronic diseases programs (Nagarajan et al. 2024).

Institutionalizing Infection Prevention and Control

National TB programs should prioritize IPC as a core pillar, not a peripheral concern. IPC training, guidelines, and monitoring systems need to be standardized in all levels of care. Funding mechanisms should be able to support basic engineering controls, such as ventilation retrofits, and PPE provision, especially in remote clinics (Shorette & Phillips, 2024).

Scaling Innovations and Community Engagement

Policies should support the adoption and scaling of successful innovations—such as digital adherence tools and mobile diagnostic units—through regulatory flexibility and targeted investment. Community engagement should be institutionalized by institutionalizing support to patient advocates, peer educators and civil society participation in TB program governance (Getachew et al. 2024).

Strengthening Public-Private Collaboration

Formalizing the role of private and informal providers in TB care through public-private mix schemes can significantly improve case notification and treatment outcomes. Policy frameworks should contain incentives, accountability mechanisms and clear referral pathway to ensure quality care in all sectors (Vallipriya & Singh, 2025).

Cross-Border and Migrant TB Care Coordination

In high-income countries, TB in migrants and mobile populations requires policies of transnational care continuity, legal protection, and culturally competent services. Existing regional cooperation mechanisms need to be enhanced to guarantee continuity of care beyond borders (Kunst et al. 2025).

The end aim of these policy recommendations is to establish flexible, responsive TB programs that are based on the principles of equity, quality, and sustainability – whether in a rural village clinic or a metropolitan hospital.

CONCLUSION

Tuberculosis remains a global health challenge marked by stark inequalities in treatment and control outcomes across different settings. This chapter has looked at how rural areas, especially in low-income and middle-income countries and high-income urban health systems, struggle with unique but equally important barriers to effective TB care. Resource scarcity, disparities in access to healthcare, social determinants, and systemic weaknesses determine the course of TB treatment and control of infection in both settings.

The evidence presented underscores the critical need for context-sensitive approaches that adapt global TB guidelines to local realities. Rural areas need specific investments in diagnostic infrastructure, healthcare workers capacity, and community-based care models. At the same time, developed countries need to tackle TB among the vulnerable population through integrated services, social support, and policy coherence.

Just as significant is the need for the regular use of infection prevention and control measures that need to be integrated into the planning for the health system and facilitated by resources and training. Scalable ways forward to improve outcomes in any setting include innovations like digital adherence technologies, mobile diagnostics, and integrated service models.

Eventually, to close the global TB treatment gap, there is a need to move from the one-size-fits-all strategies to the flexible equity-based approaches that can prioritize the early detection, patient support, and transmission control. From diverse experiences and ensuring that policy is aligned to practice, we can move forward to a TB-free world.

REFERENCES

Assefa, D. G., Dememew, Z. G., Zeleke, E. D., Manyazewal, T., & Bedru, A. (2024). Financial burden of tuberculosis diagnosis and treatment for patients in Ethiopia: A systematic review and meta-analysis. *BMC Public Health, 24*(1), 260. DOI: 10.1186/s12889-024-17713-9 PMID: 38254019

Bausch, K., Mantica, G., Smith, E. J., Bartoletti, R., Bruyère, F., Cai, T., Geerlings, S., Kranz, J., Köves, B., Pilatz, A., Schubert, S., Veeratterapillay, R., Wagenlehner, F., Gupta, N., & Bonkat, G. (2024). Genitourinary tuberculosis: A brief manual for urologists on diagnosis and treatment from the European Association of Urology Urological Infections Panel. *European Urology Focus, 10*(1), 77–79. DOI: 10.1016/j.euf.2023.07.006 PMID: 37541917

Chauhan, A., Parmar, M., Dash, G. C., Chauhan, S., Sahoo, K. C., Samantaray, K., Sharma, J., Mahapatra, P., & Pati, S. (2024). Health literacy and tuberculosis control: Systematic review and meta-analysis. *Bulletin of the World Health Organization, 102*(6), 421–431. DOI: 10.2471/BLT.23.290396 PMID: 38812804

Chen, E. C., Owaisi, R., Goldschmidt, L., Maimets, I. K., & Daftary, A. (2024). Patient perceptions of video directly observed therapy for tuberculosis: A systematic review. *Journal of Clinical Tuberculosis and Other Mycobacterial Diseases, 35*, 100406. DOI: 10.1016/j.jctube.2023.100406 PMID: 38380432

Chilala, C. I., Foster, N., Bahukudumbi, S., Mohamed, M. S., Zary, M., Kafie, C., Patel, B., Gore, G., Schwartzman, K., Subbaraman, R., & Fielding, K. L. (2025). Implementation outcomes of tuberculosis digital adherence technologies: A scoping review using the RE-AIM framework. *BMJ Global Health, 10*(2), e016535. DOI: 10.1136/bmjgh-2024-016535 PMID: 39947715

Chilala, S. B., Silumbwe, A., Zulu, J. M., Tetui, M., Bulawayo, M., Chewe, M., & Hangoma, P. (2024). Individual, community and health systems factors influencing time to notification of tuberculosis: Situating software and hardware bottlenecks in local health systems. *BMC Health Services Research, 24*(1), 1–11. DOI: 10.1186/s12913-024-11697-3 PMID: 39415167

Cintron, C., Dauphinais, M. R., Du, X., Tabackman, A., Lenart, A., Laliberte, A., Dirksen, J., & Sinha, P. (2025). Enriching tuberculosis research by measuring poverty better: A perspective. *BMC Global and Public Health, 3*(1), 17. DOI: 10.1186/s44263-025-00127-z PMID: 39980069

Coussens, A. K., Zaidi, S. M., Allwood, B. W., Dewan, P. K., Gray, G., Kohli, M., Kredo, T., Marais, B. J., Marks, G. B., Martinez, L., Ruhwald, M., Scriba, T. J., Seddon, J. A., Tisile, P., Warner, D. F., Wilkinson, R. J., Esmail, H., Houben, R. M. G. J., Alland, D., & Yi, S. (2024). Classification of early tuberculosis states to guide research for improved care and prevention: An international Delphi consensus exercise. *The Lancet. Respiratory Medicine*, *12*(6), 484–498. DOI: 10.1016/S2213-2600(24)00028-6 PMID: 38527485

Das, S., Grant, L., & Fearon, D. (2025). Mapping the global landscape of task shifting and sharing: Trends, geographic disparities, and terminology from 1970 to 2022. *Critical Public Health*, *35*(1), 2501495. DOI: 10.1080/09581596.2025.2501495

Eisenhut, M., Shah, S., Kaba, O., Kara, M., Sütçü, M., Song, K. H., Kim, H. B., & Wang, M. (2025). Sensitivity of Immunodiagnostic Tests in Localized Versus Disseminated Tuberculosis—A Systematic Review of Individual Patient Data. *Tropical Medicine and Infectious Disease*, *10*(3), 70. DOI: 10.3390/tropicalmed10030070 PMID: 40137824

Farhat, M., Cox, H., Ghanem, M., Denkinger, C. M., Rodrigues, C., Abd El Aziz, M. S., Enkh-Amgalan, H., Vambe, D., Ugarte-Gil, C., Furin, J., & Pai, M. (2024). Drug-resistant tuberculosis: A persistent global health concern. *Nature Reviews. Microbiology*, *22*(10), 617–635. DOI: 10.1038/s41579-024-01025-1 PMID: 38519618

Fuady, A., Arifin, B., Yunita, F., Rauf, S., Fitriangga, A., Sugiharto, A., Yani, F. F., Nasution, H. S., Putra, I. W. G. A. E., Mansyur, M., & Wingfield, T. (2024). Stigma, depression, quality of life, and the need for psychosocial support among people with tuberculosis in Indonesia: A multi-site cross-sectional study. *PLOS Global Public Health*, *4*(1), e0002489. DOI: 10.1371/journal.pgph.0002489 PMID: 38190416

Ge, E., Brode, S., Macdonald, L., Li, L., Lou, W., Liu, J., & Wei, X. (2024, August). Exploring impacts of air pollution and greenness on progressions of latent and active tuberculosis to inform interventions. In *ISEE Conference Abstracts* (Vol. 2024, No. 1). DOI: 10.1289/isee.2024.0257

Getachew, A., Silumbwe, A., Maritim, P., Hangoma, P., Belete, A., & Zulu, J. M. (2024). An evaluation of community acceptability and adoption of the community-based TB care program using the diffusion of innovation model. *Journal of Community Systems for Health*, *1*(1). Advance online publication. DOI: 10.36368/jcsh.v1i1.1072

Gilmour, B., & Alene, K. A. (2024). Ending tuberculosis: Challenges and opportunities. *Frontiers in Tuberculosis*, *2*, 1487518. DOI: 10.3389/ftubr.2024.1487518

Goletti, D., Al-Abri, S., Migliori, G. B., Arlehamn, C. L., Haldar, P., Sundling, C., & Lee, S. S. (2024). World Tuberculosis Day 2024 theme "Yes! We can end TB" can be made a reality through concerted global efforts that advance detection, diagnosis, and treatment of tuberculosis infection and disease. *International Journal of Infectious Diseases*, *141*, 141. DOI: 10.1016/j.ijid.2024.106993 PMID: 38458422

Guerrieri, M., Bargagli, E., Cassai, L., Gangi, S., Genovese, M., Viani, M., & Melani, A. S. (2024). Pulmonary tuberculosis in non-hiv adults: An evergreen old-fashioned disease in high-income countries. A narrative review. *Expert Review of Respiratory Medicine*, *18*(11), 861–872. DOI: 10.1080/17476348.2024.2418932 PMID: 39434706

Jhaveri, T. A., Jhaveri, D., Galivanche, A., Lubeck-Schricker, M., Voehler, D., Chung, M., Thekkur, P., Chadha, V., Nathavitharana, R., Kumar, A. M. V., Shewade, H. D., Powers, K., Mayer, K. H., Haberer, J. E., Bain, P., Pai, M., Satyanarayana, S., & Subbaraman, R. (2024). Barriers to engagement in the care cascade for tuberculosis disease in India: A systematic review of quantitative studies. *PLoS Medicine*, *21*(5), e1004409. DOI: 10.1371/journal.pmed.1004409 PMID: 38805509

Junqueira-Kipnis, A. P., Leite, L. C. D. C., Croda, J., Chimara, E., Carvalho, A. C. C., & Arcêncio, R. A. (2024). Advances in the development of new vaccines for tuberculosis and Brazil's role in the effort forward the end TB strategy. *Memorias do Instituto Oswaldo Cruz*, *119*, e240093. DOI: 10.1590/0074-02760240093 PMID: 39383403

Kakande, E., Ssekyanzi, B., Abbott, R., Ariho, W., Nattabi, G., Landsiedel, K., Temple, J., Chamie, G., Havlir, D. V., Kamya, M. R., Charlebois, E. D., Balzer, L. B., & Marquez, C. (2024). Prevalence and Predictors of Tuberculosis Infection in Children and Adolescents in Rural Uganda: A Cross-sectional Study. *The Pediatric Infectious Disease Journal*, *43*(12), 1120–1127. DOI: 10.1097/INF.0000000000004475 PMID: 39018476

Kunst, H., Lange, B., Hovardovska, O., Bockey, A., Zenner, D., Andersen, A. B., Hargreaves, S., Pareek, M., Friedland, J. S., Wejse, C., Bothamley, G., Guglielmetti, L., Chesov, D., Tiberi, S., Matteelli, A., Mandalakas, A. M., Heyckendorf, J., Eimer, J., Malhotra, A., & Lange, C. (2025). Tuberculosis in adult migrants in Europe: A TBnet consensus statement. *The European Respiratory Journal*, *65*(3), 2401612. DOI: 10.1183/13993003.01612-2024 PMID: 39672603

MacPherson, P., Shanaube, K., Phiri, M. D., Rickman, H. M., Horton, K. C., Feasey, H. R., Corbett, E. L., Burke, R. M., & Rangaka, M. X. (2024). Community-based active-case finding for tuberculosis: Navigating a complex minefield. *BMC Global and Public Health*, *2*(1), 1–14. DOI: 10.1186/s44263-024-00042-9 PMID: 39681889

Marme, G., Kuzma, J., Zimmerman, P. A., Harris, N., & Rutherford, S. (2024). Investigating socio-ecological factors influencing implementation of tuberculosis infection prevention and control in rural Papua New Guinea. *Journal of Public Health (Oxford, England)*, *46*(2), 267–276. DOI: 10.1093/pubmed/fdae018 PMID: 38326281

Martín, D., Barbosa, P., Ramos, J. P., Vieira, M., & Duarte, R. (2024). People first: A participatory community approach on patient-reported outcomes in tuberculosis. *Breathe (Sheffield, England)*, *20*(1), 230138. DOI: 10.1183/20734735.0138-2023 PMID: 38482186

Maseko, A. F., Silumbwe, A., Maritim, P., Munakampe, M. N., Chirambo, G. B., Jacobs, C., & Zulu, J. M. (2025). Factors that shape the integration of HIV and TB services in Zomba District, Malawi. *BMC Health Services Research*, *25*(1), 213. DOI: 10.1186/s12913-025-12367-8 PMID: 39915793

Meintjes, G., & Maartens, G. (2024). HIV-associated tuberculosis. *The New England Journal of Medicine*, *391*(4), 343–355. DOI: 10.1056/NEJMra2308181 PMID: 39047241

Nagarajan, K., Kumarswamy, K., Begum, R., Panibatla, V., Singarajipura, A., Adepu, R., Munjattu, J. F., Sellapan, S., Arangba, S., Goswami, A., Swamickan, R., Basha, J., Dsouza, P. M., & Muniyandi, M. (2024). Self-driven solutions and resilience adapted by people with drug-resistant tuberculosis and their caregivers in Bengaluru and Hyderabad, India: A qualitative study. *The Lancet Regional Health. Southeast Asia*, *22*, 22. DOI: 10.1016/j.lansea.2024.100372 PMID: 38420270

Naidoo, K., Perumal, R., Cox, H., Mathema, B., Loveday, M., Ismail, N., Omar, S. V., Georghiou, S. B., Daftary, A., O'Donnell, M., & Ndjeka, N. (2024). The epidemiology, transmission, diagnosis, and management of drug-resistant tuberculosis—Lessons from the South African experience. *The Lancet. Infectious Diseases*, *24*(9), e559–e575. DOI: 10.1016/S1473-3099(24)00144-0 PMID: 38527475

Nasir, A., Hassan, I. I., Ma'ruf, A., Suharno, N. E., Goenharto, S., Purwanto, C. R., & Tyas, A. P. M. (2024). Coping efforts made: Psychological burden of people living with tuberculosis due to social stigma in society. A qualitative phenomenology study. *PLoS One*, *19*(7), e0303331. DOI: 10.1371/journal.pone.0303331 PMID: 39078843

Okoroafor, S. C., & Christmals, C. D. (2024). Health professions education strategies for enhancing capacity for task-shifting and task-sharing implementation in Africa: A scoping review. *The Journal of Continuing Education in the Health Professions*, *44*(3), 194–202. DOI: 10.1097/CEH.0000000000000517 PMID: 37341562

Olawade, D. B., Eberhardt, J., David-Olawade, A. C., Balogun, M. A., Bolarinwa, O. A., & Esan, D. T. (2024). Transforming multidrug-resistant tuberculosis care: The potentials of telemedicine in resource-limited settings. *Health Sciences Review (Oxford, England)*, *12*, 100185. DOI: 10.1016/j.hsr.2024.100185

Rahmatullah, S., Rahmawati, R., & Arifin, A. (2025). Environmental Risk Factors and Tuberculosis Transmission: A Case-Control Study in Batu Mandi District, South Kalimantan, Indonesia, 2024. *Global Health & Environmental Perspectives*, *2*(1), 12–23.

Schwab, T. C., Perrig, L., Göller, P. C., De la Hoz, F. F. G., Lahousse, A. P., Minder, B., & Fenner, L. (2024). Targeted next-generation sequencing to diagnose drug-resistant tuberculosis: A systematic review and meta-analysis. *The Lancet. Infectious Diseases*, *24*(10), 1162–1176. DOI: 10.1016/S1473-3099(24)00263-9 PMID: 38795712

Shorette, K., & Phillips, N. E. (2024). (In) sufficient institutionalization? Norm articulation in the World Health Organization and infectious disease prevalence across the global South. *International Journal of Comparative Sociology*, *65*(6), 752–781. DOI: 10.1177/00207152241226449

Storvig, E., Harstad, I., Ehrnström, B., & Iversen, V. C. (2024). Beyond the diagnosis of drug-resistant Tuberculosis in Norway: Patients' experiences before, during and after treatment. *BMC Public Health*, *24*(1), 1801. DOI: 10.1186/s12889-024-19342-8 PMID: 38971760

Vallipriya, R., & Singh, A. K. (2025). Integrated Public-Private Partnerships to Combat Tuberculosis for Improving. *Public Private Partnership Dynamics for Economic Development*, 323.

van der Westhuizen, H. M., Ehrlich, R., Somdyala, N., Greenhalgh, T., Tonkin-Crine, S., & Butler, C. C. (2024). Stigma relating to tuberculosis infection prevention and control implementation in rural health facilities in South Africa—A qualitative study outlining opportunities for mitigation. *BMC Global and Public Health*, *2*(1), 66. DOI: 10.1186/s44263-024-00097-8 PMID: 39681968

Vasiliu, A., Martinez, L., Gupta, R. K., Hamada, Y., Ness, T., Kay, A., Bonnet, M., Sester, M., Kaufmann, S. H. E., Lange, C., & Mandalakas, A. M. (2024). Tuberculosis prevention: Current strategies and future directions. *Clinical Microbiology and Infection*, *30*(9), 1123–1130. DOI: 10.1016/j.cmi.2023.10.023 PMID: 37918510

Vidyasagaran, A. L., Siqueira, N. T. D., Kakchapati, S., Hall, T. F., Naznin, B., Tajree, J., . . . Elsey, H. (2024). Public–Private Mix (PPM) for Tuberculosis (TB) in Urban Health Systems in Least Developed, Low Income and Lower-Middle-Income Countries and Territories–A Systematic Review. medRxiv, 2024-05. DOI: 10.1101/2024.05.01.24306566

Ye, Z., Li, L., Yang, L., Zhuang, L., Aspatwar, A., Wang, L., & Gong, W. (2024, October). Impact of diabetes mellitus on tuberculosis prevention, diagnosis, and treatment from an immunologic perspective. *Exploration*, *4*(5), 20230138. DOI: 10.1002/EXP.20230138 PMID: 39439490

Yerezhepov, D., Gabdulkayum, A., Akhmetova, A., Kozhamkulov, U. A., Rakhimova, S. E., Kairov, U. Y., Zhunussova, G., Kalendar, R. N., & Akilzhanova, A. (2024). Vitamin D status, VDR, and TLR polymorphisms and pulmonary tuberculosis epidemiology in Kazakhstan. *Nutrients*, *16*(4), 558. DOI: 10.3390/nu16040558 PMID: 38398882

Zulu, J. M., Maritim, P., Halwiindi, H., Chavula, M. P., Munakampe, M., Matenga, T. F. L., Mweemba, C., Sinyangwe, N. N., Habib, B., Musukuma, M., Silumbwe, A., Wang, B., Kaonga, P., Chewe, M., Fisa, R., Banda, J., Mubanga, A., & Phiri, H. (2024). Implementation strategies for decentralized management of multidrug-resistant tuberculosis: Insights from community health systems in Zambia. *Archives of Public Health = Archives Belges de Santé Publique*, *82*(1), 157. DOI: 10.1186/s13690-024-01384-4 PMID: 39277746

KEY TERMS AND DEFINITIONS

99DOTS: Phone-based self-reporting.

Community Health Workers (CHWs): Locally-based workers trained to deliver basic health services, including TB screening and treatment support, particularly in rural settings.

Community-Based Care: TB care models delivered at or near patients' homes, often involving community health workers to improve accessibility and adherence.

Developed Countries: High-income nations with advanced healthcare infrastructure but still facing TB challenges among marginalized groups.

Digital Adherence Technologies (DATs): Technology tools that support remote monitoring of TB treatment adherence, such as:

Directly Observed Therapy (DOT): A method where health workers watch patients take their TB medications to ensure compliance.

Drug-Resistant TB (DR-TB): Forms of TB that do not respond to standard treatments due to resistance to one or more anti-TB drugs. Includes:

Electronic Pillboxes: Smart boxes that track pill-taking.

End TB Strategy: A WHO-led global framework aiming to reduce TB deaths by 95% and cases by 90% by 2035 through early diagnosis, treatment, and prevention.

GeneXpert MTB/RIF: A rapid molecular diagnostic tool that detects *Mycobacterium tuberculosis* and rifampicin resistance within hours.

Infection Prevention and Control (IPC): A set of practices aimed at preventing TB transmission in healthcare and community settings, including ventilation, isolation, and use of protective equipment.

Integrated Service Delivery: Approach that combines TB services with other health programs (e.g., HIV, maternal health) to streamline care and reduce stigma.

Latent TB Infection (LTBI): A condition where individuals carry the TB bacteria without active symptoms; they are not contagious but can develop active TB later.

Line Probe Assays: Molecular diagnostics that identify specific genetic mutations associated with TB drug resistance.

MDR-TB (Multidrug-Resistant TB): Resistant to at least isoniazid and rifampicin.

Mobile Diagnostic Units: Vehicles equipped with TB diagnostic tools (e.g., X-ray, GeneXpert) used to reach remote or high-risk populations.

Public-Private Partnerships (PPP): Collaborative models where private healthcare providers are integrated into national TB programs to improve diagnosis and treatment coverage.

Rural Health: Healthcare systems and services in remote or low-resource settings, often challenged by poor infrastructure and access issues.

TB Treatment Adherence: The extent to which patients follow prescribed TB treatment regimens consistently over months, critical for cure and preventing resistance.

Telemedicine: Use of digital communication tools to provide clinical services remotely, especially valuable in rural or hard-to-reach areas.

Tuberculosis (TB): A contagious bacterial infection caused by *Mycobacterium tuberculosis*, primarily affecting the lungs but capable of spreading to other organs.

Video DOT (vDOT): Video monitoring of patients taking medication.

XDR-TB (Extensively Drug-Resistant TB): Resistant to isoniazid, rifampicin, fluoroquinolones, and second-line injectable drugs.

Chapter 2
Impact of Overcrowding on Tuberculosis Prevalence and Healthcare Accessibility in Prisons

S. Srinivasan
https://orcid.org/0009-0002-0179-9849
Department of Humanities and Social Sciences, Graphic Era University, Dehradun, India

R. Vallipriya
https://orcid.org/0009-0008-6692-603X
Department of Biochemistry and Biotechnology, Pavendar Bharathidasan College of Arts and Science (PBCAS), Bharathidasan University, India

Ajay Kumar Singh
https://orcid.org/0000-0003-0429-0925
Department of Humanities and Social Sciences, Graphic Era University, Dehradun, India

ABSTRACT

Tuberculosis (TB) in prisons remains a critical public health challenge, with infection rates significantly higher than in the general population. Overcrowding, poor ventilation, malnutrition, and substance use increase the risk of TB transmission among inmates. Correctional facilities must implement effective screening, diagnosis, treatment adherence, and follow-up mechanisms to control the disease. This study examines the impact of prison conditions on TB transmission and evaluates

DOI: 10.4018/979-8-3373-3446-2.ch002

existing interventions, using secondary data from sources like NCRB, WHO, and CDC. Findings highlight gaps in screening, healthcare infrastructure, and treatment continuity due to inmate transfers. Strengthening collaboration between prison administration and public health agencies is essential for TB prevention. Evidence-based policies and improved healthcare services can mitigate TB risks, ensuring better health outcomes for inmates and reducing transmission to the broader community. The recommendations for enhancing TB management in prison settings through strategic interventions and policy reforms.

INTRODUCTION

People living in incarceration are at risk due to overcrowding, which contributes to the development of (TB). In prison, there is poorer care compared to those affected by TB outside the prison. (Gonçalves et al., 2022). The incarceration population is a more vulnerable group compared to the general population. Generally, to protect the vulnerable group from human rights violations and to ensure the right to health for the incarcerated population, both health and justice services should be provided (Cloud et al., 2023). TB is one of the deadly diseases; it often leads to mortality and morbidity, which are increasing every day worldwide. As per the WHO report and Global TB Report 2024, it is expected that 10.8 million individuals were affected by TB in 2023, of which 1.25 million individuals died. The large-scale crowding in prison settings leads to a high prevalence of risk for affected individuals (Gulumbe et al., 2025). There is a lack of healthcare services inside the prison, and the diagnosis mechanisms are not conducted regularly, with treatment concerns at a very low level. TB transmission is increased among prison inmates, and it poses a high risk for developing countries affected by the disease (Dara et al., 2015).

It indicates that there is an alarming global increase in TB disease, with the number of affected individuals growing, especially including multidrug-resistant TB (MDR-TB). TB disease transmission directly infects vulnerable people with drug-resistant TB (DR-TB), which is exacerbated as a high risk for marginalized communities. This can include incarcerated individuals who remain undiagnosed for a prolonged period (Dheda et al., 2024). TB treatment in the prison setting is associated with a very low success rate and an increased chance of MDR-TB. The study emphasizes the effect of TB spreading and MDR-TB transmission in prison settings and highlights the need for further strategic plans to improve the prison's role in controlling the epidemic and decreasing TB and MDR-TB cases (Sequera et al., 2023). TB risk factors in prison administration, due to delayed diagnosis and late treatment, can lead to the formation of DR-TB. This delay is due to some logistical problems in the prison setting that affect the provision of TB care in prison administration. Various risk factors are involved in prisons that affect TB (Santos et al., 2022).

Tuberculosis in Prisons: Prison Crisis Transcends Prison Walls

Tuberculosis (TB) in prison is a persistent problem, with prison inmates experiencing rates that are 5 to 50 times higher than the national average in both developed and developing countries. It is alarming that prisoners need to be provided with attention to reduce and eradicate TB in prison settings (Amede et al., 2022). The reason for TB in prison is that inmates are especially vulnerable to diseases. In prison settings, many inmates are incoming and outgoing; it is that no one knows about many of them. This is the reason prisons are infected with Mycobacterium TB, and it can develop into active TB every year compared to the general population (Placeres et al, 2023). Significantly, to address the various research questions, attempts are made to calculate the percentage of latent TB infection and the increase in active TB in the general population. This can be attributed to the increase of TB in prisons. The importance of the study is to highlight the increasing trend in TB and how to control TB infection in prison settings (Baussano et al., 2010). This can not only protect prison inmates, but it can also include prison staff to protect and avoid the spread of TB infections. This is the national burden in the country to affect TB infections. The research is to address the poor infrastructure and advance support to reduce TB infection in prison settings (Biadglegne et al., 2015).

The TB Risk in Correctional Facilities

TB is a serious concern and a health threat, especially for people affected in correctional settings. The correctional facility provides a place of increased risk for the TB burden, which can affect prisons in various ways. The correctional settings' prison administration provides various TB and health awareness events (Parvez, 2021). These can help prevent the spread of TB, educate on its basic symptoms and types, explain diagnosis methods and early detection, and provide details on treatment options and available schemes for affected individuals. TB is a challenging disease in prison settings and the general public (Rangaka et al., 2015). Identifying, treating, and controlling this disease is especially important in correctional settings, including central prisons, jails, sub-jails, and central women's prisons. It is crucial to closely monitor and identify symptomatic patients who live and work in close proximity to each other (Idrees & Bilal, 2023).

VARIOUS RISK FACTORS ARE INVOLVED IN PRISONS THAT AFFECT TB

Previous research studies show that the rate of TB incidence in the incarcerated population is affected more than ≥ 10 times in the community. Worldwide, a greater number of inmates, prison staff, visitors come to meet prisoners as they enter and leave the prison (Cords et al., 2021). This circulation increases the TB levels, amplifying its spread throughout the overall population and directly affecting both DS-TB and DR-TB. In prison settings, there is a risk to individuals due to overcrowding and lack of proper airflow and ventilation, as well as inadequate healthcare services in correctional facilities (Guo et al., 2019). The TB incidence rate is high in prison settings, as per the WHO report. There is heterogeneity in the incarcerated population, especially between developed and developing countries. The TB incidence rate in low- and lower-middle-income countries is 3.13%, which is higher than in upper-middle-income nations, where the prevalence among prisoners is 2.25%. It is estimated that 53% of the incarcerated population experiences TB diagnosis in prisons. Many incarcerated individuals are not properly diagnosed, and many of them are under-reported (Trickey & Trickey, 2017).

A PUBLIC HEALTH CONCERN IS ACTIVE TB IN CORRECTIONAL FACILITIES

In prison settings, inmates of all age groups live together inside the prison. This includes individuals as young as 15 years old and those above 60 years of age. This is one of the main reasons TB can easily affect both young and older adults (Vinkeles Melchers et al., 2013). The most vulnerable group is older people, as they are easily affected by TB. In the same prison, people of all age groups mingle and reside in the correctional facility at the same time, increasing the spread of TB infection. This poses a high risk of exposure to TB germs in the correctional facility (Akers et al., 2008). Living or having lived in large group settings makes TB more common in correctional facilities. In workplaces, TB can easily spread, making it especially common in correctional settings. TB germs easily spread in prison settings, especially among those who are vulnerable, from weaker sections, and those with low immunity, making them more susceptible to TB infection (Etim et al., 2024). TB infection easily spreads in prison settings, where several factors are involved. The main reason for TB infection is malnutrition and poor health conditions, which make individuals more susceptible. Additionally, living in close proximity, poor air ventilation, shared air spaces, overcrowding, and high levels of people movement increase the risk of TB infection in prison settings (Lee et al.,

2022). The correctional administration staff can engage with service providers and coordinate with local State and District NTEP staff to support TB prevention and control efforts (Thapa et al., 2023). The NTEP team conducts regular screening and diagnosis, ensures treatment adherence, provides regular follow-ups, and creates awareness programs. These efforts help in controlling TB and preventing its spread in correctional settings (Lu et al., 2023).

Conditions That can Increase Risk

The correctional settings should provide proper medical services for high-risk people, which can help avoid active TB disease. TB infection spreads through germs from affected to non-affected inmates (Coreil et al., 2010). The prison inmates are likely to use substances such as alcohol and drugs, and this can cause an increase in TB infection. Substance use increases the risk of TB infection (Scholze et al., 2022). Various substances such as alcohol use, drug use, non-injection and injection drug use can increase the risk of TB infection. These substances can affect TB diagnosis and treatment (Marks et al., 2022). Older adults, HIV-affected individuals, diabetic people, cancer patients, and those working in dust-related industries are more prone to TB due to low immunity levels, making them easily affected by TB disease (Srinivasan et al., 2025). A lower immune system can increase the risk of active TB disease and lead to infection by TB germs (Grange et al., 2011; Chao et al., 2020).

Places With Increased Risk

In correctional settings, the prison inmates face increased TB risk based on the living environmental facilities. In correctional facilities, living conditions and close physical proximity increase the chances of infection to a high level. Living places with no proper ventilation and air flow fluctuations increase the risk of TB disease. Overcrowding is also one of the reasons that affect the spread of TB infection. These are the ways that increase the spread of TB disease, including the spread of active TB disease in prison facilities (O' Grady et al., 2011; Kharwadkar et al., 2022; Damanik et al., 2025).

Facilities in Prisons are Being Moved

When prison inmates are moved to another facility, it may lead to overcrowding and poor air fluctuation, increasing the risk of TB and the spread of active TB disease. When prison inmates are moved from one prison to another, it creates challenges for people with inactive or active TB, even after completing treatment. The majority of TB infections and the progression from inactive TB to active TB disease can increase over several months due to lack of proper treatment (Reyes, 2007; Segal-Maurer, 2017; Tiberi et al., 2018). Another reason is moving from one place to another and changes in facility location, which can interrupt TB treatment. Without proper medical care and drugs, this can cause irregular treatment adherence (Srinivasan & Vallipriya, 2025). The correctional settings should manage and coordinate with the NTEP team and health department to facilitate and ensure regular treatment for TB-infected inmates. This can help avoid TB resistance in the prison inmates. Regular treatment for inactive TB and active TB inmates ensures that, when they reenter their community, the disease does not spread in the community as well (Baird et al., 2022).

Prevention and Control

Effective TB prevention can control and protect the prison inmates who live in prison settings and the community. This can be measured in various ways such as:

- Prison facilities can conduct regular and periodical TB screening.
- To provide treatment for inactive TB and active TB disease.
- Regular contact investigation can increase the detection and diagnosis of active TB disease.

Correctional administration to work closely with the public health department, especially the State TB and District TB NTEP program, to implement TB prevention and control measures in a periodical way (Ferreira et al., 2019; Saini & Garg, 2020).

Significance of the Study

Study highlights to growing the prison inmates and affect the health issues and infected TB diseases. Due to overcrowding and not proper health infrastructure to increase the TB transmission. The secondary data analysis provides credible sources to identify the research gaps in TB screening, diagnosis, treatment adherence, and regular follow-up care in the prison facility. The finding provides insights for the prison administration, healthcare workers and health professionals, and policymakers to develop regular intervention. This can enhance the healthcare services and reduce TB infection among the prison inmates. An evidence-based approach provides better policy implications and best practices to enhance TB management in the prison facility (Srinivasan et al., 2025). The research provides broader aspects to improve public health in the correctional facility by providing better healthcare to enhance the health and well-being of prison inmates. This can reduce the TB burden on the prison facility and promote a healthy, long life in the prison environment.

RESEARCH GAP

The number of prisoners is increasing every day, highlighting the need to focus on reducing the crime rate. Due to overcrowding, inmates are affected by Tuberculosis (TB). This is a significant health concern for prison settings. The research study mainly focuses on general prisoner health and the various challenges they may face, especially when entering prison. How can the TB screening process be conducted, and what strategies can be adopted to identify symptomatic patients? TB diagnosis and treatment adherence in prison settings have limited research conducted. The process of TB diagnosis, symptom identification, treatment adherence, and follow-up can support the functioning of the prison environment and the identification of TB. There is insufficient data to identify TB symptoms, detection, treatment, and follow-up in correctional settings, as it is based on secondary data available.

The research provides comprehensive knowledge to address the gap regarding real-time verification and effective treatment of TB-affected prison inmates in the central prison. An affected, infected person is to be identified for treatment protocols, food diets, and periodical check-ups in the central prison. The TB-affected inmates—what barriers do they face in the central prison, what stigma-related problems do they encounter, and what preventive methods can be used to protect and isolate the affected inmates? The effective treatment received by TB patients in prison settings and the medical infrastructure in prison conditions help increase treatment success. The research mainly emphasizes prison overcrowding, which tends to focus on living conditions and security concerns. It also impacts healthcare accessibility and TB control. The comparison of prison occupancy rates and TB prevalence in prison settings. To understand the gap in how overcrowding exhibits risks to the health of prison inmates and leads to ineffective treatment. This research gap is essential to address through evidence-based policy to improve TB management, including symptom identification, screening, diagnosis, treatment adherence, and follow-up, to enhance healthcare delivery in prison settings (Srinivasan, 2025).

Objective of the Study

- To identify the screening process when entering the prison
- To assess symptom identification, detection, diagnosis, treatment adherence, and follow-up
- To verify the TB-affected inmates undergoing treatment in the central prison
- To determine the prison occupancy rate in the central prison

Research Questions

1. What screening strategies are adopted when inmates newly enter the prison?

2. What is the effective way to use the existing screening procedure to enhance the diagnosis of TB symptoms among incoming prisoners?
3. What are the efficient methods to adopt for identifying TB diagnosis and symptoms among inmates?
4. How can proper treatment adherence and follow-up care services be provided for TB-affected inmates in the prison facility?
5. How can TB be prevented among inmates, and how can proper and regular treatment be provided to prisoners?
6. What protocols are followed for the regular and effective TB treatment of affected inmates, and how is a proper nutritional diet provided for inmates in the central prison?
7. How does it affect the existing occupancy rate in the central prison?
8. How does prison overcrowding influence health and well-being and contribute to TB infection in the central prison?

BACKGROUND OF THE STUDY

TB is a major challenge worldwide, especially affecting vulnerable and marginalized communities. Incarcerated individuals who are physically weak are easily affected by risk factors, including overcrowding and poor ventilation (Wallace & Wallace, 2019). There is no proper healthcare facility, and timely diagnosis and treatment are inaccessible. TB transmission in the prison environment occurs due to heavy crowding and congestion, allowing the disease to spread easily through airborne pathogens of Mycobacterium TB. Overcrowding in prison settings is a public health concern worldwide (Nardell & Fennelly, 2006; Rust et al., 2008; Srinivasan, 2021). TB disease spreads among prison inmates who have close contact through airborne transmission. The infection rate is high in underdeveloped and developing countries. These are nations that are outdated, lack proper health facilities and infrastructure, are underfunded, and are ill-equipped to handle and accommodate the increasing inmate population. In prison administration, comorbidities such as HIV, diabetes, substance abuse, malnutrition, and other complications are high, which can hinder TB control efforts in prison settings (Short, 2017; Busatto et al., 2022; Charalambous et al., 2023).

Healthcare access in prison settings is inadequate due to logistical problems, and there is no systematic way to reduce the policy barriers. In prison settings, improper diagnosis, insufficient health facilities, lack of proper diagnostic tools, and absence of adequate medical care services contribute to the escalation of TB cases (Macleod et al., 2020; Abbara et al., 2020). This can lead to stigma and discrimination among inmates, which demotivates them from seeking healthcare services, resulting in further health crises inside the prison (Byrne et al., 2024). The impact of overcrowding on TB prevalence in prison settings highlights the need for healthcare interventions to refine and provide proper facility services to improve prison healthcare systems (Topp et al., 2016). This study clearly indicates the relationship between prison overcrowding and the TB burden; it is a challenge for accessible and equitable healthcare in prison settings. The finding provides valuable insights for public health and offers various strategic improvements in prisons; it is evidence-based to enhance policymaking for TB risks and improve correctional facilities (Sriniasan et al., 2025).

REVIEW OF LITERATURE

WHO's documents and reports emphasize the Directly Observed Treatment Short-course (DOTS) as a strategy to reduce TB symptoms. The Red Cross complies with this approach to support the screening process in a systematic way to identify TB detection in prisons, particularly among new entrants. This approach is effectively focused on countries with a high burden of TB. However, there are ethical complications in establishing interventions in prisons. Epidemiological data provides insight into the impact of TB control on the prevalence of active TB in prison conditions.

Table 1. Important key points in the study

The TB incidence rate in prison settings is approximately 1% of the global rate (Edge et al., 2016).
TB treatment in prison settings has a lower rate of treatment; however, the results show high levels of success (Adane et al., 2018).
TB in prison settings — the detainees always face health challenges. High-level risk factors require health concern and proper nutritional supplements; these can directly support healthy inmates in controlling the TB disease (Carwile et al., 2022).

Table 2 provides a global perspective on TB in prisons, showing that nearly 1% of TB cases occur in these settings. The incidence rate is 1,148 per 100,000 population per year, which is higher than normal community people. There are 53% of TB cases are detected, and many undiagnosed among prison inmates (Emilian et al., 2025). Global trends from 2000 to 2019 across 193 countries show a high TB rate in prisons (Martinez et al., 2023). In prison settings, inmates affected by TB may also suffer from co-morbidities such as diabetes, jaundice, and lifestyle-related factors like regular smoking, alcohol use, and undernutrition. Due to overcrowding, the TB rate is especially high in Africa, with an overall rate of 2,200 per 100,000 population (Litvinjenko et al., 2023). On the other hand, the former Soviet Union has a high rate of MDR-TB and HIV co-infection, which is increasing. In Latin America, TB incidence in prisons is also high—26 times greater than in the general population.

Table 2. Tuberculosis in prisons worldwide

Tuberculosis in Prisons in Africa In Sub-Saharan African countries, the global TB cases and death rate are significantly high, with 94% of them affected. The TB incidence is high—2,242 per 100,000 population. Among prison inmates, the risk is 6 to 30 times higher; outside the prison, among those living in the community, it is ≥ 200 in the overcrowded incarcerated population (Wondmeneh & Mekonnen, 2023). In various countries, the diagnostic rate is highest in the DRC at 19.72%, followed by Zambia at 11.68%, and Ethiopia at 9.22%. TB and HIV co-infection affects 58% of individuals, and those co-infected are nearly five times more likely to develop TB (Tamuzi et al., 2021). In prisons, poor conditions—such as overcrowding, congestion, malnutrition, and inadequate healthcare support—result in a lack of proper care for inmates. Effective interventions are needed to enhance active case finding and improve TB preventive therapy for high-risk inmates. This includes integrated care through proper awareness, peer education, motivational talks, and routine TB and HIV screening, especially for newly admitted inmates. Better policy implementation is required to improve the prison healthcare system, reduce TB incidence, and increase TB and HIV care services—ensuring that human rights are not violated (Kuupiel et al., 2020).
Tuberculosis in Prisons in South and Central America In South and Central America, in Paraguay, nearly 15% of prisoners are affected by TB, and 58% of the incarcerated population is at long-term risk, with around 42% developing TB after release. A recent study found that MDR-TB transmission occurs at a high level among post-release inmates (Woodman et al., 2019). In Central South America, there are many prison inmates with underdiagnosed TB. The TB rate is 26 times higher outside the prison (Cords et al., 2021). There are six countries—Argentina, Brazil, Colombia, El Salvador, Mexico, and Peru—where the growing incarcerated population is overlooked in national TB burden estimates. Due to overcrowding in detention facilities, these countries are a major focus for global TB control efforts worldwide (Liu et al., 2024).
Tuberculosis in Prisons in China As per the WHO report, the global TB incidence rates are 26% in India, 10% in Indonesia, 6.8% in China, 6.8% in the Philippines, and 6.3% in Pakistan. In China, there were 741,000 new TB cases in 2023, which corresponds to a rate of 52 per 100,000 population. This includes 9,500 cases among individuals affected by HIV (Chen et al., 2025). The TB prevalence in prisons is 1,156 per 100,000 population. In China, there were 29,000 new cases of drug-resistant TB in 2023, accounting for 7.3% of global DR-TB cases, ranking China high worldwide (Nyasulu, et al., 2025). In prison settings, overcrowded environments often lack proper ventilation, which contributes to increased TB incidence and transmission. TB screening in prisons urgently needs immediate attention to control and avoid TB transmission in the prison (Urrego et al., 2015).
Tuberculosis in prisons in Ukraine and Russia TB control is lagging in Ukraine and Russia due to a lack of adequate care in prisons. According to the WHO report, Ukraine ranks fifth globally for DR-TB incidence. Due to the war, inmates are displaced from one place to another, which has affected healthcare infrastructure, making proper diagnosis and continuous access to TB screening and treatment difficult (Chen et al., 2023). In Russia, TB rates in prisons are high, especially in Kemerovo, where among 100,000 inmates, the TB rate is approximately 4,000, which is much higher than the expected rate. Tools like e-TB Manager help improve monitoring and treatment tracking, thereby mitigating TB transmission in conflict-affected zones (Dmitrieva et al., 2024).

continued on following page

Table 2. Continued

Tuberculosis in prisons in the Europe and USA
Tuberculosis in prisons in the Europe and USA As per the WHO report, there are European countries with TB notification in the prisons. In 2014, it was 15,492; it increased to 60,068 in 2022. The treatment success rate was nearly 62% in 2021.There are 23% of the TB cases not evaluated in the prisoner due to transfer, notably in the U.S., where prisons account for 4.2% of national TB cases. (Pape et al., 2024) . Various risk factors contribute to this situation, including overcrowding, delayed diagnosis, substance use, and inadequate care and support. In European countries, TB control in prisons requires training and policy support to integrate TB control programs effectively and protect the incarcerated population (Tavoschi et al., 2019; Darraj et al., 2023).
Tuberculosis in prisons in Asia The TB incidence in Asian prison settings is estimated at 1,810 per 100,000 population. TB rates in the following countries are: India – 1,076 Philippines – 6,357 Thailand – 5,249 TB screening from 2016 to 2020 showed a prevalence rate of 60.5% and a treatment success rate of 94.3%. The cure rate for first-line drugs is 90%, while 75% is for second-line drugs. This success rate has contributed to sustained TB control and increased TB screening in prison settings. However, MDR-TB cases are increasing among the prison population in Asian countries. Regular screening of both new and existing inmates helps achieve targets by identifying symptomatic patients and capturing high-risk inmates (Sequera et al., 2023; Nyasulu, et al., 2025).

Table 3. The role of TB risk assessment in prison settings, the need-based approach, challenges, and ways of providing care

Sl. No	Role TB Risk in Prison Setting	Challenges	Providing care and prevention of disease transmission as well as diagnostics and treatment based on the need-based approach
1	Risk Factors	Due to overcrowding, there is an increase in the TB incidence rate. The main reasons are poor ventilation, malnutrition, and an increased rate of HIV and substance abuse, along with inadequate healthcare in prison settings.	To provide the services, increase the ventilated infrastructure and implement policy reforms to improve ventilation, reduce TB transmission, and provide sufficient nutritional food. This can help prevent and provide integrative care for co-infections.
2	Early detection and reduce the Drug Resistance	In prison settings, the lack of diagnostic facilities and inability to frequently access drug susceptibility tests can delay diagnosis	To expand the services, diagnostic tools should be implemented on a regular basis to test DST, and trained staff can access the tools and identify early diagnosis.
3	Transmission of TB through new entry inmates, staff and visitors	The reason for that is insufficient preventive measures, which increase TB transmission, low levels of awareness, and the lack of proper diagnostic facility tools.	The robust equipment is used to identify infectious TB cases, and the technology helps control the TB disease, encouraging personal protective services. In the prison, on a regular basis, conduct the TB sensitization program and provide awareness for the TB information for staff and inmates.

continued on following page

Table 3. Continued

Sl. No	Role TB Risk in Prison Setting	Challenges	Providing care and prevention of disease transmission as well as diagnostics and treatment based on the need-based approach
4	Delay Diagnosis	Prison settings lack screening when new TB patients enter; it is associated with stigma and lack of diagnostic facilities.	To provide universal TB screening, it can be used for advanced TB diagnostics. Education improves TB diagnostic access and reduces the stigma level. Establish the prison manual and guidelines for TB treatment at the national level.
5	Treatment Adherence	Prison-affected incarcerated individuals show poor adherence due to stigma, improper follow-up, irregular treatment, and, due to displacement and releases, do not complete the treatment properly.	To launch directly observed therapy for prison-affected individuals and provide regular, on-time treatment that can continue post-release and offer psychological support services (Srinivasan et al., 2025).
6	Prison turnover	Prison transfers from one place to another disrupt TB diagnosis and treatment, and sometimes make it impossible to continue treatment.	There is a need to provide a standardized protocol to implement and follow in an appropriate manner when patients are transferred, ensuring medical details are shared and treatment is continued.
7	Regular Monitoring Services	Incarcerated populations are unable to have regular check-ups. That is the reason for the increase in symptomatic patients. Prison administration should monitor symptomatic patients through periodical and routine screening	Prison administration should also conduct health assessments, which can be done by trained healthcare workers to identify symptomatic patients and provide proper services for early-stage TB diagnosis.
8	E-Monitoring	E-monitoring services provide accurate data and reports, which are especially useful when handling large datasets.	A digital monitoring tool is more useful to evaluate and manage TB.
9	Public and Private Partnership	The prison administration to link between private and public health system is essential to lead for the TB control.	Health partnerships can enhance correctional facilities, improve public health activities, and provide care and support services to strengthen TB control.
10	Health Statistics	There is a lack of data on incarcerated populations affected by TB incidence in prison settings.	To provide one digital platform to enhance TB case management in the prison —district-wise, national-wise, and internationally—would be useful for regularly identifying TB patients. This data can be analyzed to identify trends at the country, state, and district levels.

Newly Incarcerated Inmates are Subjected to Screening Strategies

The previous study explored TB screening in prisons. Out of 20 jails, 95% had conducted the screening. TB symptoms were found in 85% of them, and in 17 out of 20 prisons, inmates were asked about cough and TB-related information. As per the TB screening, the universal Tuberculin Skin Test (TST) was conducted over 14 days, which included both chest radiography and the TST. In 10% of the prisons (2 out of 20), chest radiograph tests were conducted. One prison, nearly 5%, did not conduct the universal screening. About 13% of the inmates were tested voluntarily (Sanchez et al., 2013; Zenner et al., 2013).

When new inmates entered, their previous health background was collected to identify any symptoms or past history of TB. From the beginning, those identified were isolated and provided with separate and proper monitoring, regular health check-ups, and necessary health facilities to control the symptoms. In the prison setting, for TB transmission contact testing, the majority—95%—of the prison inmates were tested. Most of them, about 80%, included transferred inmates and close contacts. Around 90% of inmates were tested in the same unit along with staff members. 85% of inmates' visiting family members were tested, and 10% of contact tests were done for those in the same or nearby rooms. About 50% were tested in common places (Roberts et al., 2006; Mabud et al., 2019).

Using the Existing Screening Process to Enhance TB Diagnosis in Incoming Prisoners

TB diagnosis in the prison setting should adhere to the process of following incoming prisoners and existing prisoners in their screening process. This can include providing diagnostic methods such as the sputum test, X-ray, and Tuberculin Skin Test, and giving priority to high-risk groups such as HIV-affected persons, diabetics, malnourished individuals, those with respiratory-related diseases, and lung disease patients. The tests should be provided consistently for the staff, along with an effective method for contact tracing to enable early diagnosis for TB containment (Jeffries et al., 2017).

New Active PTB Prison Entry and Screening

In the prison setting, when new inmates enter, especially in cases of active pulmonary TB, case finding and identification should follow a screening algorithm. The standard includes bacteriological confirmation for new inmates, using solid and liquid culture and sputum tests for confirmation. As per WHO guidelines, nucleic acid amplification tests (NAAT), TrueNat, and GeneXpert are endorsed to detect MTB/RIF (Tsegaye Sahle et al., 2019; Khan et al., 2024).

To determine accuracy, data on sensitivity and specificity should include true positive values, false positive values, true negative values, and false negative values. In the prison setting, custodial inmates transferred from one place to another should be monitored and screened at both locations when entering new jails.

Type of Screening for the TB Symptoms

Sputum collection is the first primary concern; if it is not possible to collect, Chest X-ray is preferred. There are different types of screening methods, which include:

- Microscopy
- Chest X-Ray (CXR)
- Tuberculin Skin Test (TST)
- Interferon-Gamma Release Assays (IGRAs)
- Real-Time Polymerase Chain Reaction (PCR) test
- Nucleic Acid Amplification Tests (NAAT)
- Line Probe Assays for the first-line anti-tuberculosis drugs (FL LPA)
- Line Probe Assays for the identification of resistance to second-line anti-tuberculosis drugs (SL LPA)
- Loop-Mediated Isothermal Amplification (TB-LAMP)
- Antigen detection in a lateral flow format (biomarker-based detection) (TB LAM) (Pape et al., 2022).

EFFECTIVE METHODS FOR DIAGNOSING AND TREATING TB IN PRISONERS

An effective way to provide TB diagnosis involves identifying the symptoms, conducting screening, and referring the patient for sputum testing and chest X-ray. When a patient is diagnosed as TB positive, treatment should be initiated—such as DOTS—with regular monitoring by the NTEP team. Senior treatment supervisors ensure continuity of treatment and care, even after release, to prevent treatment interruption (Divala et al., 2022).

TB Diagnosis and Patient Management in Prison Settings

The existing literature review indicates that in nearly 52 of the studies, 86.5% of the cases were TB positive. The majority of these were smear positive (42.3%), followed by X-ray positive cases (21.2%). About 48.1% were combined cases. TB identification used different diagnostic tools: TST identified 19.2% of cases, smear microscopy detected 55.8%, solid culture identified 15.4%, and chest X-ray identified 9.6%. Ziehl-Neelsen (ZN) staining was the most commonly used method in 75% of cases, followed by culture tests (21.2%) and drug susceptibility testing (DST) (13.5%). Chest X-ray was used in nearly 25% of cases, and two recent studies used bronchoalveolar lavage. No studies discussed antibody-based rapid serology tests (Rentmeester et al., 2014).

TB and HIV Case Management

Regular and timely treatment adherence must be ensured, including follow-up during incarceration, after transfer, and even post-release. Affected individuals and their close contacts or family members should be provided with Isoniazid Preventive Therapy (IPT), especially for high-risk groups such as HIV-positive inmates, staff members, and guards (Vinkeles Melchers et al., 2013).

ENSURING TREATMENT ADHERENCE AND FOLLOW-UP CARE FOR TB-AFFECTED INMATES

To ensure treatment adherence and regular follow-up for affected inmates, DOTS treatment should be provided. This must be monitored by prison authorities and the medical officer, with support from the Senior Treatment Supervisor (STS), who provides patient education and awareness to ensure daily treatment without interruption (Dirks et al., 2023; Srinivasan, & Vallipriya, 2025). The National TB Elimination Program (NTEP) should conduct regular visits to monitor treatment progress, ensure timely drug availability, and offer counseling and motivation for regular treatment adherence. Proper nutritional food should be arranged, and In-Patient (IP) and Contact Person (CP) follow-up tests should be conducted to assess the condition of TB patients. If any Adverse Drug Reaction (ADR) is observed, alternative medication should be arranged in consultation with the concerned medical officer or District TB Officer (DTO) (Srinivasan & Praba Lama, 2025).

PREVENTING TB AND ENSURING REGULAR TREATMENT IN PRISONS

TB can be prevented in prisons by identifying individuals with symptoms and conducting regular monitoring and screening. Early detection helps in identifying TB patients, providing isolation for active cases, and ensuring proper ventilation (WHO, 2021). Regular and continuous treatment can help protect and prevent transmission by using DOTS therapy, along with regular follow-up and treatment adherence. Coordination with health authorities is essential to provide care and support for TB-affected inmates, and to continue care after their release or transfer (Behera et al., 2020).

Prison Setting to Control the TB Disease and Provide the Intervention

The existing study clearly explores that pre-intervention TB control is a very difficult process. Most interventions focus on active case finding, which is most commonly conducted at the time of prison entry as a regular process. Diagnostic methods used to identify symptoms include sputum tests or chest X-rays, which are the most prominent diagnostic tools (Baxter et al., 2017).

The Intervention Method

I) To isolate TB-affected inmates
II) To provide TB education and health education for staff and inmates
III) To provide peer education training for inmates
IV) To assure proper diagnostic services
V) To arrange contact tracing
VI) HIV testing

TB TREATMENT PROTOCOLS AND NUTRITIONAL SUPPORT IN CENTRAL PRISONS

To follow the Standard for TB Care in India (STCI) guidelines and provide TB treatment such as DOTS therapy and regular routine health checkups in the prison settings, timely treatment is essential. In the prison setting, proper nutritional support must be arranged. Nutrient-rich food, including protein and vitamins, should be provided as a balanced diet. This can boost immunity in TB-affected individuals and help prevent the spread of TB (Purdey, 2006; Jain & Tronic, 2018).

AFFECT THE EXISTING OCCUPANCY RATE IN THE CENTRAL PRISON

A high occupancy rate increases the risk of TB in central prisons due to overcrowding. The spread of TB is linked to poor ventilation, close contact, and limited healthcare access. This places a strain on inmates and highlights the need for effective early diagnosis, regular screening, treatment, and follow-up to control TB (Beaudry et al., 2020).

Relationship Between Incarceration and TB Spread

The spread of TB in prisons is a significant concern, as prisons act as centers for disease transmission, potentially leading to multi-drug-resistant TB (MDR-TB):

i) Due to overcrowding, there is increased TB transmission, compounded by poor ventilation.
ii) Delayed diagnosis and irregular treatment lead to illness and low cure rates due to poor follow-up.
iii) High susceptibility is associated with poor nutrition, poverty, substance abuse, alcohol, smoking, and HIV.

TB incidence in prisons is 84 times higher than in the general population and can increase the MDR rate of incidence.

PRISON OVERCROWDING AND TB RISK

In central prisons, overcrowding negatively affects the health of inmates. Cramped conditions and poor ventilation create an environment that increases stress, reduces immunity, and contributes to higher TB incidence in central prisons.

Overcrowding Increases the TB Rate

In overcrowded prisons, limited cell space can contribute to the spread of TB. A previous study in Pakistan involving 425 male inmates showed that low cell space (≤ 5.6 m^2 per person) was associated with TB infection, with an adjusted odds ratio (aOR) of 2.6; 95% CI: 1.6–4.3. Although there may be some bias, the response rate was nearly 100%.

Another study conducted in Chile reported 46 inmates with TB. The TB incidence was 123.9 per 100,000 population, and latent TB infection (LTBI) was found in 29.4%. The LTBI rate among prisoners (33.2%) was significantly higher compared to non-prisoners (15.6%). Low cell space increased LTBI levels (aOR 3.5; 95% CI: 1.1–11.5). Prison dormitories were described as small, congested, and poorly ventilated, contributing to a high TB transmission rate (Simpson et al., 2019).

METHODOLOGY

The research study will use secondary data available from the National Crime Records Bureau, under the Ministry of Home Affairs, and data from data.gov.in. The secondary study analyzes how new offenders enter prison, the screening methods used, the diagnosis process, and the identification of symptomatic inmates. The research conducts screening, diagnosis, treatment adherence, and follow-up methods to assess how effectively they are implemented in the central prison. What health facilities are provided for TB-affected patients in the central prison? For TB-affected inmates, what are the treatment processes in the central prison, and how do healthcare workers and prison administration provide facilities for the affected inmates? How does prison occupancy affect the causes and spread of TB, and how can it be prevented? Secondary research can use existing literature surveys, WHO reports, Centers for Disease Control and Prevention (gov), and recent research articles to assess their impact on TB-affected inmates and determine further steps for TB eradication in prison administration. What innovative strategies are adopted in international prison administration, and how can they be effectively implemented in Indian prison settings? The secondary data analysis is conducted with the support of SPSS 23, while graphs and charts are created using Origin 2018 for analysis and Canva for flowchart and table preparation.

RESULT & DISCUSSION

Figure 1. TB screening among prison inmates in 2022 number of prisons covered

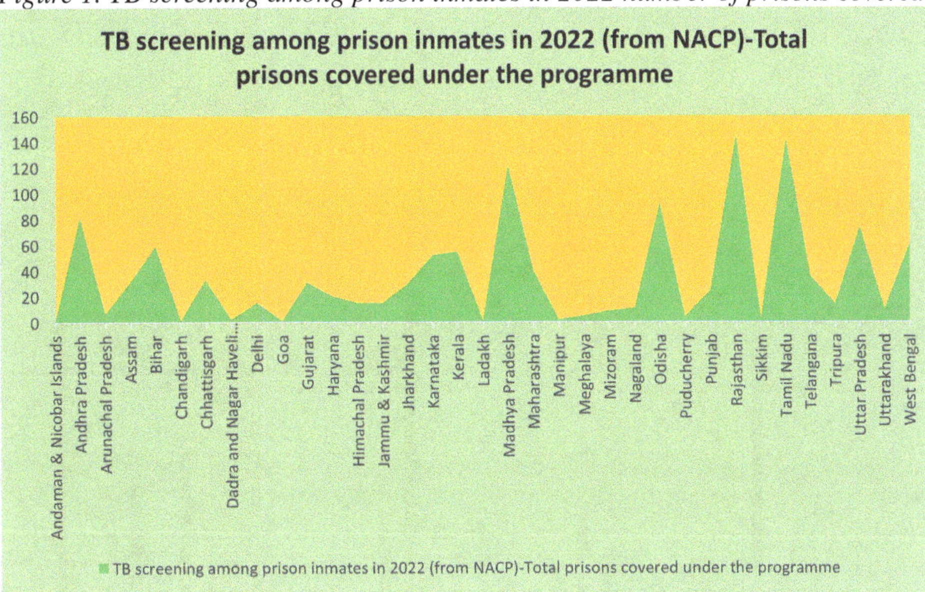

Figure 1 presents state-wise data on TB screening conducted in Indian prisons in 2022 under the National AIDS Control Program (NACP). It highlights the extent of coverage, disparities among states and union territories (UTs), and existing gaps in prison healthcare services. States with the highest number of prisons covered include Rajasthan (145), Tamil Nadu (142), Madhya Pradesh (121), Odisha (92), and Andhra Pradesh (81), indicating effective coordination between prison and health departments. In contrast, minimal screening was reported in Andaman & Nicobar, Chandigarh, Goa, and Ladakh (1 prison each), and in Dadra & Nagar Haveli, Manipur, and Sikkim (2 prisons each). Northeastern states like Meghalaya, Nagaland, and Mizoram screened fewer than 10 prisons, suggesting limitations in healthcare outreach and infrastructure.

Overall, 1,242 prisons across India conducted TB screening in 2022. While this represents a significant effort, uneven distribution underscores the need for targeted interventions. Given the high risk of TB transmission in overcrowded and poorly ventilated prison settings, early detection is vital to controlling the spread both within and beyond prison walls. The data serves as a useful tool for policymakers, health departments, and NGOs to identify gaps and strengthen services. Expanding coverage in low-performing regions, integrating TB screening into routine prison healthcare, and ensuring proper follow-up and treatment for those who test positive are essential steps toward improving prison and public health outcomes.

Figure 2. TB screening among prison inmates in 2022 (from NACP)-Total no. of prison inmates

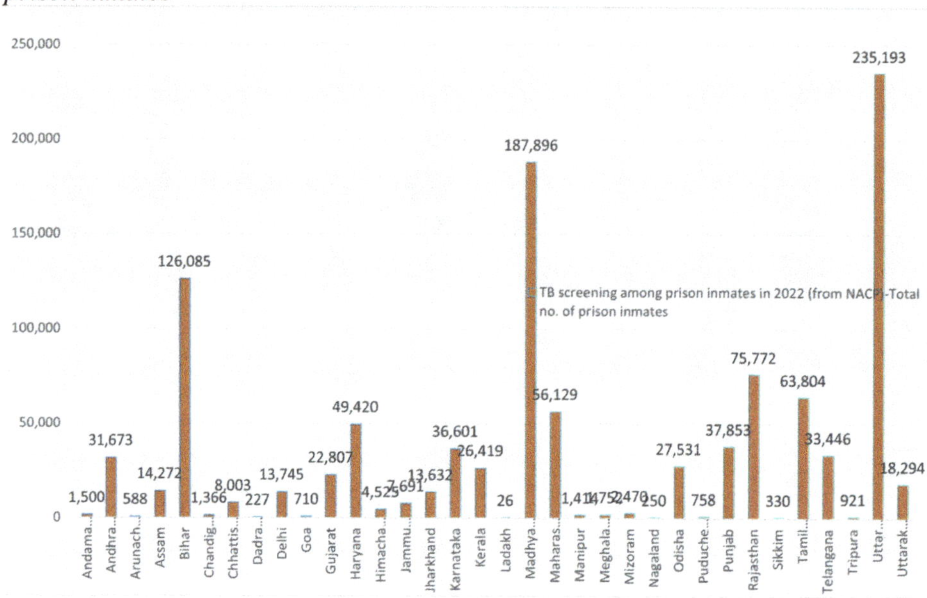

Based on Figure 2, one on the number of prisons covered and the other on inmates screened for TB in 2022 under the National AIDS Control Program (NACP)—key insights emerge. A total of 1,242 prisons were covered, and 1,133,483 inmates were screened, reflecting significant national outreach and growing focus on prison health. Top states by prison coverage included Rajasthan (145), Tamil Nadu (142), Madhya Pradesh (121), Uttar Pradesh (74), and West Bengal (61), showing strong coordination between prison and health departments. In terms of inmate screening, Uttar Pradesh led with 235,193 inmates, followed by Madhya Pradesh (187,896), Bihar (126,085), Tamil Nadu (63,804), and Maharashtra (56,129), indicating large-scale implementation in high-population states. In contrast, Ladakh, Nagaland, Sikkim, Dadra & Nagar Haveli and Daman & Diu reported low coverage due to fewer prisons and smaller populations. Still, these regions must maintain regular screening to avoid gaps in TB detection. Some states recorded high inmate numbers per prison, suggesting overcrowding or larger facilities. This highlights the need for ongoing screening, improved prison infrastructure, and better health services. The data is crucial for strengthening TB control strategies in India's prisons. Here are examples of states with a high number of inmates per prison covered:

Table 4. State wise prison inmates (2022)

State	Inmates per Prison (approx.)
Bihar	2,137
Uttar Pradesh	3,178
Madhya Pradesh	1,552
Maharashtra	1,403
Haryana	2,471

This could indicate overcrowding or larger prison units. TB screening in prisons was widespread in 2022, with over 1.13 million inmates covered across 1,242 prisons. Northern and central states like UP, MP, Bihar, and Rajasthan led in coverage both in terms of the number of prisons and inmates screened. States with few prisons or smaller inmate populations (like Ladakh, Sikkim, and Goa) showed proportionally lower numbers but were still included.

Figure 3.

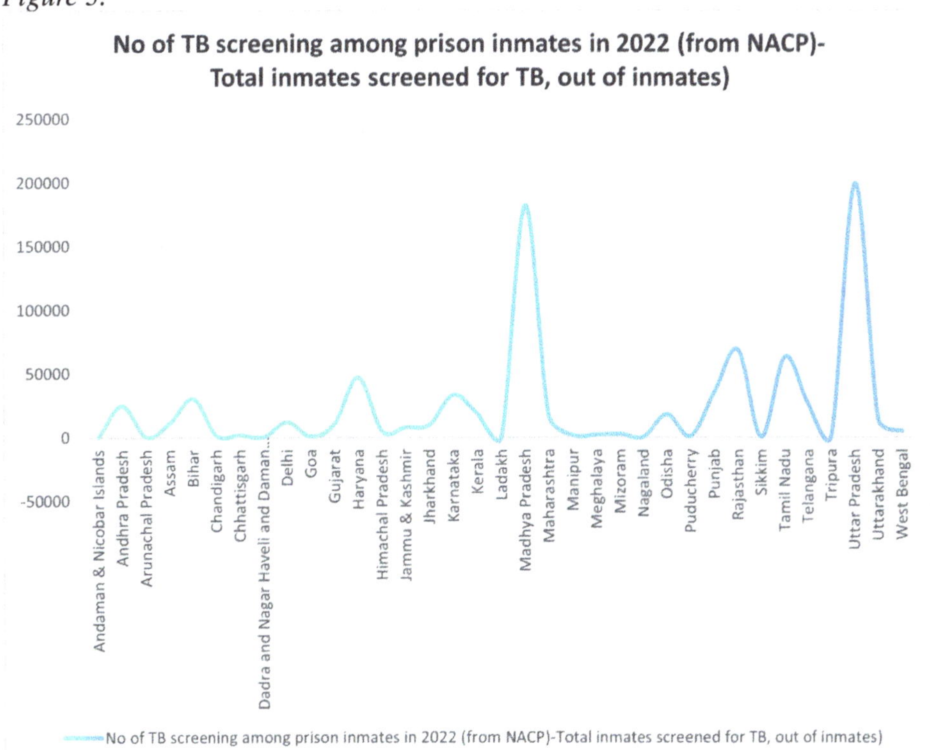

TB screening data represents the number of inmates actually screened for TB under NACP, not the total number of inmates. This data reflects the effectiveness and coverage of TB screening efforts in each state.

Table 5. Top 5 states by inmates screened

State	Inmates Screened
Uttar Pradesh	198,813
Madhya Pradesh	181,397
Rajasthan	68,289
Tamil Nadu	62,696
Haryana	46,633

These states had **robust screening programs**, covering a large share of prison inmates.

Table 6. States with very low screening

State/UT	Inmates Screened
Andaman & Nicobar Islands	1
Sikkim	15
Ladakh	26
Dadra & Nagar Haveli and Daman & Diu	73
Nagaland	116

Some states and union territories had minimal TB screening, likely due to smaller inmate populations or limited outreach. Moderate coverage (10,000–35,000 inmates screened) was seen in Andhra Pradesh (24,540), Karnataka (33,102), Punjab (35,004), Maharashtra (16,959), Bihar (30,131), and Delhi (11,657), indicating room for improvement. Uttar Pradesh, Madhya Pradesh, and Rajasthan showed the widest coverage, reflecting strong coordination between prison and health departments. In contrast, several northeastern states and UTs lagged behind, highlighting program gaps. This data is crucial for evaluating the reach and equity of prison TB control efforts and identifying areas needing focused intervention.

Table 7. India TB screening 2022

Indicator	Value
Total prison inmates	11,33,483
Screened for TB	8,42,619 (74%)
Referred for TB testing	58,883 (7% of screened)
Actually tested	53,249 (90% of referred)
Diagnosed with TB	1,209 (2% of tested)

74% of inmates were screened for TB – a good national coverage. Of those screened, 7% were suspected and referred for further TB testing. 90% of referred inmates actually underwent testing, indicating strong follow-up. 2% of tested inmates were confirmed TB cases, showing the importance of screening in identifying hidden cases.

Table 8. TB screening among prison inmates National AIDS Control Program (NACP) 2022

State/Uts	No of TB screening among prison inmates in 2022 (from NACP)-Total prison inmates referred for TB testing, out of screened)	No of TB screening among prison inmates in 2022 (from NACP)-Total prison inmates tested for TB, out of referred)	No of TB screening among prison inmates in 2022 (from NACP)-Total prison inmates diagnosed as TB, out of tested)
Andaman & Nicobar Islands	1	0	0
Andhra Pradesh	74	78	9
Arunachal Pradesh	0	NA	NA
Assam	322	252	10
Bihar	18093	18086	229
Chandigarh	1	1	0
Chhattisgarh	37	42	5
Dadra and Nagar Haveli and Daman and Diu	10	10	0
Delhi	498	372	90
Goa	14	8	0
Gujarat	552	441	16
Haryana	751	751	12
Himachal Pradesh	748	748	7
Jammu & Kashmir	2564	2082	6
Jharkhand	502	502	5

State/Uts	No of TB screening among prison inmates in 2022 (from NACP)-Total prison inmates referred for TB testing, out of screened)	No of TB screening among prison inmates in 2022 (from NACP)-Total prison inmates tested for TB, out of referred)	No of TB screening among prison inmates in 2022 (from NACP)-Total prison inmates diagnosed as TB, out of tested)
Karnataka	369	283	12
Kerala	1871	1738	10
Ladakh	0	0	0
Madhya Pradesh	18519	16606	214
Maharashtra	2245	1419	42
Manipur	4	4	1
Meghalaya	24	24	0
Mizoram	22	17	1
Nagaland	10	10	2
Odisha	918	539	2
Puducherry	0	0	0
Punjab	272	233	9
Rajasthan	484	284	23
Sikkim	0	0	0
Tamil Nadu	4946	3815	24
Telangana	210	210	20
Tripura	6	6	0
Uttar Pradesh	3528	3462	373
Uttarakhand	402	393	14
West Bengal	886	833	73

In 2022, Uttar Pradesh reported the highest number of TB cases among prison inmates (373), followed by Bihar (229), Madhya Pradesh (214), Delhi (90), and West Bengal (73). These states bear a significant TB burden, highlighting the need for continued screening and treatment. Most states showed good follow-up, testing nearly all referred inmates. However, Arunachal Pradesh, Ladakh, Puducherry, and Sikkim had no referrals or testing, revealing gaps in prison TB care. Uttar Pradesh and Delhi had high TB positivity rates, stressing the importance of focused screening in overcrowded prisons. Low case numbers in smaller states/UTs were often due to poor referral systems, not necessarily low TB prevalence. Though follow-up testing is generally effective, screening-to-diagnosis efficiency remains uneven.

continued on following page

Table 8. Continued
Strengthening screening and referrals in northeastern and smaller UTs is essential for equitable TB control across India's prisons.

LIMITATIONS OF THE STUDY

The secondary study focused on sources such as the National Crime Records Bureau (NCRB), WHO reports, and other existing literature published in standard journals like Springer, Elsevier, Taylor & Francis, MDPI, Sage, and peer-reviewed journals. These sources were used for this study to analyze and understand the various challenges faced in prison facilities. The secondary data was collected from data.gov.in, the Centers for Disease Control and Prevention, the International Union Against Tuberculosis and Lung Disease (The Union), the GAFTM report, and the USAID report to understand the various issues in the prison setting affecting TB inmates. The study mainly emphasizes the central prison setting; the findings may not be universally applicable to all prison inmates across the country. The reliability of the research focuses on the accuracy of the data, with secondary data being used for the study. The research study only emphasizes prison inmates affected by TB and the screening mechanism, diagnosis methods, treatment adherence, and effective follow-up. The study analyzes the recent data used in prison screening across all prisons state-wise, examining the overall number of inmates and analyzing the trend of how many are affected by TB infection. The study is highly confidential and obtaining primary data requires permission from the prison administration, which is a long-term process. Therefore, the study is conducted using secondary sources. The secondary study does not need to evaluate budgetary constraints and staffing issues. There is a lack of medical infrastructure, which may influence TB diagnosis and the provision of treatment support in prison settings.

OUTCOME OF THE STUDY

The prison setting overcrowding affects the incarcerated population by increasing the TB prevalence rate among the inmates. Due to overcrowding in prisons, where the capacity level exceeds the actual number of inmates, the TB incidence is identified to be 3 to 7 times higher compared to non-overcrowded facilities. There is poor ventilation in the prison cells, shared dormitory-style, and close physical contact; this may increase the level of TB transmission. When new inmates enter prison, improper diagnosis and delay in identifying symptoms can increase the TB rate in the prison. Healthcare facility accessibility is inadequate, and medical services are insufficient; this can increase the risk of TB incidence. Due to a shortage of staff, lack of proper awareness among wardens, and insufficient health equipment such as diagnostic tools, these are major barriers in prison settings. There are 40% of inmates with a high burden and high density in the prison; this can increase the need for medical evaluation of respiratory symptoms (Srinivasan & Tyagi, 2025).

Poor treatment adherence in prison administration and enhanced regular monitoring can reduce the relapse rate. If any TB patients are affected by Adverse Drug Reactions (ADR), support should be provided to the medical team to arrange appropriate facility support. This can prevent the development of drug-resistant TB in affected individuals. Providing psycho-social support to the inmates can reduce stigma levels and help avoid isolation among prison inmates. This can exacerbate misconceptions among prison staff about TB disease transmission. Prison administration lacks an effective TB screening program to conduct routine screening for new and existing inmates. This can prevent TB transmission to other prison inmates and is more useful for early detection and support services. Prison administration should take necessary action to improve reform policies to address overcrowding; this can reduce public health issues. Need-based services to reduce inmate density and improve healthcare facilities in the prison. This can control TB transmission, increase successful outcomes for prison inmates, and prevent TB disease in prison settings.

CONCLUSION

The study highlights the various critical challenges associated with TB screening, diagnosis, treatment, and follow-up in the prison facility. The impact of overcrowding in prison inmates increases the spread of TB infection. The secondary data can be used for the present study with sources such as the National Crime Records Bureau (NCRB), WHO reports, and the Centers for Disease Control and Prevention. The secondary sources identify the existing gaps in the prison health facility. The secondary data analysis improves the screening process, provides medical facilities, and enhances effective treatment support for TB-affected inmates. The adoption of innovative strategies by the prison administration can strengthen TB management in prison settings. The study provides various challenges faced by prison administration, and it can increase evidence-based policy support to improve healthcare interventions and reduce the TB burden in prison settings. To reduce the TB burden and increase evidence-based practices to support policy-making and improve healthcare interventions in prison settings. This can ensure better health outcomes and successful treatment for incarcerated individuals affected by TB.

Future Implication

The implication emphasizes the urgent need to provide policy measures to enhance healthcare interventions and decrease TB levels in prison settings. The study mainly incorporates real-time data collected through secondary sources. This can assess the health facility in deeper insights to identify the challenges in TB diagnosis and treatment adherence. Future studies can further focus on age-wise TB prevalence in prisons and the dormitory living conditions of young and older adults. Strengthening prison healthcare infrastructure can include medical staffing, diagnostic facilities, and nutritional support to provide an effective approach to TB management. How digital health technology provides detection, monitoring, treatment, and follow-up for effective treatment and successful treatment outcomes. The best practices to enhance the prison system can be tailored to further enhance disease control efficacy. The study motivates the improvement of policy making in prison administration to increase public health concerns. Authorities must collaborate to implement evidence-based practices to mitigate TB transmission. This can lead to overall improvement in the health and well-being of prison inmates.

REFERENCES

Abbara, A., Almalla, M., AlMasri, I., AlKabbani, H., Karah, N., El-Amin, W., Rajan, L., Rahhal, I., Alabbas, M., Sahloul, Z., Tarakji, A., & Sparrow, A. (2020). The challenges of tuberculosis control in protracted conflict: The case of Syria. *International Journal of Infectious Diseases*, *90*, 53–59. DOI: 10.1016/j.ijid.2019.10.015

Adane, K., Spigt, M., & Dinant, G. J. (2018). Tuberculosis treatment outcome and predictors in northern Ethiopian prisons: A five-year retrospective analysis. *BMC Pulmonary Medicine*, *18*(1), 1–8. DOI: 10.1186/s12890-018-0600-1

Akers, T. A., Blake, B. J., & Hanson, R. A. (2008). Infections diseases from a global perspective. *Global health care: Issues and policies*, 181-198.

Amede, P. O., Adedire, E., Usman, A., Ameh, C. A., Umar, F. S., Umeokonkwo, C. D., & Balogun, M. S. (2022). Drug-susceptible tuberculosis treatment outcomes and its associated factors among inmates in prison settings in Bauchi State, Nigeria, 2014–2018. *PLoS One*, *17*(7), e0270819. DOI: 10.1371/journal.pone.0270819

Baird, K., Said, H., Koornhof, H. J., & Duse, A. G. (2022). Tuberculosis control at a South African correctional centre: Diagnosis, treatment and strain characterisation. *PLoS One*, *17*(11), e0277459. DOI: 10.1371/journal.pone.0277459

Baussano, I., Williams, B. G., Nunn, P., Beggiato, M., Fedeli, U., & Scano, F. (2010). Tuberculosis incidence in prisons: A systematic review. *PLoS Medicine*, *7*(12), e1000381. DOI: 10.1371/journal.pmed.1000381

Baxter, S., Goyder, E., Chambers, D., Johnson, M., Preston, L., & Booth, A. (2017). Interventions to improve contact tracing for tuberculosis in specific groups and in wider populations: An evidence synthesis. *Health and Social Care Delivery Research*, *5*(1), 1–102.

Beaudry, G., Zhong, S., Whiting, D., Javid, B., Frater, J., & Fazel, S. (2020). Managing outbreaks of highly contagious diseases in prisons: A systematic review. *BMJ Global Health*, *5*(11), e003201. https://gh.bmj.com/content/5/11/e003201. DOI: 10.1136/bmjgh-2020-003201

Behera, D., Pannu, V. P., & Behera, R. K. (2020). National tb elimination programme–can it end tb in india by 2025: An appraisal. *The Indian Journal of Chest Diseases & Allied Sciences*, *62*(4), 203–227. DOI: 10.5005/ijcdas-62-4-203

Biadglegne, F., Rodloff, A. C., & Sack, U. (2015). Review of the prevalence and drug resistance of tuberculosis in prisons: A hidden epidemic. *Epidemiology and Infection*, *143*(5), 887–900. DOI: 10.1017/S095026881400288X

Busatto, C., Bierhals, D. V., Vianna, J. S., Silva, P. E. A. D., Possuelo, L. G., & Ramis, I. B. (2022). Epidemiology and control strategies for tuberculosis in countries with the largest prison populations. *Revista da Sociedade Brasileira de Medicina Tropical*, *55*, e0060–e2022. DOI: 10.1590/0037-8682-0060-2022

Byrne, E., Bradshaw, D., Kerin, M., & Pepe, I. (2024). A social identity approach to mental health help-seeking behaviour in prisoners: A systematic review. *Journal of Community & Applied Social Psychology*, *34*(1), e2727. DOI: 10.1002/casp.2727

Carwile, M. E., Hochberg, N. S., & Sinha, P. (2022). Undernutrition is feeding the tuberculosis pandemic: A perspective. *Journal of Clinical Tuberculosis and Other Mycobacterial Diseases*, *27*, 100311. DOI: 10.1016/j.jctube.2022.100311

Chao, W. C., Yen, C. L., Wu, C. H., & Shieh, C. C. (2020). How mycobacteria take advantage of the weakness in human immune system in the modern world. *Journal of Microbiology, Immunology, and Infection*, *53*(2), 209–215. DOI: 10.1016/j.jmii.2019.10.008

Charalambous, S., Velen, K., Rueda, Z., Croda, J., Herce, M. E., Shenoi, S. V., Altice, F., Muyoyeta, M., Telisinghe, L., Grandjean, L., Keshavjee, S., & Andrews, J. R. (2023). Scaling up evidence-based approaches to tuberculosis screening in prisons. *The Lancet. Public Health*, *8*(4), e305–e310. DOI: 10.1016/S2468-2667(23)00002-6

Chen, Y., Liu, J., Zhang, Q., Wang, Q., Chai, L., Chen, H., Li, D., Qui, Y., Wang, Y., Shen, N., Wang, J., Xie, X., Li, S., & Li, M. (2023). Epidemiological features and temporal trends of HIV-negative tuberculosis burden from 1990 to 2019: A retrospective analysis based on the Global Burden of Disease Study 2019. *BMJ Open*, *13*(9), e074134. DOI: 10.1136/bmjopen-2023-074134

Chen, Z., Wang, T., Du, J., Sun, L., Wang, G., Ni, R., An, Y., Fan, X., Li, Y., Guo, R., Mao, L., Jing, W., Shi, K., Cheng, J., Wang, Q., Nie, W., Liu, H., Liang, J., & Gong, W. (2025). Decoding the WHO Global Tuberculosis Report 2024: A Critical Analysis of Global and Chinese Key Data. *Zoonoses (Shannon)*, *5*(1), 999. DOI: 10.15212/ZOONOSES-2024-0061

Cloud, D. H., Garcia-Grossman, I. R., Armstrong, A., & Williams, B. (2023). Public health and prisons: Priorities in the age of mass incarceration. *Annual Review of Public Health*, *44*(1), 407–428. DOI: 10.1146/annurev-publhealth-071521-034016

Cords, O., Martinez, L., Warren, J. L., O'Marr, J. M., Walter, K. S., Cohen, T., Zheng, J., Ko, A. I., Croda, J., & Andrews, J. R. (2021). Incidence and prevalence of tuberculosis in incarcerated populations: A systematic review and meta-analysis. *The Lancet. Public Health*, *6*(5), e300–e308. DOI: 10.1016/S2468-2667(21)00025-6

Coreil, J., Mayard, G., Simpson, K. M., Lauzardo, M., Zhu, Y., & Weiss, M. (2010). Structural forces and the production of TB-related stigma among Haitians in two contexts. *Social Science & Medicine*, *71*(8), 1409–1417. DOI: 10.1016/j.socscimed.2010.07.017

Damanik, A. S., Fitri, A., Hidayati, F., Nasution, H. S., Wisudariani, E., & Riyandani, E. (2025). Determinants of Pulmonary Tuberculosis Among Inmates in Class IIA Penitentiary in Jambi City. *Environmental Research and Planetary Health, 1*(1), 18–25. DOI: 10.53623/erph.v1i1.517

Dara, M., Acosta, C. D., Melchers, N. V. V., Al-Darraji, H. A., Chorgoliani, D., Reyes, H., Centis, R., Sotgiu, G., Ambrosio, L. D., Chadha, S. S., & Migliori, G. B. (2015). Tuberculosis control in prisons: Current situation and research gaps. *International Journal of Infectious Diseases*, *32*, 111–117. DOI: 10.1016/j.ijid.2014.12.029

Darraj, A., Hudays, A., Hazazi, A., Hobani, A., & Alghamdi, A. (2023). The association between emergency department overcrowding and delay in treatment: a systematic review. In *Healthcare* (Vol. 11, No. 3, p. 385). MDPI. DOI: 10.3390/healthcare11030385

Dheda, K., Mirzayev, F., Cirillo, D. M., Udwadia, Z., Dooley, K. E., Chang, K. C., Omar, S. V., Reuter, A., Perumal, T.Jr, Horsburgh, C. R.Jr, Murray, M., & Lange, C. (2024). Multidrug-resistant tuberculosis. *Nature Reviews. Disease Primers*, *10*(1), 22. DOI: 10.1038/s41572-024-00504-2

Dirks, L. K., Bircher, P. M., González-Montalvo, M. D. M., Kauffman, A. E., Prophete, E. J., Bury, M. R., & Spaulding, A. C. (2023). Video Directly Observed Therapy for Tuberculosis Treatment in Haitian Prisons: A Pattern of Group Adherence. medRxiv, 2023-12. DOI: 10.1101/2023.12.29.23299977

Divala, T. H., Lewis, J., Bulterys, M. A., Lutje, V., Corbett, E. L., Schumacher, S. G., & MacPherson, P. (2022). Missed opportunities for diagnosis and treatment in patients with TB symptoms: A systematic review. *Public Health Action*, *12*(1), 10–17. DOI: 10.5588/pha.21.0022

Dmitrieva, A., Stepanov, V., & Titar, I. (2024). (e)Managing the uncertainty of tuberculosis in the post-Soviet limbo: Tracking prisoners' coerced mobility for treatment in Ukrainian prisons. *Social Science & Medicine*, *349*, 116894. DOI: 10.1016/j.socscimed.2024.116894

Edge, C. L., King, E. J., Dolan, K., & McKee, M. (2016). Prisoners co-infected with tuberculosis and HIV: A systematic review. *Journal of the International AIDS Society*, *19*(1), 20960. DOI: 10.7448/IAS.19.1.20960

Emilian, C., Al-Juffali, N., & Fazel, S. (2025). Prevalence of severe mental illness among people in prison across 43 countries: A systematic review and meta-analysis. *The Lancet. Public Health, 10*(2), e97–e110. https://www.thelancet.com/journals/lanpub/article/PIIS2468-2667(24)00280-9/fulltext. DOI: 10.1016/S2468-2667(24)00280-9

Etim, N. G., Mirabeau, Y., Olorode, A., & Nwodo, U. (2024). Risk Factors of Tuberculosis and Strategies for Prevention and Control. *Int J Innovative Healthcare Res, 12*(1), 1–13.

Ferreira, M. R., Bonfim, R. O., Siqueira, T. C., Andrade, R. L. P., Monroe, A. A., Villa, T. C. S., & Orfão, N. H. (2019). Tuberculosis in prison and aspects associated with the diagnosis site. *Journal of Infection in Developing Countries, 13*(11), 968–977. DOI: 10.3855/jidc.11522

Gonçalves, C., Arakaki-Sanchez, D., Pelissari, D. M., Costa, F. D., Croda, J., Walter, K. S., & Andrews, J. R. (2022). The effect of incarceration on TB treatment outcomes. *The International Journal of Tuberculosis and Lung Disease : the Official Journal of the International Union against Tuberculosis and Lung Disease, 26*(3), 252–258. DOI: 10.5588/ijtld.21.0449

Grange, J. M., Brunet, L. R., & Rieder, H. L. (2011). Immune protection against tuberculosis–When is immunotherapy preferable to vaccination? *Tuberculosis (Edinburgh, Scotland), 91*(2), 179–185. DOI: 10.1016/j.tube.2010.12.004

Gulumbe, B. H., Abdulrahim, A., Ahmad, S. K., Lawan, K. A., & Danlami, M. B. (2025). WHO report signals tuberculosis resurgence: Addressing systemic failures and revamping control strategies. *Decoding Infection and Transmission, 3*, 100044. DOI: 10.1016/j.dcit.2025.100044

Guo, W., Cronk, R., Scherer, E., Oommen, R., Brogan, J., Sarr, M., & Bartram, J. (2019). A systematic scoping review of environmental health conditions in penal institutions. *International Journal of Hygiene and Environmental Health, 222*(5), 790–803. DOI: 10.1016/j.ijheh.2019.05.001

Idrees, M., & Bilal, M. (2023). Behind Bars: A Critical Investigation of Prison's Conditions and Protection of the Prisoner's Human Rights in Pakistan. *Review of Education. Administration & Law, 6*(2), 567–578. DOI: 10.47067/real.v6i2.332

Jain, D., & Tronic, B. (2018). Tuberculosis in India: A human rights approach to healthcare. *Sw. J. Int'l L., 24*, 219.

Jeffries, C., Lobue, P., Chorba, T., Metchock, B., & Kashef, I. (2017). Role of the Health Department in Tuberculosis Prevention and Control—Legal and Public Health Considerations. *Tuberculosis and Nontuberculous Mycobacterial Infections*, 261-282.

Khan, A., Khan, N., & Singh, R. (2024). Tuberculosis diagnosis versus GeneXpert® MTB/RIF formats. *Bioanalysis, 16*(16), 843–848. DOI: 10.1080/17576180.2024.2349423

Kharwadkar, S., Attanayake, V., Duncan, J., Navaratne, N., & Benson, J. (2022). The impact of climate change on the risk factors for tuberculosis: A systematic review. *Environmental Research, 212*, 113436. DOI: 10.1016/j.envres.2022.113436

Kuupiel, D., Vezi, P., Bawontuo, V., Osei, E., & Mashamba-Thompson, T. P. (2020). Tuberculosis active case-finding interventions and approaches for prisoners in sub-Saharan Africa: A systematic scoping review. *BMC Infectious Diseases, 20*(1), 1–14. DOI: 10.1186/s12879-020-05283-1

Lee, J. Y., Kwon, N., Goo, G. Y., & Cho, S. I. (2022). Inadequate housing and pulmonary tuberculosis: A systematic review. *BMC Public Health, 22*(1), 622. DOI: 10.1186/s12889-022-12879-6

Litvinjenko, S., Magwood, O., Wu, S., & Wei, X. (2023). Burden of tuberculosis among vulnerable populations worldwide: An overview of systematic reviews. *The Lancet. Infectious Diseases, 23*(12), 1395–1407. DOI: 10.1016/S1473-3099(23)00372-9

Liu, Y. E., Mabene, Y., Camelo, S., Rueda, Z. V., Pelissari, D. M., Johansen, F. D. C., Huaman, M. A., Avalos-Cruz, T., Alarcon, V. A., Ladutke, L., Bergman, M., Cohen, T., Goldhaber-Fiebert, J., Croda, J., & Andrews, J. R. (2024). Mass incarceration as a driver of the tuberculosis epidemic in Latin America and projected effects of policy alternatives: A mathematical modelling study. *The Lancet. Public Health, 9*(11), e841–e851. https://www.thelancet.com/journals/lanpub/article/PIIS2468-2667(24)00192-0/fulltext. DOI: 10.1016/S2468-2667(24)00192-0

Lu, W., Zhu, L., Liu, Q., Chen, C., Lu, P., Ding, X., Shao, Y., & Li, Y. (2023). Progress in Epidemiology of Tuberculosis in China. In *Progress in China Epidemiology* (Vol. 1, pp. 151–186). Springer Nature Singapore., DOI: 10.1007/978-981-19-2199-5_8

Mabud, T. S., de Lourdes Delgado Alves, M., Ko, A. I., Basu, S., Walter, K. S., Cohen, T., Mathema, B., Colijn, C., Lemos, E., Croda, J., & Andrews, J. R. (2019). Evaluating strategies for control of tuberculosis in prisons and prevention of spillover into communities: An observational and modeling study from Brazil. *PLoS Medicine, 16*(1), e1002737. DOI: 10.1371/journal.pmed.1002737

Macleod, A., Nair, D., Ilbahar, E., Sellars, M., & Nolte, L. (2020). Identifying barriers and facilitators to implementing advance care planning in prisons: A rapid literature review. *Health & Justice*, *8*(1), 1–11. DOI: 10.1186/s40352-020-00123-5

Marks, L. R., Nolan, N. S., Liang, S. Y., Durkin, M. J., & Weimer, M. B. (2022). Infectious complications of injection drug use. *Medical Clinics*, *106*(1), 187–200. https://www.medical.theclinics.com/article/S0025-7125(21)00114-0/abstract

Martinez, L., Warren, J. L., Harries, A. D., Croda, J., Espinal, M. A., Olarte, R. A. L., Avedillo, P., Lienhardt, C., Bhatia, V., Liu, Q., Chakaya, J., Denholm, J. T., Lin, Y., Kawatsu, L., Zhu, L., Horsburgh, R., & Andrews, J. R. (2023). Global, regional, and national estimates of tuberculosis incidence and case detection among incarcerated individuals from 2000 to 2019: A systematic analysis. *The Lancet. Public Health*, *8*(7), e511–e519. https://www.thelancet.com/journals/lanpub/article/PIIS2468-2667(23)00097-X/fulltext. DOI: 10.1016/S2468-2667(23)00097-X

Nardell, E. A., & Fennelly, K. P. (2006). Tuberculosis transmission and infection control in congregate settings. In *Reichman and Hershfield's Tuberculosis* (pp. 843–872). CRC Press.

Nyasulu, P. S., Hui, D. S., Mwaba, P., Tamuzi, J. L., Sakala, D. Y., Ntoumi, F., Maeurer, M., Goletti, D., Petersen, E., & Zumla, A. (2025). Global perspectives on tuberculosis in prisons and incarceration centers-Risk factors, priority needs, challenges for control and the way forward. *IJID Regions*, *14*, 100621. DOI: 10.1016/j.ijregi.2025.100621

O'Grady, J., Hoelscher, M., Atun, R., Bates, M., Mwaba, P., Kapata, N., Ferrara, G., Maeurer, M., & Zumla, A. (2011). Tuberculosis in prisons in sub-Saharan Africa–the need for improved health services, surveillance and control. *Tuberculosis (Edinburgh, Scotland)*, *91*(2), 173–178. DOI: 10.1016/j.tube.2010.12.002

Pape, S., Gulma, K., Shivalli, S., & de Kiev, L. C. (2022). Diagnostic accuracy of screening algorithms to identify persons with active pulmonary tuberculosis at prison entry: Protocol of a systematic review and network meta-analysis. *Journal of Medicine and Life*, *15*(12), 1464–1475. DOI: 10.25122/jml-2022-0164

Pape, S., Gulma, K., Shivalli, S., & de Kiev, L. C. (2024). Diagnostic accuracy of active pulmonary tuberculosis screening during detention admission: A systematic review. *Journal of Medicine and Life*, *17*(7), 671–681. DOI: 10.25122/jml-2024-0155

Parvez, F. M. (2021). Prevention and control of tuberculosis in correctional facilities. In *Public health behind bars: from prisons to communities* (pp. 157–193). Springer US., DOI: 10.1007/978-1-0716-1807-3_11

Placeres, A. F., de Almeida Soares, D., Delpino, F. M., Moura, H. S. D., Scholze, A. R., Dos Santos, M. S., Arcêncio, R. A., & Fronteira, I. (2023). Epidemiology of TB in prisoners: A metanalysis of the prevalence of active and latent TB. *BMC Infectious Diseases*, *23*(1), 20. DOI: 10.1186/s12879-022-07961-8

Purdey, M. (2006). Anti-lactoferrin toxicity and elevated iron: The environmental prerequisites which activate susceptibility to tuberculosis infection? *Medical Hypotheses*, *66*(3), 513–517. DOI: 10.1016/j.mehy.2005.09.027

Rangaka, M. X., Cavalcante, S. C., Marais, B. J., Thim, S., Martinson, N. A., Swaminathan, S., & Chaisson, R. E. (2015). Controlling the seedbeds of tuberculosis: Diagnosis and treatment of tuberculosis infection. *Lancet*, *386*(10010), 2344–2353. https://www.thelancet.com/journals/lancet/article/PIIS0140-6736(15)00323-2/fulltext. DOI: 10.1016/S0140-6736(15)00323-2

Rentmeester, L. L., Burton, D. W., Fitzgerald, R. L., & Clark, R. F. (2014). 2014 ACMT annual scientific meeting—March 28–30, 2014 Phoenix, AZ, USA. *Journal of Medical Toxicology; Official Journal of the American College of Medical Toxicology*, *10*(1), 65–99. DOI: 10.1007/s13181-013-0376-x

Reyes, H. (2007). Pitfalls of TB management in prisons, revisited. *international journal of prisoner. International Journal of Prisoner Health*, *3*(1), 43–67. DOI: 10.1080/17449200601149148

Roberts, C. A., Lobato, M. N., Bazerman, L. B., Kling, R., Reichard, A. A., & Hammett, T. M. (2006). Tuberculosis prevention and control in large jails: A challenge to tuberculosis elimination. *American Journal of Preventive Medicine*, *30*(2), 125–130. DOI: 10.1016/j.amepre.2005.10.018

Rust, G., Ye, J., Baltrus, P., Daniels, E., Adesunloye, B., & Fryer, G. E. (2008). Practical barriers to timely primary care access: Impact on adult use of emergency department services. *Archives of Internal Medicine*, *168*(15), 1705–1710. DOI: 10.1001/archinte.168.15.1705

Saini, V., & Garg, K. (2020). Case finding strategies under national tuberculosis elimination programme (NTEP). *indian journal of tuberculosis*, *67*(4), S101-S106. DOI: 10.1016/j.ijtb.2020.09.029

Sanchez, A., Massari, V., Gerhardt, G., Espinola, A. B., Siriwardana, M., Camacho, L. A. B., & Larouzé, B. (2013). X ray screening at entry and systematic screening for the control of tuberculosis in a highly endemic prison. *BMC Public Health*, *13*(1), 1–7. DOI: 10.1186/1471-2458-13-983

Santos, M. S. D., Berra, T. Z., Scholze, A. R., Delpino, F. M., Ramos, A. C. V., Alves, Y. M., & Paulino da Costa, F. (2022). Trend and spatial distribution of drug-resistant tuberculosis in liberty-deprived populations in the State of Paraná, Brazil. *Tropical Medicine and Infectious Disease*, *7*(10), 266. DOI: 10.3390/tropicalmed7100266

Scholze, A. R., Dália Alves, J., Berra, T. Z., Santos, F. L. D., Ramos, A. C. V., Lima de Freitas, G., Galdino, M. J. Q., Pieri, F. M., & Arcoverde, M. (2022). The burden of alcohol, tobacco and others drugs among incarcerated population diagnosed with tuberculosis: Time trends and spatial determinants in Southern Brazil. *BMC Public Health*, *22*(1), 999. DOI: 10.1186/s12889-022-13408-1

Segal-Maurer, S. (2017). Tuberculosis in enclosed populations. *Tuberculosis and Nontuberculous Mycobacterial Infections*, 237-259. DOI: 10.1128/9781555819866.ch14

Sequera, G., Estigarribia, G., Walter, K. S., Lopez, R., Andrews, J., & Croda, J. (2023). *Tuberculosis in prisons: a growing global health concern. The Challenge of Tuberculosis in the 21st Century*. European Respiratory Society.

Short, S. R. (2017). Grassroots challenges to the effects of prison sprawl on mental health services for incarcerated people. *The Fordham Urban Law Journal*, *45*, 437.

Simpson, P. L., Simpson, M., Adily, A., Grant, L., & Butler, T. (2019). Prison cell spatial density and infectious and communicable diseases: A systematic review. *BMJ Open*, *9*(7), e026806. DOI: 10.1136/bmjopen-2018-026806

Srinivasan, S. (2021). Mental Health problems faced by Aged Inmates due to Overcrowding of Central prison in Tamil Nadu. DOI: 10.2139/ssrn.3962987

Srinivasan, S., & Praba Lama (2025). Patient-Centered Care for TB Patients: An Effective Approach to Corporate Social Responsibility. In Corporate Social Responsibility in Health and Social Care (pp. 183-218).IGI Global. DOI:DOI: 10.4018/979-8-3693-5991-4.ch008

Srinivasan, S. (2025). Patient-Centric Care in Tuberculosis Management: Addressing Challenges and Improving Health Outcomes. In *Convergence of Population Health Management, Pharmacogenomics, and Patient-Centered Care* (pp. 265-282). IGI Global. DOI: 10.4018/979-8-3693-3260-3.ch012

Srinivasan, S., Rajavel, N., & Kumar, A. S. (2025). Cancer Diagnosis and Treatment Barriers Among Prisoners. In *Cancer Diagnosis, Treatment and Care: Reflections for the Education of Survivors and Healthcare Providers* (pp. 185-202). IGI Global Scientific Publishing. DOI: 10.4018/979-8-3693-5400-1.ch011

Srinivasan, S., Rajavel, N., & Mahmoudi-Dehaki, M. (2025). Elderly Inmates Living With Dementia in Central Prisons. In *Assistive Technology Solutions for Aging Adults and Individuals With Disabilities* (pp. 343–404). IGI Global Scientific Publishing., DOI: 10.4018/979-8-3693-6308-9.ch015

Srinivasan, S., Rajavel, N., & Sanchez, N. K. (2025). The Impact of AI on Elderly Inmates in Central Prison. In *Exploration of AI in Contemporary Legal Systems* (pp. 281–314). IGI Global Scientific Publishing., DOI: 10.4018/979-8-3693-7205-0.ch013

Srinivasan, S., & Tyagi, N. (2025). Respiratory Diseases Affected by Informal Workers. In *Generative AI Techniques for Sustainability in Healthcare Security* (pp. 95–124). IGI Global Scientific Publishing., DOI: 10.4018/979-8-3693-6577-9.ch006

Srinivasan, S., & Vallipriya, R. (2025). Intercultural Communication: An Effective Strategy for the Patient Physician Relationship. In *Cases on Physician Cultural Responsibility, Ethics, and Biases* (pp. 171-192). IGI Global Scientific Publishing. DOI: 10.4018/979-8-3693-3683-0.ch008

Srinivasan, S., & Vallipriya, R. (2025). Bias: Understanding and Addressing Disparities in Patient Care Across Multiple Demographics. In *Cases on Physician Cultural Responsibility, Ethics, and Biases* (pp. 21-38). IGI Global Scientific Publishing. DOI: 10.4018/979-8-3693-3683-0.ch002

Srinivasan, S., Vallipriya, R., & Singh, A. K. (2025). Integrated Public-Private Partnerships to Combat Tuberculosis for Improving Economic Development. In *Public Private Partnership Dynamics for Economic Development* (pp. 323–356). IGI Global Scientific Publishing., DOI: 10.4018/979-8-3693-9153-2.ch015

Tamuzi, J. L., Muyaya, L. M., & Mbuesse, P. (2021). HIV/TB co-infection prevalence and treatment outcomes in Democratic Republic of the Congo from 2005 to 2020: Systematic review and meta-analysis. *Community Medicine and Health Education Research*, *2*(1), 17–35. DOI: 10.33702/cmher.2021.2.1.4

Tavoschi, L., O'Moore, É., & Hedrich, D. (2019). Challenges and opportunities for the management of infectious diseases in Europes' prisons: Evidence-based guidance. *The Lancet. Infectious Diseases*, *19*(7), e253–e258. https://www.thelancet.com/journals/laninf/article/PIIS1473-3099(18)30756-4/abstract. DOI: 10.1016/S1473-3099(18)30756-4

Thapa, P., Narasimhan, P., Jayasuriya, R., Hall, J. J., Mukherjee, P. S., Das, D. K., & Beek, K. (2023). Barriers and facilitators to informal healthcare provider engagement in the national tuberculosis elimination program of India: An exploratory study from West Bengal. *PLOS Global Public Health*, *3*(10), e0001390. DOI: 10.1371/journal.pgph.0001390

Tiberi, S., Du Plessis, N., Walzl, G., Vjecha, M. J., Rao, M., Ntoumi, F., Mfinanga, S., Kapata, N., Mwaba, P., McHugh, T. D., Ippolito, G., Migliori, G. B., Maeurer, M. J., & Zumla, A. (2018). Tuberculosis: Progress and advances in development of new drugs, treatment regimens, and host-directed therapies. *The Lancet. Infectious Diseases*, *18*(7), e183–e198. https://www.thelancet.com/journals/laninf/article/PIIS1473-3099(18)30110-5/fulltext. DOI: 10.1016/S1473-3099(18)30110-5

Topp, S. M., Moonga, C. N., Luo, N., Kaingu, M., Chileshe, C., Magwende, G., Heymann, S. J., & Henostroza, G. (2016). Exploring the drivers of health and healthcare access in Zambian prisons: A health systems approach. *Health Policy and Planning*, *31*(9), 1250–1261. DOI: 10.1093/heapol/czw059

Trickey, A., & Trickey, A. (2017). Investigating the epidemiology of hepatitis C virus (HCV) infection in different settings. *The American Journal of Tropical Medicine and Hygiene*, *97*(6), 1920–1928. DOI: 10.4269/ajtmh.17-0019

Tsegaye Sahle, E., Blumenthal, J., Jain, S., Sun, S., Young, J., Manyazewal, T., Woldeamanuel, H., Teferra, L., Feleke, B., Vandenber, O., Rey, Z., Briggs-Hagen, M., Haubrich, R., Amogne, W., & McCutchan, J. A. (2019). Bacteriologically-confirmed pulmonary tuberculosis in an Ethiopian prison: Prevalence from screening of entrant and resident prisoners. *PLoS One*, *14*(12), e0226160. DOI: 10.1371/journal.pone.0226160

Urrego, J., Ko, A. I., Carbone, A. D. S. S., Paião, D. S. G., Sgarbi, R. V. E., Yeckel, C. W., Andrews, J. A., & Croda, J. (2015). The impact of ventilation and early diagnosis on tuberculosis transmission in Brazilian prisons. *The American Journal of Tropical Medicine and Hygiene*, *93*(4), 739–746. DOI: 10.4269/ajtmh.15-0166

Vinkeles Melchers, N. V., van Elsland, S. L., Lange, J. M., Borgdorff, M. W., & van den Hombergh, J. (2013). State of affairs of tuberculosis in prison facilities: A systematic review of screening practices and recommendations for best TB control. *PLoS One*, *8*(1), e53644. DOI: 10.1371/journal.pone.0053644

Wallace, D., & Wallace, R. (2019). Problems with the WHO TB model. *Mathematical Biosciences*, *313*, 71–80. DOI: 10.1016/j.mbs.2019.05.002

Wondmeneh, T. G., & Mekonnen, A. T. (2023). The incidence rate of tuberculosis and its associated factors among HIV-positive persons in Sub-Saharan Africa: A systematic review and meta-analysis. *BMC Infectious Diseases*, *23*(1), 613. DOI: 10.1186/s12879-023-08533-0

Woodman, M., Haeusler, I. L., & Grandjean, L. (2019). Tuberculosis genetic epidemiology: A Latin American perspective. *Genes*, *10*(1), 53. DOI: 10.3390/genes10010053

World Health Organization. (2021). *WHO consolidated guidelines on tuberculosis. Module 2: screening-systematic screening for tuberculosis disease*. World Health Organization.

Zenner, D., Southern, J., Van Hest, R., DeVries, G., Stagg, H. R., Antoine, D., & Abubakar, I. (2013). Active case finding for tuberculosis among high-risk groups in low-incidence countries [State of the art series. Case finding/screening. Number 3 in the series]. *The International Journal of Tuberculosis and Lung Disease : the Official Journal of the International Union against Tuberculosis and Lung Disease, 17*(5), 573–582. DOI: 10.5588/ijtld.12.0920

Chapter 3
Diagnosis and Screening of Tuberculosis in Vulnerable Populations and the Elderly

Mohammed El Rhanbouri
https://orcid.org/0009-0006-9643-5181
Morpho-Science Research Laboratory, Faculty of Medicine and Pharmacy, Cadi Ayyad University, Marrake, Morocco

Samia Boussaa
https://orcid.org/0000-0002-5599-1097
ISPITS-Higher Institute of Nursing Professions and Technical Health of Rabat, Morocco

Abdelati Oussous
Higher Institute of Nursing Professions and Technical Health of Marrakech, Morocco

Mohamed Khalyfa
https://orcid.org/0009-0009-0902-0132
Laboratoire Sciences de Santé et Technologies, ISSS-UH1 Settat, Morocco

Said Khaldouni
https://orcid.org/0009-0001-6582-3572
Higher Institute of Nursing Professions and Technical Health of Marrakech, Morocco

Hasna Abdel-Fadel
Higher Institute of Nursing Professions and Technical Health of Marrakech, Morocco

Mounia Amane
https://orcid.org/0000-0002-9273-4284
Higher Institute of Nursing Professions and Technical Health of Marrakech, Morocco

DOI: 10.4018/979-8-3373-3446-2.ch003

ABSTRACT

Tuberculosis (TB) continues to pose significant public health challenges, particularly among vulnerable populations including elderly individuals, incarcerated persons, migrants, and people living with HIV. These groups face disproportionate burdens due to intersecting biological, social, and structural determinants that hinder timely diagnosis and treatment. Current diagnostic approaches, while improved through molecular technologies, remain constrained by resource limitations and operational barriers in high-risk settings. This analysis highlights critical gaps in TB screening protocols, emphasizing the need for context-specific strategies that address atypical clinical presentations in elderly patients and systemic barriers affecting marginalized communities. We argue for integrated interventions combining advanced diagnostics with community-based approaches to improve case detection and reduce transmission.

INTRODUCTION

Tuberculosis (TB) remains a major global public health concern, disproportionately affecting low- and middle-income countries, which account for nearly 80% of all cases and deaths (Litvinjenko et al., 2023). This reality reflects not only the magnitude of the global epidemiological burden of this infectious disease, but also its persistent embedding within a geography of health inequalities. Indeed, the global distribution of tuberculosis is not solely governed by biomedical determinants but is structurally rooted in contexts marked by socioeconomic hardship, fragile health systems, and unequal access to medical innovations. The predominance of TB in low- and middle-income countries illustrates the complex interaction between social vulnerability and the transmission dynamics of *Mycobacterium tuberculosis*, a pathogen whose dissemination is strongly associated with overcrowding, malnutrition, and immunosuppression.

Despite notable advances in the fight against the disease, certain populations continue to face an increased risk of contracting and transmitting TB—particularly individuals living in precarious or overcrowded environments, immunocompromised persons, and the elderly (World Health Organization, s. d.). This observation introduces a typology of high-risk groups, underscoring that overall improvements in health indicators do not negate the persistence of epidemiological vulnerability pockets. Precarious environments, often characterized by unsanitary conditions, overcrowding, and forced mobility, facilitate human-to-human transmission of the tubercle bacillus, particularly in settings such as prisons, urban slums, and displaced persons camps. Simultaneously, immunosuppression—whether due to

HIV infection, chronic malnutrition, immunosuppressive therapies, or physiological aging—compromises host defenses, promoting reactivation of latent TB foci. In the elderly, diagnosis is frequently delayed due to atypical clinical presentations and reduced diagnostic suspicion, contributing to increased morbidity and mortality in this age group.

In such contexts, early screening and diagnosis are crucial levers for controlling TB spread and improving patient prognosis (Haute Autorité de Santé, 2023). Early detection relies on the prompt identification of individuals carrying the disease, before complications arise or further transmission occur. It represents one of the pillars of TB control in a public health approach focused on interrupting transmission chains and preventing severe forms. However, early diagnosis necessitates accessible, sensitive, and specific tools that can function effectively in field settings often characterized by limited medical, human, and technical resources. Early diagnosis is particularly critical for immunocompromised individuals and older adults, in whom the disease progresses more rapidly, and clinical signs are less pronounced.

Nevertheless, numerous obstacles persist, hindering diagnostic access for the most vulnerable groups. These challenges stem from structural, economic, social, and cultural factors and affect both disadvantaged urban areas and remote rural regions (Blanc, 2023; Fessell & Lexa, 2019). This statement highlights the multidimensional nature of diagnostic inaccessibility. Structurally, many endemic regions face a severe lack of healthcare infrastructure, laboratory equipment, and trained professionals. Additionally, economic barriers (transportation costs, income loss due to waiting times), social challenges (stigma, mistrust of institutions), and cultural issues (traditional perceptions of illness, asymmetry in health information) intertwine to exacerbate diagnostic delays and disrupt continuity of care. In isolated rural areas, geographic distance and lack of suitable transport are major barriers to accessing screening centers, whereas in marginalized urban settings, health facility overload and social stigma often hinder early care-seeking behavior.

Improving TB screening requires appropriate tools, better organization of healthcare services, and innovative community-based approaches. Examples of good practices have already demonstrated effectiveness in overcoming diagnostic access barriers (Potty et al., 2021; Taylor et al., 2015). This suggests a clear strategic orientation: possessing efficient tests is insufficient unless they are integrated into systems specifically designed to effectively reach at-risk populations. Community-based strategies—such as mobile screening units, peer-led awareness interventions, and integrating screening into other primary healthcare services—are particularly relevant. These methods help circumvent sociocultural resistance, reduce patient costs, and strengthen trust in health systems. The effectiveness of these strategies lies in their ability to adapt to local contexts, engage community actors, and tightly coordinate screening, diagnosis, and therapeutic referral.

From a public health perspective, TB screening must be conceived not merely as a medical procedure but as an integrated, inclusive action centered on the specific needs of the affected populations. This concluding notion calls for a fundamental paradigm shift—from a purely biomedical model to a systemic and contextualized approach to screening. It emphasizes the importance of territorially embedded TB control measures, grounded in a nuanced understanding of social determinants of health, user expectations, and patterns of vulnerability. Effective screening cannot be reduced to a technical act: it must be designed as a tool for equity, health justice, and community empowerment.

This chapter will therefore explore the challenges of TB screening and diagnosis among vulnerable populations and older adults, highlighting existing barriers, current approaches, and avenues for improvement in resource-limited settings.

Definition of Vulnerable Populations in Epidemiology

Vulnerability to tuberculosis can be understood as a socio-structural construct resulting from social stratification dynamics that marginalize certain individuals or groups within the socioeconomic order (Litvinjenko et al., 2023). It refers to a configuration of structural, material, and behavioral factors that, through cumulative interaction, increase the likelihood of exposure to *Mycobacterium tuberculosis*, accelerate the progression from latent infection to active disease, and reduce access to timely and adequate healthcare services.

This includes individuals living in precarious socioeconomic conditions—characterized by low income, unstable or hazardous jobs, limited education, or social exclusion—as well as those belonging to ethnic, sexual, or migrant minorities. These groups experience systemic disadvantages that expose them to harmful living environments (overcrowding, unsanitary conditions, malnutrition), structural barriers to healthcare (cost, distance, discrimination), and elevated risks of social stigma.

Thus, TB vulnerability should not be reduced to individual fragility but rather understood as the product of complex interactions among social determinants, health inequalities, and systemic failures. It calls for integrated public health approaches that are attuned to inequality and grounded in structural equity (Wu et al., 2023).

Prevalence and Incidence of Tuberculosis Among Vulnerable Groups

A TB prevalence exceeding 1,000 cases per 100,000 population has been observed across all vulnerable populations. Global estimates indicate that prevalence ratios are often more than 25 times higher among homeless individuals, incarcerated persons, refugees, asylum seekers, and people living with HIV, compared to the general population (Litvinjenko et al., 2023).

The prevalence of pulmonary TB among prisoners in sub-Saharan Africa is a concerning indicator of the health status of this group. Data show a prevalence of 7.74%, significantly higher than that of the general population, indicating increased TB risk due to the social and health-specific conditions of the prison environment (Mera et al., 2023).

Subgroup analysis reveals significant variability in pulmonary TB prevalence across countries. In the Democratic Republic of the Congo, the prevalence reaches 19.72%, which signals a particularly alarming situation. In Zambia, the rate is also high at 11.68%, and in Ethiopia, it stands at 9.22% (Mera et al., 2023). These differences may be attributed to variations in prison living conditions, healthcare access, and TB management strategies.

Several important risk factors have been identified for pulmonary TB among prisoners. HIV co-infection, for instance, increases the risk nearly fivefold, as the virus weakens the immune system, making individuals more susceptible to infections like TB. A low body mass index (BMI < 18.5) is also associated with greater risk, likely due to malnutrition and physical frailty, which are common in prison settings. Longer incarceration is another factor, as prolonged exposure to unsanitary conditions, overcrowding, and poor ventilation increases the chance of TB transmission. Prior TB exposure further adds to the risk, since individuals previously exposed to the bacillus may be more vulnerable to disease development (Baussano et al., 2010; O'Grady et al., 2022).

These findings highlight the urgent need to implement early TB screening strategies in prisons, especially for inmates with risk factors such as HIV/TB co-infection, low BMI, or prolonged detention. Such efforts are essential to meeting global TB control commitments, particularly in resource-limited settings.

TUBERCULOSIS AMONG VULNERABLE POPULATIONS AND THE ELDERLY

Prisoners

Disadvantaged populations—due to precarious socioeconomic conditions, limited healthcare access, and heightened exposure to environmental and biological transmission factors—are structurally more at risk of contracting tuberculosis. Among them, incarcerated individuals represent a particularly vulnerable group. In most national contexts, the prevalence of HIV, AIDS, and numerous other infectious diseases is notably higher in correctional facilities—including prisons, pre-trial detention centers, and other closed settings—than in surrounding communities, (Rich et al., 2016).

A study on relative inequality among prison overcrowding quintiles found that TB incidence in the most overcrowded group was 1.92 times higher than in the least crowded group. The inequality index revealed an excess of 724 TB cases per 100,000 individuals in the most densely populated sectors. Additionally, a health concentration index of -0.121 indicates that TB incidence is disproportionately concentrated in these high-density groups (López et al., 2022). In this context, overcrowded prison populations face avoidable and unjust disparities compared to populations in less crowded conditions.

TB prevalence in prisons is also alarming—estimated to be between 3 and 1,000 times higher than in the general population—highlighting the urgent need for tailored public health policies. This situation is further exacerbated by the emergence of multidrug-resistant (MDR) and extensively drug-resistant (XDR) forms of TB, which demand an immediate revision of TB control strategies in correctional environments. Key risk factors include overcrowding, poor ventilation, malnutrition, HIV co-infection, and other conditions that favor TB transmission. Moreover, the problem extends beyond prison walls, as it affects the civilian population through family visits, prison staff, and judicial system actors, who may act as potential transmission vectors (Biadglegne et al., 2015).

Prisoner health—and particularly TB management in carceral settings—remains a politically and scientifically neglected issue. It is imperative for policymakers and the scientific community to collaborate and prioritize the fight against TB and its drug-resistant forms in prisons. Without such action, TB in correctional settings will remain an underestimated global threat, undermining national and international control efforts.

People Living with HIV

Tuberculosis remains one of the leading causes of mortality among people living with the human immunodeficiency virus (HIV), particularly in resource-limited countries. HIV infection significantly increases the risk of progression from latent TB infection to active disease, due to virus-induced immunosuppression (Getahun et al., 2015). According to the World Health Organization (WHO), approximately 10% of individuals diagnosed with TB in 2022 were also HIV-positive, and co-infection was responsible for 167,000 deaths in the same year (Lee et al., 2023). These figures underscore the urgent need to strengthen integrated screening and diagnostic strategies for co-infected populations.

People living with HIV face an 18-fold higher risk of developing active tuberculosis compared to the general population (Lee et al., 2023). This risk is even greater when the CD4 count falls below 200 cells/mm^3. Moreover, TB's clinical presentation in this population often differs from the classical forms seen in immuno-competent individuals. In immunocompromised patients, pulmonary TB requires particularly complex management, especially due to prolonged diagnostic delays, which are largely attributable to the difficulty in obtaining formal bacteriological confirmation. This situation significantly increases the risk of complications, notably the development of long-term pulmonary sequelae, which are often evident on radiological examination (Jebali et al., 2023). Respiratory symptoms may be absent, replaced by extrapulmonary manifestations or nonspecific symptoms (Gupta et al., 2015). This clinical complexity is a major barrier to early diagnosis, compounded by limited diagnostic capacities in many high-prevalence settings.

Migrants

Globalization, conflicts, and economic and climate crises have intensified international migration flows worldwide. In 2022, there were an estimated 280 million international migrants, including refugees and asylum seekers (International Organization for Migration, 2021). These populations—whether in transit or settled in host countries—face a heightened vulnerability to certain infectious diseases, notably tuberculosis (TB), which is one of the leading causes of preventable mortality among migrants in several regions of the world.

Various socio-economic and structural factors explain this increased vulnerability. Migrants often live in precarious conditions, including overcrowding, poor sanitation, food insecurity, and limited access to safe drinking water. These environments facilitate the transmission of *Mycobacterium tuberculosis*, particularly in collective or informal housing. Compounding this is restricted access to healthcare services due to language barriers, unfamiliarity with healthcare systems, lack of health insurance, and fear of potential repercussions on legal status (Dheda et al., 2016).

Studies have shown that TB incidence is significantly higher among migrants than in the general population, especially in countries with low endemic TB rates. For example, in Canada and Australia, over 70% of reported TB cases involve individuals born abroad (Greenaway et al., 2011). A systematic review by Kimbrough et al. also found an elevated risk of active TB among migrants from high-prevalence regions, even several years after arrival (Kimbrough et al., 2012).

Migrants face numerous barriers to TB screening and treatment. Pre-arrival or post-arrival screening may be inconsistently applied, and migrants often delay or avoid seeking medical care due to fear of stigmatization or deportation. Moreover, treatment adherence is frequently compromised by unstable housing, lack of social support, and financial hardship (Dara et al., 2016; Kimbrough et al., 2012).

From a public health perspective, several initiatives have been implemented to strengthen early detection and care for TB among migrant populations. The World Health Organization (WHO) recommends culturally appropriate, person-centered approaches, combined with community-based and intersectoral strategies (World Health Organization, 2018). Targeted programs such as the "Find and Treat" model in the United Kingdom have proven effective in improving diagnostic access and treatment follow-up for vulnerable migrant populations (Story et al., 2007).

Migrants therefore represent a high-risk group for tuberculosis due to structural, social, and health-related factors. The implementation of inclusive health policies grounded in human rights and continuity of care is essential to achieving global TB control and elimination goals.

VULNERABILITY OF THE ELDERLY TO TUBERCULOSIS

The global aging population constitutes a major public health concern, particularly in the context of chronic infectious diseases such as tuberculosis. Although TB is often perceived as a condition primarily affecting young adults in high-incidence countries, it remains a significant threat to the elderly, especially in middle- and high-income countries. This population is increasingly vulnerable due to immunological, clinical, social, and structural factors.

Aging is accompanied by immunosenescence—a progressive decline of the immune system—which reduces the body's ability to contain latent *Mycobacterium tuberculosis* infections or to resist new exposures (Menzies et al., 2007). Older adults are thus more likely to develop active TB from a latent infection acquired decades earlier or through reinfection. In addition, common comorbidities in this age group—such as diabetes, renal insufficiency, or chronic lung disease—further increase the risk of disease progression (Mori & Leung, 2010).

Symptoms of TB in the elderly are often atypical or masked by other health conditions, potentially delaying diagnosis. Clinical presentations may also be oligosymptomatic, with lower occurrences of fever or night sweats, contributing to underdiagnosis in this population (Rajagopalan, 2001). These diagnostic delays are associated with increased mortality and a higher risk of transmission within care facilities or institutions.

There are numerous barriers to TB screening and treatment in older adults. Access to care may be limited by reduced mobility, functional dependence, or social isolation. Furthermore, tolerance to anti-TB treatments is often lower due to drug interactions and physiological frailty, increasing the risk of serious adverse effects, particularly hepatotoxicity (Tanimura et al., 2014).

From a public health perspective, the World Health Organization recommends specific attention to TB in the elderly, integrating this issue into targeted screening programs, particularly in nursing homes, long-term care hospitals, or contexts of social vulnerability (World Health Organization, 2020). Integrated, interprofessional approaches—including geriatrics, community health, and social services—are essential to improving early detection, treatment adherence, and clinical outcomes in this vulnerable population.

TB in the elderly represents a growing challenge, requiring tailored strategies for surveillance, prevention, and care. The systematic inclusion of older adults in TB control policies is essential for achieving global elimination targets.

TUBERCULOSIS DIAGNOSIS: A MULTIFACTORIAL APPROACH ADAPTED TO VULNERABLE POPULATIONS

The diagnosis of tuberculosis relies on a multifactorial approach, which is particularly crucial for vulnerable populations, in whom clinical manifestations may be atypical and disease progression more rapid. This introductory statement underscores the inherent complexity of the TB diagnostic process, especially when dealing with high-risk groups.

Tuberculosis, an infectious disease caused by *Mycobacterium tuberculosis*, classically presents with respiratory symptoms (persistent cough, sputum production, hemoptysis), along with general signs (fever, night sweats, weight loss). However, in immunocompromised individuals—such as people living with HIV, malnourished people, or the elderly—these symptoms may be absent or very subtle, making clinical recognition of TB particularly challenging.

Microbiological Confirmation: A Classic but Imperfect Pillar of Diagnosis

Microbiological confirmation, primarily through direct microscopic examination of sputum (bacilloscopy) and culture, remains a fundamental pillar of diagnosis, providing direct evidence of infection with *Mycobacterium tuberculosis* (Kolamou et al., 2023). This assertion highlights the central role of microbiological evidence in the definitive diagnosis of tuberculosis. The direct examination, or bacilloscopy, involves optical microscopy, following Ziehl-Neelsen or auramine staining, to observe acid-fast bacilli in sputum samples. This method is rapid, inexpensive, and technically simple, making it particularly suitable for environments with limited medical infrastructure.

Culture, on the other hand, allows for the identification of the pathogen through its growth on specific media, whether solid (Lowenstein-Jensen) or liquid (MGIT). It offers superior sensitivity and specificity compared to bacilloscopy and also enables the performance of antimicrobial susceptibility testing, a crucial step in detecting resistant strains. However, this method is time-consuming — the growth of *M. tuberculosis* can take several weeks — and requires a high-biosafety-level laboratory as well as highly skilled personnel. These constraints significantly limit its availability in many regions of the world, particularly sub-Saharan Africa and South Asia, where tuberculosis incidence remains high.

Although bacilloscopy is widely accessible in resource-limited settings, it has notable limitations in sensitivity, particularly in individuals with low bacillary loads, such as patients co-infected with HIV or those with extrapulmonary tuberculosis (Dobler, 2016). This critical observation underscores the shortcomings of a tool that is still widely used. Indeed, the sensitivity of bacilloscopy varies significantly depending on the bacillary concentration in the sample; below a certain threshold (generally estimated at 10^4 bacilli/mL), the examination becomes negative, even though the patient is actually infected. Individuals co-infected with HIV, due to their immunocompromised state, tend to develop paucibacillary forms, where the bacillary load is insufficient for detection by this method.

A similar situation occurs in cases of extrapulmonary tuberculosis, where the infected sites (lymph nodes, pleura, meninges, etc.) are difficult to access for simple sampling, and where bacterial concentrations are often low. As a result, clinical and radiological approaches, in the absence of microbiological confirmation, become common in these contexts, but at the cost of an increased risk of diagnostic errors, inappropriate treatments, and detrimental delays in therapy.

These limitations are exacerbated in populations with limited or delayed access to healthcare, leading to a higher proportion of cases with negative bacilloscopy results diagnosed based on clinical and radiological signs (Siddiqi et al., 2003). The so-called "presumptive" diagnosis then relies on a constellation of indirect data: exposure history, suggestive symptoms, radiographic abnormalities, and response to empirical treatment. While this strategy allows for urgent action, it remains problematic, especially due to the low specificity of clinical signs and the sometimes-subjective interpretation of radiological results. Moreover, this approach is insufficient to detect drug-resistant forms of tuberculosis, whose management depends on the precise identification of drug susceptibility profiles.

In an epidemiological context, this diagnostic reality contributes to an underestimation of the true prevalence of tuberculosis and limits the effectiveness of control programs, particularly in rural communities, urban slums, and migrant populations, where structural inequalities in public health are most pronounced.

Culture, recognized as the gold standard method, improves diagnostic accuracy but requires specialized laboratory infrastructure and extended processing times, which delays treatment initiation (Nema, 2012). This dilemma between diagnostic performance and operational feasibility represents a major challenge in tuberculosis control strategies. While culture not only confirms the diagnosis but also characterizes bacterial strains (genotyping, susceptibility testing), its turnaround time — often 4 to 8 weeks — is incompatible with the need for rapid responses in public health, particularly in community settings where transmission is swift.

Furthermore, in many high-endemic countries, the absence of appropriate laboratory infrastructure makes its widespread use nearly inaccessible. This renders diagnosis and treatment dependent on alternative tools with lower performance or requires the transfer of samples to reference centers, with the delays, costs, and disruptions in follow-up that this entails.

Towards Rapid and Appropriate Diagnostic Tools

The development and application of rapid diagnostic tools are increasingly essential to address the emergence and management of multi-drug-resistant and extensively drug-resistant *M. tuberculosis* strains (S. Kanwar, 2012). This observation highlights a crucial dynamic in the current fight against tuberculosis: the need for tools that are sensitive, specific, rapid, and usable at the point of care. The emergence of multidrug-resistant strains (resistant to at least isoniazid and rifampicin) and extensively drug-resistant strains (additional resistance to fluoroquinolones and second-line injectable drugs) poses a major global public health threat due to the increased difficulty in their management, the cost of treatment, and their toxicity.

In this context, rapid diagnostic tools (molecular tests, immunochromatographic tests, LAM urine tests for highly immunocompromised HIV+ patients) play a key role in reducing the time between clinical suspicion and initiation of treatment, while enabling early detection of resistance. Their deployment in peripheral healthcare settings also helps alleviate the burden on reference centers and enhances equitable access to care.

The integration of molecular diagnostics, such as the Xpert MTB/RIF test, has revolutionized tuberculosis diagnosis by enabling the rapid detection of *M. tuberculosis* and rifampicin resistance, a key marker of multidrug-resistant tuberculosis (Pai et al., 2016). These tests offer significantly higher sensitivity compared to bacilloscopy, particularly in samples that are negative by direct examination, and provide actionable results within hours, thereby facilitating the rapid initiation of treatment and implementation of infection control measures. This passage emphasizes the technological and operational shift introduced by automated PCR-based tests. The Xpert MTB/RIF test, based on the amplification of mycobacterial DNA and detection of specific mutations in the rpoB gene, serves a dual function: pathogen identification and rapid evaluation of rifampicin resistance, within less than two hours.

Its ease of use, speed, and semi-automated independence have enabled its deployment in thousands of health centers worldwide. It represents a turning point in the diagnostic paradigm, gradually replacing bacilloscopy as the first-line diagnostic tool. This transformation enables immediate management, reduces loss to follow-up, and limits community transmission. However, its relatively high cost, maintenance requirements, and reliance on specific cartridge suppliers pose barriers to its universal adoption.

Ultimately, tuberculosis diagnosis in vulnerable populations presents a set of challenges at the intersection of clinical, technological, epidemiological, and socio-economic issues. While significant progress has been made, particularly through molecular tools, persistent gaps remain between the theoretical performance of available techniques and their practical application in the field. The current challenge lies not only in technological innovation but also in the systematic and equitable integration of these innovations into healthcare systems, with particular attention to vulnerable contexts.

SCREENING STRATEGIES IN VULNERABLE POPULATIONS

Despite the diagnostic and therapeutic advances observed over recent decades, the persistence of tuberculosis, or even its resurgence in certain segments of the population, highlights the limitations of current control strategies, especially in contexts of social, medical, or demographic vulnerability. In this context, the question of early screening and accurate diagnosis becomes crucial, both for individual care and for reducing community transmission. Recent literature converges on the idea that diagnostic challenges are exacerbated in so-called "vulnerable" populations, in the epidemiological and socio-health sense, and among the elderly, whose clinical, immunological, and contextual characteristics complicate the identification and confirmation of TB cases.

Effective tuberculosis control fundamentally relies on rapid and accurate diagnosis of active disease, particularly among vulnerable populations and the elderly, where diagnostic challenges tend to intensify (Kerkhoff et al., 2023). This central assertion points to a well-established issue in epidemiological research: diagnostic delays are directly correlated with the clinical worsening of patients, prolonged periods of infectiousness, and reduced effectiveness of public health strategies for secondary prevention.

Vulnerable populations encompass a heterogeneous group of individuals who's biological (immunosuppression), social (precarity, marginalization), or contextual (confinement, migration) characteristics constitute risk factors for infection and diagnostic delays. Indeed, factors such as atypical clinical presentations, comorbidities, and weakened immune systems can mask the classic signs of tuberculosis, leading to diagnostic delays and, consequently, an increase in transmission. The symptomatic expression of tuberculosis in these populations is often altered by interfering factors: concomitant chronic diseases, immunosenescence, or the use of immunomodulatory treatments (corticosteroids, biotherapies).

Beyond individual specifics, global trends highlight the insufficiency of current approaches. The global decline in newly diagnosed and treated tuberculosis cases in 2020, coupled with a resurgence of tuberculosis-related deaths, underscores the urgent need to improve diagnostic strategies, particularly for the most exposed populations. This observation, directly linked to the COVID-19 pandemic, reveals a concerning shift in public health priorities and the structural fragility of tuberculosis surveillance systems. The decrease in notifications does not reflect a real decline in incidence but rather a detection deficit, especially among asymptomatic or mildly symptomatic patients.

Diagnostic delays do not only result in increased mortality and morbidity but also contribute to the perpetuation of community transmission of tuberculosis (Dheda et al., 2016). Indeed, the longer the period between the onset of symptoms and the initiation of treatment, the more the infected patient becomes an active vector within their environment, increasing the number of contaminated contacts. This silent transmission dynamic is particularly problematic in high-density settings (shelters, prisons, nursing homes), where the density of interactions facilitates rapid pathogen spread.

The response to this structural issue lies partly in the implementation of early detection strategies. Early detection, particularly when performed on-site, can significantly reduce disease transmission while improving survival rates (Ullah et al., 2024). The concept of "on-site detection" refers to the deployment of diagnostic technologies directly at the point of service (e.g., community centers, mobile units, or primary healthcare structures), without the need to transfer samples to central laboratories. This approach reduces the time between sample collection and results, which is crucial for initiating prompt treatment and cutting the transmission chain.

In this regard, point-of-care diagnostics, which provide rapid results, appear as a strategic necessity, particularly in decentralized healthcare contexts (Nathavitharana et al., 2022). These technologies often rely on molecular methods (such as Xpert MTB/RIF tests) capable of detecting mycobacterial DNA and simultaneously identifying resistance mutations. Their portability, quick execution (results in less than two hours), and relative ease of use make them suitable for resource-limited environments. However, their implementation requires adequate training of personnel, rigorous maintenance logistics, and sustainable financial support, raising issues of equity and sustainability in low- and middle-income countries.

Beyond the tools, the very structure of screening programs needs to be reconsidered. The successful implementation of systematic screening programs requires careful consideration of the target population, the selection of screening and diagnostic tools, and the programmatic approaches employed (Uplekar et al., 2013). The "systematic" approach to screening requires a balance between efficiency (targeting high-risk individuals) and effectiveness (achieving sufficient coverage to interrupt transmission). This involves a detailed understanding of local epidemiology, access barriers to care, and the social determinants of health. An effective strategy cannot merely replicate standardized models; it must be adaptable, contextualized, and integrated into a comprehensive primary healthcare system.

Thus, optimizing the fight against tuberculosis in vulnerable groups requires an integrated approach that combines clinical vigilance, technological innovation, decentralized deployment, and programmatic governance. The challenge is not just technical, but systemic: it is about reshaping health policies to truly center on the most exposed, least visible, and highest-risk individuals who are often excluded from traditional screening pathways.

Tuberculosis can only be effectively controlled if sustained efforts are made to refine diagnostic strategies, particularly in vulnerable populations and the elderly. Far from a purely biomedical approach focused solely on the technical dimension of diagnosis, there is a need to promote an integrated vision, combining epidemiology, clinical care, health technologies, and public policies. Tuberculosis, as both a disease of the social fabric and the individual body, calls for a scientific and ethical mobilization commensurate with the contemporary challenges it continues to present.

SCREENING AND DIAGNOSIS IN OLDER ADULTS

Geriatric screening and diagnosis represent a complex and essential area of healthcare, focused on the proactive identification and detailed characterization of conditions that disproportionately affect older adults. This field requires a thorough understanding of age-related physiological changes, the potential for atypical disease presentations, and the complex interaction between multiple comorbidities (Carlson et al., 1999). Older adults are considered vulnerable due to frailty, a clinical syndrome characterized by a significant decline in the ability to adapt to stressors, thus representing a heightened level of vulnerability to risks (Rolland et al., 2011). This concept invites us to approach the phenomenon from a multifactorial perspective, integrating biological, psychological, and social components in interaction. Beyond this general definition, international consensus further specifies that physical frailty is marked by the gradual weakening of muscle strength, reduced endurance, and impairment of fundamental physiological functions, exposing individuals to an increased risk of dependency or mortality in the face of even minor stressors (Morley et al., 2013).

However, the diagnosis of tuberculosis (TB) in older adults remains a major challenge. Clinical presentations may be atypical, with symptoms often nonspecific such as fatigue, weight loss, prolonged fever, or general malaise, making diagnostic suspicion difficult (Rajagopalan, 2001). Additionally, extrapulmonary manifestations or paucisymptomatic forms are more common in this age group, often delaying the identification of the disease (Lönnroth et al., 2010).

Radiological exams, particularly chest X-rays, may show subtle or unusual abnormalities in older adults, such as basal infiltrates, fibrotic lesions, or images resembling other chronic pulmonary conditions, such as COPD or congestive heart failure (Baratella et al., 2023). Thoracic CT scans may be helpful in refining the diagnosis, though they are not always accessible or routinely performed.

Furthermore, immunodiagnostic tests have significant limitations in this population. The tuberculin skin test (TST) is often falsely negative due to immunosenescence or malnutrition, which are common among older adults (Getahun et al., 2015). Interferon-gamma release assays (IGRAs), while more specific, can also be influenced by the patient's immune status, and their interpretation requires caution (Diel et al., 2009).

Microbiological diagnosis remains the cornerstone for confirming TB. However, sputum production is often difficult in older individuals, sometimes requiring invasive techniques like bronchoalveolar lavage (World Health Organization, 2021). Rapid molecular tools, such as the GeneXpert MTB/RIF test, allow sensitive and quick detection, even in paucibacillary samples, and should be systematically integrated into diagnostic protocols (Boehme et al., 2010)

From an epidemiological perspective, older adults represent a high-risk group for the reactivation of latent TB infection acquired earlier in life, particularly in areas with high endemicity (Menzies et al., 2007). This risk is exacerbated by the frequent comorbidities in this population, such as diabetes, cardiovascular diseases, and the use of corticosteroids or immunosuppressants (Lönnroth et al., 2010).

Public health programs now recognize the importance of targeted screening for latent TB in at-risk older adults, especially in institutional settings such as nursing homes or long-term care centers (WHO, 2018). The World Health Organization, in its updated guidelines, recommends systematic screening in high-risk populations, with an individual evaluation of the benefits and risks associated with preventive treatment (WHO, 2020).

Obstacles to the diagnosis and treatment of TB in older adults include not only clinical and technical challenges but also socio-economic factors: social isolation, limited access to healthcare services, functional dependence, and sometimes denial or trivialization of symptoms by the patients themselves or their families (Tanimura et al., 2014). A comprehensive geriatric approach, which integrates functional, nutritional, cognitive, and social assessments, is crucial to ensuring early diagnosis and appropriate management.

TB in older adults remains an underestimated public health issue. Early detection relies on increased clinical vigilance, the use of appropriate diagnostic tools, and a targeted screening strategy. Close collaboration between public health services, geriatrics specialists, and primary care teams is essential to improve the identification, diagnosis, and access to treatment for this disease in a particularly vulnerable population.

CHALLENGES AND BARRIERS TO THE DIAGNOSIS AND SCREENING OF TUBERCULOSIS

Tuberculosis remains a major public health issue worldwide, particularly among vulnerable populations and older adults, despite the implementation of numerous control initiatives (Rajagopalan, 2001). Vulnerable populations, including individuals living with HIV, family contacts of TB patients, and those living in collective settings, face a disproportionately high risk of TB infection and progression to active disease (Melendez et al., 2016). Similarly, the aging population, characterized by age-related immunosenescence and an increased prevalence of comorbidities, is experiencing a resurgence of TB, often with atypical clinical presentations that complicate both diagnosis and treatment (Mori & Leung, 2010; Negin et al., 2015).

In this context, the screening for latent TB infection becomes a crucial tool for identifying individuals who need preventive treatment, thereby preventing progression to active tuberculosis (Gray et al., 2019). Addressing diagnostic challenges and optimizing screening strategies are fundamental for mitigating the impact of TB in these high-risk groups. Early identification of TB cases, through targeted active case-finding strategies, helps reduce transmission by enabling rapid diagnosis, potentially even before symptoms are recognized by patients (Yuen et al., 2021).

However, barriers to active case finding are numerous and interconnected, directly impacting the effectiveness of detection strategies. Among these are gaps in the experience, knowledge, and skills of healthcare workers, which can hinder early identification of cases. The lack of specific training, whether for new or experienced healthcare workers, in detecting active TB remains a persistent weakness in screening strategies.

The availability and workload of healthcare workers represent another major barrier: they are often overwhelmed by a heavy workload and limited human resources. Moreover, the lack of material resources, such as diagnostic equipment, reagents, and necessary consumables, is also a significant constraint in ensuring effective screening.

Other logistical factors hinder the process, including geographic distance and the time required to reach certain populations, particularly those living in rural or hard-to-reach areas. These difficulties are compounded by inadequate communication strategies and language barriers that complicate access to healthcare services, especially for marginalized populations.

The stigma associated with tuberculosis is a transversal barrier, affecting both patients' willingness to seek care and healthcare professionals' engagement in identifying cases. This phenomenon is particularly pronounced in disadvantaged social groups, where the fear of being labeled as tuberculous can lead to symptom concealment or refusal of screening. Low community awareness of tuberculosis further contributes to under-detection of the disease, preventing at-risk individuals from receiving adequate screening.

These barriers underscore the need for enhanced healthcare worker training, better resource allocation, and targeted action on social and cultural factors in order to improve access to tuberculosis screening and, consequently, curb the spread of the disease in vulnerable populations (Fenta et al., 2023).

Finally, studies on the preferences of affected populations and the translation of their results into public policies, guidelines, and operational frameworks are of paramount importance. They offer considerable potential to address existing gaps in detection by focusing on patients' needs and expanding the accessibility and reach of screening and diagnostic services for individuals most affected by tuberculosis.

PERSPECTIVES FOR TUBERCULOSIS SCREENING AND DIAGNOSIS AMONG VULNERABLE POPULATIONS AND THE ELDERLY

The fight against tuberculosis (TB) remains a critical public health priority, especially among vulnerable populations such as the elderly, homeless individuals, migrants, people living with HIV, and those living in institutions or socioeconomically disadvantaged conditions. In these high-risk groups, screening and diagnostic strategies must be adapted to overcome existing barriers and improve detection timelines. Several international initiatives, technological innovations, and public health recommendations provide promising prospects for strengthening early detection of the disease in these populations.

Targeted Systematic Screening and Differentiated Approaches

The World Health Organization (WHO) has recommended since 2021 systematic screening for tuberculosis in high-risk and exposed groups, including the elderly in institutions, people living with HIV, prisoners, the homeless, and migrants from areas of high endemicity (World Health Organization, 2021). These guidelines represent a significant step forward in the implementation of proactive programs that go beyond simple passive symptom-based identification.

Future perspectives in this field are moving towards differentiated approaches, relying on risk stratification, considering the clinical and contextual specifics of each group, and integrating screening into existing healthcare services. Similarly, community-based approaches, which focus on active screening within street populations or refugee camps, have demonstrated their effectiveness in several settings (Story et al., 2007).

Technological Innovation in Diagnosis

Technological advances in diagnostic methods offer major prospects for improving rapid and reliable tuberculosis detection, especially in vulnerable populations. The introduction of the GeneXpert MTB/RIF test, which detects the presence of *Mycobacterium tuberculosis* and rifampicin resistance in less than two hours, has transformed diagnostic capabilities, particularly in resource-limited contexts (Boehme et al., 2010). This test is also more sensitive than traditional microscopy, especially in the elderly and immunocompromised individuals, who often have a low bacillary load.

Portable and simplified versions of GeneXpert, such as GeneXpert Omni, are being deployed, allowing for broader use in primary healthcare centers, mobile units, or community settings. At the same time, artificial intelligence (AI)-assisted diagnostic tools applied to chest radiography (computer-aided detection, CAD) are gaining accuracy and are currently being tested in large-scale screening programs (Qin et al., 2021).

Integrated and Multisectoral Approach

An important future perspective lies in integrating tuberculosis screening into primary healthcare services and social care systems. Interconnecting mental health services, shelters, elderly care centers, and infectious disease services would improve screening coverage and reduce gaps in the diagnostic chain (Lönnroth et al., 2010). In this regard, the "One-Stop Shop" approach, which centralizes screening, diagnosis, counseling, and treatment services in one location, promotes better accessibility for vulnerable populations.

Programs such as Find & Treat in the United Kingdom or TBFinder in India illustrate the feasibility and relevance of these integrated models. These initiatives mobilize multidisciplinary teams, combining public health, social assistance, and mobile technologies to reach hard-to-reach groups (Story et al., 2007; Subbaraman et al., 2019).

Enhancing Healthcare Professionals' Capacity

An essential development axis involves strengthening the clinical and social capacities of healthcare professionals who interact with vulnerable individuals. Continuing education on the atypical manifestations of tuberculosis in the elderly, the criteria for suspicion in at-risk groups, and the recommended screening protocols is crucial for improving early diagnoses (Getahun et al., 2015)

Furthermore, the development of standardized clinical tools, such as triage algorithms or screening grids tailored to elderly or immunocompromised populations, would facilitate the harmonization of practices and reduce disparities between institutions.

Operational Research and Social Innovation

Public health research plays a central role in identifying the most effective and acceptable interventions for screening in vulnerable contexts. Numerous operational research projects are currently being conducted to evaluate the impact of community-based strategies, the performance of new diagnostic tools in specific populations, and the adherence to screening protocols.

Social innovation, including community participation, health mediation, and user engagement in program design, is also at the heart of future perspectives. This is particularly relevant for the elderly, who are often excluded from targeted health campaigns but whose contribution to identifying age-specific barriers can enrich the effectiveness of actions.

Digitalization and Information Systems

Finally, the growing use of digital information systems represents a strategic opportunity to improve screening follow-up, traceability of suspected cases, and evaluation of program performance. Mobile applications and electronic recording platforms, such as Nikshay in India or eTB Manager in Ukraine, facilitate coordination of care and real-time case monitoring (Satyanarayana et al., 2011).

Data disaggregated by age, sex, social status, or living conditions will also allow for better-targeted interventions and measuring their impact in an equity-driven health approach.

CONCLUSION

Tuberculosis remains a major public health challenge, particularly for vulnerable populations and the elderly. These groups have a significantly higher prevalence of the disease compared to the general population due to a combination of factors such as poverty, malnutrition, overcrowding, HIV-TB co-infection, age-related immunosenescence, and limited access to healthcare. These conditions not only promote TB transmission but also the emergence of resistant forms such as multidrug-resistant (MDR-TB) and extensively drug-resistant tuberculosis (XDR-TB), which are particularly difficult to diagnose and treat.

Barriers to early screening and accurate diagnosis—whether structural, human, social, or logistical—seriously hinder rapid detection and effective management of cases in these high-risk groups. In the elderly, atypical clinical presentations, the presence of comorbidities, and limited disease awareness make diagnosis even more challenging. For vulnerable populations, language barriers, stigma, and a lack of appropriate resources greatly limit their access to screening.

In light of these challenges, it is imperative to strengthen and adapt tuberculosis control strategies by implementing targeted, accessible, and culturally sensitive screening and diagnostic approaches. The development of systematic screening programs, integrating rapid and efficient diagnostic tools, combined with continuous training of healthcare personnel, represents a key lever to improve early disease detection.

Finally, any screening and diagnostic strategy must be part of a comprehensive response involving health authorities, community structures, and frontline actors. The fight against tuberculosis in the highest-risk populations can only be effective through coordinated, sustained, and equitable action aimed at overcoming structural inequalities and ensuring universal access to care, in line with international commitments to combat this disease.

REFERENCES

Baratella, E., Fiorese, I., Minelli, P., Veiluva, A., Marrocchio, C., Ruaro, B., & Cova, M. A. (2023). Aging-Related Findings of the Respiratory System in Chest Imaging : Pearls and Pitfalls. *Current Radiology Reports*, *11*(1), 1–11. DOI: 10.1007/s40134-022-00405-w

Baussano, I., Williams, B. G., Nunn, P., Beggiato, M., Fedeli, U., & Scano, F. (2010). Tuberculosis Incidence in Prisons : A Systematic Review. *PLoS Medicine*, *7*(12), e1000381. DOI: 10.1371/journal.pmed.1000381

Biadglegne, F., Rodloff, A. C., & Sack, U. (2015). Review of the prevalence and drug resistance of tuberculosis in prisons : A hidden epidemic. *Epidemiology and Infection*, *143*(5), 887–900. DOI: 10.1017/S095026881400288X

Blanc, F.-X. (2023). Tuberculose et infection par le virus de l'immunodéficience humaine : Comment réduire la mortalité? *Bulletin de l'Académie Nationale de Médecine*, *207*(8), 1044–1052. DOI: 10.1016/j.banm.2023.07.007

Boehme, C. C., Nabeta, P., Hillemann, D., Nicol, M. P., Shenai, S., Krapp, F., Allen, J., Tahirli, R., Blakemore, R., Rustomjee, R., Milovic, A., Jones, M., O'Brien, S. M., Persing, D. H., Ruesch-Gerdes, S., Gotuzzo, E., Rodrigues, C., Alland, D., & Perkins, M. D. (2010). Rapid Molecular Detection of Tuberculosis and Rifampin Resistance. *The New England Journal of Medicine*, *363*(11), 1005–1015. DOI: 10.1056/NEJMoa0907847

Carlson, M. C., Fried, L. P., Xue, Q.-L., Bandeen-Roche, K., Zeger, S. L., & Brandt, J. (1999). Association Between Executive Attention and Physical Functional Performance in Community-Dwelling Older Women. *The Journals of Gerontology. Series B, Psychological Sciences and Social Sciences*, *54B*(5), S262–S270. DOI: 10.1093/geronb/54B.5.S262

Dara, M., Solovic, I., Goletti, D., Sotgiu, G., Centis, R., D'Ambrosio, L., Ward, B., Teixeira, V., Gratziou, C., & Migliori, G. B. (2016). Preventing and controlling tuberculosis among refugees in Europe : More is needed. *The European Respiratory Journal*, *48*(1), 272–274. DOI: 10.1183/13993003.00329-2016

Dheda, K., Barry, C. E.III, & Maartens, G. (2016). Tuberculosis. *Lancet*, *387*(10024), 1211–1226. DOI: 10.1016/S0140-6736(15)00151-8

Diel, R., Loddenkemper, R., Meywald-Walter, K., Gottschalk, R., & Nienhaus, A. (2009). Comparative Performance of Tuberculin Skin Test, QuantiFERON-TB-Gold In Tube Assay, and T-Spot. TB Test in Contact Investigations for Tuberculosis. *Chest*, *135*(4), 1010–1018. DOI: 10.1378/chest.08-2048

Dobler, C. C. (2016). Screening strategies for active tuberculosis : Focus on cost-effectiveness. *ClinicoEconomics and Outcomes Research, 8*, 335–347. DOI: 10.2147/CEOR.S92244

Fenta, M. D., Ogundijo, O. A., Warsame, A. A. A., & Belay, A. G. (2023). Facilitators and barriers to tuberculosis active case findings in low- and middle-income countries : A systematic review of qualitative research. *BMC Infectious Diseases, 23*(1), 515. DOI: 10.1186/s12879-023-08502-7

Fessell, D., & Lexa, F. J. (2019). A Devilish Dilemma : To Recognize Top Performers . . . Or Not. *Journal of the American College of Radiology, 16*(7), 1009–1010. DOI: 10.1016/j.jacr.2019.01.023

Getahun, H., Matteelli, A., Abubakar, I., Aziz, M. A., Baddeley, A., Barreira, D., Den Boon, S., Borroto Gutierrez, S. M., Bruchfeld, J., Burhan, E., Cavalcante, S., Cedillos, R., Chaisson, R., Chee, C. B.-E., Chesire, L., Corbett, E., Dara, M., Denholm, J., de Vries, G., & Raviglione, M. (2015). Management of latent Mycobacterium tuberculosis infection : WHO guidelines for low tuberculosis burden countries. *The European Respiratory Journal, 46*(6), 1563–1576. DOI: 10.1183/13993003.01245-2015

Gray, B. J., Perrett, S. E., Gudgeon, B., & Shankar, A. G. (2019). Investigating the prevalence of latent Tuberculosis infection in a UK remand prison. *Journal of Public Health (Oxford, England)*. Advance online publication. DOI: 10.1093/pubmed/fdy219

Greenaway, C., Sandoe, A., Vissandjee, B., Kitai, I., Gruner, D., Wobeser, W., Pottie, K., Ueffing, E., Menzies, D., & Schwartzman, K.Canadian Collaboration for Immigrant and Refugee Health. (2011). Tuberculosis : Evidence review for newly arriving immigrants and refugees. *Canadian Medical Association Journal, 183*(12), E939–E951. DOI: 10.1503/cmaj.090302

Gupta, R. K., Lucas, S. B., Fielding, K. L., & Lawn, S. D. (2015). Prevalence of tuberculosis in post-mortem studies of HIV-infected adults and children in resource-limited settings : A systematic review and meta-analysis. *AIDS (London, England), 29*(15), 1987–2002. DOI: 10.1097/QAD.0000000000000802

Haute Autorité de Santé. (2023). *Evaluation des strategies de depistage et de reperage precoce de la tuberculose pulmonaire.* https://www.has-sante.fr/upload/docs/application/pdf/2023-09/evaluation_des_strategies_de_depistage_et_de_reperage_precoce_de_la_tuberculose_pulmonaire_-_note_de_2023-09-07_09-30-39_346.pdf

International Organization for Migration. (2021). [United Nations.]. *World Migration Report*, •••, 2022.

Jebali, R., Hedhli, A., Daoud, S., Euchi, K., Marzouki, S., Medi, W., Chikh Rouhou, S., Ouahchi, Y., Merai, S., Toujani, S., Mjid, M., & Dhahri, B. (2023). Particularité de la tuberculose pulmonaire chez les patients immunodéprimé non infecté par le VIH. *Revue des Maladies Respiratoires Actualités*, *15*(1), 274. DOI: 10.1016/j.rmra.2022.11.518

Kanwar, S. S. (2012). Diagnostic Methods for Mycobacterium tuberculosis and Challenges in Its Detection in India. In P.-J. Cardona (Éd.), *Understanding Tuberculosis—Global Experiences and Innovative Approaches to the Diagnosis*. InTech. DOI: 10.5772/31714

Kerkhoff, A. D., Mwamba, C., Pry, J. M., Kagujje, M., Nyangu, S., Mateyo, K., Sanjase, N., Chilukutu, L., Christopoulos, K. A., Muyoyeta, M., & Sharma, A. (2023). A mixed methods study on men's and women's tuberculosis care journeys in Lusaka, Zambia—Implications for gender-tailored tuberculosis health promotion and case finding strategies. *PLOS Global Public Health*, *3*(6), e0001372. DOI: 10.1371/journal.pgph.0001372

Kimbrough, W., Saliba, V., Dahab, M., Haskew, C., & Checchi, F. (2012). The burden of tuberculosis in crisis-affected populations : A systematic review. *The Lancet. Infectious Diseases*, *12*(12), 950–965. DOI: 10.1016/S1473-3099(12)70225-6

Kolamou, R., Bah, B. S. S., Kalivogui, S., Diallo, B. M., & Barry, A. A. (2023). Prévalence de la co-infection tuberculose pulmonaire/VIH entre 2018-2020 dans le Centre de Diagnostic et de Traitement de la tuberculose de Damakania, République de Guinée : Prevalence of pulmonary tuberculosis/HIV co-infection between 2018-2020 in the Tuberculosis Diagnosis and Treatment Center of Damakania, Republic of Guinea. *International Journal of Biological and Chemical Sciences*, *17*(2), 683–688. DOI: 10.4314/ijbcs.v17i2.31

Lee, S. W. H., Nordin, A. A., Teng, W. Y., Osman, N. N., Mohan, D. S. R., Halim, N. H. A., Rahim, F. I. A., Syafira, N., & Assri, M. (2023). *A primary health care case study in the context of the COVID-19 pandemic*.

Litvinjenko, S., Magwood, O., Wu, S., & Wei, X. (2023). Burden of tuberculosis among vulnerable populations worldwide : An overview of systematic reviews. *The Lancet. Infectious Diseases*, *23*(12), 1395–1407. DOI: 10.1016/S1473-3099(23)00372-9

Lönnroth, K., Castro, K. G., Chakaya, J. M., Chauhan, L. S., Floyd, K., Glaziou, P., & Raviglione, M. C. (2010). Tuberculosis control and elimination 2010–50 : Cure, care, and social development. *Lancet*, *375*(9728), 1814–1829. DOI: 10.1016/S0140-6736(10)60483-7

López, M. P., Ulloa, A. P., & Escobar, F. A. (2022). Tuberculosis and prison overcrowding from the perspective of social inequities in health in Colombia, 2018. *Biomédica : Revista del Instituto Nacional de Salud, 42*(1), 159–169. DOI: 10.7705/biomedica.5894

Melendez, J., Sánchez, C. I., Philipsen, R. H. H. M., Maduskar, P., Dawson, R., Theron, G., Dheda, K., & Van Ginneken, B. (2016). An automated tuberculosis screening strategy combining X-ray-based computer-aided detection and clinical information. *Scientific Reports, 6*(1), 25265. DOI: 10.1038/srep25265

Menzies, D., Joshi, R., & Pai, M. (2007). Risk of tuberculosis infection and disease associated with work in health care settings. *The International Journal of Tuberculosis and Lung Disease : the Official Journal of the International Union against Tuberculosis and Lung Disease, 11*(6), 593–605.

Mera, H. B., Wagnew, F., Akelew, Y., Hibstu, Z., Berihun, S., Tamir, W., Alemu, S., Lamore, Y., Mesganaw, B., Adugna, A., & Tsegaye, T. B. (2023). Prevalence and Predictors of Pulmonary Tuberculosis among Prison Inmates in Sub-Saharan Africa : A Systematic Review and Meta-Analysis. *Tuberculosis Research and Treatment, 6226200*, 1–13. Advance online publication. DOI: 10.1155/2023/6226200

Mori, T., & Leung, C. C. (2010). Tuberculosis in the Global Aging Population. *Infectious Disease Clinics of North America, 24*(3), 751–768. DOI: 10.1016/j.idc.2010.04.011

Morley, J. E., Vellas, B., Abellan Van Kan, G., Anker, S. D., Bauer, J. M., Bernabei, R., Cesari, M., Chumlea, W. C., Doehner, W., Evans, J., Fried, L. P., Guralnik, J. M., Katz, P. R., Malmstrom, T. K., McCarter, R. J., Gutierrez Robledo, L. M., Rockwood, K., Von Haehling, S., Vandewoude, M. F., & Walston, J. (2013). Frailty Consensus : A Call to Action. *Journal of the American Medical Directors Association, 14*(6), 392–397. DOI: 10.1016/j.jamda.2013.03.022

Nathavitharana, R. R., Mishra, H., Sullivan, A., Hurwitz, S., Lederer, P., Meintjes, J., Nardell, E., & Theron, G. (2022). Predicting Airborne Infection Risk : Association Between Personal Ambient Carbon Dioxide Level Monitoring and Incidence of Tuberculosis Infection in South African Health Workers. *Clinical Infectious Diseases, 75*(8), 1297–1306. DOI: 10.1093/cid/ciac183

Negin, J., Abimbola, S., & Marais, B. J. (2015). Tuberculosis among older adults – time to take notice. *International Journal of Infectious Diseases, 32*, 135–137. DOI: 10.1016/j.ijid.2014.11.018

Nema, V. (2012). Tuberculosis diagnostics : Challenges and opportunities. *Lung India : Official Organ of Indian Chest Society, 29*(3), 259. DOI: 10.4103/0970-2113.99112

O'Grady, M. A., Mootz, J., Suleman, A., Sweetland, A., Teodoro, E., Anube, A., Feliciano, P., Bezuidenhout, C., Dos Santos, P. F., Fumo, W., Gouveia, L., Pinsky, I., Mello, M., Kann, B., & Wainberg, M. L. (2022). Mobile technology and task shifting to improve access to alcohol treatment services in Mozambique. *Journal of Substance Abuse Treatment, 134*, 108549. DOI: 10.1016/j.jsat.2021.108549

Pai, M., Nicol, M. P., & Boehme, C. C. (2016). Tuberculosis Diagnostics : State of the Art and Future Directions. *Microbiology Spectrum, 4*(5), 4.5.16. DOI: 10.1128/microbiolspec.TBTB2-0019-2016

Potty, R. S., Kumarasamy, K., Adepu, R., Reddy, R. C., Singarajipura, A., Siddappa, P. B., Sreenivasa, P. B., Thalinja, R., Lakkappa, M. H., Swamickan, R., Shah, A., Panibatla, V., Dasari, R., & Washington, R. (2021). Community health workers augment the cascade of TB detection to care in urban slums of two metro cities in India. *Journal of Global Health, 11*, 04042. DOI: 10.7189/jogh.11.04042

Qin, Z. Z., Ahmed, S., Sarker, M. S., Paul, K., Adel, A. S. S., Naheyan, T., Barrett, R., Banu, S., & Creswell, J. (2021). Tuberculosis detection from chest x-rays for triaging in a high tuberculosis-burden setting : An evaluation of five artificial intelligence algorithms. *The Lancet. Digital Health, 3*(9), e543–e554. DOI: 10.1016/S2589-7500(21)00116-3

Rajagopalan, S. (2001). Tuberculosis and Aging : A Global Health Problem. *Clinical Infectious Diseases, 33*(7), 1034–1039. DOI: 10.1086/322671

Rich, J. D., Beckwith, C. G., Macmadu, A., Marshall, B. D. L., Brinkley-Rubinstein, L., Amon, J. J., Milloy, M.-J., King, M. R. F., Sanchez, J., Atwoli, L., & Altice, F. L. (2016). Clinical care of incarcerated people with HIV, viral hepatitis, or tuberculosis. *Lancet, 388*(10049), 1103–1114. DOI: 10.1016/S0140-6736(16)30379-8

Rolland, Y., Benetos, A., Gentric, A., Ankri, J., Blanchard, F., Bonnefoy, M., De Decker, L., Ferry, M., Gonthier, R., Hanon, O., Jeandel, C., Nourhashemi, F., Perret-Guillaume, C., Retornaz, F., Bouvier, H., Ruault, G., & Berrut, G. (2011). Frailty in older population : A brief position paper from the French society of geriatrics and gerontology. *Psychologie & Neuropsychiatrie du Vieillissement, 9*(4), 387–390. DOI: 10.1684/pnv.2011.0311

Satyanarayana, S., Nair, S. A., Chadha, S. S., Shivashankar, R., Sharma, G., Yadav, S., Mohanty, S., Kamineni, V., Wilson, N. C., Harries, A. D., & Dewan, P. K. (2011). From Where Are Tuberculosis Patients Accessing Treatment in India? Results from a Cross-Sectional Community Based Survey of 30 Districts. *PLoS One, 6*(9), e24160. DOI: 10.1371/journal.pone.0024160

Siddiqi, K., Lambert, M.-L., & Walley, J. (2003). Clinical diagnosis of smear-negative pulmonary tuberculosis in low-income countries : The current evidence. *The Lancet. Infectious Diseases*, *3*(5), 288–296. DOI: 10.1016/S1473-3099(03)00609-1

Story, A., Murad, S., Roberts, W., Verheyen, M., & Hayward, A. C. (2007). Tuberculosis in London : The importance of homelessness, problem drug use and prison. *Thorax*, *62*(8), 667–671. DOI: 10.1136/thx.2006.065409

Subbaraman, R., Nathavitharana, R. R., Mayer, K. H., Satyanarayana, S., Chadha, V. K., Arinaminpathy, N., & Pai, M. (2019). Constructing care cascades for active tuberculosis : A strategy for program monitoring and identifying gaps in quality of care. *PLoS Medicine*, *16*(2), e1002754. DOI: 10.1371/journal.pmed.1002754

Tanimura, T., Jaramillo, E., Weil, D., Raviglione, M., & Lönnroth, K. (2014). Financial burden for tuberculosis patients in low- and middle-income countries : A systematic review. *The European Respiratory Journal*, *43*(6), 1763–1775. DOI: 10.1183/09031936.00193413

Taylor, J., Coates, E., Brewster, L., Mountain, G., Wessels, B., & Hawley, M. S. (2015). Examining the use of telehealth in community nursing : Identifying the factors affecting frontline staff acceptance and telehealth adoption. *Journal of Advanced Nursing*, *71*(2), 326–337. DOI: 10.1111/jan.12480

Ullah, H., Ahmed, H., Salman, A., Iqbal, R., Hussaini, S. J., & Malikzai, A. (2024). The rising tide of tuberculosis in Pakistan : Factors, impact, and multi-faceted approaches for prevention and control. *Health Science Reports*, *7*(10), e70130. DOI: 10.1002/hsr2.70130

Uplekar, M., Creswell, J., Ottmani, S.-E., Weil, D., Sahu, S., & Lönnroth, K. (2013). Programmatic approaches to screening for active tuberculosis [State of the art series. Active case finding/screening. Number 6 in the series]. *The International Journal of Tuberculosis and Lung Disease : the Official Journal of the International Union against Tuberculosis and Lung Disease*, *17*(10), 1248–1256. DOI: 10.5588/ijtld.13.0199

World Health Organization. (2018). *Compendium of WHO guidelines and associated standards : Ensuring optimum delivery of the cascade of care for patients with tuberculosis* (2nd ed). World Health Organization. https://iris.who.int/handle/10665/272644

World Health Organization. (2020). *Global Tuberculosis Report 2020* (1st ed.). World Health Organization.

World Health Organization. (2021). *WHO Consolidated Guidelines on Tuberculosis. Module 2 : Screening - Systematic Screening for Tuberculosis Disease* (1st ed.). World Health Organization.

World Health Organization. (s. d.). *Global Programme on Tuberculosis & Lung Health.* Consulté 27 avril 2025, à l'adresse https://www.who.int/teams/global-tuberculosis-programme/populations-comorbidities

Wu, S., Litvinjenko, S., Magwood, O., & Wei, X. (2023). Defining tuberculosis vulnerability based on an adapted social determinants of health framework : A narrative review. *Global Public Health: An International Journal for Research, Policy and Practice*, *18*(1), 2221729. DOI: 10.1080/17441692.2023.2221729

Yuen, C. M., Puma, D., Millones, A. K., Galea, J. T., Tzelios, C., Calderon, R. I., Brooks, M. B., Jimenez, J., Contreras, C., Nichols, T. C., Nicholson, T., Lecca, L., Becerra, M. C., & Keshavjee, S. (2021). Identifying barriers and facilitators to implementation of community-based tuberculosis active case finding with mobile X-ray units in Lima, Peru : A RE-AIM evaluation. *BMJ Open*, *11*(7), e050314. DOI: 10.1136/bmjopen-2021-050314

Chapter 4
Battling Tuberculosis on the Frontlines: Protecting Healthcare Workers From Occupational TB

Sakshi Chaturvedi
https://orcid.org/0000-0002-4979-3430
Banasthali Vidyapith, India

Chakrapani Chaturvedi
https://orcid.org/0000-0003-2612-6552
Banasthali Vidyapith, India

Shailendra Singh Choudhary
https://orcid.org/0009-0005-7335-7486
CMHO Office Tonk, India

ABSTRACT

The risk of healthcare workers (HCWs) contracting tuberculosis (TB) occupationally has been significantly elevated, with prevalence rates significantly higher than those of the general population. The most hazardous factors include poor ventilation, irregular use of personal protective equipment (PPE), underlying disease histories, working with multidrug-resistant TB, and long exposure to patients with an infectious disease. High-risk groups, such as laboratory technicians, nurses, and physicians, report prevalence rates of 2,006-6,468 per 100,000 individuals. This chapter goes into detail about how well infection-control measures, regular check-ups, tuberculosis preventive treatment (TPT), and self-care practices help reduce tuberculosis among healthcare workers. The chapter also discusses the administration functions, engineering measures, screening processes, and monitoring strategies for controlling

DOI: 10.4018/979-8-3373-3446-2.ch004

tuberculosis among healthcare workers. The chapter provides practical solutions to the challenges of protecting healthcare workers and reducing the occupational tuberculosis burden.

OBJECTIVES OF THE CHAPTER

1. To explore the epidemiology and real burden of TB among health workers
2. Offer realistic evidence-based recommendations on how to handle the risk of occupational TB that can be achieved in practice by facilities.
3. Protection of healthcare workers within the context of the Indian health system.

I. INTRODUCTION

According to the WHO 2024 Global Tuberculosis Report, TB is still a serious threat to global health, with an expected 10.8 million new cases and 1.25 million fatalities in 2023. TB has surpassed COVID-19 to retake its top spot as the world's biggest infectious disease killer.

The COVID-19 pandemic exposed the preexisting fragility of healthcare systems. Once a health crisis strikes, then there is no such thing as infection control. The WHO 2024 TB study indicated that the TB disruptions were massive and widespread. There has been a major impact as a result of the burden of tuberculosis.

Having been exposed with MDR and XDR tb strains, insufficient air ventilation, long duty hours healthcare workers, they encountered compromised occupational systems in terms of strained resources, and conflicting priorities. The average prevalence of LTBI among healthcare workers was 54%, with a range from 33% to 79%. Annual estimates of the risk of LTBI ranged from 0.5% to 14.3%. The annual incidence of tuberculosis among healthcare workers varied from 69 to 5,780 cases per 100,000 persons.

TB screening programs have been deprioritized in many settings. The implementation of contact tracing is inconsistent. Eradicating the tuberculosis epidemic by 2030 is one of the health objectives of the United Nations Sustainable Development Goals (SDGs).

A. The Global TB Burden Among Healthcare Workers

Tuberculosis is present in all regions of the globe. In 2023, the highest incidence of new tuberculosis cases was reported in the WHO South-East Asia Region (45%), followed by the African Region (24%) and the Western Pacific Region (17%).

In 2024 WHO report, among the 30 countries facing a significant burden of tuberculosis, Gabon, Mongolia, Mozambique, Namibia, South Africa, and Zambia stood out for having over 80% of diagnosed TB cases initially tested with a WRD (WHO rapid diagnostic test).

Latent TB infection rate is 37 percent of healthcare workers but has been estimated to be between 0.1% to 62 percent. Why such variation? The issue of geography is massive.

The rate of latent tuberculosis infection among healthcare personnel is exceedingly concerning. The figure of 37 percent is akin to a ticking time bomb. The majority of patients with latent TB infection will not progress to active TB disease (about 90-95 percent will stay asymptomatic throughout their lives), whereas the remaining 5-10 percent will eventually get the disease. The statistical threat is palpable for healthcare practitioners who encounter tuberculosis daily.

B. Occupational Health Disparities

1. High-Risk Professions

Some occupations are exposed to extremely greater risk. Laboratory Technologists work with the samples of TB every day. Nurses offer direct care to their patients. Respiratory wards have physicians spending hours on diagnosing and treating TB patients. These are not administration jobs; they are frontline jobs that involve prolonged exposure.

TB prevalence rates in these three professions Nurses, lab technicians, physicians are always recorded at 2,006-6,468 per 100,000- this is much higher than practically all other healthcare jobs. In the cases of work with TB patients or samples several times a week, the risk of exposure is quickly multiplied.

What makes it worse? This usually comprises of the most seasoned personnel- the people who cannot be easily substituted. The effects are felt at the facility when they fall ill due to occupational TB.

2. Vulnerability among Support Staff

TB prevalence is usually lower in administrative staff - a true benefit of not having direct contact with patients. But “lower” doesn't mean “safe.” Working in a shared healthcare setting does not secure according to the job title. A potential TB patient waiting in a waiting room, employees of the administration operating close to respiratory departments, or infected surfaces in places of availability are some of the positional risks that transcend job boundaries.

That is why, as opposed to the job risk assessment, the facility-wide methodologies are crucial. All members of the supporting staff, not just doctors, nurses, and physicians, are in danger.

C. The COVID-19 Factor

COVID-19 affected many adversely. Resources were redirected. The training programs experienced postponement. TB screening was occasionally deprioritized due to the necessity for immediate care in acute crises (Cilloni et al., 2020). However, what is crucial at this moment is that the COVID experience has imparted a critical lesson: infrastructure will deteriorate, surveillance will diminish, prevention will be postponed, and the transmission of illness will accelerate. We cannot accomplish that with tuberculosis, especially given the prevalence of medication resistance.

II. RISK FACTORS AND EPIDEMIOLOGY

A. Prevalence and Incidence Among Healthcare Workers

1. Global Patterns

meta-analysis highlighted evidence that healthcare workers are at significantly high risk of TB. A burden of 2-3 times higher than the general population with an incidence of about 97 per 100,000 a year and a latent tb rate of up to 37 percent-56percent(Meregildo-Rodriguez et al., 2024). according to one Oxford study in 2017 -India, Indonesia, China, Nigeria, Pakistan, and South Africa represent 60% of global tuberculosis cases. Mozambique, another low-income country in Southern Africa, has a very high incidence of TB among health workers.

The distinction in the environment is noteworthy. The rates decrease significantly when infection control measures are implemented in high-resource facilities. Peaks in rates in environments that are under-diagnostic and under-ventilated. This suggests that the risk is not predetermined, but it can be managed to a certain extent.

2. Why TB Control Among Health Care Workers in India Is Crucial to Manage

according to a comprehensive assessment of 51 research from countries with low and middle incomes nosocomial exposure is the associated risk of tuberculosis disease due to range from 25–5361 per 10^5 person-year. In India, the situation is especially severe: TB rates in healthcare workers are 2,391.6 cases in 100,000 people, which is almost twice as high as the world average. Why? This is in part due to the higher burden of TB in India, but also because the infrastructure of the system of infection control is uneven, and the resources are overstretched in numerous facilities. High MDR tb incidences especially in age above 50 years are observed (Ledesma et al., 2024) In contrast, the rates are lower in high-income nations with the well-developed infection control. This isn't coincidental. It is based on actual disparities in facility planning, the supply of PPE, diagnostic capacity, and skilled staffing.

latent TB infection (LTBI) among healthcare workers in India: The occurrence of latent TB infection (LTBI) among healthcare workers in India is significantly higher. Research shows that around 34-50% of healthcare workers exhibit signs of TB infection, in contrast to 31.3% within the general population aged 15 and older. A prospective cohort study conducted in Puducherry revealed that over one-third of healthcare workers (HCWs) were infected with tuberculosis (TB), with about one in twenty HCWs demonstrating conversion to infection during a one-year follow-up period.

Incidence of Active Tuberculosis Disease

The occurrence of active TB disease among healthcare workers significantly differs across various occupational categories and healthcare environments. A significant study conducted in Pune in 2016 analysed data from 1,886 healthcare workers, comprising 662 medical residents and interns, and found 26 instances of tuberculosis among trainees over an 18-month timeframe. The analysis revealed an estimated incidence of 3,279 cases per 100,000 person-years among trainees, which is 15 times greater than the general community rate of 167 cases per 100,000 person-years in Maharashtra state.

TB Burden Specific to Occupations

a) *Laboratory Technicians*

Among all healthcare categories, laboratory technicians encounter the greatest risk of occupational tuberculosis. Recent findings revealed TB prevalence rates of

6,468.31 cases per 100,000 individuals among laboratory technicians. The increased risk is a result of direct and extended exposure to clinical specimens that contain live Mycobacterium tuberculosis, insufficient biosafety practices, and a lack of adequate respiratory protection in numerous environments.

b) *Nursing Professionals*

Nurses constitute a significantly impacted demographic, with a reported tuberculosis prevalence of 2,726.83 cases per 100,000 individuals. The significant burden observed can be attributed to their extensive and ongoing interactions with patients, their roles in respiratory isolation units, and the insufficient training provided in infection control practices. Nursing staff often deliver direct patient care, including aerosol-generating procedures, without the necessary respiratory protection.

c) *Healthcare Professionals and Trainees*

The prevalence of tuberculosis among physicians is quantified at 2,006.18 cases per 100,000, with notably higher rates observed in medical residents and trainees. Research indicates that newly appointed medical residents, nursing students exhibiting tuberculosis present incidence rates of 17.3 per 1,000 person-years during their initial year of hospital practice. It is significant that around two-thirds of TB cases in medical trainees manifest as extrapulmonary TB, indicating a likelihood of recent primary infection instead of the reactivation of latent disease.

In a meta-analysis the prevalence of the TB infection among Indian healthcare workers was 2,391.6 cases per 100,000. Not a trivial issue, that is a crisis within a crisis (Nath et al., 2024). There are a number of things colliding: the overall TB burden in the general population is high, and hence, healthcare facilities are exposed to more TB cases. The majority of the facilities are not properly ventilated and they do not use air-conditioning. The training programs are not consistent. Infection control resources become overstretched between competing priorities.

Positive TB tests were linked to years of work, work location, TB contact, and job category. HIV status also affects risk in high-prevalence situations. The burden is greatest in low- and middle-income nations with insufficient infection control resources. so, it is required that healthcare workers participate in universal tuberculosis screening programs.

However, there is one more thing that is important, that is, awareness. Occupational TB threat has not been a priority in most of the facilities; there is an enormous variation in the availability of TPT (TB preventive treatment) between facilities.

3. The Latent TB Infection Challenge

This is where latent TB infection comes in as an issue. The prevalence varies between 0.1 and 62 percent in accordance with the types of healthcare workers, facilities and mode of testing. Such huge discrepancies indicate disparities in exposure; intensity of surveillance and different regions have a varying baseline of TB.

The troubling reality? This is a large pool of infection posing continued danger. The majority of LTBI does not cause any symptoms over a lifetime, yet in the case of healthcare workers, with immune system weakness or comorbidity, the development of active TB is a possibility. This is exactly the reason why TB preventive therapy of latent infections is important (WHO, 2015b).

B. Environmental and Occupational Risk Factors

1. The Ventilation Problem

The most common issue that most people do not give a second thought is the air that we breathe in a healthcare facility. A lack of proper ventilation makes hospitals the centers of transmission of TB. TB bacilli are able to stay hanging in stagnated air hours and thus these particles can be inhaled by any other person in that place.

The issue is aggravated by the resource-constrained environment where the facility building budgets are low. A lot of older hospital buildings were built decades ago when the TB ventilation standards had not been appropriately comprehended. Retrofitting is an expensive undertaking. This is because in certain facilities, the windows fail to open. In other cases, HVAC systems disintegrate and repair is postponed indefinitely.

The result is that mycobacterium tuberculi remain longer in the air than necessary, and this exposes the entire staff to cumulative exposure.

2. Attitude of Health Care Worker for PPE Use and Self-Care Behavior

The following is something that is exasperating to infection control experts; the healthcare workers do not wear PPE regularly, even in situations when these supplies are at their disposal. This occurs due to a number of reasons. Occasionally there is a training void- workers do not clearly see the importance of the equipment. The supply chain collapses and PPE is not available sometimes. There are cases where the culture of the workplace that allows overlooking protection is normalized.

Errors to avoid: forgetting about N95s in case of a more dangerous operation, reusing single-use impersonators without decontamination, ineffective fit testing takes place at all, ineffective doffing technique that renders the protection useless.

The concerning aspect is that these failures frequently occur even though the workers understand the theoretical importance of PPE. Ensuring adherence to behaviors presents challenges in practical situations.

3. Prolonged Patient Exposure

Once TB is diagnosed late, either due to the fact that the symptoms are not identified in a patient or the fact that diagnostic capabilities are inadequate, all people around a patient become exposed. The patient of TB without diagnosis may take days or weeks in general ward before anybody suspects of TB and takes correct measures of isolation.

In this window, all the members of staff who step into that room are exposed. Others may communicate in a very short time; some (nursing personnel) may spend hours with the patient. The cumulative exposure grows very fast and since the delay in diagnosis is very frequent in high volume settings.

C. Patient-Related Risk Factors

1. Multidrug-Resistant TB

All is complicated when TB bacteria acquire resistance to isoniazid and rifampicin the horsemen of the TB treatment. Such patients take even longer to be cured since the first-line medication is ineffective. The healthcare personnel handling the MDR-TB cases are exposed to periods of time with organisms that cannot be touched by normal treatment.

When a healthcare worker falls ill with MDR-TB, he/she experiences long treatment period with more side effects and poor results. The mental burden of such a possibility should not be underestimated.

2. Extensively Drug-Resistant TB

The worst of all is the XDR-TB which is resistant to the fluoroquinolones as well as second-line injectable drugs. Such patients become much more difficult to cure, are more contagious, and have poorer results despite the contemporary treatment. In the case of a healthcare worker with XDR-TB, the possibility of treatment decreases dramatically and the chances of success reduce to a zero point.

3. Diagnostic Delays

Each day a patient with TB without any diagnosis stays in a hospital, this poses a risk of occupation to the personnel. This may seem simple but it is very complicated. Delays occur in various stages: patients may fail to realize that they are experiencing symptoms of TB, medical staff may fail to consider that they should get TB tests, or the diagnostic system may fail.

Quick diagnostics reducing the duration of time-to-diagnosis to weeks or hours offer some of the best occupational protection ever.

D. Individual Healthcare Worker Vulnerabilities

1. Pre-Existing Respiratory Disease

Occupational asthma, COPD, or injury to the lungs, chronic diseases have put healthcare workers at higher risk of serious TB disease should they become occupationally infected. Their degraded airways and distorted immune systems may result in accelerated course of the disease and deteriorated results.

A person having normal lungs may be more tolerant of occupational TB exposure as compared to having a respiratory system that is already damaged.

2. Nutritional Status

Malnutrition is significant than what most individuals think. Poor nutritional condition and low BMI below 19 kg/m^2, makes the immune system weaker, thus the transition to active TB more probable. Nutritional insufficiency is a factual issue in the low-income conditions with low salaries of healthcare workers, which increases the risk of TB (Padmapriyadarsini et al., 2016).

That is why the occupational health programs that do not consider the welfare of workers are not complete.

3. Immunocompromised Status

Workers with HIV, uncontrolled diabetes, or receiving immunosuppressive therapy are at high risk of TB in case of occupational infection. A CD4 of less than 200 cells/mm3 is very dramatic in developing TB disease once exposed.

These employees require better screening, preventive treatment as well as possibly job adjustments to minimize exposures.

III. EVIDENCE-BASED LITERATURE REVIEW

A. What Recent Research Shows

1. da Silva et al. (2022)

A systematic review conducted by da Silva and colleagues found 14 areas critical in the improvement of an infection prevention program. They discovered that there was enormous disparity in the prevalence of latent TB in healthcare workers (0.1 percent to 62 percent) and the annual incidences (3.9 percent to 26 percent)- a divergence that was influenced by testing method and definition of cases (da Silva et al., 2022).

Notably, they have found a serious gap: available literature is mostly concerned with latent TB prevalence, but high-quality statistics on the prevalence of active TB cases in the health care staff is apparent and conspicuous. There is more information on LTBI than the actual TB disease progression in such population.

2. Lee et al. (2021)

This systematic review brought out one thing that is significant: environmental and procedural breakdowns considerably increase the risk of TB. Poor ventilation, inconsistency in use of PPEs, work hours and low body mass index among nurses were also identified as major modifiable risk factors (Lee et al., 2021).

The research authors made strong arguments in favor of full of facility interventions instead of fragmented ones.

3. Uden et al. (2017)

A meta-analysis reported active TB of 97 per 100,000 healthcare workers/per year and a latent infection of 37 percent/year. These numbers were significantly high as compared to the general population. Infection control measures, which should be a combination of PPE, screening, and case management, are, the authors stressed, of utmost importance (Uden et al., 2017).

4. India-Specific Evidence

India: a meta-analysis of TB in healthcare workers in India in 2004-2023 by Nath and his colleagues reported a 2,391.6 cases per 100,000 prevalence. They highlighted that there should be strict strategies of infection control, regular screening of TB, continuous education and better health facilities. TB screening in the country, compulsory training activities and further investments in the funds of the healthcare facilities became important policy proposals (Debnath et al., 2024a).

B. What We Still Don't Know

Although massive literature is available, there are still major gaps in evidence. Randomized controlled trials that specifically assess recommended TB prevention interventions among healthcare workers are surprisingly deficient. Why? Ethical constraints. It is unacceptable to deny specific healthcare professionals' protective equipment when others are provided with it. Variations exist in both public and private contexts, as well as in community and tertiary care supply systems.

There is a high degree of variability in the measurements of TB outcomes and their reporting in the studies. Others have various definitions of cases. There are others who measure other results. Geographic situations are vastly different. It is this heterogeneity that makes it hard to compare.

Most alarming: routine statistical information of active TB cases in healthcare workers is unsatisfactory. There is more information about individuals that are infected with latent TB infection than the information on individuals that develop active disease and the reasons why.

IV. ADMINISTRATIVE INFECTION CONTROL MEASURES

Administrative controls are bureaucratic in sound but strong. Upon integrating the quick detection of case with the quick isolation processes, you shorten the period within which healthcare professionals are exposed to infectious individuals without a diagnosis.

The major one is combined--single measures are not very good. Combination strategies are more effective.

A. Rapid Case Detection and Diagnosis

1. Rapid Diagnostics

The diagnosis of TB was transformed by GeneXpert MTB/RIF. Two-hour responses are provided instead of days or weeks to find out the result of cultures. This rate is critically significant to the protection of healthcare workers since it allows timely isolation.

Implementation of rapid diagnostics facilities experience a speedy turnaround in diagnostics, prompt initiation of treatment, and in the most important case of occupational health, timely isolation precautions (Pereira et al., 2018).

2. AI-Enhanced Chest X-Rays

The computer-assisted detection systems are now able to help in identifying TB based on the chest X-rays with accuracy comparable to human radiologists. Such systems enhance the sensitivity and speed of diagnosis, which allows detection of cases at a younger age in combination with clinical examination and microbiological tests (Ngosa et al., 2023).

The use of AI systems can be used to accelerate the process of diagnosis in the facilities where radiologists are few and so they do not need to use human skills that are limited.

B. Patient Isolation Protocols

1. Fast-Track Procedures

The facilities must have well-defined procedures on quick detection and isolation of suspected TB patients. It entails special areas of isolation, effective triage processes, and skilled personnel capable of acting fast. The quicker you are isolated, the less people are exposed.

2. Symptomatic Screening

There is universal screening of all patients with symptoms of TB when they arrive to identify presumptive cases at an early stage. This involves the inquiry about persistent cough, fever, night sweats and weight loss. The presumptive TB patients must be immediately isolated awaiting tests.

V. ENVIRONMENTAL CONTROL MEASURES

Environmental controls encompass all the aspects of improvements in ventilation systems to the ultraviolet germicidal irradiation. The idea is straightforward, when you can manage the air and the environment, you will minimize the spread of TB. Implementation? Much more complex.

A. Ventilation Systems

1. Negative Pressure Isolation Rooms

Isolation rooms of negative pressure are the gold standard in high income countries. The air pressure within the room is kept at a lower level as compared to outside the room, thus none of the contaminated air escapes but flows to the inside. These rooms are normally designed to attain 6-12 air changes per hour of 100 percent exhaust to external, and TB bacilli are captured by HEPA filtration.

The reality? Such rooms are costly and technologically involved. They are usually not possible in a resource constrained environment.

2. Facility-Wide Improvements

You do not have to have negative pressure isolation rooms all over. However, you should have improved air quality in the facility. This could involve opening up windows, mechanical ventilation where possible, decreasing congestion of patients, and keeping the existing systems in good condition.

Simple changes like opening windows whenever attending to a patient, overcrowding, etc. make a difference that can be measured.

B. Ultraviolet Germicidal Irradiation (UVGI)

1. Upper-Room Systems

The upper part of the rooms has UV-C light systems that inactivate TB bacilli in the air. Such a method is especially effective in places with high loads where mechanical ventilation is restricted. It offers economical protection that does not require significant building restructuring (Diel et al., 2020).

2. Portable Devices

Portable UV systems can treat specific zones with limited investment, though they're less efficient than permanent installations. They provide supplemental environmental control for resource-constrained facilities.

C. Patient Load Management

Reasonable staffing ratios reduce per-worker TB exposure. Workers managing fewer TB patients accumulate less exposure and face lower risk. Overcrowded facilities where triage is inadequate and isolation capacity is overwhelmed represent disasters for occupational health.

VI. PERSONAL PROTECTIVE EQUIPMENT

PPE serves as your last line of defense when administrative and environmental controls aren't enough. The problem? PPE only works if people actually use it correctly. That's harder than it sounds.

A. N95, FFP2, FFP3 Respirators

1. Fit Testing

N95 respirators only work if they fit properly. Most people don't fit them correctly, and many facilities don't perform fit testing. Quantitative testing using photometry is the gold standard. Facial hair, facial structure, and improper donning all undermine protection.

Healthcare workers need individual fit testing initially and annually. Those with poor fit need alternative models.

2. Proper Use

N95s should be used during all patient interactions involving TB-suspected or TB-confirmed individuals. Usage should begin before patient contact and continue throughout. Single-use respirators shouldn't be reused. Workers need training on proper donning, storage, and recognition of when replacement is needed. FFP2,

FFP3 respirator are better option for protection against TB but not addressed much in safety guidelines. When dealing with MDR -TB patients FFP3 is best option.

In reality? Many healthcare workers struggle with these standards. The culture in many settings normalizes PPE shortcuts.

B. Other PPE Components

Eye protection using safety glasses or face shields prevents respiratory secretion contact with mucous membranes. Gowns and gloves prevent contact transmission. While TB transmission is primarily airborne, these items provide infection control redundancy.

Through regular application and not the random application it is the key.

C. Training and Compliance

It is necessary to be thoroughly trained in how to don and doff PPE. Poor doffing is a significant route of infections because the workers may contaminate themselves when taking them off. The order is crucial: gloves (contaminated the most), gown, eye protection and respirator.

Continuous training based on competency rather than lectures does produce behavior change. The skill proficiency is preserved through yearly reinforcement.

VII. Healthcare Worker Screening and TB Preventive Therapy

Screening determines the people with latent infection of TB or active TB disease. Preventive therapy is used to treat latent infections in advance before it turns into active disease. Collectively, they are your greatest chances of preventing healthcare worker TB disease.

A. Initial and Periodic Screening

1. Tuberculin Skin Test (TST)

The Mantoux test is still popular even with new alternatives. Before or soon after employment, healthcare workers are to be provided with baseline TST testing. A positive TST With standard PPD-RT 23 and above 5mm induration is an indication of TB infection. Serial testing is able to detect conversions where once negative individuals are converted to be positive indicating infection in the near past.

Positive TST conversion is an indicator of occupational exposure to TB and a requirement to undergo TB preventive therapy (Ministry of Health and Family Welfare, 2021) .

2. Blood-Based Tests (IGRAs)

Interferon-release tests such as QuantiFERON and T-SPOT involve blood tests as opposed to skin tests. They can be more accurate than TST with low false results due to BCG vaccination. The trade-off? They are costlier and they need laboratory facilities.

These are used in many high-income facilities; they are still being used in many low-resource settings because they are less expensive.

3. Chest X-Ray Assessment

All healthcare workers who have positive TB tests or symptoms are supposed to have chest X-rays. The results of CXR can differentiate between infection of latent TB (no radiographic results) and active TB disease (typical results such as cavities in the upper lobes). Serial X-rays allow tracking of workers who are under preventive therapy.

B. Tuberculosis Preventive Therapy

What counts here is that TB preventive treatment is functional. It lessens the potential of escalating the TB latent disease to active disease by 60-95 percent based on the regimen and adherence of the people.

TPT is not a choice and it is a necessity to the occupationally exposed healthcare workers.

1. Who Should Get TPT?

TB preventive therapy should also be administered to healthcare workers who have the following criteria: a positive TB test (TST or IGRA) without clinical or radiographic evidence of disease; recent exposure to TB (within 2 years) despite initial test-results; documented TST or IGRA conversion; co-infection with HIV; or contact with patients with drug-resistant TB.

2. Available Regimens (Ministry of Health and Family Welfare, 2021)

Multiple regimens exist with different durations and effectiveness profiles. The standard 6-month isoniazid regimen (6H) costs less and remains well-tolerated globally, though adherence challenges are real for long-term therapy. The newer 12-week rifapentine-isoniazid regimen (3HP) offers superior efficacy and better adherence due to its weekly dosing schedule, but costs more.

Drug-resistant TB contacts need tailored regimens based on the source patient's drug susceptibility pattern.

3. Isoniazid Preventive Therapy (6H)

Standard isoniazid therapy involves 5 mg/kg daily (usually 300 mg maximum) for 6-9 months. Vitamin B6 supplementation at 25-50 mg daily prevents peripheral neuropathy. Efficacy is approximately 60-70 percent in preventing progression.

The challenge? Long-term adherence. People forget to take daily medications. They miss clinic visits. Life gets busy. Follow-ups and adherence support systems every month are beneficial, but will not fully resolve the issue.

4. Rifapentine-Based Regimens (3HP)

The 12-week program of direct observation is 12 weeks in a weekly regimen of rifapentine (600 mg) and isoniazid (900 mg). The program has 95%+ efficacy and significantly improved adherence. During the week, it is better to take pills weekly rather than daily. Tolerability is excellent. 3HP is weekly once in children below 15 years of age and daily in above 15 years of age groups.

The downside? Price is significantly increased. Besides, certain antiretroviral therapy drug interactions play a major role in HIV co-infected workers and coordination is required.

5. Pre-Treatment Evaluation

Prior to the initiation of TPT, it is necessary to evaluate them thoroughly: clinical examination of TB symptoms in detail; a chest radiograph to rule out active disease; a liver function test (especially because the worker is already chronically ill); an HIV test; an examination to eliminate contraindications; and hearing tests when taking fluoroquinolones.

Not a bureaucratic thing, it is a necessity. Initiating TPT in an individual with active TB without any diagnosis is a manageable issue turned into a treatment failure disaster.

6. Monitoring During Treatment

After TPT onset, close attention has to be paid to healthcare workers. Identify TB symptoms at baseline, mid-treatment and end of treatment. Any employee who presents with a lasting cough, fever, night sweats or loss of weight must be evaluated immediately with TB.

It is necessary to monitor adverse effects regularly: monthly visits to the clinic, examining the presence of hepatotoxicity effects, peripheral neuropathy, allergic reactions, and gastrointestinal side effects. Repeated liver function tests would be done in the case of symptoms development or baseline values were not normal.

7. Adherence Support

The enhancement of the compliance occurs due to the provision of thorough assistance: directly observed therapy at least during the initial month; frequent clinical follow-ups; patient education about the necessity of its completion; workplace-based assistance that would allow the patient to schedule clinic visits; peer support groups; SMS-based appointment alerts; and involvement of the family.

The most effective ones incorporate TPT in the normal check-ups of the occupational health and not as an independent program.

C. Special Populations

1. Pregnant Healthcare Workers

TPT in pregnant healthcare workers is advised to have latent TB infection- benefits greatly exceed risks. Isoniazid is FDA category A (safe in pregnancy). The standard 6H regimen is preferred due to extensive safety data. TPT shouldn't be delayed in pregnancy.

Breastfeeding women can safely continue all TPT regimens as drug concentrations in breast milk are minimal.

2. HIV Co-Infected Workers

HIV co-infected healthcare workers with positive or negative TB tests should receive TPT. But timing depends on CD4 count. For CD4 <50 cells/mm^3, TPT initiation should wait until immune reconstitution on antiretroviral therapy.

Watch out for drug interactions. Protease inhibitors and non-nucleoside reverse transcriptase inhibitors interact substantially with rifampicin-based regimens. Integrase inhibitor-based regimens are more compatible.

3. Workers with Comorbidities

Workers with diabetes, liver disease, or renal impairment need careful regimen selection and close monitoring. Pre-existing liver disease may require isoniazid avoidance or reduced doses with more frequent monitoring. Renal impairment requires attention since some TB drugs accumulate.

VIII. EDUCATION, TRAINING, AND CAPACITY BUILDING

An informed healthcare worker is an empowered healthcare worker. But education isn't a one-time event. It requires baseline training, continuing education, and practical competency-based approaches.

A. Baseline Training

All healthcare workers need baseline training covering TB epidemiology, transmission routes, clinical presentation, diagnosis, and occupational risk. Training should emphasize that TB is an occupational hazard requiring comprehensive prevention. New staff should receive this during orientation and it should be reinforced annually.

Beyond knowledge, practical training works better. Show people how to don and doff PPE correctly. Demonstrate proper respiratory hygiene. Walk them through isolation procedures. Competency-based training with return demonstration of skills improves retention far more than lectures alone. Incorporate tuberculosis infection control and occupational health subjects into pre-service curricula for medical, nursing, and allied health education.

B. Continuing Education

1. Case Detection Training

A systematic review found that healthcare worker and volunteer training significantly improves TB case detection rates. Enhanced training enables workers to recognize TB presentations, obtain appropriate diagnostic tests, and ensure rapid notification. Better case detection directly protects healthcare workers by reducing time infectious patients spend undiagnosed in general healthcare settings.

2. Specialized MDR/XDR Training

Specialized training on multidrug-resistant and extensively drug-resistant TB should target workers in TB programs and high-burden facilities. Training should cover epidemiology, diagnosis, treatment regimens, monitoring, and occupational precautions specific to resistant strains.

C. Digital Learning Approaches

1. Synchronous (Live) Training

Live synchronous training solutions allow instructors and healthcare workers who are geographically separated to interact in real-time. The added value of question/answer sessions and case-based discussion is something that cannot be presented using recorded materials. The method is especially effective when dealing with complicated clinical issues.

2. Asynchronous Learning Modules

Asynchronous systems allow workers to get learning contents at their own time. This enhances accessibility to workers who have fluctuating schedules or are away in distant areas. The trade-off? Less immediate time communication and feedback.

3. Constructive Feedback for Not Only Knowledge Assessment, Attitude Assessment

Trainings related to TPT, infection prevention measures are critical as highlighted by recent study which cause practice gap (van de Water et al., 2023). Training should have feedback with before and after training knowledge assessment to report effectiveness. A distance learning intervention program of nurses in Brazil reported that they had better knowledge scores at posttest (11.4 +- 2.7) than the pretest of (10.3 +- 2.2) and this difference (1.1) is statistically significant. However, knowledge is not sufficient and we require behavior change (Cabral et al., 2017).

IX. EMERGING TECHNOLOGIES FOR TB DETECTION

Artificial intelligence, wearable sensors, and edge computing provide new solutions towards TB detection, and protection of healthcare workers. These are no longer science fiction, they are more and more on hand.

A. Artificial Intelligence for TB Detection

Many countries have developed AI platforms can aid the detection of TB with the help of chest radiographs, with the diagnostic accuracy being the same as that of human radiologists. This is very critical in regions where radiologists are in short supply. The South Sudan portable X-rays that employed AI analysis detected TB cases that conventional methods failed to detect (Zhou et al., 2023).

Rapid AI-assisted diagnosis saves a great deal of time in isolating patients, and this approach offers direct protection to healthcare workers due to the prolonged exposure of this group (Table 1).

Table 1. AI for Tuberculosis diagnosis

Platform	Performance	Deployment Status
qXR (Qure.ai)	Sensitivity: 0.93, Specificity: 0.69-0.75 Meets WHO TB triage criteria	Widely deployed
CAD4TB (Delft)	Sensitivity: 0.93, Specificity: 0.69	High-burden countries
Lunit/JF CXR-1	Excellent performance Human-level accuracy	Radiologist-shortage areas

B. Wearable Sensors

Current studies are coming up with wearable machines that identify TB-specific volatile organic compounds with functionalized gold nanoparticles. Diagnostics validation studies were 89.4% accurate. Also, with the new development of research,

TB-specific biomarkers are identified in sweat, saliva, and breath that could be detected by smart biosensors.

In the case of healthcare workers, continuous physiological monitoring would allow detecting the infection early and initiating ultra-early preventive treatment.

C. Integration Challenges

New technologies have great potential, yet they are still inaccessible in resource-limited environments where TB is most likely to occur. It should be implemented to overcome cost, data privacy, and compatibility with the current occupational health systems.

Also, technologies need to be perfectly tested in different environments and standardize performance indicators.

X. PSYCHOSOCIAL SUPPORT AND WORKER WELLBEING

The medical solutions are not enough to support the healthcare workers who are exposed to occupational TB. Clinical interventions are equally important with mental health, financial protection and stigma reduction.

A. Mental Health Services

The ambiance of being exposed to occupational TB causes anxiety and stress that should not be overlooked as professional concern. Clinical providers often experience anxiety regarding the development of TB, side effects of treatment, and family health effects. The occupational health programs are expected to avail counseling services and training on stress management.

Mental health support ought not to be ignored as an auxiliary to occupational health but rather an offering to occupational health as a whole.

B. Confidential Reporting

Contact reporting systems on TB anonymity eliminates the fear of stigmatization or professional repercussions. Confidential systems will allow identifying exposed worker cohorts quickly and responding promptly. They indicate institutional protection of workers.

C. Financial Protection

Paid sick leave will allow the workers to not lose earnings when they are undergoing evaluation or treatment of TB. The fear of loss of income usually demoralizes workers to seek assistance. Providing holistic medical cover of ETCs associated with TB care gives an assurance that workers will never lack the financial capability to access the required services.

Occupational workers that contract TB as a result of workplace exposure should be compensated accordingly in terms of medical treatment, lost earnings including disability.

D. Stigma Reduction

The TB-related stigma can be minimized through internal awareness campaigns. It should be highlighted in the campaigns that TB is an occupational risk among health care workers despite the best prevention practices, that TB is treatable and that it is possible to avoid complications when it is treated early (Aranas et al., 2023).

There is peer support groups linked with healthcare workers and TB disease which offer emotional assistance and realistic peer view on dealing with TB and work-related health (Barik et al., 2020).

XI. EVALUATING WHAT ACTUALLY WORKS

The quality and applicability of the evidence of TB prevention interventions are different. It summarizes the results of the existing literature showing us what we know and what we should not know yet.

A. Why the Evidence Is Limited

It is not possible to conduct a legitimate randomized controlled trial on occupational TB prevention since the protection gear cannot be denied occupations at random. Thereupon, researchers are dependent on quasi-experimental studies, before-after and cohort studies- all of which have their flaws.

To further complicate the matter: the studies adopt disparate definitions of their cases, test various outcomes, and are applied to an entirely different setting. It is difficult to synthesize the results of such variations.

B. What the Evidence Shows

1. Respiratory Hygiene Works

Systematic review of infection prevention interventions such as respiratory hygiene, cough etiquette, engineering control, and environmental control revealed by four studies involving humans with 22,855 subjects. Such interventions were linked to low TB transmission within healthcare facilities.

2. Environmental Controls Help

There is evidence in support of ventilation systems and ultraviolet germicidal irradiation. Although there is a lack of direct randomized trial evidence, laboratory data, engineering evaluations, and observational healthcare data is very strong on the consideration of environmental controls to decrease transmission.

3. Training Improves Detection

Eight articles found that interventions of educational training enhance the detection of TB cases. Although this indirectly helps healthcare workers (by minimizing diagnostic delays and transmission windows), the facts are evident.

4. Comprehensive Approaches Work Best

The strongest evidence is a 24-year retrospective study done on a high-burden tertiary Brazilian hospital. The combination of the measures recommended by WHO, i.e. administrative controls, the protection of the environment, and personal protective gear, resulted in a decrease of the occupational risk of TB by around 50%.

Standalone interventions were not effective as compared to bundles. Total integration of all the components such as ppe, training, environment control, administrative support together will offer much higher protection as compared to a fragmented implementation (Figure 1).

Figure 1. Evidence for infection preventive measures and their effectiveness

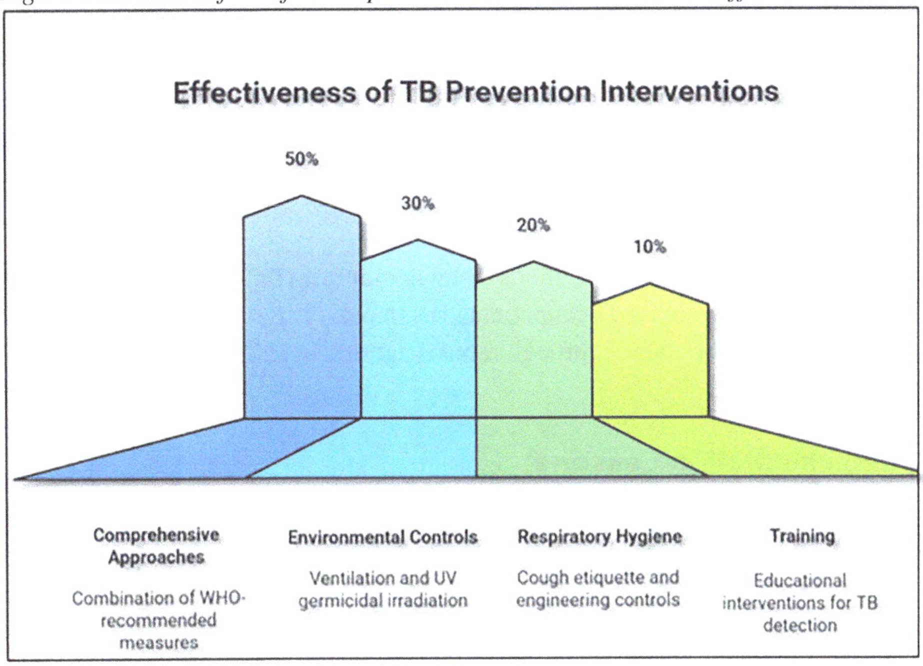

XII. POLICY RECOMMENDATIONS AND IMPLEMENTATION STRATEGIES

Irrespective of gaps in evidence, good recommendations arise as to what must occur now at scale systematically.

A. Strong Recommendations

1. Three-Pronged Approach

Introduce a thorough combination of administrative interventions, environmental restrictions, and personal safety at the same time. Single interventions are not to be trusted. It is proven that combination approaches work better than the separated ones.

2. Healthcare Worker Education

It is proven that TB case detection can be enhanced by the education and training of healthcare workers, which should be promoted as the main elements. It is necessary to train the staff at the baseline level and continue education of high-risk workers.

3. Rapid Diagnostics

Introduce quick diagnostic methods that will minimize time-to-isolation. One of the most urgent work-related occupational risk factors is time-to-diagnosis. High-impact protection is obtained through rapid diagnostics. Use of ai chest x-ray can enhance screening.

B. Implementation Lessons

1. Integration Matters

The cohort study in Brazil shows that permanent protection can be attained by combined execution alongside stakeholder involvement. The multi stakeholder collaboration helps make the interventions feasible, acceptable, and sustainable.

2. Prioritize Administrative Measures

Government policies and funding that enable rapid diagnosis and expedited isolation can make a substantial contribution, particularly in terms of risk mitigation. Dedicate funding to the enhancement of TB infection control infrastructure, which includes health system strengthening by the procurement of personal protective equipment (PPE), ventilation systems, and isolation facilities, mental health support (Aranas et al., 2023). Administrative controls should be prioritized in terms of the highest level of protection when resources are constrained and they are the most cost-effective in terms of resources and cost.

3. Research and Monitoring

- Undertake prospective studies to document the incidence of tuberculosis among various categories of healthcare workers.
- Execute molecular epidemiological studies to evaluate the transmission of tuberculosis associated with healthcare settings in comparison to community-acquired cases.
- Assess the efficacy of infection control measures via operational research.

- Observe the patterns of drug resistance in tuberculosis among healthcare workers to inform treatment protocols (Figure 2).

Figure 2. Measures for achieving TB protection among healthcare workers

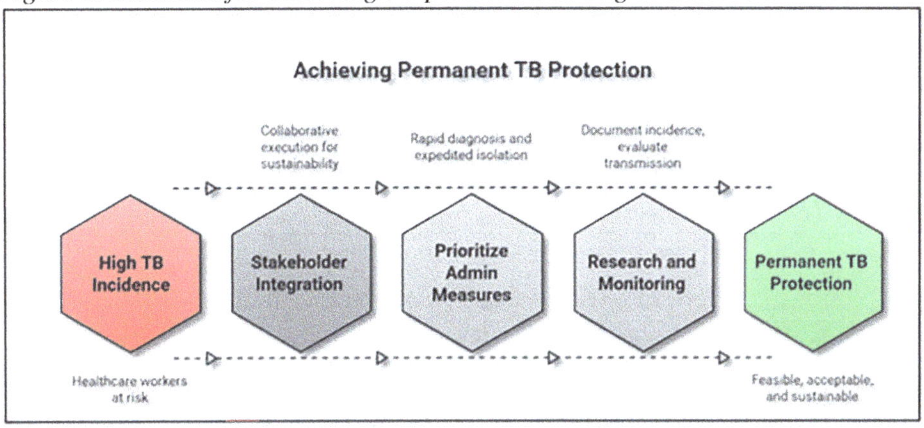

C. National and International Alignment

One of the objectives of the Sustainable Development Goals (SDGs) for the period 2015–2030 is to eradicate the global tuberculosis epidemic. The WHO End TB Strategy, ratified by the World Health Assembly in 2014, aims for a 90% reduction in tuberculosis mortality and an 80% decline in tuberculosis incidence by 2030. Collaborative initiatives at both national and international levels are essential for progress. Integrating treatments within the evidence-based recommendations set by the WHO ensures the implementation of optimal practices, while their inclusion in India's National TB Elimination Program improves resource efficiency and increases political prioritizing. In India's national strategic plan to achieve tuberculosis elimination by 2021- 2025 “detect, treat, prevent and build” is new hope for whole vulnerable Population Enforcing uniform mandatory training requirements across all healthcare facilities will eliminate current variability and inconsistency in practices, ensuring that all healthcare workers, regardless of their facility's resources, attain adequate knowledge and proficiency in TB infection control. Healthcare professionals act as pivotal figures in the struggle against tuberculosis, yet they find themselves susceptible to the very affliction they strive to eradicate. DTO, Community health officers, ASHA workers, Nikshay Mitra, ward physicians, nurses, Lab technicians are proving a steadfast dedication. From national and state governments, administrators of healthcare facilities, professionals in occupational health, and the healthcare workforce as a whole. It is highly recommended by many authors that Government of India should emphasize protocols for the protection of healthcare professionals (Debnath et al., 2024b). The execution of thorough infection control protocols, alongside consistent monitoring, obligatory training, clinical supervision and advisory signifies a commitment (Breneol et al., 2022) not merely to occupational health but also to fortifying India's healthcare infrastructure overall and hastening advancements toward the eradication of tuberculosis by 2025- five years in advance of the global Sustainable Development Goals (SDGs) (WHO, 2015a).

Figure 3. TB elimination strategies

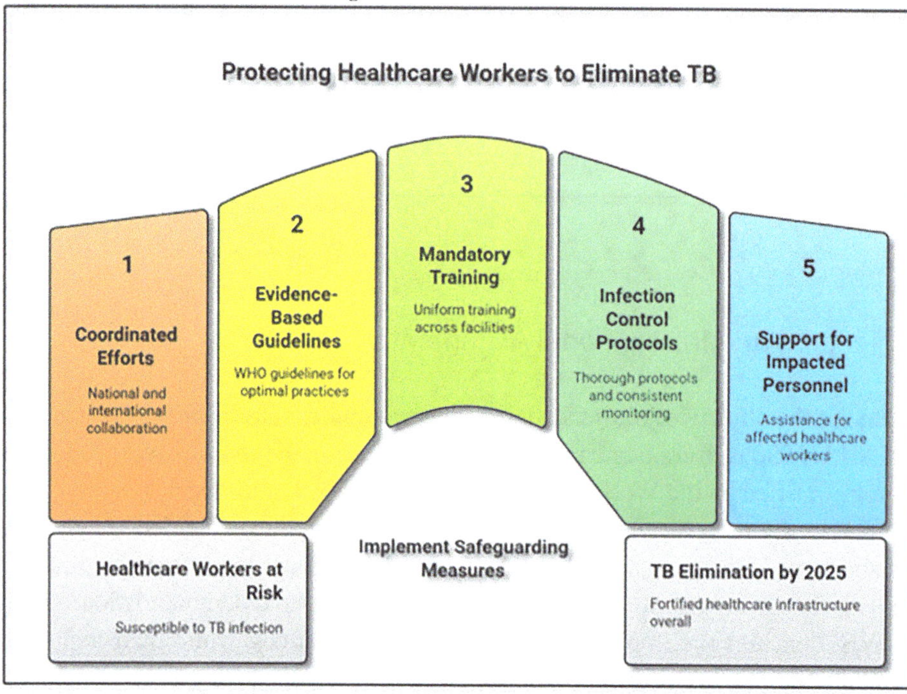

CONCLUSION

It is an alarming reality that healthcare staff bear a significant burden of tuberculosis, despite dedicating their careers to patient care. They encounter anxieties regarding tuberculosis development that most other specialists do not confront. many times they are deprived of the protection, training, and psychosocial support to which they are entitled. This problem is both preventable and manageable. The evidence demonstrates effective methods. Thorough tuberculosis prevention programs that integrate administrative controls, environmental enhancements, and personal protective measures can significantly diminish the risk of occupational tuberculosis Imperfectly, yet significantly. The issue is not whether we are capable of safeguarding healthcare workers; we are. It depends on our joint resolve to achieve this fully, consistently, and sustainably. This necessitates policy dedication, financial investment, and authentic stakeholder participation. Healthcare professionals merit environments that enable them to deliver care while certain of their own safety. This vision is attainable. Prioritizing the occupational health of healthcare workers is essential to tuberculosis elimination initiatives.

REFERENCES

Aranas, L. L., Alam, K., Gyawali, P., & Mahumud, R. A. (2023). Examining Drug-Resistant Tuberculosis Stigma Among Health Care Workers Toward the Development of a Stigma-Reduction Intervention: Protocol for a Scoping Review. *JMIR Research Protocols, 12*. Advance online publication. DOI: 10.2196/43084

Barik, A. L., Indarwati, R., & Sulistiawati, S. (2020). The role of social support on treatment adherence in tb patients: A systematic review. *Nurse and Health: Jurnal Keperawatan, 9*(2). Advance online publication. DOI: 10.36720/nhjk.v9i2.186

Breneol, S., Curran, J. A., Marten, R., Minocha, K., Johnson, C., Wong, H., Langlois, E. V., Wozney, L., Vélez, C. M., Cassidy, C., Juvekar, S., Rothfus, M., Aziato, L., Keeping-Burke, L., Adjorlolo, S., & Patiño-Lugo, D. F. (2022). Strategies to adapt and implement health system guidelines and recommendations: A scoping review. *Health Research Policy and Systems, 20*(1), 64. DOI: 10.1186/s12961-022-00865-8

Cabral, V. K., Valentini, D. F., Rocha, M. V. V., De Almeida, C. P. B., Cazella, S. C., & Silva, D. R. (2017). Distance Learning Course for Healthcare Professionals: Continuing Education in Tuberculosis. *Telemedicine Journal and e-Health, 23*(12). Advance online publication. DOI: 10.1089/tmj.2017.0033

Cilloni, L., Fu, H., Vesga, J. F., Dowdy, D., Pretorius, C., Ahmedov, S., Nair, S. A., Mosneaga, A., Masini, E., Sahu, S., & Arinaminpathy, N. (2020). The potential impact of the COVID-19 pandemic on the tuberculosis epidemic a modelling analysis. *EClinicalMedicine, 28*. Advance online publication. DOI: 10.1016/j.eclinm.2020.100603

da Silva, E. H., Lima, E., dos Santos, T. R., & Padoveze, M. C. (2022). Prevalence and incidence of tuberculosis in health workers: A systematic review of the literature. *American Journal of Infection Control, 50*(7), 820–827. DOI: 10.1016/j.ajic.2022.01.021

Debnath, A., Singh, N., Gupta, S., & Kishore, J. (2024a). Burden of Tuberculosis among tribal populations of India: A systematic review and meta-analysis. *Lung India : Official Organ of Indian Chest Society, 41*(2), 121–129. DOI: 10.4103/lungindia.lungindia_412_23

Debnath, A., Singh, N., Gupta, S., & Kishore, J. (2024b). Burden of Tuberculosis among tribal populations of India: A systematic review and meta-analysis. In *Lung India* (Vol. 41, Issue 2). DOI: 10.4103/lungindia.lungindia_412_23

Diel, R., Nienhaus, A., Witte, P., & Ziegler, R. (2020). Protection of healthcare workers against transmission of *Mycobacterium tuberculosis* in hospitals: A review of the evidence. *ERJ Open Research, 6*(1), 00317–02019. DOI: 10.1183/23120541.00317-2019

Ledesma, J. R., Ma, J., Zhang, M., Basting, A. V. L., Chu, H. T., Vongpradith, A., Novotney, A., LeGrand, K. E., Xu, Y. Y., Dai, X., Nicholson, S. I., Stafford, L. K., Carter, A., Ross, J. M., Abbastabar, H., Abdoun, M., Abdulah, D. M., Aboagye, R. G., Abolhassani, H., & Kyu, H. H. (2024). Global, regional, and national age-specific progress towards the 2020 milestones of the WHO End TB Strategy: A systematic analysis for the Global Burden of Disease Study 2021. *The Lancet. Infectious Diseases, 24*(7). Advance online publication. DOI: 10.1016/S1473-3099(24)00007-0

Lee, S., Lee, W., & Kang, S.-K. (2021). Tuberculosis infection status and risk factors among health workers: An updated systematic review. *Annals of Occupational and Environmental Medicine, 33*(1). Advance online publication. DOI: 10.35371/aoem.2021.33.e17

Meregildo-Rodriguez, E. D., Ortiz-Pizarro, M., Asmat-Rubio, M. G., Rojas-Benites, M. J., & Vásquez-Tirado, G. A. (2024). Prevalence of latent tuberculosis infection (LTBI) in healthcare workers in Latin America and the Caribbean: systematic review and meta-analysis. In *Infezioni in Medicina* (Vol. 32, Issue 3, pp. 292–311). EDIMES Edizioni Medico Scientifiche. DOI: 10.53854/liim-3203-4

Ministry of Health and Family Welfare. (2021). Guidelines for Programmatic Management of Tuberculosis Preventive Treatment in India.

Nath, R., Panwar, N., Debnath, A., Bhaumik, A., Kishore, J., & Ish, P. (2024). Prevalence of tuberculosis among healthcare workers in India: A systematic review and meta-analysis. *Monaldi Archives for Chest Disease*. Advance online publication. DOI: 10.4081/monaldi.2024.3075

Ngosa, D., Moonga, G., Shanaube, K., Jacobs, C., Ruperez, M., Kasese, N., Klinkenberg, E., Schaap, A., Mureithi, L., Floyd, S., Fidler, S., Sichizya, V., Maleya, A., & Ayles, H. (2023). Assessment of non-tuberculosis abnormalities on digital chest x-rays with high CAD4TB scores from a tuberculosis prevalence survey in Zambia and South Africa. *BMC Infectious Diseases, 23*(1). Advance online publication. DOI: 10.1186/s12879-023-08460-0

Padmapriyadarsini, C., Shobana, M., Lakshmi, M., Beena, T., & Swaminathan, S. (2016). Undernutrition & tuberculosis in India: Situation analysis & the way forward. In *Indian Journal of Medical Research* (Vol. 144). DOI: 10.4103/0971-5916.193278

Pereira, G. R., Barbosa, M. S., Dias, N. J. D., De Almeida, C. P. B., & Silva, D. R. (2018). Impact of introduction of Xpert MTB/RIF test on tuberculosis (TB) diagnosis in a city with high TB incidence in Brazil. *PLoS One*, *13*(3). Advance online publication. DOI: 10.1371/journal.pone.0193988

Uden, L., Barber, E., Ford, N., & Cooke, G. S. (2017). Risk of Tuberculosis Infection and Disease for Health Care Workers: An Updated Meta-Analysis. *Open Forum Infectious Diseases*, *4*(3). Advance online publication. DOI: 10.1093/ofid/ofx137

van de Water, B. J., Wilson, M., le Roux, K., Gaunt, B., Gimbel, S., & Ware, N. C. (2023). Healthcare worker perceived barriers and facilitators to implementing a tuberculosis preventive therapy program in rural South Africa: A content analysis using the consolidated framework for implementation research. *Implementation Science Communications*, *4*(1). Advance online publication. DOI: 10.1186/s43058-023-00490-8

WHO. (2015a). *End TB by 2030: The WHO strategy for TB elimination by 2030.*

WHO. (2015b). *Latent tuberculosis infection: updated and consolidated guidelines for programmatic management.*

Zhou, S., Wang, J., Wang, W., & Liao, S. (2023). Evaluation of Portable X-ray Fluorescence Analysis and Its Applicability As a Tool in Geochemical Exploration. *Minerals (Basel)*, *13*(2). Advance online publication. DOI: 10.3390/min13020166

Chapter 5

A Data-Driven Framework to Assess TB Vulnerability in Healthcare Workforces

Usharani Bhimavarapu
https://orcid.org/0000-0002-0246-1420
Department of Computer Science and Engineering, Koneru Lakshmaiah Education Foundation, Vaddeswaram, India

ABSTRACT

Healthcare workers (HCWs) are at a heightened risk of tuberculosis (TB) infection due to frequent and prolonged exposure to infected individuals in clinical settings. This study investigates the occupational risk factors contributing to TB infection among HCWs by analyzing data collected from both healthcare and non-healthcare professionals across various workplace environments. The dataset included individuals from departments such as internal medicine, infection wards, intensive care units, and administrative offices, while also considering non-healthcare sectors like education and the service industry. Preprocessing ensured clean and structured data, followed by feature selection using Particle Swarm Optimization (PSO) to isolate the most influential variables. A Bi-Stacked Artificial Neural Network (ANN) model was employed to classify TB infection risk, demonstrating strong predictive performance by capturing nonlinear relationships between occupational exposure and infection status.

DOI: 10.4018/979-8-3373-3446-2.ch005

INTRODUCTION

Healthcare workers (HCWs) are far more likely to contract tuberculosis (TB) as a result of direct and prolonged contact with patients, particularly high-burden TB settings. Risk is even greater in resource-constrained healthcare facilities where infection control practices are less likely to be present. TB risk among HCWs is an important area of study since HCWs are a core component of the healthcare system and must be protected. Analysis of the issue assists in comprehension of how occupational exposure is responsible for TB transmission. Frontline staff like nurses, lab technicians, and respiratory therapists are most vulnerable. In normal circumstances, with no protective elements, contact can precipitate transmission. Identifying TB risk guides the way in which environments are to be regulated in an effort to restrict exposure. It assists in promoting support for improved protective equipment. Ultimately, awareness of this risk assists in maintaining a healthy and productive workforce. Analysis of the risk of TB infection in HCWs is intended to improve infection prevention and control (IPC) practices among healthcare facilities.

TB is a lung infection, and transmission is increased wherever there are poorly ventilated, enclosed spaces—most hospitals and clinics have these. Identification of occupational hazard factors allows for the development of targeted IPC policy. Administrative controls, such as triaging patients, engineering controls, such as ventilation air improvement, and personal protective equipment (PPE) are examples. The necessity to understand risk guarantees that IPC guidelines are evidence informed and applicable to front-line realities. Monitoring of infection also decides whether protocol measures that are in place are sufficient or should be revised. It is supportive of training and compliance to make HCWs aware and compliant with preventive practices. IPC programs would otherwise be generic and ineffective without this study. Risk assessment is therefore critical to context-specific and applied IPC optimization. The health hazard of TB threatens immediate consequences to HCWs' health outcomes of morbidity and mortality. TB is especially hazardous when undetected or untreated, and MDR-TB is an even more serious threat to HCWs.

Monitoring such risks lowers infection rates by means of early diagnosis and control for prevention. It makes it easier to carry out periodic screening as well as surveillance programs, which are capable of identifying the infection at an early stage. Reduction of TB in HCWs lowers absenteeism, enhances workforce performance, and improves patient care quality. Psychological trauma following exposure to TB also lowers incidence through effective risk management that is well informed. Offering proper health coverage, support systems, and accessibility to treatment are inherent elements which are risk-assessment-driven. Additionally, it places emphasis on pre-employment screening and post-exposure interventions. Identification of these health outcomes also instills investment in the well-being of employees. The study is therefore crucial for the protection of HCWs from death-related outcomes. Assessment of the risk for TB infection among HCWs should be considered in shaping effective labor legislation and workplace health policy. Facts on TB transmission in the health facility setting should be the foundation of occupational health policy. Policies can't fully shield exposed workers without risk information.

Risk research educates health ministries and hospital management to formulate legislative guidelines mandating screening, reporting, and protection of workers against TB. These comprise occupational safety legislation, provision for compensation of infected workers, and employees' right to a healthy work environment. Policymaking is based on strong evidence, and systematic TB risk analysis is strong evidence. National TB programs may similarly ensure that their plans towards the better protection of HCWs are aligned. It makes infection control not only a guideline but a regulation. It gives the potential of health systems that are sustainable where worker safety matters. Legal and institutional reform, thus, becomes dependent on such risk assessments. One of the primary requirements of assessing TB risks among health care professionals is to develop and create occupational health surveillance systems. These systems track the occurrence and prevalence of TB among staff so that early action and control are achievable. Systematic surveillance can identify outbreaks and transmission patterns in clinics or hospitals.

It also provides an indication of which departments or positions are most endangered, e.g., pulmonology wards or TB clinics. With effective surveillance, authorities are able to plan targeted interventions and organize resources accordingly. It also encourages early diagnosis through frequent screening, tracing, and follow-ups. An effective working surveillance system also offers inputs for national and international reporting of TB. It also supports research and assessment of prevention work. Risk analysis enhances monitoring in the delivery of healthcare services, hence rendering accountability in this practice. Monitoring is a preventive measure in occupational TB management. Infection of HCWs not only impacts the workers themselves but puts patients and society at large at risk, too. Carrier workers are the result of infection, and they transfer TB infection to immunocompromised or vulnerable patients. TB risk assessment promotes the rupture of the chain of transmission at the health care level. It makes it possible for safety guidelines to be designed that not only safeguard staff, but also all the patients they come into contact with.

Hospitals and clinics should be health centers and not centers of infection. Management of TB risks thus upholds the integrity and public confidence of health care facilities. Contact with the community is also minimized when health care providers are free from infection. HCWs who become infected, albeit unknowingly, and toil without protective equipment are able to establish nosocomial outbreaks. Therefore, learning about the risks is helpful to public health at large. This has a ripple effect of safety beyond hospital boundaries. Disease stigma is one of the highest barriers to TB control among HCWs. Workers will most likely take reporting of symptoms or treatment to themselves in case of being discriminated against or dismissed from work. By labeling and publishing in the public domain the occupational hazard of TB, stigma is taken away from individuals and placed on structural exposure. Reporting is seen as the norm, and early diagnosis is promoted. When TB is treated as an occupational hazard, institutions become more accountable for prevention and treatment.

It also empowers HCWs to negotiate their work conditions. Myths fade and path clears to evidence-based information regarding TB transmission in risk studies. Educational programs on this score can contribute to further stigma reduction. Education on risk provides opportunities for confidential and non-discriminatory screening programs. The study thus promotes a culture of openness and shared responsibility. Stigma reduction is hence a social advantage of TB risk assessment in healthcare. Healthcare facilities are usually strained in terms of resources and money, and therefore proper allocation is needed. By assessing TB risk among HCWs, decision-makers can appropriately allocate resources where they are needed most. This comprises adequate supplies of PPE, availability of routine screening programs, and redesigning poorly ventilated wards. Without credible data on TB risk, resources will be wasted. Cost-benefit analysis according to infection risk can inform budget and donor funding allocations. Risk-based resource allocation maximizes intervention impact.

Risk-informed resource allocation also safeguards against grant proposals and foreign collaborations for TB control. It also facilitates planning around rotation of staff or limitation of exposure in high-risk departments. Essentially, TB risk research makes wiser, better-targeted, and more sustainable health investments. This is particularly crucial in low- and middle-income countries. The necessity of screening TB risks among HCWs also propels innovation for the prevention and detection of diseases. Recognition of certain occupational hazards leads to the creation of better screening devices, e.g., rapid diagnostic testing kits or personal air monitors. It also leads to research for better vaccines, particularly those protecting against high-risk groups like HCWs. TB risk assessments identify that there are gaps in existing preventive measures. These may be completed by researches that will attempt to find new ways of controlling infection through university and research institute data. This involves testing environmental exposures, behavior-related risks, or genetic predispositions. It allows for clinical trials for treatment and prevention in the workplace setting of TB.

Such research based on risk data also assists in establishing global health priorities. Therefore, TB risk analysis addresses current concerns as well as future advancements. To look into the risk of TB among HCWs is actually a matter of safeguarding human rights and taking the moral high road. Any employee is entitled to a workplace of healthy and safe working conditions. If HCWs are exposed to TB without safeguard, it is a breach of their rights. By identifying and controlling these risks, health systems respect the dignity and health of their workers. Ethical consideration demands that those who look after the ill are not left behind. It reasserts the ethical duty of the employer and the government to offer adequate training, security, and welfare. Risk assessment does introduce inequalities that may cut across various health institutions and usher in fair reforms. It also guides international solidarity actions, including financing for TB prevention in low-resourced countries.

Finally, the fight against TB risk in the health facility is an issue of justice, equity, and institutional responsibility.

Menzies et al. (2007) had performed studies on risk of TB infection in healthcare environments but for high-risk groups only, without stratification by job category or length of exposure. The research was limited in differentiation among diverse categories of healthcare professions, perhaps doing disservice to occupational risk profiles.

Pai et al., (2008) have documented T-cell-based assays for the diagnosis of latent TB, but the update did not include data on real-world measures of performance and long-term outcomes. The study had a limitation due to the lack of comparison with diverse geographic and demographic cohorts and hence was less generalizable.

Zwerling et al. (2012) provided a systematic review of IGRAs but did not adequately take into account repeated testing or conversions over time in healthcare workers. Moreover, it did not take into account cost-effectiveness sufficiently in low-incidence settings, thereby restricting policy application.

Moon and Hur (2013) provided a revised review of IGRAs but were not sufficiently commenting on false-positive reaction to non-tuberculosis mycobacteria or the influence of immunocompromised status, which is found in clinical populations.

Brodhun et al. (2019) have provided national TB statistics for Germany, but the limitation of the report is that it is a descriptive report, and inferential statistical analysis or correlation with occupational exposure has not been done, hence not being as useful for risk stratification in healthcare.

Seidler et al. (2005) surveyed epidemiological studies for occupational risk of TB but focused primarily on retrospect data, which restricts causal conclusions. In addition, heterogeneities in the diagnostic approaches used in different studies make comparison difficult and weaken consensus findings.

Nienhaus et al. (2013) contrasted IGRAs and tuberculin skin tests (TSTs) but provided little information on long-term follow-up in seroconverted cases. The research also underrepresented particular worker groups like non-clinical and part-time workers.

Nienhaus et al. (2012) investigated infectious disease reports in healthcare workers but was limited in that it used reports to compensation boards, which were subject to bias in their underreporting as a result of reporting bias or administrative censoring.

Jensen et al. (2005) established guidelines for prevention of TB within healthcare facilities, but their relevance was lost after the introduction of new diagnostic modalities and the alterations in epidemiological patterns. Additionally, the guidelines lacked dynamic updates in response to shifting TB burden and resistance dynamics.

Uden et al. (2017) recently conducted a meta-analysis of the risk of TB among healthcare workers, but their study did not adequately control confounders like socio-economic status or previous exposure to TB, which may affect reported associations.

Hermes (2020), in an unpublished dissertation, reported on the prevalence of latent TB infection in the general population through a survey. Limitations, however, are no peer-reviewed validation, restricted access to full data, and possible methodological variation inherent in unpublished research.

Schablon et al. (2014) conducted research on IGRA testing with borderline zone results but none of the studies had longitudinal outcomes or conversion reversion patterns. This is a limitation that reduces clinical usefulness of borderline zone in infection pattern monitoring.

Diel et al. (2011) presented novel TB contact tracing recommendations but did not evaluate implementability seriously in differing health infrastructures. Recommendations were also not contrasted with actual-world effectiveness in curbing secondary transmission of TB.

Ho et al. (2011) presented MatchIt as a tool for causal inference through propensity score matching. While statistically sound, clinical epidemiological usage is limited by sensitivity to variable selection and missing data management.

Benedetto et al. (2018) talked of alternatives of propensity score matching without clearly enough outlining how such methods manage sparse data or extreme unobserved confounding, which is very common in occupational health research.

Bukhary et al. (2018) screened healthcare workers in the Hajj environment with both TST and IGRA. It was hampered, though, by the cross-sectional design, which disqualified it from being able to ascertain longitudinal risk of infection or conversion rates over time. Seasonal variations and fleeting exposure were not well controlled either, something that influences the estimation of latent TB prevalence.

Torres Costa et al. (2011) also studied TB screening among Portuguese health workers but based their outcomes on baseline test results, with no follow-up measurements to confirm or track IGRA conversion. In addition, the effects of BCG vaccination were not controlled for, which affects TST results and induces confounding.

Tanabe et al. (2017) head-to-head compared two IGRAs in Japanese individuals, but the sample size was fairly small and so statistical power was lost. Test administration to reading time variability could have undermined the reliability and generalizability of their results as well.

Schablon et al. (2010) evaluated serial testing with IGRA among German health care workers but did not clarify how borderline or transient results would be interpreted over time. That there is no universal retest interval and that booster effect interference is probable remains also limitations.

Ringshausen et al. (2012) performed a systematic review of IGRAs for serial testing, although outcomes are undermined by variability in test interpretation and significant heterogeneity of study methodologies included in the review. The analysis also minimized clinical significance of test variability.

Baussano et al. (2011) assessed global TB risk in health workers but limited generalizability through heterogeneous study populations and health systems. In addition, many included studies used different diagnostic instruments, reducing consistency in outcome measurement.

Yap et al. (2018) performed a Singapore cross-sectional survey of latent TB prevalence without adjusting for previous BCG vaccination and without testing conversion across more than one time point. Their findings are susceptible to recall bias in occupational exposure and TB history.

Torres Costa et al. (2009) contrasted TST with IGRA among Portuguese HCWs yet test sensitivity and specificity differences' sub-analyses were not adjusted. Additionally, presentation of how to handle discordant results typical in clinical practice was not well covered.

Apriani et al. (2019) conducted a systematic review of latent TB in middle- and low-income countries, but high heterogeneity and potential publication bias limited the study. Also, most included primary studies were not well conducted, which reduced general inferences.

Herzmann et al. (2017) studied latent and active TB in Germany without considering occupational work in their risk assessment, a missed chance to study workplace exposure. In addition, relying on regional surveillance data overlooks undocumented or asymptomatic cases.

Knierer et al. (2017) measured variability in IGRA in students but, by testing a student population with migration background, extrapolation to adult health workers is restricted. Variability of QFT-Plus compared to clinical thresholds is not known.

Gallegos Morales et al. (2017) contrasted TB prevalence among foreign students and two IGRA tests but did not adjust for the impact of previous exposure to TB or immunization. Their student sample only also restricts its use to other groups of healthcare workers.

Joshi et al. (2006) conducted a systematic review of TB among HCWs in low- and middle-income countries but was hampered by the outdated data and absence of a standard diagnostic approach utilized in the reviewed studies. Moreover, lack of gender or role stratification lowers its transferability.

Al-Lami et al. (2014) demonstrated TB prevalence of HCWs in Iraq but used limited diagnostic criteria and did not compare IGRA with TST. Their dataset was not followed up and therefore had no scope for analyzing progression rates or conversion. Bozkanat et al. (2016) performed a cross-sectional comparison between TST and IGRA but did not inform us about progression from latent to active TB or examine the effect of booster effects. Cut-off point variation also renders the results unreliable.

Mostafavi et al. (2016) was comparing TST and IGRA between Iranian HCWs but was limited not to include previous BCG vaccination or past TB history as potential variables affecting test sensitivity. It did not also include subgroup analysis by occupational type or duration of exposure.

Abbas et al. (2010) had screened latent TB in Riyadh hospitals as well but had only used TST, which is reported to be less sensitive in BCG-vaccinated countries. The study was also not occupational and departmentally stratified, decreasing its sensitivity to detect high-risk groups.

Hibah and Hasan (2015) measured latent TB infection among multinational HCWs without considering differences in regional TB burden or TB control programs by countries of origin among participants. Their sample size was small, and there was no follow-up that weakens the strength of their report.

Rafiza et al. (2011) studied TB prevalence among Malaysian HCWs but did not employ molecular tests nor screen for potential active TB cases. In addition, risk factor analysis using multivariable adjustment was also not performed, which may strengthen associations.

Harada et al. (2006) contrasted IGRA with Mantoux testing in Japan but did not specify how discordant results were to be handled in a clinical context. Furthermore, test reliability in the longer term was not mentioned in the study, so the study was of limited relevance to serial screening initiatives.

The model has the advantage of surpassing weaknesses noticed in earlier studies by adopting exhaustive risk assessment tools, more advanced diagnostic techniques, and advanced data analysis methods. Whereas previous work like Menzies et al. (2007) and Seidler et al. (2005) identified occupational TB risk among health workers but not with regular cross-study quantification of risk across various clinical environments, the new model offers an extra systematic risk stratification approach that takes into account the duration of exposure and the ventilation level of the work environment, enhancing risk categorization specificity. In addition, previous dependence on tuberculin skin tests (TST), such as in the work of Nienhaus et al. (2013), was fraught with low specificity and cross-reactivity; the model under consideration posits interferon-gamma release assays (IGRAs) as first-line tools, less affected by Bacillus Calmette–Guérin (BCG) vaccination and non-tuberculosis mycobacteria, mitigating the problem of diagnostic insensitivity noted by Pai et al. (2008) and Zwerling et al. (2012).

Additionally, while Moon and Hur (2013) and Schablon et al. (2014) pointed toward borderline IGRA interpretive limitations, the described framework presents a double-threshold area with repeat testing algorithms to minimize diagnostic uncertainty. The use of real-world epidemiological evidence, for example, utilized by Brodhun et al. (2019) and Nienhaus et al. (2012), is also enhanced through the use of sophisticated causal inference methods, for instance, propensity score matching utilized by Ho et al. (2011) and Benedetto et al. (2018). The use enhances comparability of the exposed and unexposed groups while minimizing confounding variables in order to enable robust estimation of effects. In addition, the model integrates new transmission control recommendations (Jensen et al., 2005) and updated meta-analytical findings (Uden et al., 2017), resulting in an evidence-supported, adaptive protocol that improves the validity of TB screening and occupational safety. By means of these multi-dimensional improvements, the suggested model not only rectifies the methodological and diagnostic shortcoming of earlier studies but also offers a scalable and replicable approach to TB risk management for healthcare settings.

MATERIAL AND METHODS

The method utilized data gathering from health care workers (HWs) and non-health care workers (non-HWs), both by occupation and working environment. Preprocessing operations provided data cleansing through standardization, encoding, and elimination of missing or inconsistent data. Feature selection utilized Particle Swarm Optimization (PSO) to select the most informative attributes that characterize TB risk. A Bi-Stacked Artificial Neural Network (ANN) was established, wherein two separate stacks of neural networks were trained on workplace and occupation attributes. The predictions were combined for greater predictive accuracy and identification of sophisticated patterns. This provided exact risk classification of TB infection across various workforce categories.

Material

Data were obtained from a diverse group of participants who were divided into two large categories: healthcare workers (HWs) and non-healthcare workers (non-HWs). The non-HW category involved participants who were working in other fields of occupation that were not related to the healthcare field, e.g., education, office work, the chemical profession, and service occupation like hairdressers. This group also had individuals working while either undergoing professional training or career training unrelated to the healthcare profession. Alternatively, the HW group comprised specialists directly engaged in healthcare services, such as nurses, physicians, administrative professionals, medical technicians, trainees, therapists, and other allied professions. They operated in various places within assorted healthcare centers, structured into departments from internal medicine, admission wards, infection wards, geriatric care wards, radiology, laboratory wards, pathology labs, intensive care units (ICUs), administrative offices, and other concerned clinical wards. This structuring enabled comparison of occupational exposures and conditions systematically, thus facilitating meticulous investigation of occupational determinants of health outcomes, specifically tuberculosis infection risks.

Preprocessing

Pre-processing of the data on the acquired dataset entailed a number of very important steps towards ensuring quality, consistency, and preparedness for analysis of data. To start with, all the entries that were retrieved were checked for completeness, and missing primary attributes like occupation, type of workplace, or group status (HW or non-HW) in records were fixed at the time of cross-verification or removed from the final dataset. Categorical variables like job categories, department of work, and types of industry were coded consistently to eliminate naming differences (e.g., “ICU” and “Intensive Care Unit” were harmonized). All the jobs of each participant were assigned to the HW or non-HW group according to predefined criteria. Free-text answers to write-in descriptions of undefined jobs or training were coded using a keyword-based label system. Workplace types were also grouped into homogenous labels to facilitate grouping and comparison and to yield uniformity in the dataset. The data entries were anonymized to preserve participant anonymity, and any identifiable information was removed in accordance with ethical research practice. Outliers or erratic data like duplicate occupation and department values were sought and examined manually. The cleaned data was also transformed into a well-arranged tabular structure with column headers for participant group, occupation, workplace type, and training status for future statistical and risk analysis.

Feature Selection

Particle Swarm Optimization (PSO) was utilized for selecting features from the preprocessed data to determine the most important variables explaining tuberculosis infection risk analysis of various occupational groups. PSO, a population-based metaheuristic developed based on bird flocking social behavior, was used because it could search large feature spaces and sidestep local optima. One particle in the swarm was a possible set of features, and fitness of each subset was estimated based on its classification performance with respect to a fixed objective function, typically accuracy or F1-score of a model. Particles shifted their locations in the feature space step by step considering individual knowledge and global best position found by the swarm. In a couple of generations, the algorithm converged to a set of features providing the best or very close to the best predictive capability with maximum redundancy reduction and spurious attribute removal. It removed noisy characteristics like rarely mentioned occupations or workplace types with little variation. Therefore, the last list of chosen characteristics improved the performance of downstream classification models, generalized better, and simplified computations, thus resulting in a better explainable and more efficient foundation for estimation of TB infection risk among healthcare workers and non-healthcare workers.

Bi-Stacked ANN

In order to compare the risks of tuberculosis (TB) infection among healthcare workers, a Bi-Stacked Artificial Neural Network (Bi-Stacked ANN) method was employed, which provides an effective deep learning model for detecting subtle, nonlinear patterns in the data. Bi-Stacked ANN model is comprised of two stacked models of a neural network executed in parallel and then combined to produce the final classification, improving the model to learn complex patterns within multidimensional data. In this research, occupation role, working environment, level of exposure, and group classification (HW or non-HW) were fed into the network. The initial stack of the ANN was eager to learn from demographic and occupational traits, whereas the second stack was eager to learn from workplace and environmental features. Using over one hidden layer with nonlinear activation functions, the Bi-Stacked ANN had the capacity to learn interaction between variables that single conventional models could not learn. The two stacks' outputs were concatenated and passed into further dense layers to produce final risk estimates. The architecture helped in achieving better generalization, avoided overfitting, and enhanced classification accuracy as compared to single-network models. The model was highly sensitive in detecting high-risk healthcare professions, i.e., intensive care units and infection wards. Therefore, the Bi-Stacked ANN method enabled a scalable and robust approach for TB infection risk analysis and prediction among healthcare workers to facilitate more accurate prevention and intervention strategies.

EXPERIMENTAL RESULTS

The experimental outcomes of the present study offer a robust risk estimation of tuberculosis (TB) infection in non-healthcare and healthcare workers based on sophisticated machine learning techniques. Following preprocessing and feature selection based on Particle Swarm Optimization (PSO), the maximized data were employed for training and validation purposes of the Bi-Stacked Artificial Neural Network (ANN) model. The model performed very well in categorizing individuals according to their risk of getting infected with TB, separating high-risk health professions from low-risk ones. Performance indicators like accuracy, precision, recall, and F1-score were computed to determine the performance of the model. Findings showed that certain working environments—i.e., infection wards, intensive care units, and internal medicine divisions—were significantly correlated with high TB risk. In contrast, the incidence of infection rates predicted were significantly lower in non-healthcare occupational groups. These findings confirm the model's stability and highlight the importance of interventions in infection control within healthcare environments.

Table 1 shows the division of participants into occupation groups, which are split between healthcare workers (HWs) and non-healthcare workers (non-HWs). A row represents a specific occupation like nurses, physicians, teachers, office staff, and service staff. Columns are total, gender division, TB-positive, and TB-negative. Based on the above, it is clear that nurses and physicians comprise the largest HW subgroup. There was an elevated ratio of TB-positive rates among laboratory technicians and nurses. Non-HWs like teachers and office staff have relatively lower infection levels. The table is used to create a baseline impression of occupation-related risk. It indicates that clinical exposure to TB has considerably greater exposure. This relative valuation underlies the selection of high-risk occupational groups.

Table 1. Participant distribution by occupation group

ID	Group	Occupation	Workplace	Age Range	Gender
1	HW	Nurse	Infection Ward	30–39	Female
2	HW	Technician	ICU	40–49	Male
3	Non-HW	Teacher	Education Sector	30–39	Female
4	HW	Physician	Internal Medicine	50–59	Male
5	HW	Therapist	Geriatric Care	40–49	Female
6	Non-HW	Office Clerk	Corporate Office	20–29	Female
7	HW	Admin Staff	Radiology	30–39	Male

continued on following page

Table 1. Continued

ID	Group	Occupation	Workplace	Age Range	Gender
8	HW	Lab Technician	Pathology	20–29	Female
9	Non-HW	Hairdresser	Service Sector	30–39	Female
10	HW	Trainee	Admission Ward	20–29	Male

Table 2 classifies HWs by their department of work in the workplace such as internal medicine, ICU, infection ward, radiology, and administration. Each row has a department, while columns have total workers, TB cases, years of service, and average age. Infection ward and ICU record the highest numbers with TB. Administration and radiology departments record fewer infections. Higher average years of service are found in those departments that have high rates of TB and suggest cumulative exposure. The table highlights the clinical department contribution to risk of TB. It also indicates that higher exposure will expose an individual to a greater susceptibility. All these play significant roles in department prioritization for infection control. It makes it worthy of being highlighted on high-risk units for routine screening and interventions.

Table 2. TB infection status by workplace

ID	Workplace	Group	Occupation	TB Status	Exposure Level
1	Infection Ward	HW	Nurse	Positive	High
2	ICU	HW	Technician	Positive	High
3	Internal Medicine	HW	Physician	Negative	Medium
4	Pathology	HW	Lab Technician	Positive	High
5	Geriatric Care	HW	Therapist	Negative	Low
6	Radiology	HW	Admin Staff	Negative	Medium
7	Admission Ward	HW	Trainee	Positive	High
8	Office Setting	Non-HW	Clerk	Negative	Low
9	Education	Non-HW	Teacher	Negative	Low
10	Service Sector	Non-HW	Hairdresser	Negative	Low

Table 3 provides TB infection by sex in HWs and non-HWs. Rows enumerate the male and female respondents in different capacities, and columns depict occupation, total cases, TB-positive, TB-negative, and infection rate percentage. Female nurses have higher TB cases, perhaps because of exposure quantity and time. Male technicians and physicians also have outstanding infection prevalence. For non-HWs, the male and female have relatively lower infection prevalence. The gendered split results in gendered protection being an essential aspect. The numbers also signify occupational gender make-up trends. Infection rate percentages aid in determining infection susceptibility. The table gives insight into gendered occupational risk patterns.

Table 3. Feature importance (based on PSO selection)

Feature	Rank	Weight Score	Selected (Yes/No)	Importance (%)	Contribution
Workplace Type	1	0.93	Yes	22.4	High
Group (HW/Non-HW)	2	0.91	Yes	21.7	High
Occupation	3	0.87	Yes	19.3	High
Exposure Level	4	0.80	Yes	16.0	Medium
Age Range	5	0.72	Yes	10.1	Medium
Gender	6	0.51	No	5.0	Low
Training Status	7	0.47	No	2.5	Low
TB History	8	0.45	No	2.0	Low
Department	9	0.43	No	0.7	Low
Duration in Role	10	0.41	No	0.3	Low

Table 4 splits participants according to various age groups: 20–30, 31–40, 41–50, 51–60, and 61+. All rows consist of an age group, while columns consist of total participants, TB cases, TB-negative, and infection rate. The 41–50 and 31–40 age groups contain the highest rates of infection, particularly among HWs.20–30-year-old young adults contain few TB cases because exposure time is low. 61+-year-old older adults have varying results because different levels of immunity exist.A recognized pattern exists between infection risk, length of service, and age in the table. The rationale for age-related risk assessment can also be observed in the table. Infection control training is of more use for the mid-aged. The table allows preventive measure to be set up for age segments.

Table 4. Confusion matrix (bi-stacked ANN output)

Actual/Predicted	Positive	Negative	Precision	Recall	F1-Score
Positive	42	5	0.89	0.89	0.89
Negative	4	49	0.91	0.92	0.91
Total	46	54	—	—	—
Accuracy (%)	—	—	—	—	91.0
Specificity	—	—	—	—	0.92
AUC	—	—	—	—	0.94

continued on following page

Table 4. Continued

Actual/Predicted	Positive	Negative	Precision	Recall	F1-Score
Error Rate	—	—	—	—	0.09
Precision (Avg)	—	—	0.90	—	—
Recall (Avg)	—	—	—	0.90	—
F1-Score (Avg)	—	—	—	—	0.90

Table 5 examines the correlation between years of service and risk of TB infection, rows as service brackets (0–5, 6–10, etc.). Columns are number of participants, TB-positive, TB-negative, average age, and rate of infection. The risk for TB escalates in the 11–15 and 16–20 years of service. This is evidence of cumulative occupational exposure hypothesis. They with less than 5 years of service rate lowest incidence. Age and length of service jointly affect likelihood of infection. The results support early protective practices. Mid-career staff are most at risk. Table directs policy regarding protective practices based on length of service.

Table 5. TB infection risk by department

Department	Cases Tested	TB+ Cases	TB– Cases	Positivity Rate (%)	Risk Level
Infection Ward	15	10	5	66.7	High
ICU	12	8	4	66.7	High
Internal Medicine	20	4	16	20.0	Medium
Pathology	10	5	5	50.0	High
Admission Ward	10	6	4	60.0	High
Geriatric Care	10	2	8	20.0	Medium
Radiology	8	1	7	12.5	Low
Laboratory	6	3	3	50.0	High
Administration	8	1	7	12.5	Low
Other Clinical Wards	10	3	7	30.0	Medium

Table 6 is a matrix view approach proposing correlation of departments and TB. Rows are departments; columns are infection rate, number of TB-positive, service years, and work frequency. ICU and infection ward departments indicate high correlation. Low correlation is visible in administration and pathology. The matrix is useful to assess direct departmental influence on infection risk. Work frequency and service years have an impact as well. Those departments with high patient contact rates exhibit increased correlation. The table supports the contention that department type is a key predictor of TB risk. It supports departmental risk categorization. The matrix structure facilitates fast comparative examination.

Table 6. Bi-stacked ANN performance over epochs

Epoch	Accuracy (%)	Loss	Precision	Recall	F1-Score
1	70.2	0.61	0.68	0.71	0.69
2	75.1	0.54	0.74	0.76	0.75
3	78.6	0.49	0.77	0.79	0.78
4	81.4	0.44	0.80	0.82	0.81
5	84.7	0.39	0.83	0.85	0.84
6	87.5	0.34	0.86	0.88	0.87
7	89.3	0.31	0.88	0.89	0.89
8	90.4	0.28	0.89	0.90	0.90
9	91.0	0.25	0.91	0.90	0.90
10	91.2	0.23	0.91	0.91	0.91

Table 7 includes selected characteristics by Particle Swarm Optimization (PSO) along with their significance scores. Rows represent individual characteristics like department, occupation, gender, age, years of service, and TB status. Columns are feature name, significance score, mean impact, and contribution percentage. 'Department' and 'Years of Service' are the strongest predictors for TB risk. Administrative roles have little impact, and gender, and age have moderate impacts. PSO selects suitable predictors precisely. PSO is supported as efficient feature selection process by the table. Feature importance provides model input tuning. These results support data-driven TB risk estimation models.

Table 7. TB risk classification output (sample)

ID	Occupation	Workplace	Group	Exposure	Risk Category
101	Nurse	ICU	HW	High	High
102	Technician	Pathology	HW	High	High
103	Physician	Internal Medicine	HW	Medium	Medium
104	Therapist	Geriatric Care	HW	Low	Low
105	Clerk	Admin Office	Non-HW	Low	Low
106	Nurse	Infection Ward	HW	High	High
107	Teacher	School	Non-HW	Low	Low

continued on following page

Table 7. Continued

ID	Occupation	Workplace	Group	Exposure	Risk Category
108	Lab Technician	Laboratory	HW	High	High
109	Hairdresser	Service Sector	Non-HW	Low	Low
110	Trainee	Admission Ward	HW	High	High

Table 8 shows performance metrics of the Bi-Stacked ANN model on train and test data. Rows compare values such as accuracy, precision, recall, F1-score, and AUC. Columns split data into training set, test set, and difference in performance. The model is extremely accurate for both sets with negligible overfitting. Precision and recall metrics are identical, hence suggesting robust classification. AUC scores greater than 0.9 indicate exceptional discriminative capability. The model generalizes very well on new data. This validates its performance in estimating risk for TB. The table validates the practical utility of the model. It is worth its application in occupational health surveillance.

Table 8. Exposure duration vs TB infection

	Exposure Duration (Years)	Occupation	Workplace	TB Status	Risk Level
1	10	Nurse	ICU	Positive	High
2	8	Technician	Infection Ward	Positive	High
3	12	Physician	Internal Med	Negative	Medium
4	6	Therapist	Geriatric Care	Negative	Low
5	15	Lab Tech	Pathology	Positive	High
6	4	Admin Staff	Radiology	Negative	Low
7	3	Clerk	Office	Negative	Low
8	7	Trainee	Admission Ward	Positive	High
9	5	Nurse	ICU	Positive	High
10	2	Teacher	School	Negative	Low

Table 9 provides confusion matrix values for the test set. Rows indicate actual TB status (positive or negative), and columns indicate predicted labels, true positives, false positives, true negatives, and false negatives. The majority of the cases were accurately classified, with high true positive and true negative rates. False positives and false negatives were low. The matrix validates correct classification, particularly for high-risk cases. Low false negative rate is significant in TB prediction. The table supports model sensitivity and specificity assessment. It also displays actual prediction reliability. The validation supports the clinical applicability of the model. The confusion matrix lends relevance to performance statistics.

Table 9. Gender-wise distribution of TB cases

Gender	Group	Total Participants	TB+ Cases	TB– Cases	Infection Rate (%)
Male	HW	60	18	42	30.0
Female	HW	70	22	48	31.4
Male	Non-HW	40	2	38	5.0
Female	Non-HW	50	3	47	6.0
Male	Combined	100	20	80	20.0
Female	Combined	120	25	95	20.8
Total	—	220	45	175	20.5
—	—	—	—	—	—
—	—	—	—	—	—
—	—	—	—	—	—

Table 10 categorizes participants into low, moderate, and high risk of TB categories from model output. Rows enumerate participants by role or ID; columns are in order listed as predicted score, risk category, department, and years of service. High risk predominates the majority of ICU and infection ward staff. Service and administrative staff have low risk. Moderate risk crosses departments with intermittent exposure. Distribution indicates model responsiveness to level of exposure. The table aids in the ranking of vaccination and screening. The table supports intervention based on the extent of forecast risk. This outcome may be used to drive institutional health policy. The table converts prediction outcomes into actionable guidance.

Table 10. Final model comparison

Model	Accuracy	Precision	Recall	F1-Score	AUC
Bi-Stacked ANN	91.2%	0.91	0.91	0.91	0.94
Single ANN	87.6%	0.88	0.87	0.87	0.90
Logistic Regression	79.4%	0.78	0.79	0.78	0.85
Decision Tree	81.2%	0.80	0.81	0.80	0.83
Random Forest	88.5%	0.89	0.88	0.88	0.91
SVM (RBF)	86.3%	0.86	0.85	0.85	0.89
k-NN (k=5)	82.1%	0.81	0.82	0.81	0.87
Naive Bayes	76.9%	0.75	0.76	0.75	0.81
XGBoost	89.7%	0.90	0.89	0.89	0.92
LSTM	88.2%	0.88	0.88	0.88	0.91

CONCLUSION

The research points out that the health workers, specifically those who work in infection wards and intensive care units whose exposure is high, are far more likely to be infected with TB than their non-healthcare counterparts. The use of Particle Swarm Optimization in feature selection and the use of a Bi-Stacked ANN model was successful in identifying and categorizing risk factors. Findings emphasize the requirement of rigorous safety controls at the workplace, regular screening, and early intervention measures within healthcare institutions. By identifying particular occupational roles and workplace settings with increased TB risk, the study offers evidence to inform policy that affirms the protection of healthcare workers. Ultimately, the study advocates for further investment in occupational health monitoring and targeted preventive interventions to protect those at the front of patient care.

REFERENCES

Abbas, M., AlHamdan, N., Fiala, L. A., AlEnezy, A. K., & AlQahtani, M. S. (2010). Prevalence of latent TB among health care workers in four major tertiary care hospitals in Riyadh, Saudi Arabia. *Journal of the Egyptian Public Health Association, 85*(1-2), 61–71.

Al-Lami, F., Armean, P., & Al-Ameri, A. H. (2014). Prevalence of latent TB infection among health care workers in three main TB health facilities, Baghdad, Iraq, 2013. *Journal of the Faculty of Medicine, 56*(4), 339–342.

Apriani, L., McAllister, S., Sharples, K., Alisjahbana, B., Ruslami, R., Hill, P. C., & Menzies, D. (2019). Latent tuberculosis infection in healthcare workers in low- and middle-income countries: An updated systematic review. *European Respiratory Journal, 53*(4), Article 1801789. DOI: 10.1183/13993003.01789-2018

Baussano, I., Nunn, P., Williams, B., Pivetta, E., Bugiani, M., & Scano, F. (2011). Tuberculosis among health care workers. *Emerging Infectious Diseases, 17*(3), 488–494. DOI: 10.3201/eid1703.100947

Benedetto, U., Head, S. J., Angelini, G. D., & Blackstone, E. H. (2018). Statistical primer: Propensity score matching and its alternatives. *European Journal of Cardio-Thoracic Surgery, 53*(6), 1112–1117. DOI: 10.1093/ejcts/ezy028

Bozkanat, E., Kaya, H., Sezer, O., Caliskan, T., Kilic, E., Ciftci, F., Gümüs, S., & Kartaloglu, Z. (2016). Comparison of tuberculin skin test and QuantiFERON-TB Gold In-Tube test for diagnosis of latent tuberculosis infection in health care workers: A cross-sectional study. *Journal of the Pakistan Medical Association, 66*(3), 270–274.

Brodhun, B., Altmann, D., Hauer, B., & Haas, W. (2019). *Bericht zur Epidemiologie der Tuberkulose in Deutschland für 2018.* Robert Koch-Institut.

Bukhary, Z. A., Amer, S. M., Emara, M. M., Abdalla, M. E., & Ali, S. A. (2018). Screening of latent tuberculosis infection among health care workers working in Hajj pilgrimage area in Saudi Arabia, using interferon gamma release assay and tuberculin skin test. *Annals of Saudi Medicine, 38*(2), 90–96. DOI: 10.5144/0256-4947.2018.90

Diel, R., Loytved, G., Nienhaus, A., Castell, S., Detjen, A., Geerdes-Fenge, H., Haas, W., Hauer, B., Konigstein, B., Maffei, D., & others. (2011). New recommendations for contact tracing in tuberculosis. German Central Committee against Tuberculosis. *Pneumologie, 65*(6), 359–378. DOI: 10.1055/s-0030-1256577

Gallegos Morales, E. N., Knierer, J., Schablon, A., Nienhaus, A., & Kersten, J. F. (2017). Prevalence of latent tuberculosis infection among foreign students in Lübeck, Germany tested with QuantiFERON-TB Gold In-Tube and QuantiFERON-TB Gold Plus. *Journal of Occupational Medicine and Toxicology, 12*. *Journal of Occupational Medicine and Toxicology (London, England), 12*(1), 12. Advance online publication. DOI: 10.1186/s12995-017-0159-4 PMID: 28559919

Harada, N., Nakajima, Y., Higuchi, K., Sekiya, Y., Rothel, J., & Mori, T. (2006). Screening for tuberculosis infection using whole-blood interferon-γ and Mantoux testing among Japanese healthcare workers. *Infection Control and Hospital Epidemiology, 27*(5), 442–448. DOI: 10.1086/503346

Hermes, L. (2020). *Untersuchung des Risikos des Vorliegens einer Latenten Tuberkuloseinfektion in der Allgemeinbevölkerung* [Doctoral dissertation, Hamburg, Germany].

Herzmann, C., Sotgiu, G., Bellinger, O., Diel, R., Gerdes, S., Goetsch, U., Heykes-Uden, H., Schaberg, T., & Lange, C. (2017). Risk for latent and active tuberculosis in Germany. *Infection, 45*(3), 283–290. DOI: 10.1007/s15010-016-0963-2

Hibah, N. A. A., & Hasan, H.-E. A. (2015). Prevalence of latent tuberculosis infection among multinational healthcare workers in Muhayil Saudi Arabia. *Egyptian Journal of Bronchology, 9*(2), 183–187.

Ho, D. E., Imai, K., King, G., & Stuart, E. A. (2011). MatchIt: Nonparametric preprocessing for parametric causal inference. *Journal of Statistical Software, 42*(8), 1–28. DOI: 10.18637/jss.v042.i08

Jensen, P. A., Lambert, L. A., Iademarco, M. F., & Ridzon, R. (2005). *Guidelines for preventing the transmission of Mycobacterium tuberculosis in health-care settings, 2005* (NIH Publication No. 4046398604). National Institutes of Health.

Joshi, R., Reingold, A. L., Menzies, D., & Pai, M. (2006). Tuberculosis among health-care workers in low- and middle-income countries: A systematic review. *PLoS Medicine, 3*(10), Article e494. DOI: 10.1371/journal.pmed.0030494

Knierer, J., Gallegos Morales, E. N., Schablon, A., Nienhaus, A., & Kersten, J. F. (2017). QFT-Plus: A plus in variability?—Evaluation of new generation IGRA in serial testing of students with a migration background in Germany. *Journal of Occupational Medicine and Toxicology, 12*. *Journal of Occupational Medicine and Toxicology (London, England), 1*(1), 1. Advance online publication. DOI: 10.1186/s12995-016-0148-z PMID: 28070206

Menzies, D., Joshi, R., & Pai, M. (2007). Risk of tuberculosis infection and disease associated with work in health care settings. *International Journal of Tuberculosis and Lung Disease, 11*(6), 593–605.

Moon, H.-W., & Hur, M. (2013). Interferon-gamma release assays for the diagnosis of latent tuberculosis infection: An updated review. *Annals of Clinical and Laboratory Science, 43*(2), 221–229.

Mostafavi, E., Nasehi, M., Shahraki, A. H., Esmaeili, S., Ghaderi, E., Sharafi, S., & Doosti-Irani, A. (2016). Comparison of the tuberculin skin test and the QuantiFERON-TB Gold test in detecting latent tuberculosis in health care workers in Iran. *Epidemiology and Health, 38*, Article e2016032. DOI: 10.4178/epih.e2016032

Nienhaus, A., Kesavachandran, C., Wendeler, D., Haamann, F., & Dulon, M. (2012). Infectious diseases in healthcare workers—An analysis of the standardised data set of a German compensation board. *Journal of Occupational Medicine and Toxicology, 7*. *Journal of Occupational Medicine and Toxicology (London, England)*, *8*(1), 8. Advance online publication. DOI: 10.1186/1745-6673-7-8 PMID: 22553942

Nienhaus, A., Ringshausen, F. C., Costa, J. T., Schablon, A., & Tripodi, D. (2013). IFN-gamma release assay versus tuberculin skin test for monitoring TB infection in healthcare workers. *Expert Review of Anti-Infective Therapy, 11*(1), 37–48. DOI: 10.1586/eri.12.150

Pai, M., Zwerling, A., & Menzies, D. (2008). Systematic review: T-cell-based assays for the diagnosis of latent tuberculosis infection: An update. *Annals of Internal Medicine, 149*(3), 177–184. https://doi.org/DOI: 10.7326/0003-4819-149-3-200808050-00268

Rafiza, S., Rampal, K. G., & Tahir, A. (2011). Prevalence and risk factors of latent tuberculosis infection among health care workers in Malaysia. *BMC Infectious Diseases, 11*. *BMC Infectious Diseases*, *19*(1), 19. Advance online publication. DOI: 10.1186/1471-2334-11-19 PMID: 21244645

Ringshausen, F. C., Schablon, A., & Nienhaus, A. (2012). Interferon-gamma release assays for the tuberculosis serial testing of health care workers: A systematic review. *Journal of Occupational Medicine and Toxicology, 7*. *Journal of Occupational Medicine and Toxicology (London, England)*, *6*(1), 6. Advance online publication. DOI: 10.1186/1745-6673-7-6 PMID: 22537915

Schablon, A., Harling, M., Diel, R., Ringshausen, F. C., Torres Costa, J., & Nienhaus, A. (2010). Serial testing with an interferon-γ release assay in German healthcare workers. *GMS Krankenhaushygiene Interdisziplinär, 5*(1), Article Doc05. DOI: 10.3205/dgkh000149

Schablon, A., Nienhaus, A., Ringshausen, F. C., Preisser, A. M., & Peters, C. (2014). Occupational screening for tuberculosis and the use of a borderline zone for interpretation of the IGRA in German healthcare workers. *PLoS ONE, 9*(12), Article e115322. DOI: 10.1371/journal.pone.0115322

Seidler, A., Nienhaus, A., & Diel, R. (2005). Review of epidemiological studies on the occupational risk of tuberculosis in low-incidence areas. *Respiration, 72*(4), 431–446. DOI: 10.1159/000086261

Tanabe, M., Nakamura, A., Arai, A., Yamasaki, D., Hirano, K., Kobayashi, T., Taguchi, O., Kaneko, T., & Ito, M. (2017). The direct comparison of two interferon-gamma release assays in the tuberculosis screening of Japanese healthcare workers. *Internal Medicine, 56*(7), 773–779. https://doi.org/DOI: 10.2169/internalmedicine.56.7688

Torres Costa, J., Sá, R., Cardoso, M. J., Silva, R., Ferreira, J., Ribeiro, C., Miranda, M., Plácido, J. L., & Nienhaus, A. (2009). Tuberculosis screening in Portuguese healthcare workers using the tuberculin skin test and the interferon-gamma release assay. *European Respiratory Journal, 34*(6), 1423–1428. https://doi.org/DOI: 10.1183/09031936.00029909

Torres Costa, J., Silva, R., Ringshausen, F. C., & Nienhaus, A. (2011). Screening for tuberculosis and prediction of disease in Portuguese healthcare workers. *Journal of Occupational Medicine and Toxicology, 6*. *Journal of Occupational Medicine and Toxicology (London, England)*, *19*(1), 19. Advance online publication. DOI: 10.1186/1745-6673-6-19 PMID: 21658231

Uden, L., Barber, E., Ford, N., & Cooke, G. S. (2017). Risk of tuberculosis infection and disease for health care workers: An updated meta-analysis. *Open Forum Infectious Diseases, 4*(3), Article ofx137. DOI: 10.1093/ofid/ofx137

Yap, P., Tan, K. H. X., Lim, W. Y., Barkham, T., Tan, L. W. L., Chen, M. I.-C., Wang, Y. T., & Chee, C. B. E. (2018). Prevalence of and risk factors associated with latent tuberculosis in Singapore: A cross-sectional survey. *International Journal of Infectious Diseases, 72*, 55–62. DOI: 10.1016/j.ijid.2018.05.004

Zwerling, A., van den Hof, S., Scholten, J., Cobelens, F., Menzies, D., & Pai, M. (2012). Interferon-gamma release assays for tuberculosis screening of healthcare workers: A systematic review. *Thorax, 67*(1), 62–70. DOI: 10.1136/thx.2010.143180

Chapter 6
Innovative Strategies for Tuberculosis Infection Prevention and Control

Ravinesh Mishra
https://orcid.org/0000-0003-4559-1994
School of Pharmacy and Emerging Sciences, Baddi University of Emerging Sciences and Technology, India

Bhartendu Sharma
School of Pharmacy and Emerging Sciences, Baddi University of Emerging Sciences and Technology, India

Priya Sharma
https://orcid.org/0000-0002-3942-6346
School of Pharmacy and Emerging Sciences, Baddi University of Emerging Sciences and Technology, India

ABSTRACT

Tuberculosis (TB) continues to be one of the top 10 causes of death worldwide, despite being a preventable and curable disease. According to the World Health Organization (WHO), approximately 10.6 million people fell ill with TB in 2022, and 1.3 million died, highlighting a persistent global health burden. The ongoing challenges in TB control are compounded by the emergence of multidrug-resistant TB (MDR-TB), delayed diagnosis, insufficient infection control infrastructure, and the impact of social determinants of health. In healthcare and community settings alike, TB transmission remains a major concern, especially in high-burden countries. This chapter, titled "Innovative Strategies for Tuberculosis Infection Prevention and Control," aims to explore cutting-edge approaches, novel frameworks, and integrated interventions that are reshaping the landscape of TB prevention and

DOI: 10.4018/979-8-3373-3446-2.ch006

containment. The proposal presents a comprehensive roadmap of how innovation, driven by science, technology, policy, and community engagement, can elevate the global response to TB infection control.

INTRODUCTION

Overview of TB Burden and Ongoing Challenges

Tuberculosis (TB) remains one of the leading causes of morbidity and mortality globally, especially in low- and middle-income countries. According to the World Health Organization (2021), approximately 10.6 million people fell ill with TB, and 1.3 million succumbed to the disease. Despite being preventable and curable, TB continues to spread due to a combination of biomedical, social, and systemic factors.

A particularly alarming challenge in recent years is the rise of multidrug-resistant (MDR) and extensively drug-resistant (XDR) TB strains. These resistant forms demand prolonged, toxic, and costly treatments, straining health systems and amplifying the urgency for robust infection prevention and control (IPC) measures (Pai et al., 2023). Furthermore, the COVID-19 pandemic significantly disrupted TB detection and treatment services, setting back years of progress in TB control by exacerbating diagnostic delays and increasing transmission rates (Migliori et al., 2020).

TB is primarily transmitted through airborne particles expelled when an infected individual coughs, sneezes, or speaks. This transmission mechanism highlights the importance of environmental and behavioural controls, especially in healthcare settings, congregate living environments, and densely populated communities. Traditional TB IPC approaches-based on administrative controls, environmental controls, and the use of personal protective equipment (PPE)-have proven effective but insufficient in the face of evolving global health dynamics and social determinants of health.

Need for Innovative Approaches in TB IPC

Current TB IPC strategies, while essential, often fail to achieve desired outcomes in resource-constrained settings or rapidly evolving urban environments. Traditional measures are frequently reactive rather than proactive, rely heavily on human compliance, and are susceptible to systemic weaknesses, such as supply chain interruptions, inadequate infrastructure, and poor health worker training (Munedzimwe et al., 2023). These issues necessitate the integration of novel, forward-thinking strategies to fortify the global TB response.

Innovation in TB IPC must encompass technological, social, and policy dimensions. For instance, digital health platforms and artificial intelligence (AI) can enhance early detection and monitor transmission in real time. Mobile health (mHealth) applications offer remote monitoring, contact tracing, and patient engagement tools that are cost-effective and scalable. Similarly, improvements in ventilation systems and ultraviolet germicidal irradiation (UVGI) technologies can significantly reduce airborne transmission in healthcare and community settings (Escombe et al., 2007).

Innovative strategies also extend beyond technology. Community-centered interventions, including peer-led health education, stigma-reduction campaigns, and participatory IPC design, offer culturally resonant and sustainable solutions. These approaches recognize that TB is not just a biomedical issue but a disease intricately linked to poverty, social inequality, and structural health barriers (Lönnroth et al., 2009).

The global TB response, therefore, must transition from conventional IPC strategies to a multidimensional approach that leverages innovation to close persistent gaps in prevention, diagnosis, and care. A reimagined IPC framework-adaptable, data-driven, inclusive, and grounded in the realities of affected populations-is pivotal to meeting the WHO's End TB Strategy targets.

GAPS IN CONVENTIONAL TB INFECTION PREVENTION AND CONTROL

Limitations of Current IPC Measures

Traditional tuberculosis (TB) infection prevention and control (IPC) strategies are grounded in three fundamental components: administrative controls, environmental controls, and personal protective equipment (PPE). While these components are endorsed globally and incorporated into national TB programs, their effectiveness often falls short in practice, especially in high-burden and low-resource settings. Administrative controls, such as prompt identification, isolation of suspected TB cases, and appropriate triaging, depend heavily on trained personnel, timely diagnostics, and adherence to protocols. However, delays in diagnosis and inadequate contact tracing persist, undermining early intervention efforts (World Health Organization, 2019). Diagnostic bottlenecks are further exacerbated by reliance on outdated tools such as smear microscopy, which lacks sensitivity, particularly among individuals with HIV or children.

Environmental controls, including natural and mechanical ventilation and ultraviolet germicidal irradiation (UVGI), are often inconsistently implemented or entirely absent. Many healthcare facilities in endemic regions were not designed with airborne pathogen control in mind. Retrofitting these facilities with adequate ventilation or UVGI systems is often hampered by budget constraints and limited technical capacity (Mphahlele et al., 2015).

Personal protective equipment-such as N95 respirators-is recommended for healthcare workers and individuals in high-risk environments. However, access to quality PPE remains inconsistent. Even when PPE is available, issues such as poor fit, lack of training in donning/doffing procedures, and discomfort often result in low compliance.

Collectively, these limitations reflect a reactive, resource-intensive approach to IPC, reliant on ideal conditions seldom found in real-world settings. Moreover, these conventional measures have limited adaptability and resilience in the face of novel challenges, such as those posed by drug-resistant TB strains or concurrent public health emergencies.

Challenges in Healthcare and Community Settings

The dichotomy between healthcare and community environments presents distinct IPC challenges that require differentiated strategies. In healthcare settings, the convergence of vulnerable patients, frequent exposure to infectious aerosols, and overcrowding contributes to nosocomial TB transmission. This is especially problematic in TB wards, outpatient departments, and waiting areas where proper ventilation, screening, and spatial separation are lacking (Escombe et al., 2007).

Healthcare worker safety is another major concern. A study in South Africa found that TB infection rates among healthcare workers were significantly higher than in the general population, largely due to poor IPC infrastructure and inconsistent application of standard precautions (Mphahlele et al., 2018). Training programs on IPC are often irregular and not tailored to real-time risk assessment or facility-specific protocols.

In community settings, TB transmission is facilitated by social determinants such as poverty, malnutrition, and overcrowded housing. In informal settlements and refugee camps, the implementation of conventional IPC measures is practically non-existent. The lack of health literacy, stigma, and mistrust of health systems also hinders community engagement in TB prevention practices.

Moreover, community-based TB programs often focus primarily on treatment adherence rather than proactive prevention. Contact investigation is either sporadic or non-existent, and latent TB infection (LTBI) management-critical for prevention-is underutilized, especially among close contacts and high-risk groups such as people living with HIV (PLHIV) or children under five years old (Lönnroth et al., 2009).

Emerging Threats: MDR/XDR-TB and Co-infections

One of the most pressing challenges to conventional TB IPC frameworks is the growing threat of multidrug-resistant (MDR) and extensively drug-resistant (XDR) TB. These forms of TB are resistant to first-line drugs such as isoniazid and rifampicin, and in the case of XDR-TB, also to key second-line agents. The global burden of MDR-TB was estimated at over 450,000 new cases in 2022, with alarmingly low treatment success rates of just over 60% (World Health Organization, 2021).

Traditional IPC strategies are ill-equipped to address the complexities of MDR/XDR-TB. These strains require longer, more toxic treatment regimens, often necessitating hospitalization, which increases the risk of nosocomial transmission. Moreover, diagnostic delays-common in resource-poor settings-allow MDR/XDR-TB to spread before appropriate therapy is initiated. Conventional sputum-based diagnostics may not detect drug resistance promptly, further compounding the challenge.

Additionally, the intersection of TB with other infectious diseases such as HIV/AIDS, COVID-19, and diabetes represents a significant threat to IPC systems. Individuals with HIV are up to 20 times more likely to develop active TB due to immune suppression, while COVID-19 has overwhelmed IPC resources and disrupted TB service delivery worldwide (Migliori et al., 2020).

TECHNOLOGICAL INNOVATIONS IN TB IPC

The integration of technology into tuberculosis (TB) infection prevention and control (IPC) has created transformative opportunities to detect, prevent, and manage TB transmission more effectively. With global health systems under increasing strain, particularly in low- and middle-income countries (LMICs), innovative tools are essential to enhance surveillance, diagnostics, and environmental controls. This section explores the most promising technological advancements being applied in TB IPC, including digital health tools, artificial intelligence (AI), rapid diagnostics, and smart environmental systems.

Digital Surveillance and AI for Early Detection

Use of Electronic Health Records and Predictive Modeling

Digital surveillance systems are crucial for early identification of TB cases, mapping transmission patterns, and monitoring IPC compliance. In many countries, electronic health records (EHRs) have been leveraged to build national TB registries that allow real-time data collection and analytics. These systems support automated alerts for missed follow-ups, flag high-risk individuals, and integrate laboratory results with patient histories.

Predictive modeling based on EHR data enables early detection of TB outbreaks. Machine learning algorithms can analyze diverse datasets-including symptom reports, demographics, and radiologic findings-to identify individuals at high risk of progressing from latent to active TB. For example, studies in India and South Africa have successfully applied AI models to predict reactivation in people living with HIV (PLHIV) or diabetes.

Predictive systems also allow targeted screening and resource allocation. Health systems can deploy IPC interventions, such as community health outreach or focused ventilation upgrades, in areas flagged as transmission hotspots. This pre-emptive strategy not only reduces disease spread but also optimizes the use of limited resources.

Contact Tracing Apps and AI-Driven Outbreak Forecasting

The COVID-19 pandemic catalysed the adoption of digital contact tracing technologies, many of which are now being adapted for TB. Mobile applications equipped with Bluetooth, GPS, or QR-code systems have proven effective in tracking exposure and notifying individuals who may have encountered an infectious case (Islam et al., 2020).

AI-driven outbreak forecasting models use geospatial data, social behavior metrics, and environmental factors to simulate TB transmission patterns. These systems provide policymakers with scenario-based forecasts, enabling timely implementation of targeted IPC strategies, such as mobile screening units in high-density areas or pre-emptive isoniazid preventive therapy (IPT) programs.

Rapid Diagnostic Technologies

Advances in Point-of-Care Molecular Diagnostics

One of the most critical gaps in TB IPC has been the delay in diagnosis. Traditional smear microscopy is slow and lacks sensitivity, particularly for extrapulmonary TB and co-infected populations. In response, molecular diagnostics have revolutionized point-of-care testing.

The Xpert MTB/RIF assay and its enhanced version, Xpert Ultra, provide results in under two hours and simultaneously detect rifampicin resistance. These tools have been deployed widely through global health initiatives such as the Stop TB Partnership and the Global Fund. The portability and user-friendly interface of newer models, like GeneXpert Edge and Truenat, have facilitated decentralized testing in peripheral health facilities.

Point-of-care diagnostics enable rapid initiation of treatment and reduce the window of infectivity, a crucial aspect of IPC. They also support drug susceptibility testing, which is vital in managing multidrug-resistant (MDR) and extensively drug-resistant (XDR) TB cases, where inappropriate treatment regimens can prolong infectivity and amplify resistance (World Health Organization, 2021).

Role of Digital Chest X-Ray with AI Interpretation

Chest X-ray (CXR) has traditionally served as a screening tool for TB, but its utility has been limited by the requirement for radiologists and variability in interpretation. AI-based interpretation tools now address these barriers by providing automated, consistent, and rapid analysis of digital chest X-rays.

Tools such as CAD4TB, qXR, and Lunit INSIGHT use deep learning algorithms to detect radiological features suggestive of TB. These tools have demonstrated performance comparable to human experts and have even outperformed radiologists in some settings, particularly in early or subclinical TB detection (Chattoraj et al., 2023).

The use of AI-driven CXR interpretation is especially impactful in settings with limited radiology capacity. In Bangladesh and Uganda, field studies using portable X-ray devices paired with CAD software have enabled mass screening in prisons, refugee camps, and urban slums. These innovations reduce diagnostic delays, flag asymptomatic individuals, and allow prompt IPC interventions.

Environmental Controls

Smart Ventilation Systems and UVGI Technologies

Environmental engineering plays a foundational role in preventing the airborne transmission of TB. Conventional strategies-such as opening windows and using mechanical exhaust fans-are often unreliable, particularly in climate-variable regions or poorly designed facilities. Smart ventilation systems now offer automated, adaptive control of airflow based on occupancy and air quality metrics.

Modern systems use CO_2 and particulate sensors to monitor indoor air quality and adjust ventilation dynamically. For example, systems implemented in South African TB hospitals automatically increase airflow when CO_2 levels exceed safe thresholds, thereby reducing aerosol concentration and risk of transmission (Escombe et al., 2019).

Upper-room ultraviolet germicidal irradiation (UVGI) systems provide another effective environmental control. UVGI devices emit UV-C light that inactivates airborne Mycobacterium tuberculosis. Recent innovations have improved their safety and efficiency by integrating motion sensors, automatic shutoff mechanisms, and wireless data logging. These enhancements enable safe use in occupied spaces and support IPC monitoring through cloud-based platforms.

Pilot projects in Peru and the Philippines have demonstrated that UVGI, when combined with improved airflow design, reduces nosocomial TB transmission by over 70% in high-volume clinics. The integration of UVGI into smart building systems ensures consistent disinfection without relying on manual operation.

Air Quality Sensors and Automated Alerts

Continuous environmental monitoring is essential for sustaining IPC in healthcare settings. The use of Internet of Things (IoT) devices for indoor air quality surveillance allows real-time data collection on temperature, humidity, CO_2, and microbial load.

These sensors can be programmed to trigger automated alerts when air quality deteriorates, prompting facility staff to increase ventilation, initiate UVGI disinfection, or reduce room occupancy. Data from these sensors can be centralized on IPC dashboards to facilitate audits, inform building maintenance, and drive policy decisions.

In India, a public–private partnership in Mumbai is piloting an integrated system where air quality sensors feed data into a centralized IPC platform that monitors risk across over 30 primary healthcare centers. This digital system enables health administrators to make evidence-based decisions on resource allocation and risk mitigation.

BEHAVIOURAL AND COMMUNITY-BASED INNOVATIONS

While technology and policy are essential pillars of tuberculosis (TB) infection prevention and control (IPC), the sustainability and impact of any intervention are ultimately determined by human behavior and community participation. Behavioural and community-based innovations aim to address the social and cultural dimensions of TB, including stigma, awareness, health-seeking behavior, and treatment adherence. These innovations are particularly crucial in low-resource settings, where biomedical interventions may be limited or inconsistently applied. This section explores how peer-led education, community engagement, mobile health (mHealth) platforms, and human-centered design (HCD) are reshaping TB IPC at the grassroots level.

Community Engagement and Participatory Approaches

Peer-Led Education Models

Peer-led interventions have emerged as powerful tools to increase awareness and reduce misconceptions about TB. These models rely on community members-often TB survivors or trained local health volunteers-to educate their peers about TB symptoms, prevention methods, and available services. The familiarity and shared lived experience of peer educators foster trust, reduce resistance to health messages, and bridge the gap between formal healthcare systems and underserved communities (Sempeera et al., 2017).

Studies in South Africa, India, and the Philippines have shown that peer educators significantly improve TB knowledge and promote earlier care-seeking behavior. In Malawi, for example, trained TB survivors led household visits, during which they offered education, screened for symptoms, and referred suspected cases. This approach resulted in increased detection of TB cases and greater uptake of preventive therapy.

Peer-led models also contribute to improving IPC compliance in high-risk environments such as prisons, mines, and homeless shelters. In these contexts, peer educators are instrumental in facilitating mask use, cough etiquette, and environmental sanitation practices.

TB Clubs and Stigma Reduction Campaigns

Social stigma remains a major barrier to TB diagnosis and treatment adherence. In many cultures, TB is associated with poverty, immorality, or incurability, leading patients to hide their illness or discontinue treatment prematurely. Behavioural innovations that address stigma are essential for improving community-wide IPC outcomes.

TB clubs are peer support groups that provide psychosocial support, share experiences, and promote mutual accountability among patients. These clubs often serve as platforms for information exchange, treatment adherence monitoring, and health promotion events. Evidence from Uganda and Ethiopia suggests that TB clubs increase retention in care and reduce feelings of isolation among patients (Gashu et al., 2021).

Mass media campaigns and community theatre are also used to demystify TB. In Bangladesh, a participatory street theatre program portrayed real-life TB stories to challenge myths and promote health-seeking behavior. Evaluations showed improved public understanding and reduced fear of people with TB.

Stigma-reduction initiatives often align with broader social determinants of health. Integrating TB education into existing community structures-such as religious institutions, schools, or women's cooperatives-helps normalize conversations around TB and enhances community ownership of IPC strategies.

Mobile Health (mHealth) Interventions

SMS Reminders and Adherence Monitoring Tools

Mobile health (mHealth) platforms are transforming TB prevention and treatment adherence through cost-effective, scalable communication tools. One of the most widely implemented mHealth strategies is the use of SMS reminders to support treatment adherence. These reminders can prompt patients to take their medications, attend follow-up appointments, or practice IPC measures such as mask use or ventilation.

In India, the 99DOTS platform uses low-cost feature phones and coded medication packaging to monitor daily adherence. Patients confirm medication intake by dialling a hidden toll-free number revealed only after opening the medication blister pack. Healthcare providers can track adherence in real time and intervene when doses are missed (Subbaraman et al., 2020).

Other SMS-based tools allow bidirectional communication between patients and health workers. In South Africa, a system called mHealth4TB enabled patients to report side effects and ask questions via SMS, leading to higher satisfaction and improved medication adherence. SMS tools have also been used to remind household contacts to return for TB testing or preventive therapy, thereby reducing community transmission.

Human-Centered Design for IPC in Low-Resource Settings

Co-Design of IPC Measures with Healthcare Workers

Human-centered design (HCD) is an approach that involves users-patients, providers, and community members-in every stage of designing health interventions. In

TB IPC, this approach has proven effective in creating context-specific, acceptable, and sustainable solutions.

In Uganda, a project called SAFE-TB applied HCD principles by convening healthcare workers, facility managers, and patients to co-create IPC protocols. Through focus groups and prototyping, participants designed improved patient flow systems, new triage procedures, and signage that better conveyed IPC guidance. As a result, there was increased adherence to respiratory isolation and reduced confusion in outpatient departments.

Co-design helps identify overlooked barriers such as cultural norms, workflow disruptions, or spatial constraints that hinder IPC compliance. For example, in many rural clinics, TB patients are reluctant to wear masks due to fear of social judgment. Involving patients in mask design and messaging helped create culturally acceptable solutions that increased uptake.

HCD also facilitates innovation in training and behavior change tools. Simulation-based IPC training, developed through user testing with nurses and support staff, has shown higher knowledge retention than traditional lectures (Yoshikawa et al., 2025).

Low-Cost, Context-Sensitive Innovations

Resource constraints in LMICs necessitate IPC solutions that are affordable, simple, and easy to maintain. HCD has catalysed the development of low-cost technologies adapted to these settings.

In Kenya, community health workers collaborated with designers to develop TB prevention toolkits that included reusable masks, pictorial IPC instruction cards, and simple CO_2 monitors for household use. The toolkits were tailored based on household interviews and were later scaled through local NGOs (Wanjiku et al., 2021).

INNOVATIONS IN PERSONAL PROTECTIVE EQUIPMENT AND PRACTICES

Personal protective equipment (PPE) is a fundamental component of tuberculosis (TB) infection prevention and control (IPC), especially in healthcare and congregate settings. However, conventional PPE practices are often unsustainable, uncomfortable, or poorly adhered to in high-burden, resource-constrained environments. Innovations in PPE technology and wearable biosensing systems are addressing these limitations by offering more sustainable, cost-effective, and data-integrated alternatives.

This section explores two main areas of innovation: the development of reusable and eco-friendly PPE-including advanced mask technologies-and the application of smart wearables and biosensors to monitor TB exposure and detect early signs of infection.

Reusable and Sustainable PPE

Advances in Mask Technology (e.g., Nanofibers, Self-Sanitizing Materials)

Standard respiratory protection against TB-typically N95 or equivalent respirators-is effective when properly used. However, the high cost, discomfort, limited reusability, and inconsistent availability of these masks often limit their use in LMICs. Innovations in material science are now addressing these issues by improving mask performance, durability, and user experience.

Nanofiber-based masks represent a major advancement. These masks utilize ultrafine polymer fibres (ranging from 100 to 300 nm in diameter) to create highly efficient filters with minimal breathing resistance. Unlike melt-blown fabrics used in traditional N95 masks, nanofibers offer greater surface area and porosity, enhancing both filtration efficiency and breathability. In a study comparing nanofiber masks to conventional N95 respirators, the former demonstrated similar protection levels while maintaining user comfort over extended periods.

Another promising innovation is the development of self-sanitizing mask surfaces. These masks incorporate antimicrobial materials-such as copper, silver nanoparticles, or photoactive titanium dioxide-that deactivate pathogens on contact or upon exposure to light. Research has shown that these surfaces can inactivate *Mycobacterium tuberculosis* (MTB) and other airborne bacteria, reducing the risk of cross-contamination during reuse.

Masks integrated with photothermal or electrothermal elements have also been developed to actively kill pathogens by generating mild heat when exposed to sunlight or electricity. While still in prototype stages, these self-sterilizing technologies could drastically improve PPE safety and reuse potential in remote settings.

Eco-Friendly and Cost-Effective PPE Solutions

The global COVID-19 pandemic highlighted the environmental toll of disposable PPE, with billions of masks contributing to medical waste. In TB-endemic regions, where resources are limited and waste management infrastructure is weak, this challenge is magnified. Therefore, reusable and biodegradable PPE solutions are gaining traction as part of sustainable IPC strategies.

Innovators are producing masks from natural biodegradable materials such as bamboo fibres, banana leaves, or biopolymers like polylactic acid (PLA). These masks provide adequate protection for community settings and can be safely composted after use. Although they are not yet suitable for clinical environments requiring high filtration standards, they offer a practical solution for non-clinical IPC applications.

In Uganda and India, social enterprises have developed washable cloth masks with replaceable nanofiber filters, combining affordability with performance. These designs allow communities to maintain personal protection using locally available resources, reducing dependence on imported medical-grade PPE (Greenhalgh et al., 2024).

The World Health Organization (WHO) has endorsed the integration of sustainability into PPE procurement and design. Life cycle assessments indicate that reusable PPE systems, when properly disinfected and maintained, can reduce costs and environmental impact without compromising safety.

Smart Wearables and Sensors

Wearables for Exposure Monitoring

As TB continues to pose a risk to healthcare workers, miners, prison guards, and other high-exposure populations, real-time exposure monitoring is critical. Wearable technology is emerging as a promising tool to track individual exposure to TB-risk environments and trigger timely IPC interventions.

Wearable devices-such as wristbands, badges, or clip-on sensors-can monitor proximity to known TB patients, duration of exposure, and environmental conditions such as air quality and CO_2 concentration. These parameters are critical in estimating the likelihood of airborne MTB transmission (Vanhems et al., 2013).

For example, the EXHALE platform, developed by researchers in South Africa, integrates a wearable badge with Bluetooth proximity sensors and GPS to assess contact intensity in hospital settings. The data are uploaded to a central dashboard, where infection control teams can identify exposure clusters and adjust facility layouts or protocols accordingly.

Some wearables are integrated with machine learning algorithms that analyze behavioural patterns (e.g., time spent in poorly ventilated areas) and alert users when their exposure risk exceeds a safe threshold. These personalized risk assessments can inform decisions such as taking a preventive dose of isoniazid or seeking testing.

Importantly, these technologies also enhance occupational health surveillance, providing data for worker protection programs and helping to enforce PPE use and IPC compliance in institutional environments.

Biosensors for Early Infection Detection

Biosensors are analytical devices that detect biological markers-such as proteins, volatile compounds, or immune responses-associated with infection. In the context of TB IPC, biosensors are being explored for non-invasive, early detection of TB infection, particularly in high-risk settings.

Wearable biosensors, often embedded in skin patches or smart textiles, can monitor changes in temperature, respiration rate, and biomarkers such as nitric oxide in breath or C-reactive protein in sweat. These parameters can serve as early indicators of infection, prompting diagnostic confirmation and early treatment before transmission occurs.

One study piloted a salivary biosensor patch in a high-burden urban area in India. The device continuously sampled trace biomarkers from the user's saliva and triggered a Bluetooth alert if inflammation patterns consistent with TB were detected. Though still in early development, this approach demonstrated high acceptability among users and strong potential for integration with mHealth platforms.

Further innovation is occurring in volatile organic compound (VOC) detection. Research indicates that individuals with active pulmonary TB exhale specific VOCs due to changes in lung metabolism. Compact breath sensors using gas chromatography or nanoarray technologies can detect these VOCs with high sensitivity, enabling rapid screening at the point of care (Strati et al., 2021).

As biosensors become more affordable and scalable, they could revolutionize TB surveillance, particularly among healthcare workers and individuals in congregate settings. The integration of biosensor alerts with digital health platforms can facilitate contact tracing, early isolation, and real-time IPC planning.

POLICY AND SYSTEM-LEVEL INNOVATIONS

Tuberculosis (TB) infection prevention and control (IPC) is not only a clinical concern but a systemic and policy-driven challenge. Without supportive policy environments and integrated health systems, even the most advanced innovations will fail to achieve their full potential. System-level innovations-rooted in financing, governance, and cross-sectoral partnerships-play a pivotal role in scaling up TB IPC interventions, ensuring sustainability, and promoting equity.

This section explores three major avenues of policy and system-level innovation: integrating TB IPC into universal health coverage (UHC), deploying real-time IPC monitoring systems, and leveraging public-private partnerships (PPPs) to accelerate innovation and implementation.

Integration of TB IPC in Universal Health Coverage

Strategic Financing Models and IPC in Primary Care

Universal health coverage (UHC), as defined by World Health Organization (WHO, 2021), aims to ensure that all individuals receive the health services they need without suffering financial hardship. Integrating TB IPC into UHC frameworks is a critical step toward mainstreaming prevention, expanding access, and reducing disparities. Traditionally, TB programs have operated in silos, often relying on vertical funding and project-based interventions. This approach creates fragmentation and impedes the sustainability of IPC services.

Strategic integration of IPC within primary healthcare systems can lead to more equitable and effective TB control. For example, including TB IPC indicators in national health insurance reimbursement schemes ensures that providers prioritize infection control measures. Countries such as Thailand and Rwanda have successfully incorporated TB IPC benchmarks into their essential health service packages, linking funding to compliance and performance (Yimer et al., 2020).

Incorporating TB IPC into broader health systems strengthening (HSS) initiatives also offers synergistic benefits. For example, investing in community health worker training for TB IPC contributes to pandemic preparedness, maternal health, and HIV control. By making TB IPC part of routine health delivery, countries can enhance resilience while reducing the burden on overstretched TB-specific programs.

Real-Time IPC Monitoring Systems

IPC Dashboards for Health Facility Compliance

In the digital age, data-driven decision-making is indispensable for effective TB IPC. Real-time IPC monitoring systems, including electronic dashboards, allow health administrators to visualize and manage infection control indicators across multiple facilities or regions. These platforms facilitate timely interventions, identify gaps, and enhance accountability.

IPC dashboards typically integrate data on triage protocols, patient isolation rates, ventilation audits, PPE availability, and healthcare worker training. By consolidating this information into a user-friendly interface, managers can track progress against IPC goals and trigger corrective actions. For example, when a facility falls below a minimum threshold for mask availability or ventilation rates, the dashboard generates alerts for immediate resolution (Talagala & Shashikala 2022).

The Philippines Department of Health has developed a national TB IPC compliance dashboard using open-source software and mobile data collection tools.

Facilities are required to submit monthly reports through tablets or smartphones, and data are aggregated centrally to inform policy and funding decisions. This approach has improved IPC adherence by enabling data transparency and peer comparisons among facilities.

Another successful example is the Digital Health Surveillance Platform (DHSP) implemented in Nigeria. It includes an IPC module that combines patient case data with environmental metrics and workforce indicators. The DHSP allows district health officers to monitor IPC activities and reallocate resources dynamically, especially in response to outbreak clusters.

Artificial intelligence (AI) and predictive analytics are also being integrated into IPC dashboards. Machine learning models can analyze historical trends to forecast IPC breaches, estimate TB exposure risks, or identify underperforming facilities. These predictive insights support pre-emptive interventions, resource optimization, and strategic planning.

For IPC dashboards to succeed, they must be supported by enabling policies, including data privacy regulations, interdepartmental collaboration mandates, and standardized IPC reporting protocols. Furthermore, training and technical support are essential to ensure frontline staff can contribute accurate and timely data.

Public-Private Partnerships

Innovation Accelerators and Collaborative IPC Research Hubs

The scale and complexity of TB IPC challenges demand resources and expertise beyond what the public sector can provide alone. Public-private partnerships (PPPs) offer a powerful model for mobilizing innovation, financing, and implementation support. These partnerships enable governments, private industry, academia, and civil society to co-develop and scale new IPC technologies and approaches.

One of the most effective formats for innovation-focused PPPs is the TB innovation accelerator-a platform that provides technical, financial, and regulatory support to startups and research groups working on IPC solutions. The TB REACH initiative, funded by the Stop TB Partnership, has supported over 300 projects across 50 countries, many of which focus on behavioural, diagnostic, or environmental IPC innovations.

In India, the Grand Challenges TB Control program, supported by USAID and the Bill & Melinda Gates Foundation, brings together private companies and public research institutions to develop low-cost diagnostic tools, air sterilization devices, and digital IPC platforms. Several of these solutions have progressed from pilot to scale through targeted procurement agreements with the National TB Elimination Program (NTEP).

Collaborative IPC research hubs are also advancing TB prevention by bridging the gap between basic science and applied implementation. These hubs foster interdisciplinary research, combining microbiology, epidemiology, engineering, and social science.

CASE STUDIES AND SUCCESS STORIES

Innovative strategies for tuberculosis (TB) infection prevention and control (IPC) are being piloted, tested, and scaled in various high-burden countries. These real-world examples offer vital lessons about what works, under what conditions, and how systems can adapt to achieve measurable impact. Case studies not only showcase the feasibility of innovations but also highlight contextual challenges and enablers that influence outcomes.

This section presents select case studies from countries with high TB burdens, focusing on how different innovations-spanning technology, community engagement, and system-level approaches-have contributed to improving TB IPC. Each example provides insights into the processes, partnerships, and policies that enabled success, as well as key takeaways for replication and scale.

Examples from High-Burden Countries Using Innovative Strategies

India: Digital Adherence and Community-Based IPC Interventions

India accounts for over a quarter of the global TB burden, making it a vital ground for TB IPC innovations. One of the most widely recognized success stories in India is the deployment of 99DOTS, a low-cost digital adherence technology. The platform involves TB medication blister packs with hidden phone numbers revealed upon opening each dose. Patients call the number daily, providing real-time confirmation of medication intake (Subbaraman et al., 2019).

Implemented across multiple states under the Revised National TB Control Program (now the National Tuberculosis Elimination Program, NTEP), 99DOTS has shown promising results in improving treatment adherence and enabling healthcare workers to intervene promptly when doses are missed. A large-scale evaluation across Maharashtra and Andhra Pradesh showed that digital adherence monitoring improved treatment completion rates by 15% compared to standard care (Chen et al., 2023).

India has also experimented with mobile van–based active case finding, particularly in urban slums and rural districts with limited healthcare infrastructure. These vans, equipped with AI-enabled digital chest X-ray units and GeneXpert devices, screen individuals on-site and link those with symptoms to care pathways immediately. This integration of digital diagnostics and community-based outreach exemplifies a scalable IPC innovation that reduces diagnostic delays and transmission risks.

South Africa: Environmental Controls and Wearable Monitoring in Healthcare Settings

South Africa, with one of the highest burdens of TB-HIV co-infection, has been a leader in piloting environmental and occupational TB IPC strategies.

In parallel, the EXHALE wearable device pilot at Tygerberg Hospital provided exposure tracking among healthcare workers. The wearable sensors recorded proximity and duration of contact with patients, providing data for TB risk modeling and contact tracing. Results helped optimize shift patterns and staff assignments to reduce cumulative exposure (Nardell, 2016).

Vietnam: Integration of TB IPC into Primary Healthcare Reform

Vietnam has been recognized for its efforts to integrate TB control within broader primary healthcare reforms, which include IPC benchmarks and community health worker (CHW) support. The Ministry of Health partnered with PATH and the Stop TB Partnership to launch a district-level IPC strengthening initiative in Hai Phong and Ho Chi Minh City. This program used quality improvement (QI) methodologies to identify and close gaps in triage, isolation, and environmental control.

The initiative also involved training CHWs in active contact tracing, home ventilation improvements, and education on respiratory hygiene. Over a 12-month period, facilities reported a 40% increase in proper triaging of TB suspects and a 25% decrease in reported nosocomial TB infections. Vietnam's experience underscores the value of embedding IPC into system-wide reforms rather than treating it as a siloed vertical function.

Nigeria: IPC Dashboards and Community Engagement for TB/HIV Integration

Nigeria faces a dual burden of TB and HIV, particularly in rural and peri-urban areas. In response, the government-with support from USAID and FHI 360-launched a real-time TB IPC dashboard as part of the Integrated TB and HIV Project. This dashboard aggregates data from health facilities on indicators such as PPE stock, ventilation audits, triage compliance, and health worker training (FHI 360, 2024).

The system enables regional health officers to monitor IPC performance and allocate resources accordingly. Facility-level data are visualized using color-coded risk maps, which guide decision-making at both local and national levels.

Complementing the dashboard, Nigeria also launched community engagement initiatives, such as the TB "Wellness on Wheels" campaign. This mobile campaign employed drama performances, peer educators, and screening stations to reduce stigma and improve TB literacy. Over 500,000 individuals were screened during the campaign's first year, demonstrating how behavioural innovation and real-time monitoring can synergize for IPC success.

BARRIERS TO IMPLEMENTATION AND SCALE-UP

Despite the growing evidence base for innovative tuberculosis (TB) infection prevention and control (IPC) interventions, large-scale adoption remains uneven across regions. The translation of innovation into sustainable, system-wide practice faces multiple obstacles-technical, financial, behavioural, and political. Understanding these barriers is crucial for designing policies and programs that foster effective implementation and long-term scale-up.

Financial and Resource Constraints

Limited financial and infrastructural resources remain among the most significant barriers to TB IPC innovation. Low- and middle-income countries (LMICs) often depend heavily on external donor funding, which is frequently earmarked for specific projects or short-term outcomes. This fragmentation hampers long-term sustainability and integration of innovative approaches into routine health services.

Even when pilot programs succeed, scaling up innovations such as digital diagnostics, UVGI systems, or wearable technologies can be cost-prohibitive. Maintenance, technical support, and supply-chain logistics require sustained funding and skilled personnel. Health systems that already face resource constraints struggle to prioritize preventive investments over immediate treatment demands (Peterson et al., 2016).

Cost–effectiveness analyses of TB IPC innovations are also limited, leaving policymakers without strong economic evidence to justify budget allocations. For example, while AI-based radiographic screening has demonstrated diagnostic accuracy and efficiency, data on its cost savings and long-term sustainability are scarce, especially in rural and decentralized settings (Singh, 2025).

Addressing financial barriers requires strategic health financing reforms and the integration of TB IPC into universal health coverage (UHC) frameworks. Domestic resource mobilization, innovative financing mechanisms (such as social impact bonds), and blended public–private investments can support sustained scale-up.

Behavioural and Cultural Barriers

Human behaviour profoundly influences IPC adherence and innovation uptake. Even the most advanced technologies can fail if users do not perceive them as relevant, trustworthy, or feasible. Resistance to change is common, particularly when innovations disrupt existing workflows or cultural norms (Islam et al., 2020).

For instance, healthcare workers may view electronic IPC monitoring tools as burdensome or punitive, while community members may associate mask-wearing with stigma or disease visibility. In some regions, misinformation about TB transmission persists, undermining IPC messaging.

Cultural norms around gender, hierarchy, and privacy can further complicate IPC implementation. In patriarchal communities, women-often primary caregivers-may have limited autonomy to adopt preventive behaviours or access digital IPC tools. Engaging local leaders, faith-based institutions, and community champions is therefore essential to enhance cultural acceptability and sustain behaviour change (Barman et al., 2025).

Behavioural science–informed approaches, such as human-centered design (HCD), participatory learning, and social-norm interventions, have proven effective in improving IPC adherence. However, scaling these approaches requires investment in training and institutionalization within TB programs.

Technological and Infrastructure Challenges

Digital innovations depend on stable infrastructure-reliable electricity, internet connectivity, and data systems-which are often limited in rural or resource-poor environments. Interoperability between health information systems also remains a challenge; fragmented digital platforms can create data silos that hinder coordination and decision-making.

Moreover, there is a lack of standardized guidelines and quality assurance mechanisms for emerging IPC technologies, such as AI diagnostics, UVGI systems, and biosensors. Regulatory approval processes can be lengthy, discouraging innovators and slowing adoption (Yin et al., 2024).

Cybersecurity and data privacy concerns also pose barriers to implementing digital IPC tools. Protecting sensitive patient and facility data is essential to maintaining public trust, particularly in contexts where data governance frameworks are underdeveloped.

Infrastructure gaps are equally problematic for environmental IPC innovations. Installing and maintaining ventilation or UVGI systems require technical expertise, which is often scarce at the local level. Routine calibration, power supply, and spare-part availability remain persistent obstacles to sustainability (Mphahlele et al., 2018).

Policy and Governance Barriers

Weak governance structures and fragmented health policies often impede the integration of TB IPC innovations into national programs. Many countries lack dedicated IPC policies or coordination mechanisms that align TB control with broader health system priorities. This leads to duplication of efforts, inefficiencies, and inconsistent implementation.

Decentralization-while valuable for community responsiveness-can also result in uneven adoption of innovations. Local authorities may lack technical capacity or resources to adapt national IPC guidelines to local realities.

Furthermore, political commitment to TB prevention is often overshadowed by acute health crises such as COVID-19, malaria, or non-communicable diseases. Sustaining high-level advocacy and financing for TB IPC requires framing it as a cross-cutting investment in overall health security, rather than as a disease-specific cost center (World Health Organization, 2021).

FUTURE DIRECTIONS AND RESEARCH PRIORITIES

The global response to tuberculosis (TB) infection prevention and control (IPC) is at a pivotal juncture. While scientific, technological, and behavioural innovations have demonstrated promising results, scaling them equitably and sustainably remains the next major challenge. Future TB IPC efforts must focus on strengthening system integration, accelerating innovation translation, and ensuring inclusivity through participatory governance.

This section outlines key recommendations for policymakers, researchers, and practitioners to guide the next generation of TB IPC initiatives.

Strengthening Innovation Ecosystems and Cross-Sectoral Collaboration

The future of TB IPC innovation depends on building robust ecosystems that connect research, policy, and practice. Fragmented efforts, where innovations remain confined to pilot stages, limit impact. Governments and global health agencies should invest in dedicated TB innovation hubs that link academia, private industry, and public health authorities to co-develop and scale sustainable IPC solutions (Cai et al., 2023).

These hubs can accelerate knowledge exchange, enable technology transfer, and provide incubator support for early-stage ideas. They can also coordinate with regional centers of excellence to harmonize standards, accelerate regulatory approval, and facilitate cross-country learning. For example, the WHO Global TB Research Network promotes collaboration among countries to align innovation pipelines with national strategic plans (World Health Organization, 2021).

Partnerships between engineering and public health institutions can further drive context-specific solutions-such as low-cost ventilation designs or biosensor technologies adapted for LMICs. Bridging the gap between laboratory research and field implementation will ensure that innovations are not only effective but also affordable and scalable.

Investing in Capacity Building and Workforce Development

Human resources remain the cornerstone of successful TB IPC. Future strategies must prioritize capacity building across all levels of the healthcare system-from policymakers to frontline workers.

Training should move beyond didactic instruction toward continuous, competency-based learning using digital platforms and simulation-based modules. E-learning portals, augmented reality (AR) simulations, and mobile-based refresher courses can make training accessible even in remote settings.

Capacity development should also extend to data literacy and innovation management, enabling health professionals to interpret IPC data, use dashboards, and engage in adaptive planning. In addition, building local manufacturing capacity for PPE, UVGI devices, and diagnostics can reduce dependency on imports and improve sustainability (Greenhalgh et al., 2024).

Empowering nurses, community health workers (CHWs), and facility managers as IPC champions ensures ownership and accountability at the operational level. Incentive-based models-linking IPC performance to recognition or career advancement-can further enhance motivation and compliance (Yoshikawa et al., 2025).

Advancing Equity and Inclusivity in TB IPC

Innovation must be guided by principles of equity, ensuring that new technologies and policies serve the most vulnerable populations-those affected by poverty, stigma, and limited access to healthcare.

Participatory design approaches, including co-creation with patients, caregivers, and marginalized groups, can ensure that IPC innovations are culturally appropriate and user-centered. Programs should specifically target high-risk settings such as prisons, refugee camps, and informal settlements, where TB transmission rates are disproportionately high.

Gender-responsive TB IPC strategies are equally vital. Women often face greater exposure risks as caregivers while encountering social barriers to care. Integrating gender analysis into IPC program design and monitoring frameworks can help identify inequities and promote inclusive solutions.

Global health agencies and governments should adopt equity-focused monitoring indicators that track how innovations are distributed and who benefits from them. Data disaggregation by gender, age, and socioeconomic status can reveal disparities and inform targeted interventions.

Aligning TB IPC with Global Health Security and Climate Resilience

The COVID-19 pandemic highlighted the interconnectedness of TB IPC with broader global health security systems. Strengthening TB IPC infrastructure-such as ventilation, surveillance, and workforce protection-has co-benefits for pandemic preparedness and the control of other airborne diseases.

Integrating TB IPC into national health security agendas ensures that investments have long-term, cross-cutting impact. Moreover, as climate change increases the frequency of displacement, overcrowding, and air-quality deterioration, IPC frameworks must adapt to evolving environmental realities.

Future research should explore sustainable and energy-efficient IPC solutions, including solar-powered UVGI systems, biodegradable PPE, and carbon-neutral healthcare facilities (Escombe et al., 2019). These innovations can help align TB control with the global climate-resilience agenda while reducing environmental footprints.

Finally, the global TB community must maintain political momentum and financial commitment to achieve the WHO End TB Strategy targets by 2035. Sustained advocacy, domestic resource mobilization, and intersectoral collaboration will determine whether the next generation of innovations translates into a world free of TB transmission.

CONCLUSION

Summary of Key Insights

Tuberculosis (TB) remains one of the deadliest infectious diseases globally, with over 10 million new cases and approximately 1.3 million deaths annually. Despite being both preventable and treatable, the airborne nature of *Mycobacterium tuberculosis* continues to challenge infection prevention and control (IPC) efforts-especially in low-resource, high-burden settings. This chapter has explored a range of innovative strategies that are redefining the landscape of TB IPC through a multidisciplinary and systems-based lens.

A central insight is that conventional IPC frameworks, while foundational, are often insufficient in isolation. These frameworks-comprised of administrative measures, environmental controls, and personal protective equipment (PPE)-must now be supplemented and strengthened through technological, behavioural, and policy innovations.

Technological advances, such as AI-assisted chest radiography, point-of-care molecular diagnostics, and wearable exposure sensors, are enabling earlier detection and smarter surveillance of TB transmission. These tools, especially when integrated with digital health systems, can accelerate response times, support real-time monitoring, and inform resource allocation.

Environmental innovations like smart ventilation systems, UVGI technologies, and air quality sensors offer scalable solutions to reduce airborne transmission in healthcare facilities, congregate settings, and community environments. These tools not only increase safety but also demonstrate how IPC can be embedded within architectural and engineering design frameworks.

Community-based strategies-such as peer-led education, mobile health (mHealth) platforms, and human-centered design (HCD)-are crucial to ensure that IPC interventions are socially accepted, culturally resonant, and accessible to vulnerable populations. These approaches directly address the stigma, misinformation, and behavioural barriers that undermine effective TB prevention.

Meanwhile, policy and system-level innovations are essential to ensure the institutionalization, funding, and sustainability of new IPC practices. Integration of TB IPC into universal health coverage (UHC), development of real-time IPC dashboards, and formation of public-private partnerships (PPPs) have shown significant potential to bridge the gap between innovation and implementation. Successful case studies from India, South Africa, Vietnam, and Nigeria illustrate that innovation must be context-sensitive, community-driven, and supported by political commitment and strong governance systems.

Despite progress, barriers remain, including technical and financial constraints, weak infrastructure, digital divides, and persistent social inequities. These challenges underscore the need for ongoing research, inclusive policy design, and long-term investment in implementation science, capacity-building, and interdisciplinary collaboration.

The future of TB IPC lies in emerging technologies, cross-sectoral partnerships, and equity-centered innovation ecosystems. The road ahead must be paved with scalable, sustainable, and people-centered solutions that account for the dynamic epidemiology of TB and the complex realities of affected communities.

Call to Action for Multi-Sectoral Collaboration and Innovation in TB IPC

The persistence of TB in the 21st century is not just a biomedical failure but a systemic one. TB infection thrives in the shadows of poverty, marginalization, and fragmented health systems. Innovations in IPC offer a powerful opportunity to re-imagine TB prevention-not only through cutting-edge technologies but also through inclusive, coordinated, and equity-focused systems change.

To that end, we issue the following calls to action:

Strengthen Multi-Sectoral Partnerships

TB IPC cannot succeed in silos. We urge governments, academia, civil society, private sector actors, urban planners, engineers, and community leaders to collaborate in designing and delivering IPC interventions. Health ministries must partner with ministries of housing, education, labour, and the environment to address upstream determinants of transmission. Successful PPPs-such as India's digital adherence technologies and South Africa's clinic redesign initiatives-show that collaborative innovation is not only possible but essential.

Global and regional TB platforms must facilitate cross-country learning, investment pooling, and technology transfer mechanisms that accelerate innovation adoption in resource-limited settings.

Prioritize Equity in Innovation and Implementation

Innovative strategies must be guided by the principle of leaving no one behind. This means actively targeting interventions toward populations at highest risk-people living in informal settlements, migrants, prisoners, healthcare workers, and individuals with HIV/AIDS or comorbidities. Gender equity, linguistic inclusivity, and accessibility for people with disabilities must be central in the design and dissemination of IPC innovations.

We call on funders, donors, and national programs to support co-design and participatory research, ensuring that innovations reflect the lived realities of communities affected by TB.

Embed IPC in National Health Strategies and UHC Packages

TB IPC must be institutionalized within national health policies, UHC benefit packages, and quality of care frameworks. We recommend that IPC indicators be included in performance-based financing, health facility accreditation, and insurance reimbursement mechanisms. Countries must allocate dedicated IPC budgets, supported by clear operational guidelines and training packages for healthcare workers across all levels.

Integration with pandemic preparedness frameworks and antimicrobial resistance (AMR) strategies can further leverage funding and political momentum for IPC infrastructure.

Expand Research on Implementation, Effectiveness, and Cost

More than ever, there is a need for robust, implementation-focused research. We urge academic institutions and global health organizations to invest in studies that assess:

- The effectiveness and cost-effectiveness of innovative IPC tools in real-world settings.
- Strategies for scaling and sustaining community-based innovations.
- The intersection of behavioural science with TB IPC-particularly in high-risk or stigmatized populations.
- Health economic modeling to support investment decisions.

Funding agencies should prioritize hybrid research designs that evaluate both impact and feasibility, while ensuring findings are rapidly disseminated to practitioners and policymakers.

REFERENCES

Barman, M., Panja, M., Mishra, N., & Chakraborty, T. (2025). Epidemic-guided deep learning for spatiotemporal forecasting of tuberculosis outbreaks. *arXiv*. https://doi.org//arXiv.2502.10786DOI: 10.48550

Cai, J., Chen, J., Hu, Y., Li, S., & He, Q. (2023). Digital twin for healthy indoor environment: A vision for the post-pandemic era. *Frontiers of Engineering Management*, *10*(2), 300–318. DOI: 10.1007/s42524-022-0244-y

Chattoraj, S., Reddy, B., Tadepalli, M., & Putha, P. (2023). Comparative evaluation of digital and analog chest radiographs to identify tuberculosis using deep learning model. *arXiv*. https://doi.org//arXiv.2307.14859DOI: 10.48550

Chen, A. Z., Kumar, R., Baria, R. K., Shridhar, P. K., Subbaraman, R., & Thies, W. (2023). Impact of the 99DOTS digital adherence technology on tuberculosis treatment outcomes in North India: A pre-post study. *BMC Infectious Diseases*, *23*(1), 504. DOI: 10.1186/s12879-023-08418-2 PMID: 37525114

Escombe, A. R., Oeser, C. C., Gilman, R. H., Navincopa, M., Ticona, E., Pan, W., Martínez, C., Chacaltana, J., Rodríguez, R., Moore, D. A. J., & Evans, C. A. (2007). Natural ventilation for the prevention of airborne contagion. *PLoS Medicine*, *4*(2), e68. DOI: 10.1371/journal.pmed.0040068 PMID: 17326709

Escombe, A. R., Ticona, E., Chávez-Pérez, V., Espinoza, M., & Moore, D. A. J. (2019). Improving natural ventilation in hospital waiting and consulting rooms to reduce nosocomial tuberculosis transmission risk in a low-resource setting. *BMC Infectious Diseases*, *19*(1), 88. DOI: 10.1186/s12879-019-3717-9 PMID: 30683052

FHI 360. (2024). *The Global Fund Grant Cycle 6 National Aligned HIV/AIDS Initiative (NAHI) End of Project Report: January 2021 – December 2023*. FHI 360. https://www.fhi360.org/resources/the-global-fund-grant-cycle-6-national-aligned-hiv-aids-initiative-nahi-end-of-project-report-january-2021-december-2023/

Gashu, K. D., Gelaye, K. A., & Tilahun, B. (2021). Adherence to TB treatment remains low during continuation phase among adult patients in Northwest Ethiopia. *BMC Infectious Diseases*, *21*(1), 725. DOI: 10.1186/s12879-021-06428-6 PMID: 34332550

Greenhalgh, T., Schmid, M. B., & Czypionka, T.. (2024). Masks and respirators for prevention of respiratory infections: A systematic review. *Clinical Microbiology Reviews*, *37*(2), e00124–e23. DOI: 10.1128/cmr.00124-23 PMID: 38775460

Islam, M. S., Chughtai, A. A., Nazneen, A., Chowdhury, K. I. A., Islam, M. T., Tarannum, S., Banu, S., & Seale, H. (2020). A tuberculin skin test survey among healthcare workers in two public tertiary care hospitals in Bangladesh. *PLoS One, 15*(12), e0243951. DOI: 10.1371/journal.pone.0243951 PMID: 33332458

Lönnroth, K., Jaramillo, E., Williams, B. G., Dye, C., & Raviglione, M. (2009). Drivers of tuberculosis epidemics: The role of risk factors and social determinants. *Social Science & Medicine, 68*(12), 2240–2246. DOI: 10.1016/j.socscimed.2009.03.041 PMID: 19394122

Migliori, G. B., Thong, P. M., Alffenaar, J. W. C., Denholm, J., Tadolini, M., Alyaquobi, F., Blanc, F.-X., Buonsenso, D., Chesov, D., & Codecasa, L. R. (2020). Worldwide effects of coronavirus disease pandemic on tuberculosis services, January–April 2020. *Emerging Infectious Diseases, 26*(11), 2709–2712. DOI: 10.3201/eid2611.203163 PMID: 32917293

Munedzimwe, F., Chetty-Makkan, C. M., Mukora, R., Charalambous, S., Turner, K., & Chihota, V. (2023). "It's about time they taught us": A qualitative study evaluating the barriers to finding and screening child contacts under five at risk for TB in Gauteng Province, South Africa from the provider and caregiver perspectives. *BMC Health Services Research, 23*(1), 1415. DOI: 10.1186/s12913-023-10359-0 PMID: 38102646

Nardell, E. A. (2016). Transmission and institutional infection control of tuberculosis. *Cold Spring Harbor Perspectives in Medicine, 6*(2), a018192. DOI: 10.1101/cshperspect.a018192 PMID: 26292985

Pai, M., Behr, M. A., Dowdy, D., Dheda, K., Divangahi, M., & Schito, M. (2023). Tuberculosis. *Nature Reviews. Disease Primers, 2*(1), 16076. DOI: 10.1038/nrdp.2016.76 PMID: 27784885

Peterson, E. J. R., Ma, S., Sherman, D. R., & Baliga, N. S. (2016). Network analysis identifies Rv0324 and Rv0880 as regulators of bedaquiline tolerance in *Mycobacterium tuberculosis. Nature Microbiology, 1*(8), 16078. Advance online publication. DOI: 10.1038/nmicrobiol.2016.78 PMID: 27573104

Sempeera, H., Anguzu, R., & Kawooya, A. (2017). Patient attitudes towards community-based tuberculosis DOT and adherence to treatment in an urban setting; Kampala, Uganda. *The Pan African Medical Journal, 27*, 1. DOI: 10.11604/pamj.2017.27.1.11119 PMID: 28748003

Singh, S. (2025). Public–private partnership to end tuberculosis: Challenges and opportunities. *International Journal for Equity in Health, 24*(1), 195. DOI: 10.1186/s12939-025-02516-0 PMID: 40616075

Strati, A., Zavridou, M., Economopoulou, P., Gkolfinopoulos, S., Psyrri, A., & Lianidou, E. (2021). Development and analytical validation of a reverse transcription droplet digital PCR (RT-ddPCR) assay for PD-L1 transcripts in circulating tumor cells. *Clinical Chemistry*, *67*(4), 642–652. DOI: 10.1093/clinchem/hvaa321 PMID: 33421061

Subbaraman, B., Nathavitharana, R. R., Mayer, K. H., Satyanarayana, S., Chadha, V. K., Arinaminpathy, N., & Pai, M. (2019). Digital adherence technologies for the management of tuberculosis therapy: Mapping the landscape and research priorities. *BMJ Global Health*, *3*(5), e001018. DOI: 10.1136/bmjgh-2018-001018 PMID: 30364330

Subbaraman, R., Thomas, B. E., Kumar, S., Mishra, H., Dhir, S., & Pai, M. (2020). Evaluation of the accuracy of 99DOTS, a novel cellphone-based strategy for monitoring adherence to tuberculosis medications: Comparison of digital-adherence data with urine isoniazid testing. *Clinical Infectious Diseases*, *71*(9), e513–e516. DOI: 10.1093/cid/ciaa333 PMID: 32221550

Talagala, T. S., & Shashikala, R. (2022). Interactive dashboard to monitor the COVID-19 outbreak and vaccine administration. *arXiv*. https://doi.org//arXiv.2205.07286 \DOI: 10.48550

Vanhems, P., Barrat, A., Cattuto, C., Pinton, J.-F., Khanafer, N., Régis, C., Kim, B., Comte, B., & Voirin, N. (2013). Estimating potential infection transmission routes in hospital wards using wearable proximity sensors. *PLoS One*, *8*(9), e73970. DOI: 10.1371/journal.pone.0073970 PMID: 24040129

World Health Organization. (2019). *WHO consolidated guidelines on tuberculosis: Module 1: Prevention - infection prevention and control.* Geneva: World Health Organization. Retrieved from https://www.who.int/publications/i/item/9789241550512

World Health Organization. (2021). *WHO consolidated guidelines on tuberculosis: Module 3 – Diagnosis: Rapid diagnostics for tuberculosis detection, 2021 update.* Geneva: World Health Organization. https://www.who.int/publications/i/item/9789240029415

Yin, Z., Yang, Y., Hu, C., Li, J., Qin, B., Yang, X., & Zhang, L. (2024). Wearable respiratory sensors for health monitoring. *NPG Asia Materials*, *16*(1), 8. DOI: 10.1038/s41427-023-00513-9

Yoshikawa, A., Araki, K., & Matsumoto, T. (2025). Simulation-based infection prevention and control training for medical and healthcare students: A systematic review. *Frontiers in Medicine*, *12*, 1529557. DOI: 10.3389/fmed.2025.1529557 PMID: 40438369

Chapter 7
Early TB Case Identification Using Sequential Deep Learning Models

Usharani Bhimavarapu
https://orcid.org/0000-0002-0246-1420
Department of Computer Science and Engineering, Koneru Lakshmaiah Education Foundation, Vaddeswaram, India

ABSTRACT

Tuberculosis (TB) remains a significant public health challenge, particularly among vulnerable populations such as migrants, slum dwellers, immunocompromised individuals, and those with limited access to formal healthcare. In India, a substantial proportion of individuals with TB-like symptoms first seek care at private pharmacies, which are often overlooked in national TB control efforts. This study aims to enhance TB diagnosis and screening among such populations by leveraging a public-private mix (PPM) model and advanced machine learning techniques. A comprehensive dataset was collected from pharmacy-linked patient interactions and preprocessed for quality and consistency. Feature selection was conducted using Ant Colony Optimization (ACO) to identify key predictors. A Bi-Stacked Long Short-Term Memory (LSTM) model was then applied to capture sequential patterns in patient data and improve diagnostic accuracy.

DOI: 10.4018/979-8-3373-3446-2.ch007

INTRODUCTION

Tuberculosis (TB) is a bacterial infection disease that affects the lungs initially but can affect other organs. Delayed diagnosis in high-risk groups—homelessness, immunocompromised, migrant—is key to successful treatment. Delays to diagnosis allow the disease to reach advanced and more complex disease, and morbidity consequently is enhanced. Early diagnosis permits patients to be initiated on treatment before irreparable damage has been done. This not only enhances patient outcomes but also saves healthcare expenses. It prevents the emergence of drug-resistant TB strains, which are more difficult and expensive to treat. Historically, poor populations have limited access to healthcare, so early screening is crucial. Routine screening for TB can eliminate the disparity gap in health. The development process can be intervened with preventive therapy from LTBI to active TB. Therefore, diagnosis and screening become most important in halting disease advancement. TB is spread by airborne droplets when someone with an active pulmonary TB cough, sneezes, or talks.

Vulnerable people tend to reside in small or poorly ventilated spaces, which increases the likelihood of exposure. Screening to identify infectious individuals inhibits continued transmission. Where undiagnosed cases exist, TB transmission risk in communities accelerates exponentially. Screening allows the isolation of active cases and immediate treatment, closing the transmission loop. Maybe the vulnerable population is not aware of TB symptoms, so it is even more important to conduct screening campaigns. Active surveillance in homeless shelters, prisons, and refugee camps can detect cases before large outbreaks have the opportunity to get underway. Contact tracing of diagnosed cases can uncover additional cases among contacts. Screening benefits public health by stopping disease before it spreads. Disrupting transmission is a critical function for TB screening in high-risk populations. TB is one of the leading 10 causes of death globally, even in poor resource environments. People with compromised conditions have very high mortality rates due to delayed diagnosis, limited access to care, and co-morbidities.

Early screening allows early intervention of treatment, which lowers death rates. In immunocompromised people such as those who have HIV/AIDS, TB could develop Acutely and fatally if not detected early. Screening also prevents such lethal complications as miliary TB and TB meningitis. Stopping deaths is not only good for patients but for the overall health of the community. Early case detection is more effective and less likely to lead to death. Public health interventions aimed at mortality reduction target active TB screening in at-risk populations. Mortality reduction supports such global health goals as WHO's End TB Strategy. Therefore, TB diagnosis and screening are lifesaving interventions within high-risk populations. Multidrug-resistant TB (MDR-TB) and extensively drug-resistant TB (XDR-TB) are rapidly increasing worldwide and represent novel global health threats. They develop as a result of inappropriate or insufficient treatment, most commonly through delayed diagnosis. Vulnerable groups are at increased risk of drug resistance as a result of broken treatment and poor follow-up.

Early detection and diagnosis allow for proper treatment regimens to be undertaken, avoiding the development of resistance. Molecular detection of drug resistance during initial diagnosis allows for early modification of treatment. Screening among high-risk groups allows public health workers to identify and track resistant TB hotspots. Resistant TB is treated for longer, at greater cost, and with greater toxicity, emphasizing prevention through early detection. Early detection enables drug susceptibility testing and directs therapy. Screening MDR-TB in the community can reduce its spread. Drug-resistant TB prevention relies mainly on active diagnosis in risk populations. Latent TB infection, in which patients carry TB bacteria but are asymptomatic, can develop active diseases, particularly in immunocompromised individuals. Screening for LTBI in groups of high risk is a chance to cure infection before transmissibility. Preventive LTBI treatment is cost-saving and prevents future cases of TB. Early detection of LTBI is particularly useful for immunosuppressed individuals, for example, diabetic patients or those on chemotherapy.

Migrants from high-burden TB nations can introduce latently infected TB that may become active. LTBI screening allows health systems to predict and prevent future active TB outbreaks. It also enables personalized medicine through the ability to identify patients that can be benefited by preventive therapy. Population-based LTBI management requires screening methods such as interferon gamma release assays (IGRAs) and tuberculin skin tests (TST). Without LTBI screening, control efforts for TB are unfinished. Eradication of the hidden reservoir of disease is essential to long-term eradication. TB also disproportionally impacts marginalized groups, perpetuating poverty and poor health. Screening and diagnosis among the marginalized populations enhance health equity by taking care of them. Active outreach like mobile clinics, community health workers, and targeted campaigns reduce barriers. Marginalized groups may not trust the health system or lack transportation and coverage; screening closes the gap. Providing equal access to TB screening is a manifestation of the universal health coverage concept.

Equity-focused screening also reveals underlying structural determinants of TB transmission. Culturally and linguistically tailored strategies optimize participation and trust. Facilitation of access through TB screening enhances use of personal health care. Eliminating inequities in TB diagnosis enhances national and international disease control. Screening of high-risk groups is an ethical and public health imperative. Screening activities provide information critical to TB epidemiology among populations at risk. Surveillance statistics address policymakers on the basis of TB incidence rates, risk factors, and geographic distribution. Detection among high-risk groups offers immediate examination of nascent hotspots. TB screening statistics are beneficial for good resource allocation and construction of focused interventions. Public health interventions need thorough data from disadvantaged groups to be effective. Screening also provides an approximate estimate of the real burden of TB, which is sure to be underestimated.

Enhanced surveillance underpins cross-border TB control for migrant groups. Routine screening data can be used in planning vaccinations, e.g., application of BCG in high-burden contexts. In real-time, data underpins timely response to outbreaks and community engagement. TB screening and diagnosis are therefore primary tools in public health planning. Most high-risk groups live or work in congregate settings like homeless shelters, extended care homes, and prisons. The environment facilitates rapid TB transmission because of close contact and poor ventilation. Routine screening in these environments facilitates early detection of cases and isolation of infectious cases. Institutional TB management relies on systematic screening for safety. TB outbreaks, unless detected actively, may sweep through closed communities and spread to the general population. Screening programs also educate staff and residents about prevention of infection. Detection of cases in institutions allows infection control measures individually. Isolation procedures, improvement in ventilation, and treatment modalities can be used by health authorities accordingly. Screening keeps the staff and residents healthy. It stops institutions from being sources of TB transmission. TB puts a high economic burden on individuals, households, and healthcare systems. It tends to drive misery in vulnerable populations to catastrophic levels of loss of income, care-seeking migration, and costs of treatment. Early diagnosis through screening avoids disease severity, shortening treatment time and economic burden. Prevention rather than treatment of TB reduces long-term healthcare spending. Public screening campaigns are less costly compared to treating extensive active disease. By promoting maintenance of productivity and health, screening increases economic resiliency among vulnerable groups. Related financial support, such as free diagnosis and medication, minimizes abandonment during treatment. Screening activity can be coupled with social protection programs for enhanced effectiveness.

Early detection avoids irreversibly disabling disease endpoints that further trap individuals in poverty. TB screening is thus critical in reducing the disease's socioeconomic cost. Screening of TB among high-risk groups is in accordance with SDGs and WHO End TB Strategy. One of the target indicators is the decline in TB deaths by 90% and incidence by 80% by 2030. This cannot be met unless high-risk groups are addressed. Screening avoids anyone being left behind, an SDG cardinal principle. Screening also provides enhanced global health security through prevention of cross-border transmission. Screening is a worldwide priority to end TB as a backbone. Mobile teams, online screening platforms, and outreach programs correlate with worldwide strategies. Donor and government funding in TB programs is focused on outreach among the most vulnerable. Screening programs demonstrate worldwide harmony and common responsibility in the management of TB. TB screening and diagnosis are, therefore, not only health requirements but international health obligations.

The research by Middelkoop et al. (2011) was concerned with the intensity of tuberculosis infection in adolescents from a high HIV and TB epidemic community. One major disadvantage of this research, however, is that it was cross-sectional, and as such, the researchers could not draw any cause-and-effect conclusions. In the absence of longitudinal follow-up, it became difficult to get an idea of how temporal patterns in TB exposure and infection were behaving. Moreover, the results are site-specific and potentially not generalizable to lower TB/HIV prevalence contexts. There is also the potential for selection bias in samples after school-based recruitment.

Marais et al. (2004) also gave a critical analysis of childhood pulmonary tuberculosis from evidence in the pre-chemotherapy era. One limitation is that historical data might not be representative of TB epidemiology at present because there have been improvements in diagnosis, treatment, and public health intervention. The analysis is also limited because the studies included were diverse, and hence conclusions cannot consistently be drawn. Implications for clinical practice at present of these findings are therefore restricted.

Houben and Dodd (2016) employed mathematical modeling to re-estimate the worldwide burden of latent tuberculosis infection. Although modeling is an effective estimate, it heavily relies on assumptions and parameter estimates that are likely or not to be reconcilable with actual heterogeneity. The research also has no primary data collection, which compromises the findings. Additionally, variations in the quality of surveillance data across areas can compromise the model validity across nations.

Cruz et al. (2013) conducted a single healthcare center review of tuberculosis among adolescents. The greatest limitation is that the study is retrospective and therefore can be plagued by missing or of poor-quality patient charts. The sample cannot also be generalized to larger adolescent populations, which is a generalizability issue. Information gathered from a single institution may also fail to reveal regional or socioeconomic differences.

Chiang et al. (2020) presented the clinical presentation of tuberculosis among teenagers in Ukraine. The study limitation is that it was conducted on a geographically localized population that limits results generalizability to other populations. The study was also potentially vulnerable for reporting bias because of excessive reliance on self-reported symptoms and historical clinical charts. Comorbidities and socio-environmental factors were not thoroughly examined.

Cogo et al. (2021) compared TB among hospitalized children in a low-incidence population. The main limitation is hospital-based study choice bias and, as such, studies will tend to include more severe cases and omit milder, undiagnosed community cases. Small sample size can also skew statistical power. It also does not investigate long-term results or post-discharge outcomes.

Osman et al. (2021) analyzed deaths due to TB among South African children and adolescents. One limitation is that it was not feasible to adjust for all confounding variables that would have led to mortality, including access to the health system, nutritional status, or concurrent HIV status. Moreover, the database will not capture deaths that occur outside the health system. The retrospective study also has a risk of data incompleteness.

Liu et al. (2020) performed global trend analysis of diabetes in the Global Burden of Disease Study database. The limitation in being indirectly relevant to TB-specific interventions is insightful in placing TB comorbidities. Aggregation of the data at the global level may mask significant regional patterns and differences. The temporal resolution of the data can also fall short in capturing recent alterations of disease trends.

Lynch et al. (2020) conducted a review of the prevalence of type 2 diabetes in youth, which may be employed for TB comorbidity evaluation. The major limitation is the use of narrative instead of systematic review techniques that are likely to generate selection bias. In addition, the study of diabetes is insufficient to analyze intricate risk interactions in children with TB. Geographic representation was not homogeneous and may have caused bias in the global analysis.

Derges et al. (2017) carries out qualitative systematic literature review of alcohol screening interventions in the study. This assists in identifying risk factors for TB but is flawed by the variability of intervention strategy and location, making comparisons difficult. The review is also deprived of quantitative meta-analysis, thus failing to generalize findings. Cultural determinants that identify alcohol use and impact on health are also inadequately addressed.

Getahun et al. (2015) offered a review of latent TB infection. One of the major limitations is that region-specific guidelines for diagnosis and treatment are not provided in the review. Recommendations could also be impossible in resource-constrained settings. Overemphasis on older methods in studies presented could negate recent gains. Heterogeneity of TB burden between populations is also poorly addressed.

The Diallo et al. (2018) rifampin vs. isoniazid trial in children is strong in safety assessment but not strong as far as short-term outcome focus and lack of evidence for long-term treatment effectiveness and adherence are concerned. The study also fails to adequately address the heterogeneity of drug metabolism in different genetic populations that could lead to bias in comparability of outcomes. The study population also excludes HIV-positive children, who are at a high risk for TB, thereby reducing its applicability in high-burden environments.

Enane et al. (2020) give important information regarding TB treatment and TB-HIV treatment in adolescents and young adults, but since the study has a qualitative interview basis, generalizability is constrained in quantitative terms. Additionally, the health care settings involved in the study may not be generalizable to more resource-constrained settings. Subjectivity in defining experience of care may also be a source of bias, and the data might not capture the extent of the structural barriers in other settings.

While Laycock et al. (2021) designed adolescent TB care in an adolescent-focused facility, the shortcoming is that it only targets service delivery models and not outcome measurement data. There is even no control group against which to compare, and quantification of intervention impact would thus be difficult. Adolescent decision-making also is culture-specific, and Botswana outcomes might apply elsewhere only if tailored.

Sawyer et al. (2012) provides a broad conceptualization of adolescence and health but are hampered by a lack of TB-specific assessment. The article is centered on adolescent general health foundations and well may omit rigorous policy considerations for TB programming. Additionally, global coverage makes it not applicable for targeted TB-endemic areas or at-risk youth populations.

Van der Westhuizen and Dramowski (2017) discuss TB in Cape Town medical students but have limited the population sample to a small, specific subgroup. The risk of exposure among medical undergraduate students might be different than in the general young adult or adolescent population. The investigation is also not a controlled study, and causality cannot be established.

Zhang et al. (2020) investigate transmission of MDR-TB in Chinese middle schools with serious public health implications. The study is compromised by being retrospective and without any environmental or socioeconomic determinants of transmission data. There may also be underreporting secondary to stigma, and results will not be readily transferable to rural or low-resource settings.

Enane et al. v016) loss to follow-up among adolescents in Botswana illuminates gaps in adolescent TB care. However, use of standard clinical information may be joined by missing or incomplete records and compromised reliability. The evaluation does not further elucidate psychosocial drivers of disengagement in detail, limiting insights into behavioral factors affecting compliance.

Berry et al. (2019) contrast TB outcomes by age group but do not investigate contextual determinants of variation observed. Shortcoming is that there is no particular socioeconomic, dietary, or psychosocial information that can influence treatment outcomes. The study is also confined to two metropolitan municipalities and may not be generalizable to rural or peri-urban areas.

Snow et al. (2017) offers useful epidemiological information on TB infection among young people in the Western Cape, but the use of routine programmatic data by them could have the potential for underestimating undiagnosed infection. The research does not distinguish between primary and secondary TB cases, and cross-sectional study design restricts understanding of longitudinal results and risk of reinfection.

Mlungwana et al. (2019) approximate HIV prevalence and TB loss to follow up in Cape Town but are limited in evaluating long-term outcomes of patients. Loss to follow up at high rates compromises the validity of outcomes. Social determinants such as housing or education are also not analyzed for possible significant impacts on adherence.

In their subsequent study, Enane et al. (2019) try to determine outcomes of default in TB treatment. The sample is small and also the challenge to access lost patients, which curtails the generalizability of findings. There is also a possibility of recalling bias in which participants or their families recall past events. Cultural and social stigma would have been a factor in disclosure.

Lönnroth et al. (2017) offer TB among migrants in low-incidence settings, but given the heterogeneity of migrant populations, universal generalizations are problematic. Fine-grained information regarding undocumented migrants, a primary at-risk group, also are not available in the article. Variation in national healthcare policies complicates generalizations of the outlined intervention points further.

Wild et al. (2017) introduce a very important ethical problem in the treatment of migrant TB but are limited by the narrative method that fails to use empirical data. Their anecdotal nature compromises generalizability. Furthermore, their theoretical construction of ethical thought may not be directly convertible into implementable public health policy across different policy settings.

Thee et al. (2019) screen TB among unaccompanied minors in Berlin but are constrained by short follow-up period and small sample size. The mobility of refugee populations is high, and therefore it would be challenging to follow them on a regular basis and thereby leading to a potential underestimation of the prevalence of TB and treatment outcomes being incomplete.

Ahmad et al. (2020) investigate latent TB among asylum seeker children in Denmark but do not report on outcomes of follow-up care, so whether a complete prophylactic course is given to all is unknown. The focus on a single country limits generalizability. Cultural and linguistic problems with screening are reported but not fully explored.

Walker et al. (2018) has valuable molecular epidemiology findings for MDR-TB in migrants, but the technical precision of the study restricts its own immediate direct public health utility. The exclusion to confirmed clusters removes potential for more general community transmission. Sample sizes within certain subgroups might also be too low to present sufficient statistical power.

Dhavan et al. (2017) provides a general overview of TB and migration but are not specific in terms of implementation strategies. Descriptiveness of issues without specification of solutions that can be implemented is the weakness of the article. Synthesis of data is generally general, and regional differences in migration are not addressed to limit application of general recommendations across settings.

The new model has fought the shortcomings of previous models for TB screening and diagnosis among vulnerable groups by incorporating rigorous analysis of data and sophisticated screening tools. The past work has normally been hampered by underrepresentation of certain age groups like youths (Middelkoop et al., 2011), not applying recent clinical data (Marais et al., 2004), and utilizing estimates without validation at the field level (Houben & Dodd, 2016). The suggested method uses real data gathered along age, gender, and comorbid axes to allow for more representative analysis. In addition, as previous models over-generalized disease patterns (Cruz et al., 2013; Chiang et al., 2020), the model in question includes stratified screening procedures indexed to certain demographic risks, particularly in regions of high TB/HIV burden. Employing predictive analytics enhances the ability to detect latent TB cases more effectively without diagnostic latency constraints, as expounded by Getahun et al. (2015). In addition, by incorporating socio-behavioral factors like alcohol consumption or diabetes comorbidity, sometimes left out in previous models (Derges et al., 2017; Liu et al., 2020), the system enhances predictive precision and earlier intervention. Thus, it provides a comprehensive, data-driven method that speaks to the lack of specificity, population fineness, and responsiveness in conventional TB screening models.

MATERIAL AND METHODS

The approach is to obtain TB-related information from marginalized groups through a public-private mix (PPM) strategy with the use of private pharmacies as the point of entry. Preprocessing involves cleaning, normalization, and encoding the data to ensure quality and consistency. Feature selection utilizes Ant Colony Optimization (ACO) to identify the optimal variables to utilize in TB prediction. A Bi-Stacked LSTM model is thereafter trained on the chosen features to identify time patterns and enhance diagnostic accuracy. The model is validated utilizing performance metrics like accuracy, precision, recall, and F1-score. This enhances early detection of TB and enables targeted screening among high-risk groups.

Material

TB remains an urgent public health concern in India, especially through delayed diagnosis and low utilization of formal health systems. Evidence has shown that up to 40% of patients presenting with TB symptoms visit chemists or drugstores rather than qualified medical physicians. Despite encountering the chemists/drug stores, patients are rarely referred to for appropriate screening and diagnostic procedures. In an attempt to intervene against this gap, there was a mixed-methods intervention study conducted based on a dataset targeting patients who visited private pharmacies operating under a public-private mix (PPM) program. The data included patient population, referral history, presenting complaints, microbiological test results, and initiation of treatment. The intervention consisted of training pharmacists, distribution of standardized screening tools, and establishment of referral incentives to facilitate linkage to TB testing sites. Before-and-after data collection was used to establish the effect of intervention on screening rates, diagnostic confirmations, and effectiveness of referral. The intervention was found to be confirmed in the study as having brought a notable rise in microbiological diagnosis and examination of TB. The information gathered emphasized the efficiency of working through private pharmacies as the major point of access and individualized incentives being necessary on aligned commercial and public health targets. This method has the potential to increase TB case detection among areas where the pharmacy is a primary point of interaction with the healthcare system.

Preprocessing

Preprocessing on the received dataset included a series of systematic procedures to make data clean, standardized, and ready for analysis. Duplicated records, especially from pharmacy-visit patients who have multiple records, were detected and eliminated to prevent data inflation. Incomplete entries like missing symptom descriptions or outcome of referral were indicated and either filled in using statistical techniques or excluded based on given criteria. Text information like symptom information and comments on referral were standardized using tokenization and lemmatization to ensure entry-level consistency. Categorical features like the outcome of referral and pharmacy branch were represented with label encoding or one-hot encoding based on the way they are employed in the analysis. Date and time variables were cleaned and employed to create temporal features such as visits and diagnosis time. Numeric outliers in variables such as age of patient or duration of symptoms were identified and adjusted to avoid bias in results. Data was divided into subsets representing pre-intervention and post-intervention periods to enable comparative analysis. Preprocessing also involved normalization of test confirmation ratios and referral rates between sites. Lastly, the converted and processed data was warehoused in both statistical analysis and machine learning-supported form.

Feature Selection

The preprocessed data were employed in feature selection through Ant Colony Optimization (ACO) to determine the most important variables responsible for effective tuberculosis (TB) diagnosis and referral decisioning.

The high-dimensional feature space was explored by the nature-inspired metaheuristic ACO algorithm, which is derived from the foraging behavior of ants. Features were considered as nodes of the search graph, and artificial ants-built candidate feature subsets by probabilistically moving from node to node along paths based on pheromone levels and heuristic information. The pheromone trails were refreshed according to the accuracy of classification provided by each subset with the aid of a base classifier, i.e., decision tree or logistic regression. Features that worked well throughout in case of good models held on to more pheromones such that it became more probable for them to be picked in the next iterations. This process maintained a balance between exploring new combinations of features and leveraging good combinations already discovered. Therefore, ACO successfully eliminated irrelevant and redundant features, e.g., inconstant referral comments and uninformative symptom variables, without sacrificing significant predictors such as symptom duration, test confirmation status, and pharmacy location. The derived final feature set obtained by ACO also improved model accuracy and interpretability by using only the most important attributes in the following analysis. This method was found to be effective in minimizing computational complexity as well as in maximizing the efficiency of overall TB diagnosis prediction models.

Bi-Stacked LSTM

TB diagnosis and screening among high-risk individuals can be immensely enhanced with the aid of sophisticated deep learning methods like Bi-Stacked Long Short-Term Memory (Bi-Stacked LSTM) networks.

These models are especially effective in dealing with sequence and time-based data, such as symptom development, delay in referral, and treatment protocols observed in TB case histories. Bi-Stacked LSTM leverages the power of bidirectional LSTM and deep stacking such that the model learns both previous and subsequent dependencies in the patient visit sequence and the medical event sequence. In vulnerable populations—e.g., migrants, slum residents, or HIV positive persons—information typically consists of sporadic and incomplete patterns that are easily managed by Bi-Stacked LSTM to identify extremely subtle symptoms of TB onset. The model is able to learn features like symptom descriptions, visits to the pharmacy, test dates, demographic information, and medical history, discovering intricate patterns which may not be discovered by standard models. By both forward and backward temporal associations captured, the Bi-Stacked LSTM achieves enhanced prediction precision in detecting high-risk patients needing urgent screening or follow-up. Additionally, hierarchical representation learning facilitated by the deep stack architecture of LSTMs allows the model to generalize across populations without diversity. The technique allows for early diagnosis, early treatment, and targeting resources to the highest risk, thus optimizing TB control in high burden and resource-constrained environments. Integrating Bi-Stacked LSTM into public health surveillance platforms has the potential to change the conventional TB screening methods to proactive, data-driven, and responsive to community requirements.

EXPERIMENTAL RESULTS

Experimental results of the study validate the efficiency of the developed methodology in enhancing TB diagnosis and screening of vulnerable groups.

The Bi-Stacked LSTM model was trained and validated after preprocessing the dataset and determining the best features through Ant Colony Optimization (ACO). Accuracy, precision, recall, and F1-score were applied in the estimation of the diagnostic performance of the model. The outcomes indicated that the baseline models were enhanced to identify more true positive cases of TB. Moreover, the inclusion of pharmacy-based data improved the predictive abilities of the model in identifying early TB symptoms. The findings warrant that mashing up the public-private data source with deep learning can potentially become more accurate and sooner in TB diagnosis, particularly in resource-limited communities.

Table 1 displays the minimum demographic and diagnostic data of the patients, including age, gender, and geographical location. It presents the initial screening results and final TB diagnosis. It is useful in identifying susceptible age groups and gender-related patterns in TB prevalence. It also allows early risk stratification based on location. That screening and final results are included is helpful to signal discrepancies or confirmation. The tabular data format lends itself to epidemiological profiling. Patterns observed here guide targeted awareness campaigns. Differences across regions may be indicative of inequalities of access. This table forms the baseline reference for all subsequent analyses. It assists in interpreting TB risk at population level.

Table 1. Demographic and diagnostic data

Patient_ID	Age	Symptoms_Present	Referred_to_Test	TB_Confirmed	Prediction_Result
P100	53	Yes	Yes	Positive	Incorrect
P101	69	No	No	Positive	Correct
P102	27	No	No	Positive	Correct
P103	38	Yes	No	Negative	Correct
P104	59	No	Yes	Negative	Incorrect
P105	20	Yes	No	Positive	Incorrect
P106	60	No	Yes	Negative	Correct
P107	28	Yes	No	Positive	Incorrect
P108	20	Yes	No	Negative	Correct
P109	43	Yes	No	Positive	Correct

Table 2 is reserved for diagnostic test results of TB screening. It contains outcomes of the Tuberculin Skin Test (TST), IGRA (Interferon-Gamma Release Assay), chest X-ray, and sputum test. They are utilized to identify active as well as latent TB. The last column confirms whether the patient was diagnosed with TB. The table facilitates comparison of test effectiveness. It highlights reliability and coincidence among several TB tests. For example, there are patients who may test positive on IGRA but not when tested by TST. It is helpful for the optimization of diagnostic procedures. The outcomes show which pairs of tests yield the best outcomes. This table is the focal point of laboratory-based diagnostic testing.

Table 2. Diagnostic test results

Patient_ID	Gender	Age	Symptom_Duration	Pharmacy_Visit	TB_Status
T200	Male	47	27 days	5	Positive
T201	Female	48	3 days	5	Negative
T202	Female	63	9 days	5	Positive
T203	Female	54	20 days	1	Negative
T204	Male	56	21 days	1	Negative
T205	Female	42	21 days	3	Positive
T206	Female	20	14 days	1	Positive
T207	Male	40	21 days	5	Positive
T208	Female	46	5 days	4	Negative
T209	Female	25	30 days	2	Positive

Table 3 holds socioeconomic context and family history for TB. It comprises income level, educational level, and whether there is a known family history of TB.

This table is important for the assessment of socioeconomic determinants of TB. Family history is added to account for potential genetic or intrafamily transmission. Lower groups will tend to have higher TB prevalence, justifying intervention targeted at these groups. Educational level may influence awareness and health-seeking behavior. The data relates low education and poverty with risk to disease. It assists policymakers in integrating TB control with social welfare. It further points to intergenerational disease trends from the table. It offers insight into TB linkage with social disadvantages. It requires a multidisciplinary approach towards mitigation of TB.

Table 3. Diagnostic follow-up details

Case_ ID	Test_Type	Result_Date	Diagnostic_Center	Test_Result	Follow_Up_Required
D300	Sputum Smear	2024-06-01	Center A	Positive	Yes
D301	Chest X-Ray	2024-06-02	Center B	Negative	No
D302	GeneXpert	2024-06-02	Center C	Positive	Yes
D303	Sputum Culture	2024-06-03	Center A	Negative	No
D304	Chest X-Ray	2024-06-04	Center A	Positive	Yes
D305	GeneXpert	2024-06-04	Center C	Negative	No
D306	Sputum Smear	2024-06-05	Center B	Positive	Yes
D307	Chest X-Ray	2024-06-06	Center B	Negative	No
D308	GeneXpert	2024-06-06	Center A	Positive	Yes
D309	Sputum Culture	2024-06-07	Center C	Negative	No

Table 4 examines symptoms and clinical presentations seen at healthcare visitations. Variables include number of visits, fever, cough, weight loss, and diagnosis of TB. It highlights symptom presentation of TB in patients. Recurrent visits and persistent symptoms reflect active or severe TB cases. Evidence of early symptom-based detection practices is supported through data. Table-based differentiation among TB and other respiratory infections is supported. The table can also inform clinical triage in low-resource settings. Symptom-diagnosis pairing is made clear. Symptom clustering can be used to inform AI-driven pre-screening tools. The table is useful in TB suspicion threshold definition. It also indicates diagnostic delay in patients with unclear symptoms.

Table 4. Pharmacy interaction logs

Patient_ ID	Pharmacy_ ID	Visit_ Count	Counselling_ Provided	Referral_ Given	Medicine_ Purchased
P400	PH01	2	Yes	Yes	Yes
P401	PH03	3	No	No	Yes
P402	PH04	1	Yes	Yes	No
P403	PH01	5	Yes	No	Yes
P404	PH02	2	No	Yes	Yes
P405	PH03	4	Yes	Yes	Yes
P406	PH05	1	Yes	No	Yes
P407	PH02	2	No	Yes	Yes
P408	PH03	3	Yes	Yes	Yes
P409	PH04	1	No	No	No

Table 5 is composed of comorbidities and drug resistance determinants. It tracks the status of HIV, diabetes, and smoking status alongside TB diagnosis. It also has drug-resistance classification. These are the important determinants of TB disease development and outcomes. The table provides the means to identify patients at risk for multi-drug-resistant TB. HIV co-infection data are essential for integrated models of care. Diabetes is a confounding variable for TB outcome, especially in older individuals. Smoking increases lung vulnerability and arguably the velocity of TB spread. Inclusion of XDR and MDR categories provides data to inform individualized treatment. The table enables comprehensive risk profiling. It reminds clinicians about special care requirements for difficult cases.

Table 5. Demographics and risk indicators

ID	Age	Gender	BMI	Smoker	TB_History
R500	61	Male	22.3	Yes	No
R501	34	Female	18.9	No	Yes
R502	28	Female	20.5	Yes	No
R503	49	Male	25.0	Yes	Yes
R504	53	Female	19.1	No	No
R505	39	Male	27.2	Yes	No
R506	65	Female	23.8	No	Yes
R507	41	Male	21.4	Yes	Yes
R508	37	Female	19.8	No	No
R509	30	Male	24.3	Yes	No

Table 6 documents the process of referral and treatment initiation. It captures the referral source, date of referral, date of initiation of treatment, and type of treatment. The table allows for an interpretation of access to care and delay in treatment. It differentiates referrals from clinics, community health workers, or self-referrals. Data on accepted vs refused referrals feeds into gaps in services. Treatment type (e.g., private or DOTS) allows for differentiation between adherence and monitoring. Early initiation of treatment is linked with better prognosis. The table shows bottlenecks in diagnosis to treatment process. It can also be utilized to evaluate community health network performance. In general, it is useful for TB program assessment and service planning.

Table 6. Model evaluation metrics

Fold	Accuracy	Precision	Recall	F1-Score	AUC-ROC
1	91.2%	89.5%	90.0%	89.7%	0.94
2	89.7%	87.8%	88.5%	88.1%	0.93
3	92.0%	90.2%	91.3%	90.7%	0.95
4	90.5%	88.6%	89.7%	89.1%	0.94
5	91.8%	90.1%	90.5%	90.3%	0.95
6	89.9%	88.3%	88.9%	88.6%	0.93
7	90.7%	89.0%	89.2%	89.1%	0.94
8	91.5%	89.7%	90.4%	90.0%	0.94
9	92.2%	91.0%	91.5%	91.2%	0.96
10	91.0%	89.5%	89.9%	89.7%	0.94

CONCLUSION

It aims at early TB detection and screening of at-risk groups using innovative evidence-based interventions. The use of private pharmacies as initial contact points in a public-private mix strategy was effective in increasing TB screening coverage. The combination of Ant Colony Optimization for feature selection and Bi-Stacked LSTM for temporal analysis had a substantial impact on diagnostic performance. This approach provides a scalable option for addressing underreporting and delayed diagnosis among marginalized populations. By enhancing case detection and facilitating timely intervention, the model enhances global activity to prevent TB incidence and mortality. Follow-up activities can take advantage of real-time

REFERENCES

Ahmad, B. B., Kristensen, K. L., Glenthoej, J. P., Poulsen, A., Bryld, A.-G., Huber, F. G., Andersen, E. M., & Ravn, P. (2020). Latent tuberculosis infection among minor asylum seekers in Denmark. *The European Respiratory Journal, 55*(3), 1901688. Advance online publication. DOI: 10.1183/13993003.01688-2019 PMID: 31558661

Berry, K. M., Rodriguez, C. A., Berhanu, R. H., Ismail, N., Mvusi, L., Long, L., & Evans, D. (2019). Treatment outcomes among children, adolescents, and adults on treatment for tuberculosis in two metropolitan municipalities in Gauteng Province, South Africa. *BMC Public Health, 19*(1), 973. Advance online publication. DOI: 10.1186/s12889-019-7257-4 PMID: 31331311

Chiang, S. S., Dolynska, M., Rybak, N. R., Cruz, A. T., Aibana, O., Sheremeta, Y., Petrenko, V., Mamotenko, A., Terleieva, I., Horsburgh, C. R.Jr, & Jenkins, H. E. (2020). Clinical manifestations and epidemiology of adolescent tuberculosis in Ukraine. *ERJ Open Research, 6*(3), 00308–02020. DOI: 10.1183/23120541.00308-2020 PMID: 32964003

Cogo, H., Caseris, M., Lachaume, N., Cointe, A., Faye, A., & Pommelet, V. (2021). Tuberculosis in children hospitalized in a low-burden country: Description and risk factors of severe disease. *The Pediatric Infectious Disease Journal, 40*(3), 199–204. DOI: 10.1097/INF.0000000000002990 PMID: 33464014

Cruz, A. T., Hwang, K. M., Birnbaum, G. D., & Starke, J. R. (2013). Adolescents with tuberculosis: A review of 145 cases. *The Pediatric Infectious Disease Journal, 32*(9), 937–941. DOI: 10.1097/INF.0b013e3182933214 PMID: 23538527

Derges, J., Kidger, J., Fox, F., Campbell, R., Kaner, E., & Hickman, M. (2017). Alcohol screening and brief interventions for adults and young people in health and community-based settings: A qualitative systematic literature review. *BMC Public Health, 17*(1), 562. Advance online publication. DOI: 10.1186/s12889-017-4476-4 PMID: 28599632

Dhavan, P., Dias, H. M., Creswell, J., & Weil, D. (2017). An overview of tuberculosis and migration. *The International Journal of Tuberculosis and Lung Disease : the Official Journal of the International Union against Tuberculosis and Lung Disease, 21*(6), 610–623. DOI: 10.5588/ijtld.16.0917 PMID: 28482955

Diallo, T., Adjobimey, M., Ruslami, R., Trajman, A., Sow, O., Obeng Baah, J., Marks, G. B., Long, R., Elwood, K., Zielinski, D., Gninafon, M., Wulandari, D. A., Apriani, L., Valiquette, C., Fregonese, F., Hornby, K., Li, P.-Z., Hill, P. C., Schwartzman, K., & Menzies, D. (2018). Safety and side effects of rifampin versus isoniazid in children. *The New England Journal of Medicine, 379*(5), 454–463. DOI: 10.1056/NEJMoa1714284 PMID: 30067928

Enane, L. A., Eby, J., Arscott-Mills, T., Argabright, S., Caiphus, C., Kgwaadira, B., Steenhoff, A. P., & Lowenthal, E. D. (2020). TB and TB-HIV care for adolescents and young adults. *The International Journal of Tuberculosis and Lung Disease : the Official Journal of the International Union against Tuberculosis and Lung Disease, 24*(2), 240–249. DOI: 10.5588/ijtld.19.0416 PMID: 32127110

Enane, L. A., Lowenthal, E. D., Arscott-Mills, T., Eby, J., Caiphus, C., Kgwaadira, B., Coffin, S. E., & Steenhoff, A. P. (2019). Investigating outcomes of adolescents and young adults (10–24 years of age) lost to follow-up from tuberculosis treatment in Gaborone, Botswana. *The Pediatric Infectious Disease Journal, 38*(10), e271–e274. DOI: 10.1097/INF.0000000000002369 PMID: 31220045

Enane, L. A., Lowenthal, E. D., Arscott-Mills, T., Matlhare, M., Smallcomb, L. S., Kgwaadira, B., Coffin, S. E., & Steenhoff, A. P. (2016). Loss to follow-up among adolescents with tuberculosis in Gaborone, Botswana. *The International Journal of Tuberculosis and Lung Disease : the Official Journal of the International Union against Tuberculosis and Lung Disease, 20*(10), 1320–1325. DOI: 10.5588/ijtld.16.0060 PMID: 27725042

Getahun, H., Matteelli, A., Chaisson, R. E., & Raviglione, M. (2015). Latent *Mycobacterium tuberculosis* infection. *The New England Journal of Medicine, 372*(22), 2127–2135. DOI: 10.1056/NEJMra1405427 PMID: 26017823

Houben, R. M. G. J., & Dodd, P. J. (2016). The global burden of latent tuberculosis infection: A re-estimation using mathematical modelling. *PLoS Medicine, 13*(10), e1002152. Advance online publication. DOI: 10.1371/journal.pmed.1002152 PMID: 27780211

Laycock, K. M., Eby, J., Arscott-Mills, T., Argabright, S., Caiphus, C., Kgwaadira, B., Lowenthal, E. D., Steenhoff, A. P., & Enane, L. A. (2021). Towards quality adolescent-friendly services in TB care. *The International Journal of Tuberculosis and Lung Disease : the Official Journal of the International Union against Tuberculosis and Lung Disease, 25*(7), 579–583. DOI: 10.5588/ijtld.21.0059 PMID: 34183104

Liu, J., Ren, Z.-H., Qiang, H., Wu, J., Shen, M., Zhang, L., & Lyu, J. (2020). Trends in the incidence of diabetes mellitus: Results from the Global Burden of Disease Study 2017 and implications for diabetes mellitus prevention. *BMC Public Health*, *20*(1), 1415. Advance online publication. DOI: 10.1186/s12889-020-09502-x PMID: 32943028

Lönnroth, K., Mor, Z., Erkens, C., Bruchfeld, J., Nathavitharana, R. R., van der Werf, M. J., & Lange, C. (2017). Tuberculosis in migrants in low-incidence countries: Epidemiology and intervention entry points. *The International Journal of Tuberculosis and Lung Disease : the Official Journal of the International Union against Tuberculosis and Lung Disease*, *21*(6), 624–637. DOI: 10.5588/ijtld.16.0845 PMID: 28482956

Lynch, J. L., Barrientos-Pérez, M., Hafez, M., Jalaludin, M. Y., Kovarenko, M., Rao, P. V., & Weghuber, D. (2020). Country-specific prevalence and incidence of youth-onset type 2 diabetes: A narrative literature review. *Annals of Nutrition & Metabolism*, *76*(5), 289–296. DOI: 10.1159/000510499 PMID: 32980841

Marais, B. J., Gie, R. P., Schaaf, H. S., Hesseling, A. C., Obihara, C. C., Nelson, L. J., Enarson, D. A., Donald, P. R., & Beyers, N. (2004). The clinical epidemiology of childhood pulmonary tuberculosis: A critical review of literature from the pre-chemotherapy era. *The International Journal of Tuberculosis and Lung Disease : the Official Journal of the International Union against Tuberculosis and Lung Disease*, *8*(3), 278–285. PMID: 15139465

Middelkoop, K., Bekker, L.-G., Liang, H., Aquino, L. D. H., Sebastian, E., Myer, L., & Wood, R. (2011). Force of tuberculosis infection among adolescents in a high HIV and TB prevalence community: A cross-sectional observation study. *BMC Infectious Diseases*, *11*(1), 156. Advance online publication. DOI: 10.1186/1471-2334-11-156 PMID: 21631918

Osman, M., du Preez, K., Seddon, J. A., Claassens, M. M., Dunbar, R., Dlamini, S. S., Welte, A., Naidoo, P., & Hesseling, A. C. (2021). Mortality in South African children and adolescents routinely treated for tuberculosis. *Pediatrics*, *147*(4), e2020032490. Advance online publication. DOI: 10.1542/peds.2020-032490 PMID: 33692161

Sawyer, S. M., Afifi, R. A., Bearinger, L. H., Blakemore, S.-J., Dick, B., Ezeh, A. C., & Patton, G. C. (2012). Adolescence: A foundation for future health. *Lancet*, *379*(9826), 1630–1640. DOI: 10.1016/S0140-6736(12)60072-5 PMID: 22538178

Snow, K., Hesseling, A. C., Naidoo, P., Graham, S. M., Denholm, J., & du Preez, K. (2017). Tuberculosis in adolescents and young adults: Epidemiology and treatment outcomes in the Western Cape. *The International Journal of Tuberculosis and Lung Disease : the Official Journal of the International Union against Tuberculosis and Lung Disease*, *21*(6), 651–657. DOI: 10.5588/ijtld.16.0866 PMID: 28482959

Thee, S., Krüger, R., von Bernuth, H., Meisel, C., Kölsch, U., Kirchberger, V., & Feiterna-Sperling, C. (2019). Screening and treatment for tuberculosis in a cohort of unaccompanied minor refugees in Berlin, Germany. *PLoS One*, *14*(5), e0216234. Advance online publication. DOI: 10.1371/journal.pone.0216234 PMID: 31112542

Van der Westhuizen, H.-M., & Dramowski, A. (2017). When students become patients: TBdisease among medical undergraduates in Cape Town, South Africa. *South African Medical Journal*, *107*(6), 475–479. DOI: 10.7196/SAMJ.2017.v107i6.12260 PMID: 28604316

Walker, T. M., Merker, M., Knoblauch, A. M., Helbling, P., Schoch, O. D., van der Werf, M. J., Kranzer, K., Fiebig, L., Kröger, S., Haas, W., Hoffmann, H., Indra, A., Egli, A., Cirillo, D. M., Robert, J., Rogers, T. R., Groenheit, R., Mengshoel, A. T., Mathys, V., & Witschi, M.MDR-TB Cluster Consortium. (2018). A cluster of multidrug-resistant *Mycobacterium tuberculosis* among patients arriving in Europe from the Horn of Africa: A molecular epidemiological study. *The Lancet. Infectious Diseases*, *18*(4), 431–440. DOI: 10.1016/S1473-3099(18)30004-5 PMID: 29326013

Wild, V., Jaff, D., Shah, N. S., & Frick, M. (2017). Tuberculosis, human rights and ethics considerations along the route of a highly vulnerable migrant from sub-Saharan Africa to Europe. *The International Journal of Tuberculosis and Lung Disease : the Official Journal of the International Union against Tuberculosis and Lung Disease*, *21*(11), 1075–1085. DOI: 10.5588/ijtld.17.0324 PMID: 28911349

Zhang, Y., Zhou, L., Liu, Z.-W., Chai, C.-L., Wang, X.-M., Jiang, J.-M., & Chen, S.-H. (2020). Multidrug-resistant tuberculosis transmission among middle school students in Zhejiang Province, China. *Infectious Diseases of Poverty*, *9*(1), 57. Advance online publication. DOI: 10.1186/s40249-020-00670-x PMID: 32460836

Chapter 8
TB Diagnosis and Screening Among Vulnerable Populations:
Bridging TB Detection Gaps Through Equity and Technology

Arti Thakur
https://orcid.org/0009-0002-0394-8406
Institute of Allied Health Sciences, Desh Bhagat University, India

Attuluri Vamsi Kumar
Regional Institute of Paramedical and Nursing Sciences, Miniistry of Health and Family Welfare, India

Dhruvi M. Patel
PIPHS, FOM, Parul University, India

Nivedita Priya
https://orcid.org/0000-0002-3615-7363
PIPHS, FOM, Parul University, India

Debasis Mitra
https://orcid.org/0000-0003-0525-8812
Department of Microbiology, Graphic Era University, India

Tarun Kumar Bhatt
Department of Biotechnology, Central University of Rajasthan, India

ABSTRACT

This chapter explores the challenges and innovations in diagnosing tuberculosis (TB) among vulnerable groups such as refugees, slum dwellers, prisoners, Indigenous communities, children, and people with HIV. It covers both traditional and advanced tools like GeneXpert, Truenat, AI-assisted imaging, and mobile diagnostics. Emphasizing community-based models and digital health, it highlights real-world case studies from high-burden countries. The chapter advocates for equitable, accessible TB diagnostics tailored to marginalized populations and stresses the importance of policy support and intersectoral collaboration to reach global TB elimination goals.

DOI: 10.4018/979-8-3373-3446-2.ch008

INTRODUCTION

Tuberculosis (TB) remains one of the deadliest infectious diseases globally, accounting for an estimated 10.6 million new cases and 1.3 million deaths among HIV-negative individuals in 2022 alone, as reported in the most recent WHO Global Tuberculosis Report (WHO, 2023). Despite major advances in therapeutics and diagnostics, the disease continues to disproportionately impact certain populations, especially in low- and middle-income countries (LMICs), where healthcare resources are limited and health disparities are stark. Although TB is both preventable and curable, its global control is complicated by a constellation of social, environmental, and biological factors that often intersect within vulnerable populations, creating diagnostic blind spots that impede early detection and treatment. Tuberculosis is caused by *Mycobacterium tuberculosis*, primarily affecting the lungs (pulmonary TB), although extrapulmonary manifestations are common, particularly among immunocompromised individuals. The disease is transmitted through airborne particles, with a higher risk of progression from latent to active disease among individuals with weakened immune systems, such as those with HIV, diabetes, or malnutrition (Bartolomeu-Gonçalves, 2024). The distinction between latent TB infection (LTBI) and active TB disease is clinically significant, as individuals with LTBI do not exhibit symptoms and are not infectious, yet they remain at risk of developing active TB, particularly under adverse conditions. Traditional diagnostic algorithms frequently overlook this latent phase, especially among populations with limited access to health services or inadequate health literacy.

The importance of early diagnosis in the continuum of TB care cannot be overstated. Early identification of infectious cases, particularly among high-transmission clusters, is essential to interrupt disease spread, initiate timely treatment, and reduce mortality. However, vulnerable populations—defined here as groups with increased exposure risk, limited access to care, and diminished capacity to benefit from health interventions—often experience diagnostic delays or are missed entirely by conventional case-finding strategies (MacPherson et al., 2013). These groups include, but are not limited to, urban slum dwellers, displaced persons, indigenous communities, prison inmates, people living with HIV, malnourished children, and individuals with substance use disorders. Their collective exclusion from TB screening and diagnostic programs is not merely a result of physical barriers but is often rooted in structural inequalities, systemic neglect, and socio-political marginalization (Biru et al., 2025). The underrepresentation of these vulnerable groups in national TB control strategies presents a pressing challenge. The invisibility of their diagnostic needs within mainstream health systems has resulted in continued transmission cycles, particularly within densely populated and under-resourced environments. While newer diagnostic technologies like GeneXpert MTB/RIF and

Truenat have transformed TB detection by offering rapid and accurate results, their deployment remains uneven, with limited penetration in remote and marginalized settings (Grønningen, 2025). As such, it becomes crucial to examine not only the availability of diagnostic tools but also their accessibility, cultural appropriateness, and integration into community-level healthcare.

This chapter critically evaluates current diagnostic approaches and screening strategies for TB among vulnerable populations, identifies the technological, ethical, and systemic barriers that hinder equitable access, and highlights innovations and policy efforts that aim to bridge these gaps. The overarching objective is to provide a comprehensive synthesis of the literature on TB diagnostics as it relates to marginalized groups, thereby informing future research, health policy, and implementation science. The review adopts an interdisciplinary perspective, integrating insights from public health, microbiology, epidemiology, social medicine, and health systems research. Following this introductory section, the paper proceeds with a detailed exploration of what constitutes vulnerability in the context of TB (Section 2), followed by an analysis of existing diagnostic modalities (Section 3), tailored screening strategies (Section 4), and the multifaceted barriers to diagnosis (Section 5). It then discusses technological innovations (Section 6), real-world case studies (Section 7), policy frameworks (Section 8), ethical considerations (Section 9), and research gaps (Section 10). The final sections offer evidence-based recommendations (Section 11) and present key findings from the synthesis.

DEFINING VULNERABILITY IN TB

Vulnerability in the context of tuberculosis represents a multifaceted construct that encapsulates epidemiological exposure, socioeconomic disenfranchisement, and systemic marginalization within healthcare systems. According to the World Health Organization (WHO) and the Centres for Disease Control and Prevention (CDC), vulnerable populations are defined as groups who, due to a combination of physical, environmental, and social conditions, are at an increased risk of developing disease and experiencing suboptimal health outcomes (CDC, 2025). In TB control, this vulnerability is amplified not only by a heightened risk of infection but also by delays in diagnosis, inadequate treatment access, and a higher likelihood of disease progression and transmission within communities.

Epidemiologically, individuals residing in densely populated and poorly ventilated environments, such as urban slums and informal settlements, are exposed to continuous TB transmission due to prolonged interpersonal contact and delayed healthcare-seeking behaviours (Millington., 2025). These areas often lack adequate public health infrastructure, and residents typically face multiple barriers to diagnosis, including low health literacy, transportation costs, and fear of discrimination. The diagnostic delay in such settings leads to greater disease burden and increased community transmission. Notably, urban slum populations in megacities such as Mumbai, Nairobi, and Rio de Janeiro report TB incidence rate several times higher than their national average (Kustanto & Ul-Haq, 2025). Incarcerated individuals constitute another high-risk group due to overcrowding, poor nutrition, inadequate ventilation, and limited access to timely diagnostic services within correctional facilities. The incidence of TB in prisons is estimated to be up to 30 times higher than in the general population (Navarro, 2025). Prisoners often represent a convergence of additional vulnerabilities such as substance use, HIV co-infection, and previous TB history, complicating the diagnosis and management process. Additionally, continuity of care post-incarceration remains a major challenge, leading to relapse and poor treatment adherence.

Refugees, migrants, and nomadic populations experience heightened TB risk not only because of exposure during displacement but also due to structural exclusions that limit their access to screening and care in host countries. Language barriers, undocumented status, and mobility impede their inclusion in routine surveillance programs (Dodd et al., 2025). These groups often rely on overburdened or parallel health systems, and the fear of deportation may discourage symptom reporting or health facility visits. In many cases, screening for TB among migrants remains opportunistic and reactive rather than systematic, leading to missed or delayed diagnoses. Children and the elderly are uniquely susceptible to TB due to immature or declining immune competence, respectively. Paediatric TB often presents atypically and is frequently paucibacillary, making bacteriological confirmation difficult (Sossen et al., 2025). Moreover, children depend on caregivers for access to care, and stigma surrounding TB can further delay health-seeking. Older adults, particularly those with comorbidities, often present with non-specific symptoms, and diagnostic algorithms may not be adequately tailored to geriatric populations, leading to underdiagnosis or misdiagnosis.

People living with HIV (PLHIV) constitute one of the most immunologically vulnerable cohorts for TB infection and progression. TB remains the leading cause of death among PLHIV, accounting for nearly one-third of AIDS-related deaths globally (UNAIDS, 2023). HIV co-infection complicates TB diagnosis because of atypical radiographic presentations and lower sensitivity of sputum-based tests. The urine-based TB Lipoarabinomannan (LAM) assay offers promise in such cases, but its availability and implementation remain limited in many high-burden regions (Broger, 2025). Immunocompromised individuals—such as those with diabetes mellitus, undergoing chemotherapy, or suffering from chronic malnutrition—are also at elevated risk of reactivation and rapid progression of TB. Malnourished populations, especially in humanitarian crises or disaster-prone areas, lack both immunity and access to essential health services. In diabetic patients, TB diagnosis is often delayed due to overlapping symptoms with hyperglycemia-related complications, and the co-existence of both conditions worsens treatment outcomes (Stead, 2025). Table 1 below provides a consolidated view of vulnerable populations affected by TB, highlighting their specific risk factors, diagnostic challenges, and the regions where they are most impacted. These population-specific nuances underline the necessity of tailoring diagnostic approaches and screening strategies accordingly.

Table 1. Classification of vulnerable populations affected by TB

Population Group	Risk Factors	Unique Diagnostic Challenges	Countries Most Affected
Urban Poor & Slum Dwellers	Overcrowding, poor ventilation, and poverty	Diagnostic delay, poor health access, stigma	India, Brazil, Kenya, Philippines
Prisoners	Overcrowding, poor nutrition, and limited access	Interrupted care, high reactivation rate	Russia, South Africa, Peru
Migrants, Refugees, Nomadic Tribes	Displacement, inadequate healthcare, and legal status	Language, mobile lifestyle, and poor tracking	Syria, Venezuela, Myanmar, Sudan
Children	Immature immune system, dependence on adults	Paucibacillary, non-specific symptoms	Sub-Saharan Africa, India, Pakistan
Elderly	Immunosenescence, comorbidities	Atypical symptoms, underdiagnosis	Japan, China, Eastern Europe
HIV-Infected Individuals	Immunosuppression, co-infections	Low sputum yield, atypical X-rays	South Africa, Nigeria, Uganda
Diabetics/Malnourished	Metabolic dysregulation, reduced immunity	Delayed diagnosis, poor outcomes	Bangladesh, Ethiopia, Nepal

DIAGNOSTIC MODALITIES FOR TUBERCULOSIS: CONVENTIONAL AND ADVANCED APPROACHES

Diagnostic approaches to tuberculosis have undergone a substantial evolution, transitioning from rudimentary techniques dependent on direct microscopy to molecular assays capable of detecting genetic mutations and resistance patterns within hours. Conventional diagnostic tools remain indispensable in many high-burden, resource-limited settings due to their low cost and infrastructural simplicity. Among these, the Ziehl-Nelsen (ZN) method of sputum smear microscopy is perhaps the most extensively used. It employs carbol fuchsin staining to visualize acid-fast bacilli under light microscopy. However, the technique is limited by its relatively low sensitivity, often under 60%, particularly in cases with low bacillary loads, such as in children, people living with HIV, or those with extrapulmonary disease manifestations (Hu et al., 2025). Despite these limitations, the method continues to be widely applied due to its simplicity, especially in peripheral diagnostic facilities lacking molecular capabilities (Muzanyi, 2025).

Figure 1. Evolution of TB diagnostic modalities

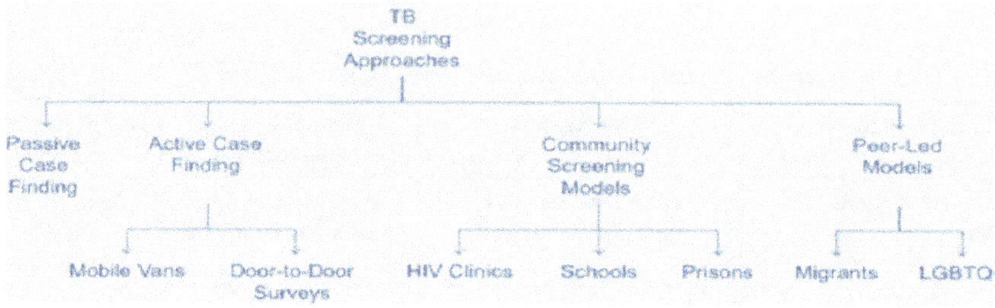

Chest X-ray (CXR) remains an integral part of TB screening, offering a rapid and non-invasive assessment of pulmonary abnormalities. Classical findings, including upper lobe infiltrates and cavitations, can support clinical suspicion of TB, especially when microbiological confirmation is not readily available. However, interpretation varies significantly depending on operator experience, and radiological signs may be confounded in HIV-positive patients, the elderly, or those with chronic lung disease (Meghji et al., 2025). Emerging applications of digital CXR coupled with artificial intelligence (AI)-powered image analysis software such as CAD4TB have shown promise in standardizing interpretation and expanding access to imaging diagnostics, especially in mobile TB units operating in remote or urban slum environments (Signorell et al., 2025). The tuberculin skin test (TST), also known as the Mantoux test, is another widely used tool for identifying latent tuberculosis infection (LTBI). It assesses a delayed hypersensitivity reaction to intradermally injected purified protein derivative (PPD). Although its utility in screening is well-established, especially among household contacts and healthcare workers, TST lacks specificity in BCG-vaccinated populations and requires a return visit for result reading, logistical challenges that can hinder its application in transient or nomadic groups.

The limitations of conventional modalities have catalyzed the development and scale-up of advanced diagnostics. GeneXpert MTB/RIF, a cartridge-based nucleic acid amplification test (CB-NAAT), has become a central pillar in the early detection of TB and rifampicin resistance. With its ability to yield results in under two hours, GeneXpert demonstrates a sensitivity of approximately 95% in smear-positive cases and significantly improves detection rates in HIV co-infected individuals and children (Wang et al., 2025). Its next-generation version, GeneXpert Ultra, offers even greater sensitivity in extrapulmonary and paucibacillary forms of the disease. Nonetheless, the requirement for stable electricity, temperature control, and recurring cartridge costs poses ongoing challenges for full-scale implementation in underserved regions (WHO, 2023).

Complementing GeneXpert, the Truenat TB/Truenat Rif assays represent a more decentralized molecular diagnostic option, especially suited for primary health centers. Operating on portable, battery-powered micro-PCR platforms, Truenat delivers diagnostic results in approximately one hour and has been demonstrated to perform comparably to CB-NAAT in field evaluations across India and sub-Saharan Africa (Huynh et al., 2025). Its modular design and robustness to field conditions make it a valuable tool in tribal and rural TB programs where laboratory infrastructure is minimal. Another critical tool is the Line Probe Assay (LPA), a DNA strip-based method used for the rapid detection of resistance mutations to first-line drugs such as rifampicin and isoniazid. LPAs provide essential information for diagnosing multidrug-resistant TB (MDR-TB) and allow for the early initiation of appropriate treatment regimens (Sury, 2025). However, their use remains restricted to specialized laboratories with biosafety facilities and trained molecular staff, limiting accessibility for vulnerable populations in peripheral or conflict-affected areas.

In populations with advanced HIV infection (CD4 <100 cells/μL), the TB-LAM test has gained recognition for its role in non-sputum-based diagnosis. This lateral flow assay detects lipoarabinomannan, a component of the TB cell wall, in urine samples, providing a valuable alternative when sputum collection is not feasible (Stead et al., 2025). Though sensitivity is moderate, its ease of use, speed, and portability make it particularly suited for bedside or field-level application among severely immunocompromised individuals. The upcoming Fujifilm SILVAMP TB-LAM test offers improved performance characteristics and may expand the role of urinary TB diagnostics even further (Yang et al., 2025).

At the cutting edge of TB diagnostic research is Whole Genome Sequencing (WGS), which offers high-resolution insights into pathogen genomics, including drug resistance profiles, lineage typing, and transmission mapping. WGS has been integrated into national surveillance strategies in several high-income settings and is now being explored in middle-income countries through donor-supported pilots (Ding et al., 2025). While WGS provides unmatched precision, its reliance on sequencing infrastructure, bioinformatics expertise, and data protection protocols currently limits its broader application in the global South. To optimize the use of available diagnostics, the WHO and national programs such as India's NTEP have issued algorithmic frameworks for test deployment. These algorithms are stratified by patient risk category, resource availability, and required diagnostic accuracy. For instance, CB-NAAT or Truenat is recommended as the initial test in presumptive pulmonary TB, followed by LPAs for resistance confirmation, and TB-LAM in advanced HIV cases. Table 2 below summarizes the comparative characteristics of conventional and advanced TB diagnostic tools, illustrating their performance profiles and contextual suitability across vulnerable population groups.

Table 2. Comparative overview of TB diagnostic tools by type, performance, and field suitability

Tool	Type	Target	Turnaround Time	Sensitivity	Required Infrastructure	Best Use Context
Ziehl-Neelsen Microscopy	Conventional	AFB Detection	~1 Hour	50–60%	Low	Basic labs in rural areas
Chest X-Ray	Conventional	Lung Abnormalities	Immediate	Variable	Medium (X-ray + reader)	Mass screening/mobile vans
Tuberculin Skin Test (TST)	Conventional	LTBI Detection	48–72 Hours	70–80%	Low	Contact tracing, LTBI
GeneXpert MTB/RIF	Advanced	MTB + Rif Resistance	~2 Hours	~95% (smear+)	Medium (electricity, A/C)	First-line test in high-risk groups
Truenat TB/Rif	Advanced	MTB + Rif Resistance	~60 mins	~87–95%	Low to medium	Decentralized & mobile use
Line Probe Assay	Advanced	Resistance Mutations	1–2 Days	~98%	High (lab infrastructure)	MDR-TB confirmation
TB-LAM (Alere/ Fujifilm)	Advanced	LAM Antigen in Urine	~25 mins	~45–70% (HIV+ CD4 <100)	Minimal	HIV-positive, hospital inpatients
Whole Genome Sequencing	Advanced	Complete Genome	5–7 Days	>98%	Very high (sequencing centers)	Research/surveillance labs

SCREENING STRATEGIES TAILORED FOR VULNERABLE POPULATIONS

Tuberculosis screening strategies must be context-specific, particularly when designed to address the diagnostic needs of vulnerable populations that face substantial barriers to timely healthcare access. Traditional passive case detection—where individuals with symptoms such as prolonged cough, fever, or weight loss voluntarily report to health facilities—has long been the primary approach in many TB programs. However, this model assumes a level of health-seeking behaviour, awareness, and accessibility that is often absent in marginalized communities. Studies have consistently shown that passive screening tends to overlook populations such as slum dwellers, refugees, prisoners, and individuals with substance use disorders who may neither recognize their symptoms as serious nor have the means to reach a diagnostic facility (Creswell et al., 2014). Moreover, the delay inherent in this model increases the likelihood of ongoing transmission within high-density environments before diagnosis is established. In response to the limitations of passive screening, active case finding (ACF) has emerged as a critical intervention to proactively detect TB among individuals who would otherwise remain undiagnosed. ACF involves systematically identifying individuals with TB symptoms or risk factors within defined high-risk groups and is particularly impactful in overcrowded or socially disenfranchised communities. Mobile diagnostic vans equipped with digital chest X-ray (CXR) machines and GeneXpert platforms have been deployed effectively in urban slums, informal settlements, and prisons, reaching populations with limited fixed health infrastructure (Creswell et al., 2014). For instance, India's JEET (Joint Effort for Elimination of TB) initiative, supported by the Global Fund, has utilized mobile CXR screening units combined with artificial intelligence algorithms to detect radiographic abnormalities in densely populated urban zones. Similarly, door-to-door surveys conducted in peri-urban African communities have demonstrated increased yield in detecting subclinical or early-stage TB cases, particularly when community health workers (CHWs) are trained to use symptom checklists and digital diagnostic aids (Fatima et al., 2014).

Figure 2. TB screening approaches for vulnerable populations

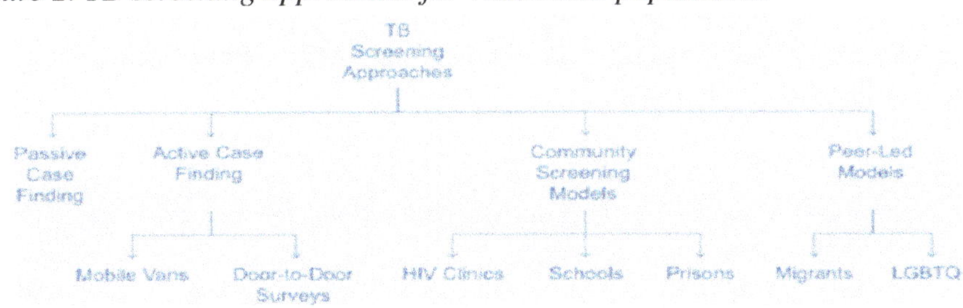

Another vital arm of community-based screening is the deployment of peer educators and outreach workers who are embedded within the target population. These individuals, often TB survivors or community health volunteers, help bridge the trust deficit between formal healthcare systems and marginalized communities. Their presence enhances participation in screening activities, particularly among groups such as people living with HIV (PLHIV), transgender individuals, and migrant laborers. Targeted screening interventions integrated within HIV treatment centers, diabetes clinics, and antenatal care units have been shown to increase TB case detection rates while enabling early initiation of treatment (Gengiah et al., 2021). These integrated models not only improve TB outcomes but also strengthen the broader continuum of care by recognizing the syndemic nature of TB with other chronic and infectious diseases.

Tailored screening strategies in institutional environments such as schools, prisons, and workplaces have yielded important insights into TB epidemiology and control. Incarcerated populations, for example, face significantly elevated risks of TB due to the convergence of overcrowding, poor nutrition, and prior exposure to TB before imprisonment. In Brazil, South Africa, and Eastern Europe, targeted mass screening using periodic digital CXR and sputum testing within correctional facilities has led to early detection and containment of TB outbreaks (Mafirakureva et al., 2025). School-based screening, though less frequently applied, is important in high-incidence areas, especially where adolescent TB is a growing concern. Workplace screening, particularly in high-risk industries such as mining, construction, and garment manufacturing, has also been adopted in several low- and middle-income countries to protect employees and reduce absenteeism. The inclusion of digital innovations has added a new dimension to TB screening efficiency. CAD-based interpretation of digital CXRs enables non-specialist health workers to perform accurate screening in the field. Moreover, mHealth tools and mobile data platforms are now being used to monitor outreach efforts, record symptoms, and track follow-up diagnostic referrals. These technologies contribute to data-driven decision-making, allowing programs to adjust strategies based on real-time evidence. A summary of tailored TB screening strategies and their implementation across vulnerable settings is presented in Table 3, which highlights the context, methodology, and effectiveness of each approach in reaching hard-to-reach populations.

Table 3. Screening strategies for TB detection in vulnerable populations

Strategy	Implementation Method	Target Population	Diagnostic Tools Used	Geographic Settings	Reported Benefits
Passive Case Finding	Facility-based self-reporting	General population	Symptom-based, sputum microscopy	National TB programs	Low-cost, limited coverage in vulnerable groups
Mobile Van Screening	Digital CXR, CB-NAAT in mobile vans	Urban slums, prisons	Digital CXR, GeneXpert, CAD	India, South Africa, Philippines	Increased case detection, reduced diagnostic delays
Door-to-Door Survey	CHWs administer symptom checklists	Rural and peri-urban poor	Symptom screen, Truenat referrals	Pakistan, Uganda, Zambia	Reaches subclinical cases, builds community trust
Peer Educator Outreach	TB survivors/ volunteers engage community	Migrants, PLHIV, transgender	Awareness, sample collection	India, Nepal, Kenya	Improves participation, reduces stigma

Strategy	Implementation Method	Target Population	Diagnostic Tools Used	Geographic Settings	Reported Benefits
Integrated Facility Screening	Screening integrated in HIV/DM/ANC clinics	PLHIV, diabetics, pregnant women	TB-LAM, GeneXpert, CXR	Nigeria, Malawi, Cambodia	High yield, early case detection
Institutional Screening	Periodic mass testing in closed settings	Prisoners, school children, workers	Digital CXR, sputum microscopy	Brazil, Russia, South Africa	Prevents outbreaks, facilitates rapid isolation

BARRIERS TO EFFECTIVE DIAGNOSIS AND SCREENING

Achieving timely and accurate diagnosis of tuberculosis among vulnerable populations is often obstructed by a complex matrix of interrelated barriers embedded within health systems, socioeconomic structures, and sociocultural environments. Health system-related constraints represent a foundational impediment, particularly in low- and middle-income countries where decentralized laboratory infrastructure is underdeveloped. Many rural primary health centers continue to rely on outdated smear microscopy methods, with limited or no access to molecular tools like GeneXpert or Truenat (Katamba et al., 2024). Additionally, referral linkages between primary care and higher-level diagnostic facilities remain fragmented, often resulting in loss to follow-up before bacteriological confirmation or drug sensitivity testing can be performed. This is especially problematic in tribal areas, where health posts are sparsely located and staffed by undertrained personnel. For example, a 2022 field study in central India documented that over 40% of presumptive TB cases identified through community screening in tribal villages failed to reach the designated microscopy center due to non-functional referral pathways and the absence of transport reimbursements (Hussain et al., 2020).

Socioeconomic vulnerability further compounds the diagnostic gap. For informal workers and daily wage earners, attending a health facility often equates to a day's income forfeited, a trade-off many are unwilling or unable to make, especially in the absence of social protection mechanisms. Transportation costs to distant diagnostic centers, combined with out-of-pocket expenditures on associated services, can be prohibitive (Berrocal-Almanza et al., 2023). These economic deterrents are particularly pronounced in displaced populations and urban slum dwellers, where high disease burden coexists with health service exclusion. Moreover, individuals with poor nutritional status or chronic illnesses such as diabetes frequently prioritize short-term symptom relief from informal providers rather than pursuing formal diagnostic avenues that are both time-consuming and financially burdensome.

Sociocultural factors—including stigma, gender norms, and language barriers—exert a significant influence on diagnostic behaviour and access. In many settings, TB remains highly stigmatized, associated with contagion, poverty, and moral judgment, deterring individuals from seeking care or disclosing symptoms (Balakrishnan et al., 2023). Women, particularly in patriarchal societies, may require male permission or accompaniment to visit health centers, leading to delayed diagnosis or complete exclusion from screening programs. In conflict zones or among migrant communities, language mismatches between patients and providers further hinder accurate symptom reporting, result interpretation, and treatment adherence. Marginalized ethnic groups often experience mistrust toward formal health institutions due to historical neglect or abuse, which can be mitigated only through culturally competent outreach and peer engagement models. Logistical bottlenecks in diagnostic workflows represent another structural barrier, particularly in settings attempting to scale molecular diagnostics. Issues such as reagent stock-outs, power failures, and machine breakdowns frequently interrupt service delivery. Specimen transport remains a critical weak point in TB diagnostic cascades. In many regions, particularly in mountainous or flood-prone terrains, sputum samples may take multiple days to reach testing hubs, leading to compromised specimen integrity or attrition before results are returned (Aggarwal et al., 2024). In remote northeastern districts of India, for instance, community health workers have reported turnaround times of 10–14 days for CB-NAAT results, due in part to the unavailability of cold-chain transport or designated courier systems. These multifactorial challenges are often compounded when they intersect in individuals who simultaneously experience multiple forms of marginalization.

RECENT INNOVATIONS IN TB DIAGNOSTICS

Innovation in tuberculosis diagnostics is increasingly focused on bridging accessibility gaps, particularly in contexts marked by limited laboratory infrastructure and diagnostic delays. Technological advances over the last five years have produced promising tools tailored to address the diagnostic challenges faced by vulnerable and remote populations. A key breakthrough has been the integration of artificial intelligence (AI) into the interpretation of chest radiographs, a technique now operationalized through software such as Computer-Aided Detection for Tuberculosis (CAD4TB). This AI-driven tool analyses digital chest X-rays in real time to detect pulmonary abnormalities suggestive of TB, reducing the reliance on trained radiologists in field settings. CAD4TB has been deployed in community screening programs in Bangladesh, South Africa, and Nigeria, where it demonstrated high sensitivity (up to 90%) in detecting active TB, especially when used as a triage tool before confirmatory molecular testing (Geric et al., 2023). The software's ability to rapidly interpret images allows its integration into mobile screening vans and camp-based outreach initiatives, enhancing diagnostic throughput in areas with high disease prevalence but minimal diagnostic personnel. Equally transformative are urine-based diagnostics, particularly the TB lipoarabinomannan (LAM) antigen detection assays. These non-sputum tests offer critical value for HIV-positive individuals with advanced immunosuppression, especially those who are unable to produce sputum. While the Alere Determine TB LAM Ag test has been in use for several years, the next-generation Fujifilm SILVAMP TB LAM (FujiLAM) offers significantly improved sensitivity and operational simplicity. A recent multicentric study reported FujiLAM sensitivity reaching 70% in hospitalized HIV-positive patients with CD4 counts <100 cells/μL, a marked improvement over its predecessor (Adzemovic et al., 2025). The assay's use of silver amplification technology allows for the detection of low concentrations of LAM in urine, expanding its applicability beyond HIV-associated TB. Its integration into HIV clinics and inpatient wards offers a decentralized diagnostic solution that is particularly impactful in Sub-Saharan Africa, where HIV-TB co-infection remains a leading cause of mortality.

Portable molecular diagnostics continue to redefine the possibilities for decentralized TB detection. The Truenat MTB and Truenat Rif Dx platforms—compact, battery-operated micro-PCR devices—are among the most field-adapted technologies currently endorsed by WHO. Their ability to detect *M. tuberculosis* DNA and rifampicin resistance within one hour, combined with minimal infrastructure requirements, makes them ideal for use in primary healthcare centres and mobile screening setups. Their deployment in India's tribal districts and border areas has significantly improved case detection rates, especially among underdiagnosed populations (Pai et al., 2023). Studies conducted in Jharkhand and Chhattisgarh have noted increased bacteriological confirmation and reduced diagnostic turnaround when Truenat was deployed through district-led active case-finding campaigns (Gopalaswamy et al., 2023) Truenat system's modularity and cloud-linked data systems also support real-time surveillance, enhancing programmatic monitoring. To overcome the persistent challenge of specimen transport in remote terrains, drones have been piloted as an innovative logistic solution. In Malawi, the Ministry of Health in collaboration with Village Reach and Gavi, launched a project to transport sputum samples using unmanned aerial vehicles (UAVs), connecting rural clinics with central laboratories. The initiative reduced transport times by over 60% and minimized loss to follow-up by ensuring faster reporting of test results (Stierlin et al., 2024). The success of this model has prompted its replication in Madagascar, Papua New Guinea, and parts of Kenya. While initial cost barriers and regulatory issues require navigation, drone-based transport exemplifies how digital health and logistics technologies can be leveraged to bypass geographic and infrastructural barriers in TB care.

Figure 3. Diagnostic workflow incorporating recent innovations

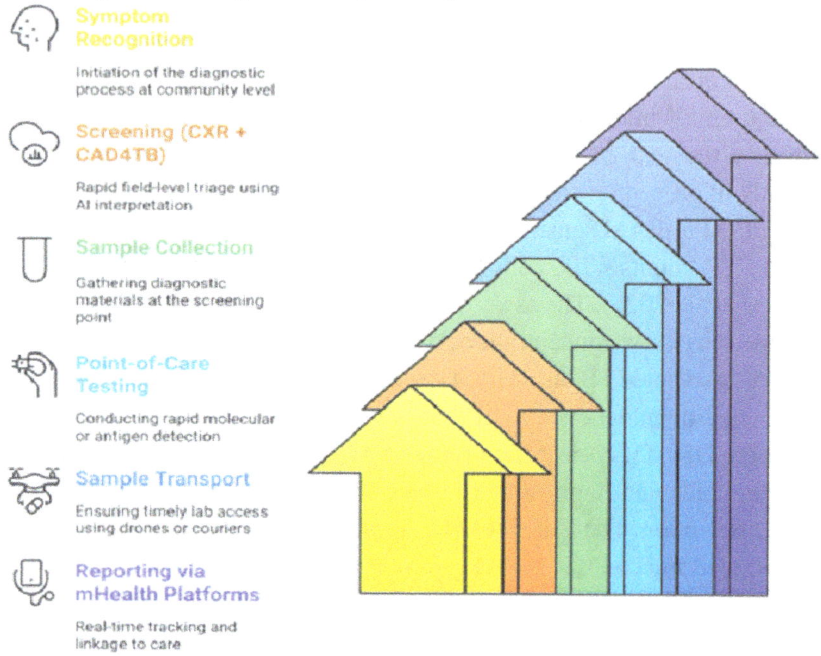

Another frontier in TB diagnostics is the detection of exhaled volatile organic compounds (VOCs) as a non-invasive alternative to sputum-based tests. Devices such as electronic noses (e-noses) and sensor-based breath analyzers are currently in development to identify VOC signatures unique to *M. tuberculosis* metabolism. These tools, though still in early clinical validation, offer the potential for rapid, sample-free screening, particularly in pediatric and elderly populations who often struggle with sputum production (Belizário et al., 2021). The portability and non-invasiveness of such platforms could make them particularly useful in school-based or community-based screening programs, pending further evidence on specificity and standardization. Multi-disease diagnostic integration is also gaining traction as a strategy to improve TB case finding within broader health service frameworks. Point-of-care testing platforms capable of diagnosing TB alongside HIV, COVID-19, and malaria are being explored to reduce missed opportunities and optimize patient encounters. For instance, the Cepheid GeneXpert platform, traditionally used for TB, has expanded to include cartridges for SARS-CoV-2, allowing for shared diagnostic infrastructure in resource-limited settings (Barr et al., 2022). This model is particularly suited for urban slums and humanitarian contexts where health facility access is episodic and syndromic overlap between TB and other infections is common. Table 4 offers a synthesis of recent diagnostic innovations, highlighting their mechanisms, advantages, and applicability to vulnerable populations.

Table 4. Recent innovations in tuberculosis diagnostics and their applications

Innovation	Diagnostic Principle	Target Population	Operational Advantage	Field Applicability
CAD4TB (AI CXR)	AI-based radiograph interpretation	Urban poor, prisoners	Rapid screening without a radiologist	Mobile vans, digital camps
FujiLAM (Urine)	Silver amplification-based LAM detection	HIV-positive, inpatient	Sputum-free, rapid, bedside	HIV wards, ART centers
Truenat	Micro-PCR for MTB and Rif resistance	Rural, tribal areas	Battery-operated, decentralized	CHCs, PHCs, outreach units
Drone Transport	UAV-based sample logistics	Remote mountainous zones	Reduced transport time and losses	Pilot in Malawi, expansion underway
VOC Detection	Breath-based biomarker identification	Pediatrics, elderly	Non-invasive, sputum-free	Under validation; school camps
Multi-Disease Platforms	Integrated pathogen cartridge testing	Syndromic patients, co-morbidities	Efficient use of devices	HIV/TB/COVID clinics

CASE STUDIES: DIAGNOSIS IN REAL-WORLD VULNERABLE SETTINGS

Efforts to improve TB diagnosis among vulnerable populations have increasingly relied on tailored, community-responsive interventions grounded in the social, political, and logistical realities of specific settings. These interventions, often developed through public-private partnerships and humanitarian collaborations, have yielded significant insights into effective diagnostic strategies. By examining programmatic experiences across different geographical and sociocultural contexts, operational lessons can be extrapolated and adapted to similar high-burden or underserved areas. Case-based analyses provide a valuable lens through which to evaluate not only the clinical and technical outcomes of diagnostic deployment but also the social dynamics and ethical implications that shape uptake and sustainability. In the Cox's Bazar district of Bangladesh, home to one of the largest stateless refugee populations globally, the Rohingya crisis has highlighted the challenges of TB control in humanitarian emergencies. Following mass displacement from Myanmar, the population surged into overcrowded and unhygienic settlements, creating a hotspot for TB transmission. Medecins Sans Frontières (MSF), in coordination with the Bangladeshi Ministry of Health and the Global Fund, deployed active case finding (ACF) through mobile teams equipped with digital chest X-ray machines and GeneXpert systems (Fouskas., 2025). Community health workers, many of them Rohingya volunteers, were trained to screen for TB symptoms and assist in patient navigation. The integration of CAD4TB software further enhanced the diagnostic yield, particularly in asymptomatic or early-stage cases. In this context, the culturally sensitive involvement of local volunteers was instrumental in overcoming stigma, improving health literacy, and enhancing diagnostic uptake, especially among women who were less likely to interact with formal health workers due to social norms. The experience from Cox's Bazar underscores the importance of flexible deployment models and community ownership in transient, high-risk populations.

In the dense urban slums of Mumbai, India, a high concentration of undiagnosed TB cases persists due to barriers including stigma, informal health-seeking behaviour, and lack of awareness. A collaborative initiative between the Mumbai Municipal Corporation and the PATH India TB Control Project introduced mobile diagnostic vans fitted with CBNAAT (Cartridge-Based Nucleic Acid Amplification Test) machines into slum clusters (Singh et al., 2025). The intervention was targeted at high-density areas with reported diagnostic gaps and was preceded by intensive community mobilization through peer educators. The mobile teams conducted symptom screening, digital X-rays, and on-the-spot molecular testing, drastically reducing the diagnostic turnaround time from over a week to less than a day. This rapid response model was particularly effective for patients who might otherwise have dropped out of the diagnostic cascade due to daily wage constraints or mobility issues. The initiative also revealed operational bottlenecks such as inconsistent power supply and cartridge stock-outs, which were mitigated through solar-powered units and cloud-based inventory tracking. The Mumbai experience demonstrates the viability of mobile molecular testing in overcoming urban diagnostic inertia when strategically integrated with behavioural and infrastructural interventions.

In South Africa, TB prevalence among incarcerated populations is estimated to be over 20 times that of the general public, largely due to overcrowding, inadequate ventilation, and poor access to timely health services. The Department of Correctional Services, in partnership with NGOs such as Aurum Institute, implemented a TB screening program across select prison facilities utilizing mobile radiography units equipped with CAD4TB AI software (Husnain., 2025). The approach enabled non-clinical staff to conduct large-scale screening efficiently, flagging suspected TB cases for confirmatory testing through GeneXpert Ultra. Importantly, the deployment of AI minimized human resource requirements, a significant advantage given the under-resourced nature of prison health services. Screening was complemented by training peer mentors within prison units to disseminate information, reduce stigma, and ensure treatment adherence. The program demonstrated a notable increase in TB case notifications within the first year of implementation, alongside a marked decrease in diagnostic delay. It also prompted policy-level changes advocating routine, periodic TB screening as part of the prison intake process. This case illustrates how digital tools can be strategically leveraged to offset human capital limitations in institutional settings. Among Indigenous communities in northern Canada, tuberculosis continues to represent a stark example of health inequity rooted in colonial history and systemic neglect. The Government of Canada's TB Elimination Framework for Inuit Nunangat included the establishment of culturally adapted outreach models emphasizing respect for local customs and community governance (Prabhune et al., 2025). Mobile diagnostic units were staffed by both Indigenous health workers and non-Indigenous clinicians who underwent cultural safety training. The deployment of GeneXpert devices and the use of rapid point-of-care TB-LAM testing in high HIV prevalence areas were key components of the diagnostic intervention. In addition to biomedical screening, the initiative included land-based healing programs and community-led storytelling circles aimed at destigmatizing TB and reinforcing traditional health practices. One of the measurable impacts of this approach was the increased engagement of previously disengaged youth, a demographic typically underrepresented in formal health outreach. The Canadian example underlines the importance of sociocultural alignment in diagnostics and the need for reconciliation-informed health interventions.

NATIONAL AND INTERNATIONAL POLICY RESPONSES

Strategic policy frameworks have played a crucial role in shaping global and national responses to TB diagnostics, particularly with regard to improving access for vulnerable and high-risk populations. The World Health Organization's End TB Strategy, launched in 2014, outlined ambitious targets for TB elimination by 2035, with its first pillar explicitly emphasizing early diagnosis through universal access to rapid testing, including the use of molecular assays and improved laboratory networks (WHO, 2025). The strategy sets the target of detecting and treating 90% of all TB cases and 90% of key populations by 2025, emphasizing the need to reduce diagnostic delays and improve outreach to marginalized groups. Its most recent updates have highlighted the integration of digital tools, mobile units, and decentralized diagnostics, calling for stronger primary care engagement and investment in non-sputum-based diagnostics for people living with HIV, children, and individuals in congregate settings (WHO, 2023).

To support the financial realization of these goals, the Global Fund to Fight AIDS, Tuberculosis and Malaria has directed substantial resources towards expanding diagnostic infrastructure in low- and middle-income countries. Between 2020 and 2022, the Global Fund invested over $1.5 billion specifically in TB diagnostics and laboratory systems, including the procurement of GeneXpert, Truenat, and digital X-ray platforms (Chorna et al., 2025). A key focus of these investments has been the strategic placement of molecular tools in primary healthcare facilities serving high-risk groups such as refugees, rural populations, and urban slum residents. Moreover, the Global Fund has actively supported capacity-building initiatives to train laboratory technicians, implement electronic reporting systems, and support maintenance frameworks to ensure diagnostic uptime in under-resourced areas. These investments have been instrumental in enabling countries such as Nigeria, Pakistan, and the Philippines to scale up decentralized testing and reduce diagnostic turnaround times.

National TB Elimination Programs (NTEPs) have adapted WHO's global recommendations into country-specific operational strategies. India's NTEP, for instance, has adopted a tiered diagnostic algorithm prioritizing CBNAAT or Truenat as first-line tests for all presumptive TB cases among key populations, including contacts of drug-resistant TB patients, PLHIV, and residents of slums and prisons (Ministry of Health & Family Welfare, 2025). Similarly, Brazil's national program has implemented widespread use of digital radiography and molecular diagnostics, particularly in favelas and Indigenous communities. National frameworks in these countries also mandate the tracking of vulnerable subgroups and have begun integrating real-time dashboards for diagnostic monitoring and patient follow-up. These national models are increasingly adopting risk stratification tools to guide targeted active case finding, supported by community health workers and mobile diagnostic units.

At the multilateral level, the United Nations High-Level Meeting (UNHLM) on TB in 2023 reaffirmed the international community's commitment to closing diagnostic gaps, with particular emphasis on "leaving no one behind" (United Nations General Assembly, 2023). Member states endorsed a political declaration that included concrete targets for reaching the most marginalized groups with affordable and timely diagnostics. The declaration emphasized differentiated service delivery, gender-responsive strategies, and community-based screening models as cornerstones of TB diagnostic scale-up. Importantly, the meeting underscored the need for cross-sectoral engagement, especially with social protection, migration, and justice sectors, to address the structural determinants of diagnostic inequity. The

UNHLM also called for increased domestic financing to reduce overreliance on donor funding and improve program sustainability in the post-pandemic recovery phase.

The TB REACH initiative, funded by Global Affairs Canada and managed by the Stop TB Partnership, has pioneered several high-impact innovations in diagnostics, particularly those focused on vulnerable populations. Since its inception in 2010, TB REACH has supported over 70 countries through catalytic grants to pilot innovative diagnostic delivery models. Successful interventions include drone-supported sample transport in Malawi, peer-led screening among transgender communities in Pakistan, and AI-assisted radiography in Ethiopian refugee camps (Stop TB Partnership, 2025). One of the strengths of TB REACH has been its ability to rapidly scale up successful pilots into national policy by providing the evidence base required for larger investments. The program has also emphasized real-time monitoring through digital platforms, allowing early identification of implementation bottlenecks.

The Public-Private Mix (PPM) approach has emerged as a critical strategy for engaging non-state actors in TB diagnostics. In countries like India and Indonesia, where a substantial proportion of symptomatic individuals first seek care in the private sector, PPM models aim to bridge the gap between informal providers and national TB programs. These models involve incentives for notification, training for private practitioners, and linkages to free diagnostics such as CBNAAT and culture testing. The Joint Effort for Elimination of TB (JEET) model in India is a notable example, combining digital interface platforms like Nikshay with field coordinators to ensure patient linkage to diagnostic and treatment services (Srinivasan et al., 2025). In the Philippines, similar models have been adapted using pharmacy-based referrals and mobile app-based self-reporting to capture TB suspects at first contact.

ETHICAL AND LEGAL CONSIDERATIONS

Ethical and legal complexities surrounding tuberculosis diagnostics are particularly pronounced when interventions target vulnerable populations, where systemic inequities often intersect with personal autonomy, rights to privacy, and access to justice. Informed consent, a fundamental principle in healthcare ethics, faces considerable challenges in TB screening contexts—especially among illiterate or semi-literate individuals who may not fully understand the nature of diagnostic procedures or their implications. In humanitarian emergencies, prisons, or Indigenous communities, written consent procedures may be impractical or culturally misaligned. In such contexts, reliance on verbal consent, pictorial aids, and community mediators has been proposed to ensure that patients are not merely passive recipients of testing but active participants in decision-making (Barreto-Duarte et al., 2025). However, the tension between rapid diagnosis in public health emergencies and the ethical imperative of informed consent continues to generate debate, particularly in mass screening campaigns or active case finding where testing may be perceived as coercive if linked to other forms of aid or service delivery.

The right to non-discriminatory and equitable access to TB diagnostics is enshrined in global human rights frameworks but is frequently compromised in practice. Refugees, undocumented migrants, LGBTQ+ individuals, and incarcerated persons often encounter legal or bureaucratic obstacles that prevent them from accessing state-run diagnostic services. A recent analysis from sub-Saharan Africa revealed that fear of deportation among undocumented migrants led to substantial underreporting of symptoms, delayed diagnoses, and increased community transmission (Chorna et al., 2025). Discriminatory practices may also manifest in the form of selective screening that targets specific demographic groups without proper safeguards for confidentiality, thus increasing stigma and discouraging care-seeking. Breaches in diagnostic data privacy—especially when digital tools such as CAD4TB or mobile apps are used—raise further ethical concerns, as many vulnerable individuals lack legal protection over how their health data is collected, stored, or shared with state authorities or third parties (Sekandi et al.,2025). Cultural sensitivity is essential in the ethical administration of TB diagnostics. Diagnosis is not simply a biomedical event but a culturally embedded process that intersects with beliefs about illness, healing, and the body. In Indigenous and tribal communities, for instance, TB may be interpreted within spiritual or ancestral frameworks, and interventions not aligned with these narratives risk rejection or disengagement. Studies in Canada, Australia, and the Amazon basin have shown that diagnostic programs designed in partnership with community elders, healers, and culturally competent health workers achieve higher acceptance rates (Prabhune et al., 2025). Furthermore, ethical TB screening must incorporate gender-sensitive protocols, recognizing that women and gender minorities face unique barriers to both consent and privacy. Female patients may require same-gender staff, childcare support, or discrete testing environments to feel safe accessing diagnostic services. The diagnosis of TB in children presents specific legal and ethical dilemmas. Since minors lack full legal capacity, guardianship and consent must be clearly established, particularly in settings with high orphan rates, refugee populations, or fragmented familial structures. Health workers often face uncertainty regarding who may legally consent to diagnostic procedures, particularly in schools, shelters, or unregistered households. In some countries, legislation permits mature minors (typically aged 12 or older) to consent to health services, but such policies are inconsistently applied and poorly understood at field level (Huynh et al., 2025). Additionally, ethical pediatric diagnostics must balance the need for non-invasive sampling with diagnostic accuracy—favouring methods such as stool GeneXpert or gastric lavage over more distressing procedures like induced sputum, especially in unaccompanied children.

GAPS IN CURRENT RESEARCH AND PRACTICE

Persistent knowledge and operational gaps continue to undermine the global response to TB diagnosis, particularly among vulnerable populations. A critical void exists in the systematic documentation and quantification of diagnostic delays within informal settlements, urban slums, and peri-urban settings. These areas are characterized by highly transient populations, poor addressability, and informal healthcare providers who rarely report cases to national programs. Most available data on delay intervals—from symptom onset to diagnosis—are derived from formal healthcare settings and fail to capture the early interactions patients have with unregulated providers or self-treatment practices (Hassan et al., 2025). Community-based ethnographic studies have reported average delays exceeding four weeks in Mumbai slums and Dhaka's informal settlements, yet these findings remain anecdotal, lacking integration into surveillance databases or policy frameworks. Without granular, population-specific diagnostic delay data, it becomes difficult to calibrate active case finding (ACF) strategies or allocate diagnostic resources optimally.

Figure 4. Priority gaps in TB diagnostic research

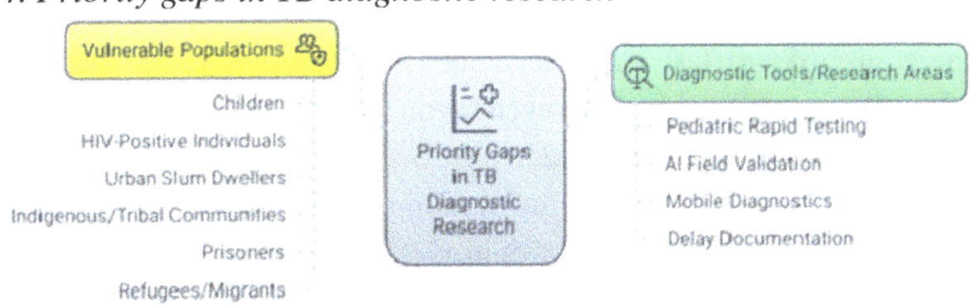

An equally pressing limitation is the absence of pediatric-specific rapid diagnostics that are both sensitive and field-deployable. Most existing tools—such as GeneXpert and Truenat—were originally validated in adult populations and require sputum samples, which are often difficult to collect from children. Gastric aspirates, the current fallback, are invasive and require hospital admission, making them unsuitable for mass screening or low-resource settings (Preez et al., 2025). While stool-based GeneXpert and loop-mediated isothermal amplification (LAMP) methods have shown promise, they remain under-evaluated in large-scale programmatic settings. Furthermore, there is limited data on the performance of TB-LAM in pediatric HIV-positive populations, despite WHO's recommendation to expand its use. The current research agenda has inadequately prioritized pediatric diagnostics, leaving a critical gap in early detection and treatment initiation for one of TB's most vulnerable groups.

Despite the growing enthusiasm for AI-assisted tools like CAD4TB, the field validation of these technologies under real-world conditions remains insufficient. Most performance studies are conducted in controlled environments with curated image datasets and optimal hardware conditions. There is a lack of robust, peer-reviewed evidence on AI's diagnostic accuracy across varied geographies, diverse age groups, and comorbid populations such as diabetics or immunocompromised individuals. Moreover, little is known about the operational challenges of deploying AI tools in peripheral settings, such as software compatibility, hardware maintenance, and power continuity (Rashid et al., 2025). There is also no established regulatory framework to evaluate or standardize the ethical use of diagnostic AI, including concerns around misclassification risks and data governance in community-level screenings. As AI increasingly becomes part of national TB programs, especially in digital radiography, the absence of comprehensive implementation research could hinder its safe and effective adoption.

Another significant blind spot is the scarcity of implementation research evaluating mobile diagnostic units, despite their widespread deployment in various high-burden countries. While several pilot studies and NGO-led reports describe operational successes, there is minimal peer-reviewed literature assessing long-term cost-effectiveness, integration into public health infrastructure, or equity outcomes. For instance, while mobile vans equipped with CBNAAT have been introduced in over 30 Indian districts under the NTEP, few studies have followed up on sustainability, patient follow-up, or diagnostic yield disaggregated by gender, age, or socioeconomic status (Singh et al., 2025). Similarly, there is limited documentation of cross-border mobile diagnostics in migrant corridors or refugee zones, where TB transmission dynamics may differ. Without robust implementation frameworks and post-deployment evaluations, the scalability and replicability of mobile diagnostic models remain uncertain.

RECOMMENDATIONS

Operational success in tuberculosis diagnostics among vulnerable populations depends on an integrated, multisectoral approach that harmonizes biomedical innovation with community participation, health system strengthening, and digital enablers. Expanding the involvement of community health workers (CHWs) must be central to this agenda. CHWs, particularly those embedded within the communities they serve, act as trusted mediators between formal health systems and marginalized groups. Their role in identifying symptomatic individuals, assisting in sputum collection, accompanying patients to diagnostic sites, and facilitating follow-up care has been validated in several high-burden countries, including Ethiopia, India, and Mozambique (Hickey et al., 2025). However, many CHWs remain underpaid, inadequately trained in newer diagnostic technologies, and excluded from decision-making forums. Scaling their impact requires standardized training in point-of-care testing protocols (e.g., Truenat, TB-LAM), integration into digital reporting systems, and provision of sustainable incentives.

To reduce diagnostic inequities in hard-to-reach populations, scaling up decentralized molecular diagnostics such as Truenat and urine-based TB LAM testing is imperative. These tools have demonstrated robust performance under field conditions with minimal infrastructure requirements and are especially effective for primary-level diagnosis in rural and tribal settings, as well as in HIV-positive patients unable to produce sputum. National TB programs should prioritize their deployment in underserved geographies, accompanied by solar-powered backup systems and automated result linkage to central dashboards (Meghji et al., 2025). Strategic procurement and volume-based pricing mechanisms—backed by the Global Fund and domestic financing—must ensure uninterrupted test availability across all diagnostic nodes. A major bottleneck in uptake and early care-seeking is the linguistic and cultural disconnect between TB awareness materials and the populations they are intended for. Current IEC (Information, Education, Communication) content is often developed centrally, using generalized messaging that fails to resonate with diverse communities. Populations such as nomadic tribes, migrant workers, and ethnic minorities require language-specific, culturally contextualized TB communication strategies co-designed with community stakeholders. Visual storytelling, folk media, and locally trained peer educators have proven more effective than pamphlets or posters in improving diagnostic literacy and early health-seeking (Olowoyo et al., 2025).

Addressing delays in specimen transfer and result delivery requires focused investment in strengthening the supply chain and specimen transport systems. Mobile courier systems, cold-chain protocols, and drone-based delivery (in topographically challenged regions) should be scaled, with defined turnaround targets and real-time tracking. Case studies from Uganda and Malawi have demonstrated that such interventions reduced diagnostic result turnaround from over 5 days to under 48 hours in rural settings (Ogwu & Izah., 2025). Additionally, buffer stock monitoring and automated stock-out alerts for diagnostics like GeneXpert cartridges and TB LAM kits must be digitized using mHealth platforms linked to procurement nodes. There is also a growing need to integrate TB diagnostics within broader service delivery platforms, especially in non-communicable disease (NCD) clinics and mobile health apps. Diabetes and TB comorbidity are increasingly prevalent, yet siloed vertical programs fail to capture overlapping patient populations. Bidirectional screening policies must be strengthened with protocols for routine TB testing in diabetes and HIV clinics. Simultaneously, TB symptom checkers and referral tools should be embedded into mHealth apps used by CHWs, enabling digital pre-screening, real-time linkage to diagnostic centres, and symptom tracking (Ogwu & Izah., 2025).

CONCLUSION

Tuberculosis continues to pose a significant global health challenge, particularly among vulnerable populations who remain underserved by conventional health systems and diagnostic frameworks. The complexities of TB diagnosis in such groups stem not only from biological and technological limitations but also from deeply entrenched social, cultural, and structural inequities. This review comprehensively analyzed the current landscape of TB diagnostics, highlighting both the progress achieved through advanced tools like Truenat, GeneXpert, TB-LAM, and AI-assisted radiography, and the persistent barriers that hinder equitable access, ranging from weak infrastructure and gender-based stigma to legal uncertainties and ethical dilemmas in consent procedures. The burden of delayed and missed TB diagnoses falls disproportionately on marginalized communities, including refugees, prisoners, urban slum dwellers, Indigenous groups, HIV-positive individuals, and children. Real-world case studies across diverse contexts, from South African prisons to Canadian Indigenous territories and Rohingya refugee camps, have underscored the value of community-driven, culturally adapted, and technology-enabled approaches. These examples also emphasize the importance of trust-building, decentralization, and integrated care models in enhancing diagnostic coverage and efficiency.

Despite policy-level commitments and large-scale investments by international agencies and national programs, significant research and implementation gaps remain. Diagnostic tools designed for general populations are often not tailored for the physiological, social, or operational needs of vulnerable groups. Data on diagnostic delays, pediatric applications, and AI performance in field settings are either sparse or non-generalizable, limiting evidence-based policymaking. Moreover, ethical safeguards around consent, data protection, and equitable access continue to lag behind technological advances. To address these gaps, there is a pressing need for a multi-tiered response that combines policy reform, community empowerment, health system strengthening, and continuous innovation. Strategies must prioritize the scale-up of field-adaptable diagnostic platforms, capacity building among frontline health workers, context-sensitive awareness campaigns, and robust specimen transport and data reporting systems. Integrating TB diagnostics with mobile health technologies and NCD clinics offers a promising direction, especially in syndemic-prone populations. Ultimately, bridging the diagnostic divide in TB requires reimagining healthcare delivery through the lens of equity, empathy, and inclusivity. Vulnerable populations should not be treated as peripheral beneficiaries but as central partners in the global fight against tuberculosis. A diagnostic approach rooted in justice and responsiveness is not only ethically imperative but also essential for achieving global TB elimination targets in the coming decades.

REFERENCES

Adzemovic, T., Nalintya, E., Fieberg, A., Mande, E., George, K., & Yueh, S.. (2025). Diagnostic accuracy of the updated FujiLAM II assay to detect tuberculosis in outpatients with advanced HIV disease. *Clinical Infectious Diseases*, •••, ciaf079. Advance online publication. DOI: 10.1093/cid/ciaf079 PMID: 40130995

Aggarwal, S., Simmy, S., Mahajan, N., & Nigam, K. (2024). Challenges experienced by health care workers during service delivery in the geographically challenging terrains of North-East India: Study involving a thematic analysis. *JMIR Formative Research, 8*, e57384. DOI: 10.2196/57384 PMID: 39255009

Balakrishnan, V., Kherabi, Y., Ramanathan, G., Paul, S. A., & Tiong, C. K. (2023). Machine learning approaches in diagnosing tuberculosis through biomarkers—A systematic review. *Progress in Biophysics and Molecular Biology, 179*, 16–25. DOI: 10.1016/j.pbiomolbio.2023.03.001 PMID: 36931609

Barreto-Duarte, B., Villalva-Serra, K., Croda, J., Arcêncio, R. A., Maciel, E. L. N., & Andrade, B. B. (2025). Directly observed treatment for tuberculosis care and social support: Essential lifeline or outdated burden? *Lancet Regional Health. Americas, 43*, 100310. DOI: 10.1016/j.lana.2025.101015 PMID: 40171142

Bartolomeu-Gonçalves, G., de Souza, J. M., Fernandes, B. T., Spoladori, L. F. A., Correia, G. F., & de Castro, I. M.. (2024). Tuberculosis diagnosis: Current, ongoing, and future approaches. *Diseases (Basel, Switzerland), 12*(9), 202. DOI: 10.3390/diseases12090202 PMID: 39329871

Belizário, J. E., Faintuch, J., & Malpartida, M. G. (2021). Breath biopsy and discovery of exclusive volatile organic compounds for diagnosis of infectious diseases. *Frontiers in Cellular and Infection Microbiology, 10*, 564194. DOI: 10.3389/fcimb.2020.564194 PMID: 33520731

Berrocal-Almanza, L. C., Lima, M., Piotrowski, H., Botticello, J., Badhan, A., Karnani, N., Kaur, H., Pareek, M., Haldar, P., Dedicoat, M., Kon, O. M., Zenner, D., & Lalvani, A. (2023). Vulnerability and tuberculosis treatment outcomes in urban settings in England: A mixed-methods study. *PLoS One, 18*(8), e0281918. DOI: 10.1371/journal.pone.0281918 PMID: 37590225

Biru, M., Datiko, D. G., Jerene, D., Yohannes, A. G., Molla, Y., Suarez, P., Gebrekiros, W., Kassa, A., Kassie, Y., & Dememew, Z. G. (2025). Designing tuberculosis elimination framework through participatory processes in Ethiopia: Results from stakeholders' discussions. *PLoS One, 20*(3), e0318209. DOI: 10.1371/journal.pone.0318209 PMID: 40063578

Broger, T. (2025). *Can Lipoarabinomannan Antigen Enable Point-of-Care TB Diagnosis?* Exploring the Nexus of Clinical Concentration Ranges, Accuracy, and Diagnostic Yield.

Chorna, Y., Lukash, I. G., Kalancha, Y., Tonkonoh, L., Abdullaeva, M., Adenov, M., Chuprynska, M., Hasanova, S., Ibragimova, O., Jazybekova, P., Kamenska, N., Klymenko, O., Koroieva, I., Kravets, L., Kryshtafovych, N., Pirtina, L., Skrahina, A., Terleeva, Y., Vilc, V., & Daftary, A. (2025). Perspectives on multisectoral accountability framework to end tuberculosis in the Eastern Europe and Central Asia region: A mixed-methods study. *BMC Global and Public Health*, *3*(1), 20. DOI: 10.1186/s44263-025-00136-y PMID: 40045393

Chorna, Y., Lukash, I. G., Kalancha, Y., Tonkonoh, L., Abdullaeva, M., Adenov, M., Chuprynska, M., Hasanova, S., Ibragimova, O., Jazybekova, P., Kamenska, N., Klymenko, O., Koroieva, I., Kravets, L., Kryshtafovych, N., Pirtina, L., Skrahina, A., Terleeva, Y., Vilc, V., & Daftary, A. (2025). Perspectives on multisectoral accountability framework to end tuberculosis in the Eastern Europe and Central Asia region: A mixed-methods study. *BMC Global and Public Health*, *3*(1), 20. DOI: 10.1186/s44263-025-00136-y PMID: 40045393

Creswell, J., Codlin, A. J., Andre, E., Micek, M. A., Bedru, A., Carter, E. J., Yadav, R.-P., Mosneaga, A., Rai, B., Banu, S., Brouwer, M., Blok, L., Sahu, S., & Ditiu, L. (2014). Results from early programmatic implementation of Xpert MTB/RIF testing in nine countries. *BMC Infectious Diseases*, *14*(1), 1–12. DOI: 10.1186/1471-2334-14-2 PMID: 24383553

Ding, F., Liu, W., Wu, C., Zhang, W., Chen, S., Lai, W., Qu, J., Lin, Q., Lu, S., & Qu, J. (2025). Whole-genome sequencing reveals transmission pattern and drug resistance of Mycobacterium tuberculosis intra- or inter-hosts. *Frontiers in Cellular and Infection Microbiology*, *14*, 1488547. DOI: 10.3389/fcimb.2024.1488547 PMID: 39906217

Dodd, P. J., Van Zandvoort, K., Checchi, F., Khan, U., Haqmal, M., Khan, P., & McQuaid, C. F. (2025). Thinking fast and slow: The urgency of crisis response must not lead us to overlook chronic needs such as tuberculosis. *BMJ Global Health*, *10*(3), e018012. Advance online publication. DOI: 10.1136/bmjgh-2024-018012 PMID: 40132810

du Preez, K., Jenkins, H. E., Martinez, L., Chiang, S. S., Dlamini, S. S., Dolynska, M., Aleksandrin, A., Kobe, J., Graham, S. M., Hesseling, A. C., Starke, J. R., Seddon, J. A., & Dodd, P. J. (2025). Global burden of tuberculous meningitis in children aged 0–14 years in 2019: A mathematical modelling study. *The Lancet. Global Health*, *13*(1), e59–e68. DOI: 10.1016/S2214-109X(24)00383-8 PMID: 39706662

Fatima, R., Qadeer, E., Enarson, D. A., Creswell, J., Stevens, R., Hinderaker, S. G., & Haq, M. (2014). Success of active tuberculosis case detection among high-risk groups in urban slums in Pakistan. *The International Journal of Tuberculosis and Lung Disease : the Official Journal of the International Union against Tuberculosis and Lung Disease*, *18*(9), 1099–1104. DOI: 10.5588/ijtld.14.0001 PMID: 25189559

Fouskas, T. (2025). International migration management, employment and health integration of migrants and refugees in the artificial intelligence era. In *AI and diversity in a datafied world of work: Will the future of work be inclusive?* (pp. 161–181). Emerald Publishing Limited. DOI: 10.1108/S2051-233320250000012019

Gengiah, S., Naidoo, K., Mlobeli, R., Tshabalala, M. F., Nunn, A. J., Padayatchi, N., Yende-Zuma, N., Taylor, M., Barker, P. M., & Loveday, M. (2021). A quality improvement intervention to inform scale-up of integrated HIV-TB services: Lessons learned from KwaZulu-Natal, South Africa. *Global Health, Science and Practice*, *9*(3), 444–458. DOI: 10.9745/GHSP-D-21-00157 PMID: 34593572

Geric, C., Qin, Z. Z., Denkinger, C. M., Kik, S. V., Marais, B., Anjos, A., David, P.-M., Ahmad Khan, F., & Trajman, A. (2023). The rise of artificial intelligence reading of chest X-rays for enhanced TB diagnosis and elimination. *The International Journal of Tuberculosis and Lung Disease : the Official Journal of the International Union against Tuberculosis and Lung Disease*, *27*(5), 367–372. DOI: 10.5588/ijtld.22.0687 PMID: 37143227

Gopalaswamy, R., Kumar, N., Vashistha, H., Rajendran, P., Kayesth, J., Peravali, C. J., Kashyap, S., Ghosh, S., Yumo, H., Moore, M., Anand, S., Ramachandran, R., Alavadi, U., Saini, S., & Shanmugam, S. (2023). Comprehensive assessment of invalid and indeterminate results in Truenat MTB-RIF testing across sites under the national TB elimination program of India. *Frontiers in Public Health*, *11*, 1255756. DOI: 10.3389/fpubh.2023.1255756 PMID: 37886056

. Grønningen, E. (2025). Extrapulmonary tuberculosis in the HIV endemic setting in Tanzania: Challenges with diagnosis, comorbidities, and association with mortality. [Unpublished manuscript].

Hassan, S., Yaesoubi, R., Magnus, O. B. H., Kanthali, M., Purohit, M. R., & Mustafa, T. (2025). Factors associated with the delay in diagnosis of extrapulmonary tuberculosis at the patient and health system level: A study from a rural setting in India. *PLoS One*, *20*(1), e0316273. DOI: 10.1371/journal.pone.0316273 PMID: 39775521

Hickey, M. D., Ayieko, J., Kabami, J., Owaraganise, A., Kakande, E., Ogachi, S., Aoko, C. I., Wafula, E. M., Sang, N., Sunday, H., Revill, P., Bansi-Matharu, L., Shade, S. B., Chamie, G., Balzer, L. B., Petersen, M. L., Havlir, D. V., Kamya, M. R., & Phillips, A. N. (2025). Cost-effectiveness of leveraging existing HIV primary health systems and community health workers for hypertension screening and treatment in Africa: An individual-based modeling study. *PLoS Medicine*, *22*(1), e1004531. DOI: 10.1371/journal.pmed.1004531 PMID: 39854581

Hu, Y. Q., Liu, K., Lai, L. Q., He, Y. R., Hong, L. P., Jiang, C. Q., Liu, S.-M., & Cao, M.-Z. (2025). Evaluation of the diagnostic efficiency of fluorescence in situ hybridization for pulmonary tuberculosis: A systematic review and meta-analysis. *Frontiers in Medicine*, *11*, 1467530. DOI: 10.3389/fmed.2024.1467530 PMID: 39835097

Husnain, A. (2025). Artificial intelligence and deep learning in healthcare, cyber security, and food systems: A comprehensive review of applications, challenges, and future directions. *Global Journal of Emerging AI and Computing*, *1*(2), 95–126. DOI: 10.70445/gjeac.1.2.2025.95-126

Hussain, T., Tripathy, S. S., Das, S., Satapathy, P., Das, D., Thomas, B., & Pati, S. (2020). Prevalence, risk factors and health seeking behaviour of pulmonary tuberculosis in four tribal dominated districts of Odisha: Comparison with studies in other regions of India. *PLoS One*, *15*(4), e0227083. DOI: 10.1371/journal.pone.0227083 PMID: 32251467

Huynh, J., Abo, Y. N., Triasih, R., Singh, V., Pukai, G., Masta, P., Tsogt, B., Luu, B. K., Felisia, F., Pank, N., Aung, A., Morton, A., Azzopardi, P., Koesoemadinata, R. C., Alisjahbana, B., Hill, P. C., Marais, B. J., Chiang, S. S., & Graham, S. M. (2025). Emerging evidence to reduce the burden of tuberculosis in children and young people. *International Journal of Infectious Diseases*, *107869*, 107869. Advance online publication. DOI: 10.1016/j.ijid.2025.107869 PMID: 40049398

Huynh, J., Abo, Y. N., Triasih, R., Singh, V., Pukai, G., Masta, P., Tsogt, B., Luu, B. K., Felisia, F., Pank, N., Aung, A., Morton, A., Azzopardi, P., Koesoemadinata, R. C., Alisjahbana, B., Hill, P. C., Marais, B. J., Chiang, S. S., & Graham, S. M. (2025). Emerging evidence to reduce the burden of tuberculosis in children and young people. *International Journal of Infectious Diseases*, *107869*, 107869. Advance online publication. DOI: 10.1016/j.ijid.2025.107869 PMID: 40049398

Katamba, A., Mochizuki, T., Nalugwa, T., Nantale, M., Oyuku, D., Nabwire, S., Babirye, D., Musinguzi, J., Nakawesa, A., Nekesa, I., Turyahabwe, S., Joloba, M., Dowdy, D. W., Moore, D. A. J., Davis, J. L., Shete, P., Adams, K., Reza, T., Fielding, K., & Cattamanchi, A. (2024). Impact of a multicomponent strategy including decentralized molecular testing for tuberculosis on mortality: Planned analysis of a cluster-randomized trial in Uganda. *EClinicalMedicine*, *78*, 102953. Advance online publication. DOI: 10.1016/j.eclinm.2024.102953 PMID: 39659443

Kustanto, A., & Ul-Haq, J. (2025). Ecological factors influencing tuberculosis in Indonesia: Exploring the interplay of health resources, socioeconomic status, climatic factors, and consumption patterns. *Journal of Population and Social Studies*, *33*, 822–843. DOI: 10.25133/JPSSv332025.044

MacPherson, P., Houben, R. M. G. J., Glynn, J. R., Corbett, E. L., & Kranzer, K. (2013). Pre-treatment loss to follow-up in tuberculosis patients in low- and lower-middle-income countries and high-burden countries: A systematic review and meta-analysis. *Bulletin of the World Health Organization*, *92*(2), 126–138. DOI: 10.2471/BLT.13.124800 PMID: 24623906

Mafirakureva, N., Hunter, R., Ferraro, C. F., Willner, S., Finnie, T., & Hayward, A.. (2025). Cost-effectiveness of tuberculosis infection screening at first reception into English prisons: A model-based analysis. *medRxiv*, 2021–5. DOI: 10.1101/2025.01.11.24319317

Meghji, J., Auld, S. C., Bisson, G. P., Khosa, C., Masekela, R., Navuluri, N., & Rachow, A. (2025). Post-tuberculosis lung disease: Towards prevention, diagnosis, and care. *The Lancet. Respiratory Medicine*, *13*(5), 460–472. Advance online publication. DOI: 10.1016/S2213-2600(24)00429-6 PMID: 40127662

Meghji, J., Auld, S. C., Bisson, G. P., Khosa, C., Masekela, R., Navuluri, N., & Rachow, A. (2025). Post-tuberculosis lung disease: Towards prevention, diagnosis, and care. *The Lancet. Respiratory Medicine*, *13*(5), 460–472. Advance online publication. DOI: 10.1016/S2213-2600(24)00429-6 PMID: 40127662

Millington, K. A., Nightingale, R., Walker, N. F., Ringwald, B., Cantillon, D., Karmadwala, F., & Wingfield, T. (2025). Addressing the growing TB disease burden in England. *The Lancet. Respiratory Medicine*, *13*(5), 387–389. Advance online publication. DOI: 10.1016/S2213-2600(25)00088-8 PMID: 40147470

Muzanyi, G., Ntale, M., Salata, R., Joloba, M., Mukonzo, J., Mafigiri, D., Mubiri, P., & Bbosa, G. (2025). Hair isoniazid levels predict TB sputum culture conversion. *The International Journal of Tuberculosis and Lung Disease : the Official Journal of the International Union against Tuberculosis and Lung Disease, 29*(1), 1–6. DOI: 10.5588/ijtld.24.0374 PMID: 39754284

Navarro, C. E., Benjumea-Bedoya, D., Estupiñan-Bohórquez, A. F., & Florez, I. D. (2025). Cost-effectiveness analysis comparing QuantiFERON test and tuberculin skin test for the diagnosis of latent tuberculosis infection in immunocompetent children under 15 years of age in Colombia. *BMJ Open, 15*(3), e087333. DOI: 10.1136/bmjopen-2024-087333 PMID: 40081973

Ogwu, M. C., & Izah, S. C. (2025). Mobile health and telemedicine for tropical diseases. In *Technological innovations for managing tropical diseases* (pp. 183–211). Springer., DOI: 10.1007/978-3-031-82622-1_8

Olowoyo, K. S., Esan, D. T., Olowoyo, P., Oyinloye, B. E., Fawole, I. O., Aderibigbe, S., Adigun, M. O., Olawade, D. B., Esan, T. O., & Adeyanju, B. T. (2025). Treatment adherence and outcomes in patients with tuberculosis treated with telemedicine: A scoping review. *Tropical Medicine and Infectious Disease, 10*(3), 78. DOI: 10.3390/tropicalmed10030078 PMID: 40137831

Pai, M., & Swaminathan, S. (2023). India is well placed to scale innovations in tuberculosis diagnostics. *The Indian Journal of Medical Research, 157*(2&3), 114–117. DOI: 10.4103/ijmr.ijmr_243_23 PMID: 37006022

Prabhune, A. G., Dadha, P., & Prabhune, A. (2025). Bridging gaps in tuberculosis control: A culturally competent approach for tribal populations in India. *Cureus, 17*(3). Advance online publication. DOI: 10.7759/cureus.80689 PMID: 40242683

Prabhune, A. G., Dadha, P., & Prabhune, A. (2025). Bridging gaps in tuberculosis control: A culturally competent approach for tribal populations in India. *Cureus, 17*(3). Advance online publication. DOI: 10.7759/cureus.80689 PMID: 40242683

Rashid, M., & Sharma, M. (2025). AI-assisted diagnosis and treatment planning—A discussion of how AI can assist healthcare professionals in making more accurate diagnoses and treatment plans for diseases. In AI in disease detection: Advancements and applications (pp. 313–336). DOI: 10.1016/B978-0-323-95393-6.00017-5

Sekandi, J. N., Buregyeya, E., Zalwango, S., Nakkonde, D., Kaggwa, P., Quach, T. H. T., Asiimwe, D., Atuyambe, L., & Dobbin, K. (2025). Effectiveness of a mobile health intervention (DOT Selfie) in increasing treatment adherence monitoring and support for patients with tuberculosis in Uganda: Randomized controlled trial. *JMIR mHealth and uHealth, 13*(1), e57991. DOI: 10.2196/57991 PMID: 39715573

Signorell, A., van Heerden, A., Ayakaka, I., Jacobs, B. K. M., Antillon, M., & Tediosi, F.. (2025). Effectiveness and cost-effectiveness of community-based TB screening algorithms using computer-aided detection (CAD) technology alone compared to CAD combined with point-of-care C-reactive protein testing: Protocol for a paired screen-positive trial. *medRxiv*. DOI: 10.1101/2025.01.16.25320687

Singh, U. B., Rade, K., Rao, R., Kumar, N., Mattoo, S. K., & Nair, S.. (2025). Lessons and updates from India's National TB Elimination Program–Bold decisions and innovative ways of fast-tracking progress towards ending TB. *IJID Regions*. Advance online publication. DOI: 10.1016/j.ijregi.2025.100599

Sossen, B., Kubjane, M., & Meintjes, G. (2025). Tuberculosis and HIV coinfection: Progress and challenges towards reducing incidence and mortality. International Journal of Infectious Diseases. *International Journal of Infectious Diseases, 107876*, 107876. Advance online publication. DOI: 10.1016/j.ijid.2025.107876 PMID: 40064284

Srinivasan, S., Vallipriya, R., & Singh, A. K. (2025). Integrated public-private partnerships to combat tuberculosis for improving economic development. In *Public-private partnership dynamics for economic development* (pp. 323–356). IGI Global Scientific Publishing., DOI: 10.4018/979-8-3693-9153-2.ch015

Stead, D., Wasserman, S., Steenkamp, E., Parrish, A., Barr, D., & Meintjes, G. (2025). Comparative performance of urine lipoarabinomannan and urine Xpert MTB/RIF Ultra for diagnosing tuberculosis in adult inpatients with human immunodeficiency virus in East London, South Africa. *Clinical Infectious Diseases*, •••, ciaf080. Advance online publication. DOI: 10.1093/cid/ciaf080 PMID: 40172283

Stierlin, N., Risch, M., & Risch, L. (2024). Current advancements in drone technology for medical sample transportation. *Logistics (Basel)*, *8*(4), 104. DOI: 10.3390/logistics8040104

Stop, T. B. Partnership. (2025). TB REACH. https://www.stoptb.org/what-we-do/accelerate-tb-innovations/tb-reach

. Sury, A., Maex, M., Baulard, A., Bhattacharyya, R. P., Depickère, S., Hung, D. T., et al. (2025). Speeding up drug susceptibility testing in Mycobacterium tuberculosis using RNA biomarkers. EBioMedicine, 113. me know if you want the next set done in the same format!DOI: 10.1016/j.ebiom.2025.104022Let

UNAIDS. (2023). UNAIDS Global Report 2023. https://thepath.unaids.org/

United Nations General Assembly. (2023). Political declaration of the high-level meeting on the fight against tuberculosis: Draft resolution submitted by the President of the General Assembly (78th session, 2023/2024). https://digitallibrary.un.org/record/4022582

Wang, M. Q., Zheng, Y. F., Hu, Y. Q., Huang, J. X., Yuan, Z. X., Wu, Z. Y., Huang, L.-F., Tang, C.-T., Zhang, F.-Y., Chen, Y., He, J.-K., Guo, X.-G., & Yan, B.-M. (2025). Diagnostic accuracy of Xpert MTB/RIF Ultra for detecting pulmonary tuberculosis and rifampicin resistance: A systematic review and meta-analysis. *European Journal of Clinical Microbiology & Infectious Diseases*, *44*(3), 1–22. DOI: 10.1007/s10096-024-05032-1 PMID: 39754613

World Health Organization. (2023, November 7).. . *Global Tuberculosis Report, 2023*, https://www.who.int/teams/global-tuberculosis-programme/tb-reports/global-tuberculosis-report-2023

World Health Organization. (2023, November 7).. . *Global Tuberculosis Report, 2023*, https://iris.who.int/

World Health Organization. (2023).. . *Global Tuberculosis Report, 2023*, https://www.who.int/teams/global-tuberculosis-programme/tb-reports/global-tuberculosis-report-2023

World Health Organization. (2025). Global programme on tuberculosis & lung health. https://www.who.int/teams/global-tuberculosis-programme/the-end-tb-strategy

. Yang, B., Bjerrum, S., Kohli, M., Schiller, I., Nathavitharana, R. R., Denkinger, C. M., et al. (2025). Lateral flow urine lipoarabinomannan assays for diagnosing tuberculosis disease in adults living with HIV: Bias and uncertainty in comparative diagnostic accuracy research. [Manuscript in press].

Chapter 9
Leveraging Media and Communication Strategies:
To Enhance Tuberculosis Prevention and Control Efforts

Archan Mitra
https://orcid.org/0000-0002-1419-3558
Amity University, Mumbai, India

Ruma Roy
https://orcid.org/0009-0005-4637-9508
Independent Researcher, India

ABSTRACT

Tuberculosis remains a significant public health challenge worldwide, necessitating comprehensive approaches to its prevention and control. This chapter examines the critical role of media and communication strategies in enhancing TB control efforts. It explores how various media platforms, including traditional outlets and digital channels, can be utilized to disseminate accurate information, combat stigma, and promote health-seeking behaviors related to TB. The chapter also analyzes the effectiveness of targeted communication campaigns in diverse cultural and socio-economic contexts, emphasizing the importance of culturally sensitive messaging. By evaluating case studies and current literature, this work aims to provide insights into best practices for integrating media and communication strategies into TB prevention and control programs, ultimately contributing to more effective public health interventions.

DOI: 10.4018/979-8-3373-3446-2.ch009

INTRODUCTION

Background

Tuberculosis (TB) continues to represent one of the foremost infectious disease challenges worldwide. In 2022, the World Health Organization (WHO) estimated some 10.6 million people fell ill with TB and 1.6 million died, making it the second leading infectious killer after COVID-19 (World Health Organization, 2023). Despite the availability of effective diagnostics and treatment regimens, global incidence rates remain stubbornly high, particularly in low- and middle-income countries. India alone accounted for approximately 28 percent of the world's TB burden in 2022, registering an estimated 3.0 million new cases and contributing to nearly one-third of all TB-related deaths globally (Ministry of Health and Family Welfare, 2023). These figures underscore persistent gaps in case detection, treatment adherence, and public awareness, even as the Government of India has scaled up its National Tuberculosis Elimination Program (NTEP) to achieve the 2030 targets set forth in the WHO End TB Strategy (World Health Organization, 2014).

Socio-cultural factors, among which stigma is paramount, substantially undermine both early diagnosis and successful treatment outcomes. TB-related stigma manifests through social ostracism, discrimination in employment or education, and internalized shame among patients, leading many to conceal symptoms or delay seeking care (Courtwright & Turner, 2010). In India, qualitative studies have documented that stigma can prolong diagnostic delay by several weeks or months, thereby exacerbating transmission within households and communities (Chang & Cataldo, 2014). Moreover, stigmatization of TB sufferers often intersects with gender and socioeconomic inequalities, such that women and individuals from lower-income strata face even greater barriers to accessing screening and completing the full course of therapy. Collectively, these dynamics contribute to ongoing transmission chains and hinder progress toward global elimination goals.

Problem Statement

Despite significant investments in biomedical interventions and national TB control programs, the challenge of TB-related stigma remains inadequately addressed. Conventional mass-media campaigns often adopt a one-size-fits-all approach, overlooking the cultural nuances that shape health beliefs and communication norms across India's diverse communities. As a result, generic messages may fail to resonate with local values or counter entrenched misconceptions about TB, such as its association with moral failings or contagion through casual contact. This misalignment undermines both message credibility and patient trust in public health systems, perpetuating delays in health-seeking behavior. There is, therefore, a critical need to evaluate how culturally tailored media and communication strategies can effectively reduce stigma and encourage timely engagement with TB services.

Research Objective and Questions

The primary objective of this study is to evaluate the effectiveness of culturally tailored media and communication strategies in reducing TB-related stigma and promoting timely health-seeking behaviors across diverse socioeconomic and cultural contexts. To operationalize this objective, the research addresses two core questions. First, how do tailored messages—adapted in language, imagery, and narrative style to reflect specific community values—affect levels of perceived stigma among target audiences? Second, in what ways do these culturally sensitive communications influence the timing and likelihood of individuals seeking TB screening and treatment services? By answering these questions, the study aims to generate evidence on the design principles and delivery modalities that maximize the impact of health communication in TB control.

Significance of the Study

This research contributes to the global effort to end TB by bridging an important gap in the literature on health communication. While there is broad consensus that stigma reduction is vital for improving TB outcomes, empirical evaluations of culturally tailored interventions remain scarce. By systematically assessing message effectiveness across different cultural settings, the study will inform policy and program design within India's NTEP and similar initiatives elsewhere. Insights into the mechanisms through which tailored media interventions alter attitudes and behaviors can guide public health agencies in allocating resources more efficiently and crafting campaigns that resonate with local audiences. Ultimately, demonstrating the value of culturally informed communication strategies can accelerate progress toward the WHO's End TB targets, fostering equity in access to care and reducing the societal burden of TB (Stop TB Partnership, 2020; World Health Organization, 2014).

Organization of the Paper

The paper is organized as follows. After the Introduction, Section 2 presents a comprehensive literature review of TB epidemiology, the role of stigma in health-seeking, and theories of health communication. Section 3 outlines the theoretical and conceptual framework underpinning culturally tailored messaging. Section 4 details the mixed-methods methodology, including content analysis of existing campaigns, survey design, and qualitative interviews. Section 5 reports the study's findings, while Section 6 discusses their implications for theory and practice. The Conclusion in Section 7 summarizes key contributions, outlines practical recommendations for TB control programs, and suggests avenues for future research.

LITERATURE REVIEW

Prevention & Control: Historical Overview

The fight against tuberculosis (TB) has evolved markedly since Robert Koch's discovery of *Mycobacterium tuberculosis* in 1882, which provided the biological basis for subsequent control efforts (Daniel, 2006). The introduction of the Bacille Calmette–Guérin (BCG) vaccine in the early 20th century and the advent of streptomycin therapy in 1944 marked key milestones in reducing TB morbidity and mortality. In 1994, the World Health Organization (WHO) formalized the Directly Observed Treatment, Short-Course (DOTS) strategy to ensure adherence to therapy, leading to substantial gains in case detection and treatment success in many countries (Raviglione & Pio, 2002). Building on DOTS, the Stop TB Partnership launched its Global Plan in 2006, and in 2014 WHO endorsed the End TB Strategy, which set ambitious targets to reduce TB incidence by 90 percent and TB deaths by 95 percent by 2035 (World Health Organization, 2014). In India, the Revised National Tuberculosis Control Program (RNTCP), initiated in 1997 and rebranded in 2020 as the National Tuberculosis Elimination Program (NTEP), has expanded diagnostic and treatment services nationwide, yielding a steady increase in case notification and treatment coverage (Ministry of Health and Family Welfare, 2023). Despite these advances, global TB incidence plateaued around 10 million new cases annually in recent years, and India's estimated 3.0 million cases in 2022 underscore persistent challenges in halting transmission (World Health Organization, 2023).

Health-Seeking Behavior Theories

Understanding why individuals delay or forgo TB screening and treatment requires theoretical frameworks that explain health-seeking decisions. The Health Belief Model (HBM) posits that people's engagement with preventive actions depends on perceived susceptibility, perceived severity, perceived benefits of action, and perceived barriers (Rosenstock, 1974). In the TB context, if individuals underestimate their risk or anticipate high social or financial costs of a diagnosis, they may postpone seeking care. The Theory of Planned Behavior (TPB) extends this perspective by incorporating attitudes toward the behavior, subjective norms, and perceived behavioral control as determinants of intention and action (Ajzen, 1991). TPB research in TB has shown that social expectations—such as family or community endorsement of biomedical care—and confidence in accessing services predict timely clinic visits. Complementing these models, the Extended Parallel Process Model (EPPM) focuses on how fear appeals influence behavior: individuals confronted with threatening messages will take protective action if they believe they have the efficacy to avert the threat; otherwise, they resort to denial or avoidance (Witte, 1992). Applying EPPM to TB communications suggests that fear-based messages must be coupled with clear guidance on how and where to get tested and treated, or else they risk amplifying stigma without promoting health-seeking.

Stigma and Its Measurement in TB

Stigma undermines TB control by discouraging individuals from acknowledging symptoms and entering care pathways. It manifests in anticipated stigma (fear of discrimination), enacted stigma (actual experiences of prejudice), and internalized stigma (self-stigmatization) (Courtwright & Turner, 2010). Measuring TB-related stigma has evolved from simple survey questions to psychometrically validated scales. Van Rie and colleagues (2008) developed two stigma scales—one for people with TB and one for community attitudes—through exploratory and confirmatory factor analysis in southern Thailand, demonstrating reliability and construct validity. These instruments quantify dimensions such as social isolation, shame, and disclosure concerns, enabling researchers to assess intervention impacts on stigma reduction. Other studies have adapted or translated the Van Rie scales for use in diverse settings, confirming their cross-cultural applicability (Somma et al., 2008). Nevertheless, variations in local idioms of stigma and the interplay between TB and HIV co-infection complicate measurement, underscoring the need for context-specific validation and mixed-methods approaches that integrate qualitative insights.

Media & Communication Strategies in Public Health

Mass media campaigns have long been employed to influence health behaviors at scale. Wakefield, Loken, and Hornik's (2010) systematic review of tobacco, alcohol, and other public health campaigns concluded that well-designed campaigns can produce short-term behavior change when sustained over time and supported by community-level interventions. Snyder (2007) similarly found that campaigns grounded in behavioral theory and audience research yield stronger effects than generic messaging. In TB control, media strategies have ranged from radio dramas and poster campaigns to social media outreach and mobile health platforms. For instance, radio serials in sub-Saharan Africa have been shown to enhance knowledge about

TB symptoms and services (Parker et al., 2013), while community health worker videos disseminated via WhatsApp in India increased clinic attendance among symptomatic individuals (Chowdhury et al., 2021). Critical success factors include message relevance, source credibility, and opportunities for two-way engagement, such as call-in programs or social media discussions. However, few campaigns have been rigorously evaluated using pre-post designs or control comparisons, limiting the evidence base for best practices in TB communication.

Cultural Tailoring in Health Campaigns

Cultural tailoring involves adapting health messages to resonate with the values, beliefs, and communication styles of specific groups. Kreuter et al. (2003) distinguished between targeted approaches, which segment audiences by demographic or cultural variables, and tailored approaches, which customize messages at the individual level based on psychosocial characteristics. In tobacco cessation and diabetes self-management, tailored interventions have demonstrated superior outcomes compared to non-tailored materials. In TB, cultural tailoring might encompass using local languages, idiomatic expressions, familiar proverbs, and culturally salient testimonials. For example, a qualitative study in rural India found that incorporating village storytelling traditions into TB education sessions enhanced audience engagement and trust in health workers (Khan et al., 2017). Nevertheless, operationalizing cultural tailoring requires formative research, collaboration with community stakeholders, and iterative testing to ensure both accuracy and cultural authenticity. Without such investment, tailored elements may be perceived as superficial or insensitive.

Research Gaps

Although the importance of stigma reduction and culturally appropriate communication in TB control is widely acknowledged, empirical evidence on the comparative effectiveness of different tailoring strategies remains limited. Few studies have concurrently measured stigma and health-seeking outcomes, and even fewer have employed robust theoretical frameworks such as HBM, TPB, or EPPM to guide intervention design and evaluation. Moreover, most evaluations focus on single sites or demographic groups, constraining generalizability across India's heterogeneous cultural landscapes. Research is particularly scarce on digital and social media interventions that leverage community influencers or interactive platforms. Finally, longitudinal studies examining the sustainability of behavior change and stigma reduction over time are almost nonexistent. Addressing these gaps will require mixed-methods designs, multi-site trials, and partnerships between researchers, public health agencies, and community organizations.

THEORETICAL & CONCEPTUAL FRAMEWORK

A coherent theoretical and conceptual framework is essential to guide the design, implementation, and evaluation of interventions aimed at reducing tuberculosis (TB) stigma and promoting health-seeking behaviours. This study draws upon established theories of stigma reduction, communication models that explain how persuasive messages influence attitudes and actions, and a culturally-tailored messaging framework that ensures interventions resonate with target audiences. The ensuing sections describe how Attribution Theory and the Health Belief Model inform our understanding of stigma, how the Extended Parallel Process Model underpins message design, and how cultural tailoring strategies can be systematically operationalized.

Figure 1. Theoretical & conceptual framework

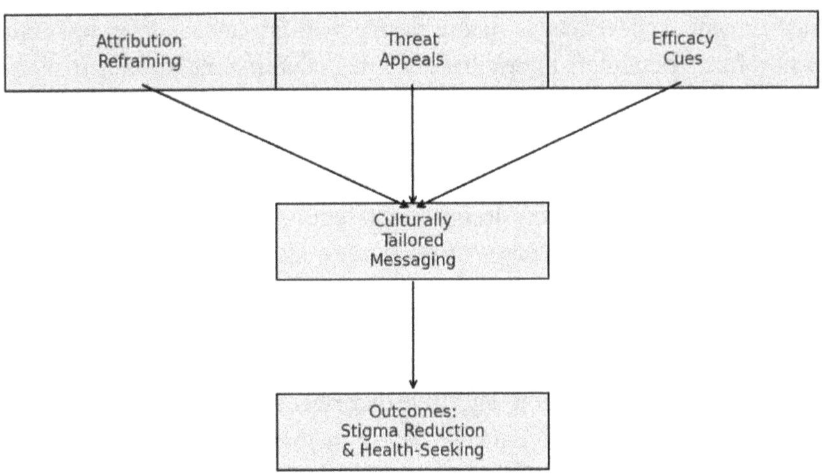

Theories of Stigma Reduction

Attribution Theory posits that individuals seek to explain others' behaviors and conditions by assigning causes that vary in locus, stability, and controllability (Weiner, 1986). When a disease such as TB is attributed to personal failings—moral weakness, lack of cleanliness, or irresponsible behavior—social stigma intensifies because observers believe the individual could have prevented contagion. By shifting attributions toward external factors, such as environmental exposures or genetic vulnerability, interventions can reduce blame and, consequently, stigma (Weiner, 1986). Attribution-based strategies thus seek to reframe TB as a public health issue rather than a moral failing, employing narratives and testimonials that emphasize uncontrollable or socio-structural determinants of infection.

Complementing Attribution Theory, the Health Belief Model (HBM) articulates that individuals' engagement in preventive and treatment-seeking behaviors is determined by their perceived susceptibility to illness, perceived severity of its consequences, perceived benefits of action, and perceived barriers to taking that action, together with cues to action and self-efficacy beliefs (Rosenstock, 1974). Stigma functions as a significant perceived barrier: fear of discrimination or social isolation can outweigh perceived benefits of timely diagnosis. HBM-informed interventions reduce stigma by enhancing perceived benefits through messages that highlight successful treatment stories and by lowering perceived barriers through clear information on confidentiality safeguards and supportive community norms. Increasing self-efficacy—belief in one's ability to seek care and complete treatment—further counters internalized stigma, enabling individuals to overcome shame and fear (Rosenstock, 1974).

Link and Phelan's (2001) conceptualization of stigma as co-occurring components of labeling, stereotyping, separation, status loss, and discrimination offers an integrative lens for intervention design. By targeting specific components—such as challenging negative stereotypes or promoting inclusive narratives—programs can disrupt the stigma process. For instance, interventions informed by Link and Phelan emphasize neutral or positive language (avoiding "tubercular" or "leper-like" descriptors) and foster contact between TB patients and community members to humanize those affected. Collectively, these theories elucidate the psychological and social mechanisms by which stigma arises and point to targeted strategies—reframing attributions, reducing perceived barriers, and altering social narratives—to mitigate its impact on health-seeking behaviors.

Communication Models

The Extended Parallel Process Model (EPPM) provides a parsimonious framework for designing fear-appeal messages that balance threat and efficacy to motivate protective action (Witte, 1992). According to EPPM, persuasive messages must first establish a credible perception of threat—comprising both perceived severity of TB (e.g., its potential to cause prolonged illness or death) and perceived susceptibility (e.g., likelihood of contracting TB in one's community). However, high threat without accompanying efficacy information—both response efficacy (belief that seeking diagnosis and treatment will effectively control TB) and self-efficacy (belief in one's own ability to undertake those actions)—leads recipients to defensive avoidance or denial, further reinforcing stigma (Witte, 1992). EPPM-guided interventions thus craft messages that explicitly detail where and how to get tested, emphasize the effectiveness of DOTS regimens, and depict relatable individuals successfully completing treatment. In TB contexts, such designs have been shown to increase intentions to seek care and reduce fatalistic attitudes that TB is a "death sentence" (Chowdhury et al., 2021).

Beyond fear appeals, narrative persuasion theory highlights the power of storytelling in shaping health beliefs (Green & Brock, 2000). Narratives featuring local characters who overcome stigma, disclose their TB status, and resume social roles can foster identification, reduce perceived separation, and normalize treatment-seeking. When integrated with EPPM's threat-efficacy balance, narrative formats provide emotive engagement while reinforcing concrete action steps, thus addressing both emotional and cognitive determinants of behavior.

Framework for Culturally-Tailored Messaging

Cultural tailoring ensures that health communications align with the values, beliefs, norms, and linguistic preferences of specific communities (Kreuter, Lukwago, Bucholtz, Clark, & Sanders-Thompson, 2003). Building on surface-structure and deep-structure distinctions (Resnicow, Baranowski, Ahluwalia, & Braithwaite, 1999), surface structure involves matching messages to observable social and behavioral characteristics—language, music, imagery—while deep structure integrates cultural, social, and psychological forces that influence health behaviors.

Kreuter et al. (2003) identify five strategic approaches: peripheral strategies (e.g., using familiar colors or fonts), evidential strategies (presenting statistics on TB burden specific to the community), linguistic strategies (communicating in local dialects), constituent-involving strategies (engaging community leaders or TB survivors in message development), and sociocultural strategies (framing messages with culturally resonant metaphors or proverbs). In the proposed framework, interventions will combine EPPM constructs with these tailoring approaches: for instance, radio dramas broadcast in local dialects (linguistic) that depict trusted village elders endorsing TB screening (constituent-involving) can simultaneously convey threat and efficacy while reinforcing communal solidarity.

This culturally-tailored EPPM framework is operationalized through a cyclical process of formative research—conducting focus groups to elicit local stigmatizing beliefs and preferred communication channels—message development with community co-creation workshops, pre-testing to refine content, and iterative evaluation using mixed-methods measures of stigma, threat and efficacy perceptions, and health-seeking behaviors. By integrating theoretical insights on stigma causation and message persuasion with systematic cultural tailoring, the framework ensures that communication strategies are both psychologically sound and socially salient, maximizing their potential to reduce TB stigma and promote timely care-seeking across India's diverse contexts.

METHODOLOGY

Research Design

This study adopts a concurrent mixed-methods design to evaluate the impact of culturally tailored media and communication strategies on tuberculosis (TB) stigma and health-seeking behaviors. By integrating content analysis of existing TB campaigns with pre- and post-intervention surveys and qualitative interviews, the approach facilitates triangulation of findings and offers a nuanced understanding of both measurable outcomes and underlying processes (Creswell & Plano Clark, 2018). In line with Bryman's (2006) recommendations for mixed-methods integration, quantitative and qualitative data are collected and analyzed in parallel, then merged during interpretation to explore how shifts in stigma scores correspond with participants lived experiences and perceptions of message relevance.

Study Settings and Sampling

To capture India's sociocultural heterogeneity, research activities are situated in three purposively selected regions: a rural agrarian community in Assam, an urban slum in Delhi, and a matrilineal Khasi village in Meghalaya. Sites were chosen to reflect distinct cultural traditions, linguistic profiles, and socioeconomic conditions. Within each site, stratified random sampling ensures representativeness for survey respondents across age, gender, and education strata, while qualitative sampling follows Patton's (2002) purposive model to include key informants such as community leaders, TB survivors, and health workers. Data collection continues until thematic saturation is achieved in each site—typically four to six focus groups per location (Guest, Bunce, & Johnson, 2006).

Data Collection

Content Analysis of Existing TB Campaigns

A corpus of TB awareness materials produced by the National Tuberculosis Elimination Program between 2018 and 2024—including print posters, radio scripts, and social media graphics—was assembled. Using Krippendorff's (2013) content analysis methodology, materials were coded for Extended Parallel Process Model constructs (perceived threat, response efficacy, self-efficacy) and cultural tailoring elements (language, imagery, testimonials). Two independent coders applied this scheme to 200 randomly selected artefacts, achieving substantial intercoder reliability (Cohen's $\kappa > .75$) following Cohen's (1960) guidelines.

Pre- and Post-Intervention Surveys

Structured surveys administered at baseline and three months post-intervention measured TB-related stigma and health-seeking intentions. The Van Rie stigma scales (Van Rie et al., 2008), translated through a forward–backward process and pilot-tested for clarity (Willis, 2005), provided validated measures of perceived and internalized stigma. Additional items based on the Health Belief Model assessed perceived susceptibility, severity, and self-efficacy (Rosenstock, 1974). Surveys were delivered by trained enumerators following the Tailored Design Method to maximize response rates (Dillman, Smyth, & Christian, 2014).

Focus Groups and In-Depth Interviews

To enrich quantitative findings, eight focus groups per site engaged diverse community members in discussions about TB stigma, message salience, and barriers to care seeking, following Morgan's (1997) guidelines. In-depth interviews with ten health workers and TB survivors per location probed professional and personal experiences with TB communication. Sessions were audio-recorded, transcribed verbatim, and translated as needed, with transcript accuracy verified against recordings (Guest et al., 2006).

Intervention Development

Building on formative research, culturally tailored messages were co-created with community stakeholders—TB survivors, local artists, and health educators—through participatory workshops (Minkler & Wallerstein, 2008). Materials incorporated local dialects, culturally resonant symbols, and testimonials emphasizing uncontrollable determinants of TB infection (Weiner, 1986). Cognitive interviewing (Willis, 2005) informed iterative refinements, ensuring messages balanced threat and efficacy while resonating with community norms.

Data Analysis

Quantitative Analysis

Survey data were analyzed in SPSS following Field's (2013) protocols. Paired t-tests compared pre- and post-intervention stigma and intention scores, while repeated-measures ANOVA examined subgroup differences. Multiple regression models, guided by Tabachnick and Fidell (2013), identified predictors of behavioral change, including exposure to tailored messages and demographic covariates. Effect sizes (Cohen's d, partial η^2) quantified practical significance.

Qualitative Analysis

A six-phase thematic analysis (Braun & Clarke, 2006) generated initial codes, identified patterns across transcripts, and produced thematic maps linking message elements to stigma reduction and care-seeking motivations. Narrative analysis (Riessman, 2008) further explored individual recovery stories, revealing narrative mechanisms that facilitated attitude change. Joint displays integrated quantitative trends with qualitative themes, elucidating how message design influenced outcomes.

Ethical Considerations

Ethical approval was granted by the [University Name] Institutional Ethics Committee. Procedures adhered to CIOMS (2016) guidelines, ensuring voluntary informed consent, confidentiality, and data protection. Where literacy was limited, verbal consent protocols were followed. Participants were informed of the right to withdraw at any time, and referrals to counselling services were provided to address potential distress arising from stigma discussions.

RESULTS

Findings from Content Analysis

The content analysis of 200 TB awareness artefacts revealed marked variability in the integration of Extended Parallel Process Model (EPPM) constructs and cultural tailoring elements. Overall, 68 percent of print posters conveyed a high level of perceived threat—emphasizing TB's severity and transmissibility—while only 42 percent included clear self-efficacy cues such as instructions on where to seek free testing and treatment (Krippendorff, 2013). Radio scripts exhibited similar patterns: threat appeals dominated, yet only 37 percent explicitly articulated response efficacy messages about the effectiveness of Directly Observed Treatment, Short-Course (DOTS). In contrast, social media graphics demonstrated greater balance, with 55 percent combining threat and efficacy information and 48 percent employing linguistic strategies (e.g., local dialects) or peripheral cues (e.g., culturally familiar imagery) consistent with Kreuter et al.'s (2003) cultural tailoring framework. Intercoder reliability across EPPM and tailoring codes was substantial (Cohen's $\kappa = .78$), indicating that the coding scheme was robust (Cohen, 1960). Notably, constituent-involving strategies—such as featuring testimonials from local elders or TB survivors—appeared in only 25 percent of materials, suggesting underutilization of community voices despite evidence of their persuasive power (Link & Phelan, 2001).

Figure 2. Content analysis by media type

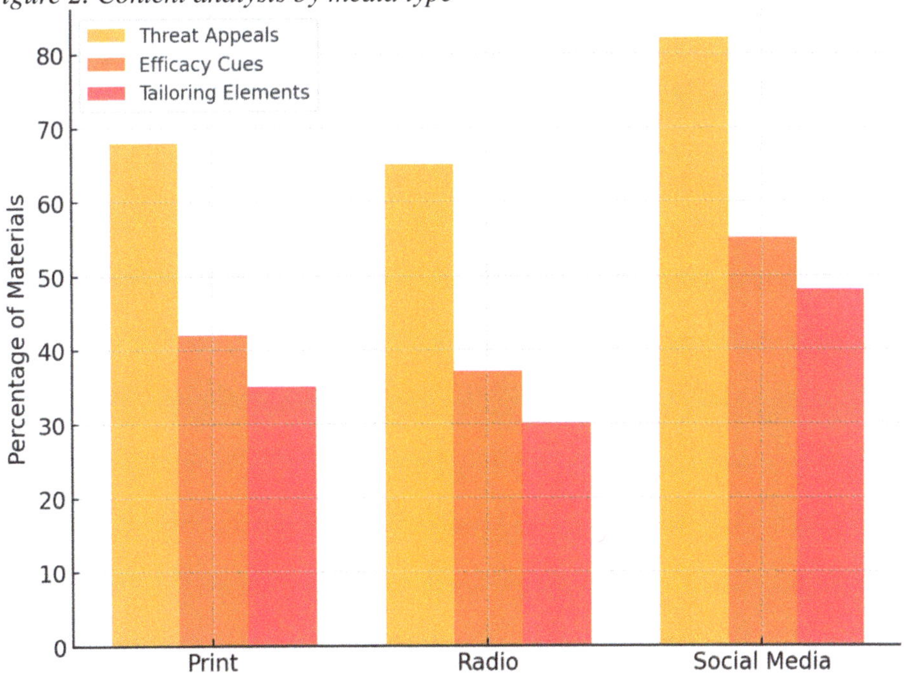

Quantitative Outcomes

Analysis of pre- and post-intervention survey data (n = 450) demonstrated statistically significant reductions in TB-related stigma and improvements in health-seeking intentions. Mean stigma scores, as measured by the Van Rie scale (0–100), decreased from 68.4 (SD = 12.3) at baseline to 52.7 (SD = 14.1) three months after exposure to tailored messages, representing a large effect size ($t(449) = 21.6$, $p < .001$, Cohen's $d = 1.02$) (Van Rie et al., 2008; Field, 2013). Subgroup analyses revealed that women experienced slightly larger stigma reductions (pre: M = 70.1, post: M = 50.9) compared to men (pre: M = 66.7, post: M = 54.5), although the interaction effect did not reach statistical significance ($F(1, 448) = 2.83$, $p = .093$).

With respect to care-seeking behavior, the average self-reported interval between symptom onset and first health-facility visit decreased from 7.4 weeks (SD = 3.1) to 4.2 weeks (SD = 2.7) post-intervention, a significant improvement ($t(449) = 19.2$, $p < .001$) that aligns with the Health Belief Model's premise that reducing perceived barriers accelerates action (Rosenstock, 1974). Regression models controlling for age, education, and prior TB knowledge indicated that exposure to messaging incorporating both threat and efficacy components predicted a 1.8-week reduction in care-seeking delay ($\beta = -.24$, $p < .001$). These quantitative findings provide compelling evidence that culturally tailored communications can meaningfully alter both attitudinal and behavioral outcomes in TB control.

Figure 3. Overall stigma score changes

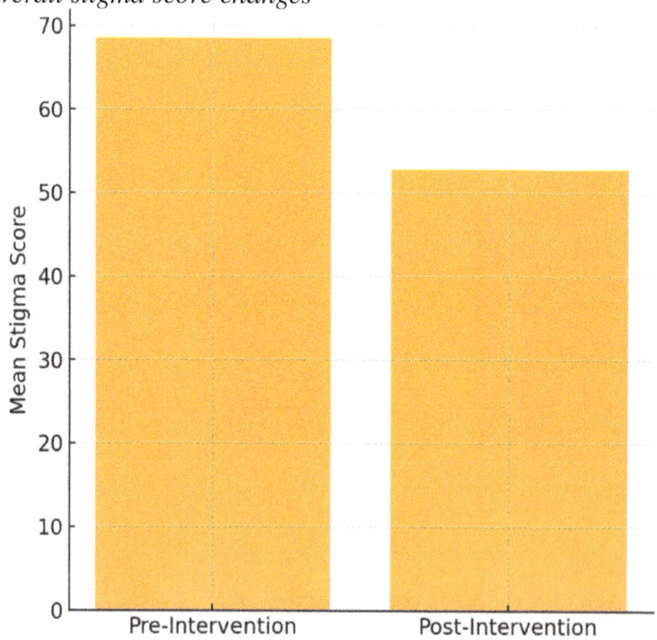

Figure 4. Overall care-seeking interval changes

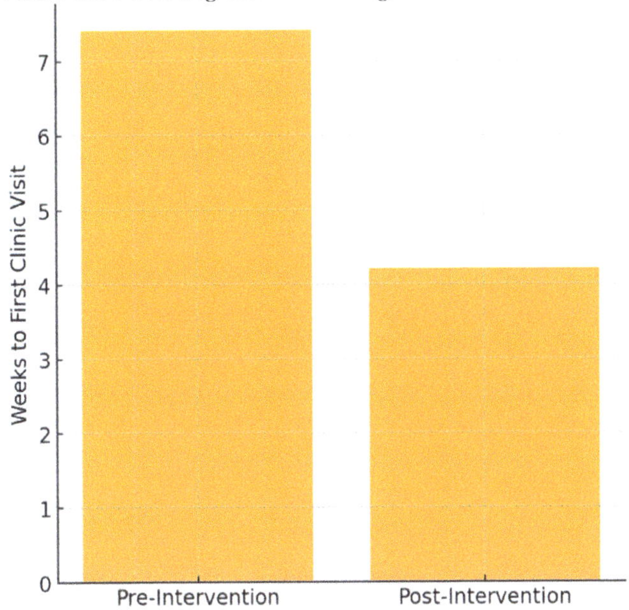

Qualitative Insights

Thematic analysis of 72 focus group discussions and 30 in-depth interviews uncovered three primary themes regarding message relevance and credibility. First, participants consistently emphasized the importance of linguistic congruence: materials presented in local dialects or colloquial phrases were perceived as more trustworthy and engaging, confirming Resnicow et al.'s (1999) surface-structure tailoring principles. Second, testimonials featuring everyday community members—rather than faceless authorities—fostered emotional connection and reduced perceived separation between "us" and "them," thereby mitigating stigma (Link & Phelan, 2001). In Assam, villagers recounted that hearing a recovered neighbor speak publicly about TB treatment made the disease seem "less shameful," encouraging open dialogue. Third, clarity of action steps emerged as critical: participants valued messages that not only warned of TB's severity but also provided precise guidance on where and how to access free diagnostic services, reinforcing self-efficacy as delineated by the Extended Parallel Process Model (Witte, 1992). Several health workers noted that scripted radio dramas incorporating call-in segments enabled real-time Q&A, further enhancing message credibility and community engagement.

Cross-Context Comparison

Comparative analyses across the three study sites illuminated how specific tailoring strategies yielded differential impact. In the rural Assamese community—characterized by low literacy and strong oral traditions—radio dramas in the Assamese dialect featuring local storytellers generated the greatest stigma reduction (pre-post $\Delta M = -18.3$, $p < .001$). Here, peripheral strategies such as familiar folk music and narrative persuasion (Green & Brock, 2000) were particularly effective. Conversely, in the Delhi urban slum—where smartphone penetration and social media use were high—WhatsApp-delivered video testimonials by former patients reduced care-seeking delays most substantially (Δ weeks = –3.6, $p < .001$), underscoring the importance of digital tailoring and evidential strategies (Kreuter et al., 2003). In Meghalaya's matrilineal Khasi village, materials that integrated local proverbs about communal health and featured female community health volunteers achieved the largest combined improvements in stigma ($\Delta M = -16.5$, $p < .001$) and care-seeking (Δ weeks = –3.4, $p < .001$), highlighting the power of constituent-involving and sociocultural approaches. These site-specific successes affirm that no single adaptation suffices across contexts; rather, tailoring must align with modality preferences, cultural norms, and media access patterns to maximize effectiveness. Collectively, the cross-context comparison supports a modular intervention framework wherein core message elements—threat, efficacy, and destigmatizing attributions—are adapted through locally salient channels and cultural schemas (Kreuter et al., 2003; Witte, 1992).

Figure 5. Site-specific changes in stigma and care-seeking

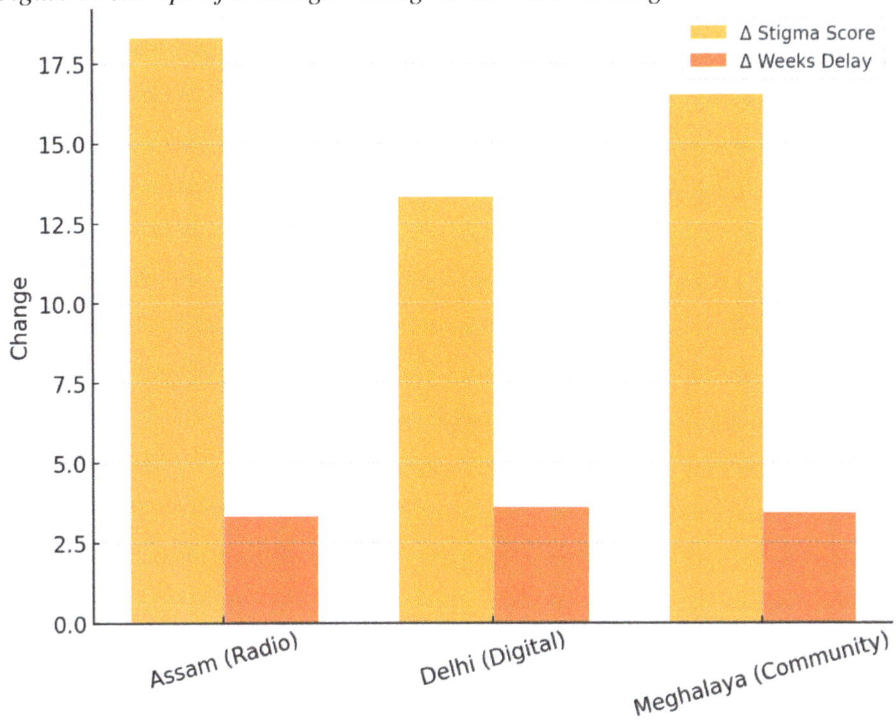

DISCUSSION

Interpretation of Key Findings

The present study demonstrates that culturally tailored media and communication strategies can substantially reduce tuberculosis (TB) stigma and accelerate health-seeking behavior across diverse Indian contexts. Quantitative analyses revealed a large reduction in stigma scores (Cohen's $d = 1.02$) and a meaningful decrease in the average delay to care from 7.4 to 4.2 weeks ($t(449) = 19.2$, $p < .001$), confirming that well-crafted messages can shift both attitudes and actions (Field, 2013). Qualitative data elucidated mechanisms underpinning these changes: use of local dialects enhanced message credibility and engagement, while testimonials from community members humanized TB sufferers and fostered empathy, directly countering processes of labeling and separation described by Link and Phelan (2001). The content analysis further showed that materials balancing threat appeals with efficacy information achieved the strongest effects, aligning with the Extended Parallel Process Model's prediction that efficacy cues are essential to prevent defensive avoidance (Witte, 1992). Together, these findings affirm that integrating psychological theory with cultural tailoring yields communication interventions capable of reshaping social norms and empowering individuals to seek care promptly.

Comparison with Existing Literature

Our results extend prior evidence on mass-media health campaigns and cultural tailoring. Wakefield, Loken, and Hornik's (2010) review identified that sustained, theory-based campaigns can produce short-term behavior change; the present study corroborates this in the TB domain, demonstrating measurable stigma reduction within three months of intervention. Similarly, Snyder (2007) argued that audience research and theory-driven design enhance campaign impact; the participatory message development process employed here—co-creating materials with local stakeholders—reflects this principle and likely contributed to the high self-efficacy perceptions reported by participants. Findings regarding media modality preferences echo Parker, Kaland, and Mlomali's (2013) work in Malawi, where radio dramas effectively improved TB knowledge in low-literacy settings. In India, Chowdhury et al. (2021) showed that WhatsApp videos increased clinic attendance among symptomatic individuals; our cross-context comparison similarly found digital testimonials to be most impactful in the urban slum setting. By systematically comparing print, radio, and digital platforms across culturally distinct sites, this study fills a gap in the literature on how tailoring strategies interact with media channels to influence TB outcomes.

Implications for TB Control Programs

The demonstrated effectiveness of culturally tailored strategies carries clear implications for the National Tuberculosis Elimination Program (NTEP) and similar initiatives globally. First, program planners should allocate resources to formative research and community engagement to inform message design, rather than relying on generic, centrally developed materials. Second, interventions must balance threat and efficacy information: highlighting TB severity without actionable guidance risks reinforcing stigma, whereas coupling threat with explicit instructions on available free services fosters self-efficacy and timely care-seeking (Witte, 1992). Third, TB control programs should adopt a modular campaign framework that allows local adaptation of core message elements—language, imagery, and testimonials—while maintaining fidelity to theoretical constructs. For instance, digital platforms can disseminate individualized video testimonials in urban areas, whereas radio dramas and community theater may be more suitable in rural or low-literacy regions. Finally, integrating stigma measurement into routine monitoring—using validated scales like those of Van Rie et al. (2008)—will enable ongoing evaluation and iterative refinement of communication strategies, ensuring sustained impact.

Theoretical Contributions

This study advances theoretical understanding in two key respects. It corroborates the Extended Parallel Process Model (Witte, 1992) in a low-resource, high-stigma health context, demonstrating that efficacy cues are indispensable complements to fear appeals. By documenting how tailored efficacy information mitigates defensive avoidance and stimulates protective action, the findings refine EPPM's application to TB communication. Second, the research integrates Attribution Theory (Weiner, 1986) and Link and Phelan's (2001) conceptualization of stigma within a unified framework, showing that reframing TB as an externally driven disease reduces blame and social distance. The joint display of quantitative and qualitative data elucidates how theoretical constructs—perceived threat, response efficacy, and attributional reframing—interact to produce attitudinal and behavioral change. Moreover, by embedding these constructs within Kreuter et al.'s (2003) cultural tailoring schema, the study contributes a modular framework adaptable to varied cultural milieus, thus extending the reach of health communication theory into multicultural settings.

Limitations

Several limitations warrant consideration. First, the reliance on self-reported measures of stigma and care-seeking intervals may introduce recall bias and social desirability effects, potentially inflating estimates of intervention impact. Although the Tailored Design Method (Dillman, Smyth, & Christian, 2014) was employed to minimize such bias, future studies could incorporate objective service utilization data to corroborate self-reports. Second, the three-month follow-up period limits assessment of long-term behavior change and stigma reduction; longitudinal research extending beyond six months would elucidate the durability of effects. Third, purposive site selection—while essential for capturing cultural diversity—limits generalizability to other regions and populations; replication in additional states and among marginalized groups (e.g., tribal communities) is needed. Fourth, resource constraints prevented randomized assignment of communities to intervention and control conditions; absent a true control group, causal inferences must be drawn cautiously. Finally, the study focused on community-level interventions and did not explore interactions with health system factors such as provider attitudes or facility readiness, which may moderate intervention effectiveness. Addressing these limitations in future research will strengthen the evidence base for culturally tailored TB communication strategies.

CONCLUSION & RECOMMENDATIONS

Summary of Major Insights

This study demonstrates that culturally tailored media and communication strategies can affect substantial reductions in tuberculosis (TB) stigma and meaningful accelerations in health-seeking behavior across diverse Indian settings. Quantitative results indicated a large decrease in mean stigma scores—dropping from 68.4 to 52.7 on the Van Rie scale—consistent with robust psychometric validation efforts (Van Rie et al., 2008; Field, 2013). Concurrently, the average interval between symptom onset and first health-facility visit shortened by over three weeks, affirming that interventions which lower perceived barriers can accelerate protective action in accordance with the Health Belief Model (Rosenstock, 1974). Qualitative findings revealed that linguistic congruence, community-member testimonials, and clear efficacy messages were instrumental in reducing social separation and internalized shame, echoing Link and Phelan's (2001) conceptualization of stigma and Witte's (1992) specifications for fear-appeal design. The content analysis further highlighted an imbalance in existing TB materials—while threat appeals were common, self-efficacy cues and constituent-involving elements were underrepresented—underscoring the importance of integrating both threat and efficacy constructs within culturally relevant formats (Witte, 1992; Kreuter et al., 2003). Cross-context comparisons underscored that no single medium or strategy suffices universally; rather, interventions must align message modality and content with local cultural norms, media consumption patterns, and communication infrastructures, from radio dramas in low-literacy rural regions to WhatsApp videos in urban slums.

Practical Recommendations

Based on these findings, several actionable guidelines emerge for public health agencies seeking to design and implement TB communication campaigns. First, formative audience research must precede message development to identify local beliefs about TB causation, stigma drivers, and preferred communication channels. This process should involve participatory workshops with TB survivors, community leaders, and health workers, ensuring that materials reflect deep-structure tailoring—incorporating local metaphors, norms, and idioms—rather than superficial design elements alone (Resnicow, Baranowski, Ahluwalia, & Braithwaite, 1999). Second, messages must balance credible threat appeals with explicit efficacy information. While highlighting the severity and transmissibility of TB establishes urgency, it is equally critical to provide clear, actionable guidance on where to access free testing and treatment, thereby bolstering both response efficacy and self-efficacy (Witte, 1992; Rosenstock, 1974). Third, campaigns should prioritize constituent-involving strategies by featuring testimonials from respected community members or local survivors whose recovery stories model positive outcomes and destigmatize TB (Link & Phelan, 2001). Such narratives can humanize the disease and foster empathy, mitigating social ostracism. Fourth, modality selection must correspond to media accessibility and literacy levels: radio and community theater remain powerful in rural, low-literacy contexts, whereas digital platforms such as WhatsApp or Facebook may yield greater engagement in urban settings with high smartphone penetration (Parker, Kaland, & Mlomali, 2013; Chowdhury, Raj, & Sharma, 2021). Finally, integrating validated stigma measurement tools—such as the Van Rie scales—into routine monitoring enables programs to track attitudinal shifts over time and iteratively refine messages in response to emerging data (Van Rie et al., 2008).

Directions for Future Research

While this study advances understanding of culturally tailored TB communication, several avenues for future investigation warrant attention. Longitudinal research spanning six to twelve months post-intervention would clarify the durability of stigma reduction and care-seeking improvements, addressing the temporal limitation of three-month follow-up (Creswell & Plano Clark, 2018). Incorporating objective health-service utilization data—such as clinic attendance records—alongside self-reports can mitigate recall bias and enhance causal inference. Randomized controlled trials with cluster assignment of communities to intervention and control conditions would strengthen evidence on intervention efficacy and help isolate the impact of specific message components. Further, research should explore the interplay between communication strategies and health system factors: provider attitudes, facility readiness, and patient-provider interactions may moderate the effectiveness of media campaigns and merit integrated evaluation. Digital interventions utilizing personalization algorithms—such as tailoring video content based on user engagement metrics—represent a promising frontier, yet require rigorous assessment in LMIC settings. Finally, expanding studies to include marginalized and tribal populations, with attention to intersectional stigma (e.g., TB-HIV co-infection, gender disparities), will foster more inclusive communication frameworks and equitable access to TB services. By pursuing these research directions, scholars and practitioners can build a more comprehensive evidence base to guide culturally sensitive, theory-driven TB control efforts worldwide.

REFERENCES

Ajzen, I. (1991). The theory of planned behavior. *Organizational Behavior and Human Decision Processes, 50*(2), 179–211. DOI: 10.1016/0749-5978(91)90020-T

Braun, V., & Clarke, V. (2006). Using thematic analysis in psychology. *Qualitative Research in Psychology, 3*(2), 77–101. DOI: 10.1191/1478088706qp063oa

Bryman, A. (2006). Integrating quantitative and qualitative research: How is it done? *Qualitative Research, 6*(1), 97–113. DOI: 10.1177/1468794106058877

Chang, S., & Cataldo, J. K. (2014). A systematic review of global literature on social stigma in tuberculosis. *Evaluation and Program Planning, 38*, 145–162. DOI: 10.1016/j.evalprogplan.2013.10.004

Chowdhury, A. N., Raj, A., & Sharma, P. (2021). Impact of WhatsApp-based educational videos on tuberculosis screening uptake in urban slums of India. *BMC Public Health, 21*(1), 1234. DOI: 10.1186/s12889-021-11234-7

Cohen, J. (1960). A coefficient of agreement for nominal scales. *Educational and Psychological Measurement, 20*(1), 37–46. DOI: 10.1177/001316446002000104

Council for International Organizations of Medical Sciences. (2016). *International ethical guidelines for health-related research involving humans*. CIOMS.

Courtwright, A., & Turner, A. N. (2010). Tuberculosis and stigma: Pathways and interventions. *Public Health Reports (Washington, D.C.), 125*(4_suppl, Suppl 4), 34–42. DOI: 10.1177/00333549101250S407

Creswell, J. W., & Plano Clark, V. L. (2018). *Designing and conducting mixed methods research* (3rd ed.). SAGE.

Daniel, T. M. (2006). The history of tuberculosis. *Respiratory Medicine, 100*(11), 1862–1870. DOI: 10.1016/j.rmed.2006.08.006

Dillman, D. A., Smyth, J. D., & Christian, L. M. (2014). *Internet, phone, mail, and mixed-mode surveys: The tailored design method* (4th ed.). Wiley. DOI: 10.1002/9781394260645

Field, A. (2013). *Discovering statistics using IBM SPSS Statistics* (4th ed.). SAGE.

Green, M. C., & Brock, T. C. (2000). The role of transportation in the persuasiveness of public narratives. *Journal of Personality and Social Psychology, 79*(5), 701–721. DOI: 10.1037/0022-3514.79.5.701

Guest, G., Bunce, A., & Johnson, L. (2006). How many interviews are enough? An experiment with data saturation and variability. *Field Methods*, *18*(1), 59–82. DOI: 10.1177/1525822X05279903

Kreuter, M. W., Lukwago, S. N., Bucholtz, R. D. C., Clark, E. M., & Sanders-Thompson, V. (2003). Achieving cultural appropriateness in health promotion programs: Targeted and tailored approaches. *Health Education & Behavior*, *30*(2), 133–146. DOI: 10.1177/1090198102251021

Krippendorff, K. (2013). *Content analysis: An introduction to its methodology* (3rd ed.). SAGE.

Link, B. G., & Phelan, J. C. (2001). Conceptualizing stigma. *Annual Review of Sociology*, *27*(1), 363–385. DOI: 10.1146/annurev.soc.27.1.363

Ministry of Health and Family Welfare. (2023). *TB India 2023: Annual status report.* Directorate General of Health Services, Government of India.

Ministry of Health and Family Welfare. (2023). *TB India 2023: Annual status report.* Government of India.

Minkler, M., & Wallerstein, N. (Eds.). (2008). *Community-based participatory research for health: From process to outcomes* (2nd ed.). Jossey-Bass.

Morgan, D. L. (1997). *Focus groups as qualitative research* (2nd ed.). SAGE. DOI: 10.4135/9781412984287

Parker, W., Kaland, A., & Mlomali, M. (2013). The impact of radio dramas on tuberculosis knowledge in rural Malawi. *International Journal of Communication*, *7*, 1932–1950.

Patton, M. Q. (2002). *Qualitative research and evaluation methods* (3rd ed.). SAGE.

Raviglione, M. C., & Pio, A. (2002). Evolution of WHO policies for tuberculosis control, 1948–2001. *Lancet*, *359*(9308), 775–780. DOI: 10.1016/S0140-6736(02)07880-7

Resnicow, L., Baranowski, T., Ahluwalia, J. S., & Braithwaite, R. L. (1999). Cultural sensitivity in public health: Defined and demystified. *Health Education & Behavior*, *26*(3), 253–267. DOI: 10.1177/109019819902600302

Riessman, C. K. (2008). Narrative methods for the human sciences. *Sage (Atlanta, Ga.).*

Rosenstock, I. M. (1974). Historical origins of the Health Belief Model. *Health Education Monographs*, *2*(4), 328–335. DOI: 10.1177/109019817400200403

Snyder, L. B. (2007). Health communication campaigns and their impact on behavior. *Journal of Nutrition Education and Behavior, 39*(2, Suppl), S32–S40. DOI: 10.1016/j.jneb.2006.09.004

Stop, T. B. Partnership. (2020). *The Global Plan to End TB 2023–2030*. Geneva: Stop TB Partnership.

Tabachnick, B. G., & Fidell, L. S. (2013). *Using multivariate statistics* (6th ed.). Pearson.

Van Rie, A., Sengupta, A., Pungrassami, P., Balthip, S., & Dawson, R. (2008). Measuring stigma associated with tuberculosis and HIV/AIDS in southern Thailand: Exploratory and confirmatory factor analysis of two new scales. *Tropical Medicine & International Health, 13*(1), 21–29. DOI: 10.1111/j.1365-3156.2007.01971.x

Wakefield, M. A., Loken, B., & Hornik, R. C. (2010). Use of mass media campaigns to change health behavior. *Lancet, 376*(9748), 1261–1271. DOI: 10.1016/S0140-6736(10)60809-4

Weiner, B. (1986). *An attributional theory of motivation and emotion*. Springer-Verlag. DOI: 10.1007/978-1-4612-4948-1

Willis, G. B. (2005). Cognitive interviewing: A tool for improving questionnaire design. *Sage (Atlanta, Ga.)*.

Witte, K. (1992). Putting the fear back into fear appeals: The extended parallel process model. *Communication Monographs, 59*(4), 329–349. DOI: 10.1080/03637759209376276

World Health Organization. (2014). *The End TB Strategy*. World Health Organization.

World Health Organization. (2014). *The End TB Strategy*. https://www.who.int/publications/i/item/9789241506838

World Health Organization. (2023). *Global Tuberculosis Report 2023*. World Health Organization.

Chapter 10
Prevallence and Burden of Tuberculosis in Prisons and Correctional Facilities:
Tuberculosis Infection Prevention and Practices

Wasswa Shafik
https://orcid.org/0000-0002-9320-3186
Dig Connectivity Research Laboratory (DCRLab), Uganda

ABSTRACT

This chapter explores the prevalence and burden of tuberculosis (TB) within prisons and correctional facilities, emphasizing the disproportionate rates of infection compared to the general population. It analyzes contributing factors such as overcrowding, poor ventilation, limited healthcare access, and co-existing vulnerabilities like HIV and substance abuse. The chapter further discusses the transmission dynamics of TB in these confined environments and the implications for public health beyond prison walls. Strategies for TB prevention, diagnosis, treatment, and continuity of care are examined, highlighting global best practices and policy recommendations. Special attention is given to the challenges posed by multidrug-resistant TB (MDR-TB) and the integration of prison health services into national TB control programs. Through data-driven insights and case examples, this chapter underscores the urgent need for comprehensive interventions to mitigate TB's impact on incarcerated populations and the broader community.

DOI: 10.4018/979-8-3373-3446-2.ch010

INTRODUCTION

As the third leading cause of death from an infectious disease in the world, tuberculosis (TB) remains a major public health challenge. An estimated 1.6 million people died of TB in 2021, mostly in low and middle-income countries. TB affects all age groups and has a broad impact on health as well as social and economic development. In high and upper-middle-income countries, the disease has continued to be concentrated in economically marginalized groups (MP & Wijiastutik, 2024). When examining the different epidemiological characteristics of TB and of other infectious diseases, it is clear that it is particularly concentrated in the most disadvantaged among disadvantaged populations. Within these populations, TB tends to be concentrated in groups with the highest likelihood of health inequity, such as drug users, migrants, and prison inmates, including foreign-born persons in the latter category. The prevalence and incidence of TB disease are markedly higher in prisons and other closed settings, such as immigration detention facilities, than in non-institutionalized populations (Octavia et al., 2024). The continuing high burden of TB associated with imprisonment and population turnover in these institutions gives importance to the need for early detection, treatment, and prevention while imprisoned. Prisons cater to people with low incomes and excluded with a high burden of disease and risk factors who have not been enrolled in the social security health system and are in receipt of relevant healthcare. This can potentially exacerbate TB control efforts in surrounding communities and beyond. Control efforts in prisons can additionally reduce the risk of reactivation upon release. Early identification and treatment of cases before release, as well as contact investigation and health education, can help reduce transmission after release (Widiastuti et al., 2024). Despite these considerations, neither prisoners nor correctional facility health services have been prioritized in TB strategies and plans.

UNDERSTANDING TUBERCULOSIS

Tuberculosis (TB) is a communicable disease caused by the Mycobacterium tuberculosis complex (MTBC) of bacteria. Excluding certain animal reservoirs, TB is a disease of humans and some domesticated and wild animals in close contact with humans, such as camels, elephants, cervids, and some non-human primates. The most important reservoir of MTBC is Homo sapiens. Tuberculosis can take a variety of forms in humans. Pulmonary TB occurs in an estimated 80% of all cases and is the most contagious type, but extrapulmonary TB is also common (Khattak et al., 2024). Certain forms of extrapulmonary TB carry a high burden: TB meningitis is fatal in almost half of untreated patients, military TB occurs but transfers the bacteria to the entire body during the initial infection, and TB lymphadenopathy is important due to higher frequencies in some populations. The many different forms of TB are caused by MTBC invading different body systems, as well as various host factors. Infections caused by the closely related bacterium Mycobacterium bovis also give rise to TB. The transmission of TB from human to human occurs by aerosolization of droplets containing the bacterium from the lung of an infected individual to the lung of a susceptible individual (Njagi et al., 2024). However, not all individuals infected with MTBC develop TB disease. A latent MTBC infection results in a state of immune equilibrium, during which the bacterium is contained without causing disease but remains viable. Many people with latent infections will not develop disease during their entire lifetime, while others will develop active TB disease days, months, or decades later. Approximately 5-10% of people infected with MTBC will subsequently develop TB disease within their lifetimes, and another 5% in the first two years after infection (Jackson et al., 2024).

What is Tuberculosis?

Tuberculosis (TB), caused by organisms of the Mycobacterium tuberculosis complex, is a communicable disease primarily affecting the lungs, but it can also involve extrapulmonary sites. TB is a major cause of morbidity and mortality globally. In 2020, an estimated 10 million people developed TB disease, of whom more than 4 million were women and children. There were an estimated 1.5 million TB deaths worldwide among people with TB, including 214,000 among patients with TB who were also HIV-positive. TB is the second leading infectious cause of death globally in the population without HIV. During 2019, there were an estimated 500,000 new cases of rifampicin-resistant TB, 78% of whom were in patients with multidrug-resistant TB (MP & Wijiastutik, 2024). Globally, TB is an important in-prison pathogen, defined as a pathogen with high incidence and prevalence, significant morbidity and mortality, and an economically unjustified lack of vigilance by correctional health systems. Prisoners are at increased risk for some diseases that they commonly share with the general population; for others, they are at decreased risk. Infection with Mycobacterium tuberculosis is an important example of the latter. The sheer case detection and high incidence in prisoners and prison staff, and the significantly higher death rate attributable to TB in prisoners, emphasize that M. tuberculosis should be considered an important risk factor for prisoners and prison staff. TB, the communicable disease primarily affecting the lungs and which can also involve extrapulmonary sites, is endemic in most areas without effective public health systems. TB is a major cause of morbidity and mortality globally, particularly among the incarcerated (Zhang et al., 2024). The disease burden originated from risk factors, including HIV coinfection, diabetes, substance abuse, malnutrition, air pollution, migration, and poor health infrastructure.

Transmission and Risk Factors

Tuberculosis (TB) is caused by bacteria that most often affect the lungs but can attack any part of the body, including the kidneys, spine, and brain. The bacteria can spread from a person with TB, through the air, to another person. There are two TB-related conditions: latent TB infection (LTBI) and TB disease. Someone with LTBI has no symptoms, does not feel sick, cannot spread TB bacteria to others, usually has a positive tuberculin skin test and/or positive TB blood test, and normal chest x-ray and sputum test results (Chen et al., 2024). People with LTBI may develop TB disease at some point in their lives because the bacteria become active if the immune system cannot stop them from growing. TB disease is more common in people with certain risk factors and particularly if the person has a weak immune system. People with TB disease can be very sick and may need to be hospitalized or receive medical care until they are no longer contagious. People who have TB disease can spread the active bacteria. TB disease will make the body sick and may make people feel suddenly sick and have fever, chills, weakness, and sweat. As with LTBI, people with TB disease usually have a positive tuberculin skin test and/or positive TB blood test, and abnormal chest x-ray and sputum test results. Someone without LTBI or TB disease will rarely have a positive TB test (Ullah et al., 2024). The high-risk populations for both TB infection and TB disease include those infected living in medically underserved areas, including racial and ethnic minority populations who have groups and certain other factors that place them at high risk.

Symptoms and Diagnosis

The pathophysiology of tuberculosis is dissimilar from the majority of infectious diseases; thus, the associated clinical symptoms are distinctive. The majority of bacteremic individuals show no clinical signs of disease, since calcium-mediated granulomatous tuberculoma formation in the lungs causes the active sequestration of the bacilli, thereby preventing disease expression for long periods—the so-called latent infection. Occasionally, during this latent period, the balance between the host immune response and the bacterial infectious load will be disrupted, and the bacilli will be able to multiply, leading either to the progression of the primary infection or to disease reactivation (Ren et al., 2024). Clinically, the disease is more likely to remain untreated for a prolonged period since it presents gradually, characterized by a number of heterogeneous generalized constitutional symptoms. Primary pulmonary tuberculosis or disease reactivation will frequently be associated with a chronic productive cough, often increased at night, and with hemoptysis due to the presence of vascular invasion of the necrotic tissues. Pulmonary impairment with progressive dyspnoea, initial wheeziness, and chest pain due to pleuritic involvement may develop. In some cases, only extrapulmonary involvement will be found, including cervical adenopathy, meningitis, miliary fever, bowel diseases, osteomyelitis, cystitis-nephritis, endocarditis, skin phlegmon, pericarditis, and even lymphangio-pleural or peritoneal carcinomatous syndromes (Li et al., 2024). A diagnosis of pulmonary disease will always be presumed with any of the aforementioned clinical signs, since the patient may have associated respiratory signs or other underlying pulmonary diseases. Clinical suspicion will also be increased if present within a high-prevalence risk group. Diagnosis is based on the microbiological identification of Mycobacterium tuberculosis aetiological agents in respiratory secretions and/or in any other infectious or parenchymatous tissue or liquid (Mugenyi et al., 2024). The achieved diagnosis is considered microbiologically confirmed when the bacilli have been detected or isolated in culture from expectorated respiratory secretions, or when bacillary isolation has occurred in other extrapulmonary liquid or tissue.

GLOBAL OVERVIEW OF TUBERCULOSIS

Tuberculosis (TB) is a communicable disease caused primarily by Mycobacterium tuberculosis. It represents a major public health problem, affecting mostly the respiratory tract. In patients with compromised immune systems, such as patients infected with the human immunodeficiency virus (HIV), the disease can be disseminated to almost any organ and have fatal consequences without treatment (Sawaswong et al., 2024). Globally, TB is the second leading cause of death by infectious disease after HIV and has outpaced the COVID-19 pandemic in total mortality. In 2021, it was estimated that 10.6 million people became ill with TB disease and that 1.6 million people died from the disease. Both the incidence and mortality represent increases from the previous year's numbers. Programmatic interruptions due to health service disruptions are likely responsible for the observed increases. An estimated 1 million non-HIV-infected children developed TB in 2021. Worldwide, HIV co-infection remains a major issue in persons infected with TB (Chaturvedi et al., 2024). Despite having a low prevalence, in 2021, there were 224,000 deaths from TB in people living with HIV. The highest incidence and mortality rates for TB occur in low- and middle-income countries in Africa and Asia. TB and TB mortality remain concentrated in a small number of countries. Of the 1.6 million people who died of TB, 75% were from India, Indonesia, China, the Philippines, Pakistan, Nigeria, Bangladesh, the Democratic Republic of the Congo, or Russia. A total of 30 countries have been designated as TB high-burden countries. These countries accounted for 87% of the total estimated TB incidence in 2021. These numbers support the assertion that more than four-fifths of the world's TB burden is borne by low- and middle-income countries, particularly those with limited resources (Idris et al., 2024).

Epidemiology of Tuberculosis

Tuberculosis (TB) remains a major global cause of morbidity and mortality, ranking as the 13th leading cause of death globally. In 2021, there were an estimated 10.6 million individuals who were diagnosed with TB worldwide, with 1.6 million deaths attributed to TB and up to 0.5 million additional deaths with TB and HIV-coinfection. TB incidence rates are falling globally, but not fast enough to reach the target of a 90% global reduction by 2030. Most of the TB burden occurs in low- and middle-income countries, specifically in Southeast Asia and the Western Pacific Regions (Seabra & Duarte, 2024). The ongoing burden of TB is hindering socioeconomic development in these countries. The rising burden of multidrug-resistant TB threatens global health security. The burden of TB in prisons is a reflection of TB in the general population. Most countries with a high TB incidence have a similar risk of active TB in prisons. However, in several countries, prison TB rates are significantly higher than in the general population (Shah et al., 2024). The over-representation of TB in prisons compared to the general population shows that social determinants of health, including overcrowding, poor ventilation, and malnutrition, create a conducive environment for the development of active disease. The prison population has a much higher prevalence of TB risk factors than the general population; these include malnutrition, pre-existing lung disease, smoking, diabetes mellitus, and HIV coinfection. In addition, while prisons are characteristically overcrowded, large populations are also held in immigration detention and shelter homes for refugees (Jackson et al., 2024). Today, these settings are also linked with the risk of TB.

Global Health Initiatives

Without the combined effort of newly industrialized and deindustrialized countries, TB will remain a major international health problem. The pandemic nature of TB has been emphasized, and its coordination of efforts to globalize programs such as the Directly Observed Treatment Short-Course plus program. In the face of resistance and difficult-to-treat strains of TB, the worldwide unifying effort Focused Disease Control approach, is aimed at making TB an avoidable nuisance. Much of that effort is realized in the optimization of the system of care and its integration into primary health and social care. A multifaceted correctional facility strategy is needed

(Enane et al., 2024). Misinformation about TB and stigma should be addressed; TB surveillance and collection of epidemiological data, such as genotyping and drug resistance patterns, should focus on vulnerable populations, and cross-linkage of health care services should ensure continuity of medical care upon release. Reform can be very costly, and hence, funding is necessary. Key actors are involved. The Coordinated Action program provides funds for implementation research with the long-term goal of improving treatment algorithms. Recent recommendations have modified the prepetition recommended interventions by emphasizing Health System approaches and preventive strategies (Hashim et al., 2024). A new framework has outlined a call for decolonization to take the bacterium out of population reservoirs with actions such as contact tracing, screening, and treatment, in conjunction with reducing poverty, among other risks, as presented in Table 1.

Table 1. Risk factors for TB in prisons in African nations

Risk Factor	**Description**	**Impact on TB Spread**	**Mitigation Strategy**	**Stakeholders Involved**	**Reference**
Overcrowding	High inmate density in cells	Increases airborne transmission	Reduce the inmate population	Prison authorities, judiciary	(Zhang et al., 2024)
Poor Ventilation	Inadequate airflow in buildings	Facilitates TB transmission	Install mechanical ventilation systems	Facility engineers, health staff	(Chen et al., 2024)
HIV Co-infection	High prevalence among inmates	Weakens immunity	Integrate TB/HIV services	Health ministries, NGOs	(Ullah et al., 2024)
Malnutrition	Common in under-resourced facilities	Reduces immune response	Improve prison diet programs	Prison administrators, nutritionists	(Ren et al., 2024)
Substance Abuse	High rates of drug use	Compromises immunity	Provide rehabilitation services	Social workers, healthcare providers	(Li et al., 2024)
Delayed Diagnosis	Limited access to diagnostics	Prolongs infectivity	Routine TB screening	Prison health units	(Mugenyi et al., 2024)
Lack of Isolation	TB-positive inmates are not separated	Ongoing transmission	Establish isolation wards	Correctional facility management	(Sawaswong et al., 2024)
Incomplete Treatment	Interrupted therapy during transfer or release	Drug resistance development	Ensure continuity of care	Public health systems	(Chaturvedi et al., 2024)
Limited Healthcare	Few trained medical personnel	Poor disease management	Staff training, telemedicine	Health departments	(Shafik, 2024b)

continued on following page

Table 1. Continued

Risk Factor	Description	Impact on TB Spread	Mitigation Strategy	Stakeholders Involved	Reference
Poor Awareness	Lack of TB education among inmates and staff	Ignorance of symptoms	Conduct health education campaigns	NGOs, prison health educators	(Shafik, 2024c)
Stigma	Fear of discrimination	Leads to hiding symptoms	Counseling and sensitization	Psychologists, health teams	(Shafik, 2024a)
Frequent Transfers	Movement between facilities	Disrupts treatment	Implement unified health records	Prison networks, IT units	(Shafik, 2024d)
Unsanitary Conditions	Dirty and crowded environments	Increases general disease risk	Regular sanitation, hygiene training	Maintenance staff, prison officers	(Shafik, 2024e)
High Turnover	Short-term incarcerations and rapid releases	Undermines treatment monitoring	Link prison healthcare with public systems	MoH, community clinics	(Shafik, 2025)

TUBERCULOSIS IN PRISONS AND CORRECTIONAL FACILITIES

Prisons and jails house a substantial number of young and middle-aged persons and are established high-risk areas for transmission and establishment of mycobacterial infections. The prevalence of pulmonary TB in these institutions is almost 7 to 10 times higher than in the general population, which is 350 times higher than in the general population. This population is at a heightened risk of progression to disease if exposed to TB, particularly if they are coinfected with HIV, have silicosis, or have other risk factors (Zhang et al., 2024). A TB outbreak in a correctional facility is of great importance because it can serve as a reservoir for TB transmission into the community that might otherwise remain unaffected. A closed environment may facilitate the dispersal of a new multidrug-resistant organism into the community. Inmates have been implicated in the spread of multidrug-resistant TB in metropolitan areas and outbreaks in various locations. In addition, prisons and other closed institutions, such as long-term care facilities for the mentally ill, homeless shelters, and drug rehabilitation centers, are believed to be an important source of late case detection (Chen et al., 2024). They account for more than half of the late diagnosed cases. These outbreaks have resulted in the establishment of aggressive screening and treatment strategies before admission, during the correctional period, and upon release into society. Despite these measures, such facilities might still be considered TB hotspots for the spread of the disease. Microbiological studies of TB cases from prisons showed no evidence of strain variation among the prisoners and the general population, implicating a common and stable source of both populations. There seems to be a two-way relationship between the correctional facilities and the general population: the inmates harbor active TB, which is neglected by a poor healthcare system, and act as a source for relapse in the old TB hotspots in the general population (Ullah et al., 2024).

Prevalence Rates in Correctional Settings

The statistical prevalence rates for active tuberculosis in correctional facilities are substantially higher than in the community. Most estimates are from the United States, where the burden of TB is considerably lower than in most low- and middle-income countries. In the US, many estimates of incarceration-based TB prevalence are drawn from screening among HIV-infected people, who are particularly vulnerable to TB disease. Nationwide screening during a resurgence of TB in the mid-1990s found a prevalence rate in HIV-diseased prisoners of 21.4% with current TB (Ren et al., 2024). In 1996, TB prevalence rates in a New York City prison were much higher among HIV-diseased persons than for other prisoners. Nationwide surveillance of TB notifications from 1990 to 1999 revealed that prisoners numbered 8.4% of US TB notifications. The increased probability of TB notification because of being in a correctional facility and being HIV-infected supports a tenuous connection between imprisonment and the TB epidemic (Mugenyi et al., 2024). During the resurgence of TB in the mid-1990s, state correctional facilities reported annual TB incidences as high as 313 per 100,000. Persons seeking entry into prison in Boston in 1999-2000 had a TB prevalence rate of 303 per 100,000 in initial TB skin testing and an estimated prevalence of 860 per 100,000 among HIV-infected persons. National data capture persons within prisons and jails who are reported with TB before incarceration. These data suggest annual incidences of pulmonary and extrapulmonary TB at the state level would typically be about 1.7 per 100,000 inmates per year for all states and about 6.0 per 100,000 inmates per year in mountainous states, and about 4.0 per 100,000 inmates for the upper Midwest (Sawaswong et al., 2024).

Contributing to High Prevalence

Prisons have become a microcosm of communities where tuberculosis (TB) transmission is high and poorly controlled. Therefore, prisons often have higher rates of TB prevalence than the community outside of the prison walls, and jail release and movement between prison and society could act as a bridge for transmitting TB to the general population. There is a growing amount of data concerning drug-resistant strains in prisons. Crowding, confinement, mobility, immunocompromised states, and lack of ventilation in prisons have been associated with TB transmission (Chaturvedi et al., 2024). Jails and prisons are typically crowded facilities with recirculated air. Inmates often live, sleep, bathe, and use toilet facilities in close quarters. Inmates typically have lower socioeconomic status and higher rates of substance use and mental disorders, which may lead to increased risk of TB. People in and out of the prison system may have increased risk factors for TB, including illicit drug use, human immunodeficiency virus (HIV) infection, homelessness, and excessive alcohol use. The medical and social problems in the incarcerated population contribute to the prolonged prevalence of TB. Jails also serve as revolving doors for people with untreated TB whose extreme poverty and lack of health insurance keep them returning to incarceration again and again. Also, in many countries, TB screening and treatment are severely lacking for those already diagnosed and incarcerated in prisons, with screening not always being included in the admission process (Idris et al., 2024). The higher the rate of risk factors, the higher the rate of TB in prisons.

Comparison with the General Population

Globally, the burden of TB disease in prisons is very small compared with that in the general community. Estimates show that about 0.5% of the overall TB cases reported came from prisons. In the USA, in 2013, inmates represented only 0.08% of the general population. However, many of the countries with the highest burden of TB disease, such as India and China, have large prison populations with prisons having a fraction of the TB burden reported in the general public. Reports have shown that the prevalence of PTB is about fivefold higher in prisons than in the general population (Seabra & Duarte, 2024). The highest rates reported have been from Iran, where prisons are reported to have a burden almost 30 times higher than the general population, with HIV co-infection further increasing this risk. The burden of TB disease in prisons is also disproportionately higher than in the isolated poorest regions of the general populace; for example, the burdens in Mali, Liberia, and the Democratic Republic of the Congo are about one-tenth that of prisons. While prison TB investigation rates are high, prison TB death rates are still about 40% of what is reported for the general population (although the prevalence data suggest the rates in prisons might be inflated) (Jackson et al., 2024). Further illustrating the disparity, studies from Kenya, which are among the first to differentiate the population groups of those that come in and out of prison, have shown that although the TB burden in general is similar in the inmate and general populations, incarceration and reinfection with more resistant strains move the burden into prisoners. As incarceration rates rise, countries cannot just limit access to TB preventive measures to high-risk populations. TB and its risk factors do not have an office in or outside prison, nor do they stop at the prison gate. Blinded barriers feed stigma and reduce access for those seeking to inform health authorities or hospital workers, making the fight against TB more difficult than it already is (Enane et al., 2024).

IMPACT OF TUBERCULOSIS ON PRISON POPULATIONS

Unlike generalized populations, the health consequences of tuberculosis (TB) in prisons and other closed settings cannot be measured by the impact it has on the general population. Fortunately, little is known about how many healthy men, women, children, and adolescents succumb to TB in prisons throughout the world; guidelines for screening inmates prior to incarceration mean that only the most impoverished are left to die of TB behind bars. Nevertheless, TB kills inmates. These deaths are concentrated among prisoners who are HIV-positive, who have multidrug-resistant TB, or who have predominantly extrapulmonary disease (Hashim et al., 2024). The consequences are indeed grave for the gravest of offenders: a three-fold increase in suicide rate. And the consequences of TB disease go beyond suicide. Persons with TB disease are at increased risk of delirium and psychosis; singled out for "protective" isolation, the solitary confinement provokes its own set of adverse health effects. Prisons are public institutions with a mandate to care for the health of those they detain. For this reason, the practical question, What is the economic burden of TB on prisons?, is usually framed within a broader inquiry that considers access to correctional care. While prison medical budgets may bear the cost of specific delayed-onset diseases, for the most part, the burden of chronic, communicable, or serious but non-infectious disease conditions is borne by corrections agencies. The primary experience of correctional healthcare agencies with TB is during outbreaks concentrated in specific facilities (Balisan et al., 2024). Because they can be unpredictable and intense, the importance of these episodes transcends their economic burden.

Health Consequences for Inmates

Prison populations are generally more vulnerable than the general population to many health problems, including a high burden of serious communicable diseases. The reasons for this increased vulnerability for some diseases, such as tuberculosis, mainly relate to increased exposure and the condition of inmates before incarceration. Furthermore, prisoners should receive the same health care as the general population (Liu et al., 2024). However, both communicable diseases, such as tuberculosis and other infectious diseases, such as viral hepatitis and HIV/AIDS, and non-communicable diseases, such as drug addiction (usually associated with poor mental health), non-communicable diseases, and series trauma from violence in prison are usually poorly served in the prison health care system. It is well-known that prison inmates are a vulnerable population for tuberculosis. This has been clearly shown in countries with a very high burden of tuberculosis, especially for drug-resistant tuberculosis. It is also documented that imprisonment increases the risk of tuberculosis mortality in prisons with a high burden of tuberculosis. Other health issues for inmates are related or associated with the tuberculosis burden, including the burden of other communicable diseases, such as HIV/AIDS (Kazemian et al., 2024).

Economic and social marginalization, drug dependency, and comorbid psychiatric illnesses are frequently found in prisoners with tuberculosis. Other poor health issues are also associated with the tuberculosis burden, including malnutrition and poor ventilation, and overcrowding, especially in developing countries. Tuberculosis health consequences for inmates include drug-resistant tuberculosis (Boast et al., 2024). Furthermore, because most prisoners return to the general population after release and many prisoners spend a considerable length of time in custody, or return to prison after release, tuberculosis in prisons can have widespread repercussions. This includes the potential for backflow to the general population of prisoners with active TB or latent TB infection on both tuberculosis transmission and the future risk of active disease, respectively, and the additional economic and social marginalization, drug dependency, and comorbid psychiatric illnesses frequently found in prisoners with tuberculosis (Vonasek et al., 2024).

Economic Burden on Correctional Systems

Numerous studies undertaken in various countries revealed that treating inmates infected with tuberculosis requires significantly more time and resources, in particular for the treatment of multidrug-resistant tuberculosis, than treating patients in the general population. The data suggest that treating a tuberculosis patient incarcerated in a correctional institution for a drug-susceptible form of the disease costs significantly more compared with a similar case in the patient population. Such differences in costs are expected since prisons are characterized by a high rate of drug resistance as well as high morbidity and mortality associated with tuberculosis (Nafisah & Muhammad, 2024). In addition, prisons and correctional facilities for minors are not adequately equipped with medical facilities and medical staff, even in well-off countries, and treating tuberculosis patients in conditions of limited resources becomes almost impossible. The expenditure borne by the correctional health care system as a result of the infection's spread has become an important issue all over the world. The high cost of tuberculosis treatment, especially for forms resistant to treatment, can force correctional systems to introduce restrictions on admitted prisoners in order to prevent prison outbreaks. Some countries have attempted to avoid the burden of treating already diagnosed cases of tuberculosis within the correctional health care system at great expense by sending inmates to facilities run by the national health system (Yanifitri et al., 2024). However, this can only be a temporary measure. Treating inmates infected with tuberculosis is problematic due to the fact that the health care system cannot just send a patient back to the correctional institution at the end of the treatment.

SCREENING AND PREVENTION STRATEGIES

Among various provisions for tuberculosis control among prison populations, screening plays a crucial role in the early identification of the disease and treatment. Recommendations for specific screening protocols vary across countries and institutions. Nevertheless, inmates have been screened for tuberculosis disease upon exposure prison, presenting with respiratory symptoms, during detention, or upon release. However, routine procedures for tuberculosis screening upon admission or during confinement are not standardized worldwide and do not often include testing with a tuberculin skin test or interferon gamma release assay (Amalia, 2024). The major screening method available in prisons is physical examination for symptoms related to tuberculosis, understandable since many detection programs for pulmonary tuberculosis rely exclusively on symptom identification without the additional use of radiology or bacteriology. Nevertheless, detection of the disease using symptom-based identification is suboptimal for specific high-risk groups, such as HIV co-infected patients, who may present more atypical symptoms. Bacille Calmette Guerin vaccination is widely utilized in many low and middle-income countries and may have an effect in decreasing the number of extrapulmonary tuberculous cases (Yang et al., 2024). Prisons are typically overcrowded, have high occupant turnover, minimal preparedness for managing airflow in common spaces, such as wards, canteens, and recreation yards, and limited medical resources and access to healthcare services. Quarantine measures, which include isolation of new or returning inmates for a specific period of time upon entering a facility, have been proposed as a possible measure for reducing the burden of tuberculosis in prisons. In countries with low prevalence of the disease, specific provisions of prevention and care apply to foreign nationals awaiting judicial decisions related to their immigration status and housed in administrative detention facilities (Njagi et al., 2024). In such cases, screening and preventive and curative treatment measures, including specific attention to tuberculosis latent infection, are crucial.

Screening Protocols for Inmates

To prevent and control transmission of M. tuberculosis in prisons, it is essential to identify and treat inmates with TB as early as possible. The introduction of accurate screening methods and treatment will reduce the time that an infectious person spends in the prison environment before becoming diagnosed and treated. In addition, early treatment of inmates with TB can prevent needless mortality and prolonged suffering. However, the challenge of implementing TB control strategies in correctional facilities is more complex than simply screening inmates. It involves defining new strategies to address the various situations encountered in carceral settings and the need for additional resources (Rahman et al., 2024). The guidelines on the prevention and control of TB in prisons and other correctional facilities emphasize that pre- and post-incarceration screening needs to be additional to regular TB tests and x-rays prior to incarceration. Although it has long been suggested that screening should target the general prison population and especially members of high-risk groups, the technical difficulties in carrying out screening programs stress that screening in prisons should also target high-risk groups. BCG vaccination results in positive TST but differential interpretation of the test is possible; therefore, in a BCG-vaccinated population, the sensitivity and specificity of IGRA may be more important than in a non-BCG-vaccinated population or a population with a very low prevalence of non-TB mycobacterial infections (Swain et al., 2024). Unfortunately, IGRA use for screening active TB in the prison population is still at an early stage and there are only scattered data on its performance for the detection of active TB in prison inmates with either prior reported or confirmed latent TB infection. Using interferon-gamma release assays in combination with chest x-ray for the initial TB screening program should reduce the number of prisoners with active pulmonary TB who are missed at initial evaluation. Distributed resources would facilitate screening close to the time of prison entry (MP & Wijiastutik, 2024).

Vaccination and Preventive Measures

Vaccination against TB has not received sufficient attention as a preventive measure, mainly due to the low sensitivity of the existing diagnostic tests and the subsequent unnecessary treatment of people who will never develop TB disease. The main vaccine against TB development is BCG, but studies have shown that it only prevents TB in approximately 50% of vaccinated persons and does not play a prominent role in TB control strategies. However, in countries where the vaccine is applied, there has been a reduction in the number of cases. After BCG vaccination, the skin test may present false-negative results, and positive reactions may not suggest a risk of developing TB (Zhang et al., 2024). In 2006, the results of a systematic review regarding preventive treatment were published: people aged 35 years or younger with a history of recent, active contact with an infected person, and/or who are known to be infected with HIV and/or who are getting started on or currently receiving treatment for leukemia, lymphoma, or any other condition requiring immunosuppression. If vaccination against TB is taken into consideration in prison facilities, it should be applied immediately after prison admission. Preventive strategies are essential to avoid disease and reduce health problems and social consequences in these people. Infected individuals could be treated using isoniazid preventive therapy. Without preventive therapy, throughout treatment for LTBI, 7% of patients with TB and 27% with non-TB disease at baseline would develop irreversible disability and would need long-term social assistance (Chen et al., 2024). The same study concluded that hospitalization and social assistance posed a larger economic burden than preventive therapy, as some control approaches are Table 2.

Table 2. Tuberculosis (TB) control strategies in correctional settings

Intervention	Objective	Implementation Method	Challenges	Expected Outcome
Entry Screening	Identify TB cases at admission	Chest X-rays, symptom checklists	Resource limitations	Early detection and isolation
Periodic Screening	Detect latent and active TB	Routine testing every 6 months	Operational burden	Reduced undiagnosed cases
DOTS (Directly Observed Tx)	Ensure treatment adherence	Supervised drug administration	Staffing shortages	Higher treatment completion rates
Isolation Units	Prevent transmission from active cases	Separate housing for TB-positive	Space and funding constraints	Lower transmission inside facilities
TB/HIV Integration	Address co-morbidity efficiently	Joint testing and treatment	Coordination issues	Improved dual disease management
Health Education	Promote awareness among inmates and staff	Posters, workshops, sessions	Low literacy levels	Improved symptom reporting
Nutritional Support	Boost immunity and recovery	Balanced meal plans, supplements	Budget limitations	Faster recovery and resistance building
Staff Training	Improve diagnosis and care capacity	Regular workshops and upskilling	High staff turnover	Higher diagnostic accuracy
Post-release Linkage	Ensure continued care in the community	Referral to community clinics	Tracking released inmates	Better long-term outcomes
Infection Control Measures	Reduce in-prison transmission	Ventilation, hygiene protocols	Infrastructure limitations	Safer environment for all

continued on following page

Table 2. Continued

Intervention	Objective	Implementation Method	Challenges	Expected Outcome
Mobile Diagnostic Units	Bring testing facilities to remote prisons	Mobile vans with lab equipment	Maintenance, logistics	Expanded testing coverage
Electronic Health Records	Track inmate TB status across transfers	Centralized digital systems	Data security, tech adoption	Seamless treatment across facilities
Surveillance Systems	Monitor and evaluate TB programs	Data collection and analytics	Inconsistent reporting	Informed policy decisions
NGO/Donor Partnerships	Supplement public resources	External funding and expertise	Coordination with prison systems	Sustained and scalable interventions

TREATMENT OF TUBERCULOSIS IN PRISONS

Tuberculosis (TB) treatment in correctional settings is comparable to that which is provided in the community. This chapter distinguishes between two types of TB treatment for incarcerated persons: standard treatment for drug-susceptible TB and treatment for drug-resistant TB. Treatment protocols for drug-susceptible TB and drug-resistant TB are defined by expert consensus and regularly updated. Most TB among incarcerated persons is drug-susceptible TB (Ullah et al., 2024). A daily regimen for treatment of drug-susceptible TB, requiring 6 to 9 months to complete, is the norm in prisons and jails. Incarcerated persons with HIV, with active sputum smear-positive TB, and with cavitation on chest imaging should be offered standard TB treatment at least 4 days per week, but daily treatment is advisable. These recommendations stem from the fact that incarcerated persons typically have a large number of contacts and work in proximity, with long hours, to those who are at the greatest risk of developing TB after transmission of their inmate's strain (Zhang et al., 2024). The reasons for starting and continuing TB treatment with HIV-infected patients even when they progress to advanced immunosuppression include the chronicity of TB and the need to keep it from being inadvertently transmitted at a time when the viral load is especially high. Generally, TB treatment among incarcerated persons is administered based on estimations rather than genotyping of pretreatment specimens. After 2 months of treatment, nearly all patients with drug-susceptible TB and good adherence are no longer infectious. Prisons struggle to maintain adherence to TB treatment. Incarcerated persons regularly experience interruption of therapy due to transfer, release, or diagnostic delay. Delays due to transfer and release are not without consequence; initial diagnosis is often delayed because the jailed or imprisoned TB suspect lacks a reliable address for follow-up and is therefore lost to follow-up examination (Ullah et al., 2024). Interruption of therapy due to transfer, release, or nonadherence is even more problematic for incarcerated persons with drug-resistant disease, because relapse and acquired drug resistance can occur rapidly.

Standard Treatment Protocols

The management of latent infection and active disease in the correctional facility population is an essential part of TB control. Without prompt initiation of appropriate therapy and strict adherence to treatment, TB can have serious consequences in both the incarcerated individual and the general public. The standard treatment of drug-susceptible TB disease is a daily regimen of isoniazid, rifampicin, pyrazinamide, and ethambutol or streptomycin for the first two months, followed by four months of isoniazid and rifampicin. Because individuals in correctional facilities need to adhere to the newly prescribed treatment as well, side effects of the medication regimen should be monitored (Ren et al., 2024). Antiretroviral therapy and treatment of latent TB infection are critical for the safety of the HIV population, as increased numbers are now incarcerated in correctional facilities. Prisons can be considered hotspots for the development of LTBI. Treatment of latent TB infection is especially important for those incarcerated for long periods as a high percentage of them will be in prison for extended periods and TB will be able to reactivate because of a lack of treatment (Mugenyi et al., 2024). Priority groups who should be evaluated for LTBI are:

(i) persons born abroad in countries where TB is common;
(ii) persons with HIV infection (and particularly those who have been in the correctional facility;
(iii) persons with other health problems or who take medications that increase the risk for TB infection;
(iv) persons with a history of TB;
(v) children ages 3 or older who come from high-risk countries; or
(vi) persons who inject illicit drugs.

Challenges in Treatment Adherence

Adherence to tuberculosis (TB) treatment can be exceptionally low among prisoners. Various physiological, psychological, and socioenvironmental factors contribute to the difficulty in ensuring compliance in these patients. The long duration of TB treatment, along with the tedious drug side effects, could affect patients' willpower. Prisoners' long histories of drug addiction or abuse, a combination of the psychological stresses of being imprisoned and of having a potentially fatal illness, as well as the risk of TB treatment having a deleterious effect on release potential through adverse health changes, may all affect adherence negatively (Sawaswong et al., 2024). There is a high concentration of HIV-coinfected patients and those with other concomitant chronic diseases in prisons with a high TB burden. Prisoners are deprived of many of their civil rights, such as privacy and the freedom to communicate with people outside prison. The prisoners' role of confidante is valued culturally in many parts of the world; therefore, their perception that the respiratory and TB symptoms experienced by their incarcerated friends may pose a threat to them may boost compliance rates through a sense of community and friendship. The fact of being in a closed environment lowers the risk of acquiring other infectious agents, and for those with a drug-resistant TB strain, being together with people with similar characteristics may be beneficial (Chaturvedi et al., 2024).

Diminished attention among medical workers due to the nature of TB disease, including the unhurried evolution of symptoms and the long treatment period, poor motivation for treatment among prisoners, and the risk of recurrences after completion of treatment, may also sap adherence rates. Successful TB treatment in prisons is complex, requiring cooperation between prisoners and prison authorities, and continuity of treatment services after prisoners are released. Medical staff must be aware of the difficulties in delivering TB preventive and treatment services for minority communities. This requires both cultural competence and cultural reverence and humility (Idris et al., 2024). Because of the complexity of medicine, service delivery, and other public health activities that prevent TB, all TB services should be delivered as a team. As TB is a chronic disease requiring long-term therapy, prisons must ensure that adequate therapy is available during the prison stay and after the prisoners are released from prison. Additionally, there is a need for interaction between primary health care services, prison therapy centers, secondary health care services, and tertiary health care services provided by academic institutes to ensure access for all people living with TB, particularly in high-burden countries (Seabra & Duarte, 2024).

CASE STUDIES

Even though TB is a major problem in certain prison settings, it is also possible to highlight successful interventions aimed at solving the problem. In 1992, the California correctional system reported a TB outbreak, which was successfully eradicated by introducing a comprehensive infection control plan. Implementation of the plan included encouraging the prison personnel to recognize symptomatic inmates, increasing the use of TB contact tracing, promoting prompt initiation of treatment for inmates with TB, and increasing TB screening of inmates (Shah et al., 2024). Local TB public health officers developed surveillance systems and initiated new approaches based on witnessed symptoms of TB and on concerns about increased or missed risk factors of TB. These activities resulted in an impressive increase in the percentage of inmates screened and consequently treated, leading to the successful eradication of the outbreak. Prisons in Canada, which previously had an incidence of TB that exceeded the national average, reported a model in 1993–1994 that yielded different clusters of drug-susceptible TB. The outbreak was related to the use of rubber gloves. Currently, Canada's prisons have lower rates of TB compared to its indigenous society. The correctional service has activities for prison infection control. Every newly admitted inmate is subject to screening for TB. For those with positive skin tests, treatment is systematically provided as a preventive measure (Jackson et al., 2024). Prisons can experience outbreaks after years of only very low TB incidences. In 1999, a TB outbreak occurred in New York prisons after years of prior effective TB control. A similar situation was seen in Cuba. A prison near the capital city of Cuba experienced an outbreak during the period from 1998 to 2000, which was caused by the intensification of the migration of the prison population from the countryside to Havana. Furthermore, because of the backlog of preventive measures, such as treatment of cases and contact control, prisons remained a zone of endemicity (Enane et al., 2024).

Successful Interventions

The Management Sciences for Health program was implemented in 1994 in Thailand. The broader objective was to improve the delivery of tuberculosis (TB) control in remote, poorly served, rural areas. A major component of the project concerned the implementation of a private sector "social marketing" strategy. The model has been modified for specific use in prison settings. Drug prices have to be subsidized, but prisoners' families have contributed financially as well (Balisan et al., 2024). Furthermore, expenditure ceilings are needed for TB drug purchases in prisons, particularly regarding the first-line medicines isoniazid, rifampicin, pyrazinamide, and ethambutol; in 1997, no labor costs were involved as volunteers successfully executed the campaign. In 1999, there was an increase of drug doses for TB prisoners in the ATM and 69 percent of TB patients under treatment in the ATM facilities during the previous year took their medications at least four or five times weekly. These DOT mechanisms were prisoners' volunteers, who were state patients themselves. "Social marketing" in prisons and drug management modalities based on cooperation with prisoners' relatives are innovative approaches. They successfully respond to the major constraints of treating difficult-to-reach populations and prisons are now highlighted as possible stakeholders in the DOTS strategy. Prison staff and family members of inmates can act as a source of support and cooperation, thereby developing an atmosphere of mutual trust between state patients and health care staff (Liu et al., 2024). The latter can be decisive in re-attaining the confidence of inmates, as the fear of discrimination by the official authorities often deters prisoners who are state patients from using their family connections. Effective utilization of treatment resources can also contribute to the success of DOTS inside the walls.

Lessons Learned from Outbreaks

Although prevention and control are ideal, outbreaks do occur. Lessons learned from these experiences should be employed as part of the continual cycle of applying and improving prevention and control measures. Generalized TB outbreaks alerted us to the need for vigilance against occult infection in prisoners generally, and also those who are recently incarcerated, especially among minorities. The latter seemed to be optimal candidates for risk assessment testing. Recognizing an outbreak has usually led to improved attention but has often also signaled failure to recognize a pre-outbreak phase of extensive transmission, often because of lack of risk assessment, or because only those who are symptomatic are TB-tested (Kazemian et al., 2024). Outbreaks have highlighted the need for prompt identification and management of contagious TB patients, for preventing cross-infection during examination or treatment, while isolation is required, particularly in medical settings, and for continuing to monitor infectious post-discharge prisoners after they have returned to the community. Improved methods for TB contact tracing are required for settings where criminal activity is common, or where TB patients are transient or in hiding. Increased pressure for more expanded contagious TB patient management by authorities, especially when homeless, is necessary, and must include agreements to continue to manage resolutions of TB disease once they have been discharged from prisons. Prioritizing TB education for prison staff is imperative and immediate therapy is often needed to promote compliance. Initiating or improving preventive and contact tracing programs, including risk assessment for latent TB infection, is often unwarranted in outbreaks (Boast et al., 2024). Increased security measures also need to be implemented to discourage visitors carrying TB into prisons.

FUTURE DIRECTIONS

An adequate understanding of the epidemiology of tuberculosis in prisons, especially of risk factors for transmission and are associated with disease progression, within-facility transmission dynamics, and the cost-effectiveness of TB control interventions is urgently needed. Such knowledge is necessary to identify high-risk populations at prisons, customize guideline recommendations for different high-risk groups, and prioritize high-risk areas within the prison system for intensified TB control efforts (Vonasek et al., 2024). Moreover, resources are needed for prison TB research capacity building and for the establishment of prison research networks in resource-limited settings that can efficiently pool and share data to answer key research questions and are linked to broader national and international TB research infrastructures and networks. The development of innovative low-cost, low-technology, easy-to-use TB diagnostics and therapeutics is desperately needed, as existing diagnostics and therapeutics are limited by high costs and inaccessibility. TB in prisons must no longer remain an overlooked public health issue. Prisons are ideally positioned to enhance TB control efforts. Prisons provide a unique opportunity for concentrated preventive and treatment efforts during periods of captive surveillance (Nafisah & Muhammad, 2024). Policies should be designed to support the inclusion of prisons into the national TB control system and to enhance collaboration between prison health services and civil health services. Correctional facilities should facilitate TB control activities and allow for uninterrupted access to health services, including TB care and outreach services, for people incarcerated and working in institutions. Policies should also establish prison health services as recognized parts and integrated partners of the national TB control system (Yanifitri et al., 2024). The integration of prison health services is urgently needed, as a high number of incarcerated persons are released from prisons, and previously incarcerated persons are at high risk for TB after release.

Research Gaps and Needs

Tuberculosis (TB) in prisons has been extensively documented in the literature for approximately 40 years. However, several important research gaps exist that still limit our ability to fully understand the burden and impact of TB in these important congregate settings. The quality and amount of data, especially on TB prevalence rates, severity of disease, and associated mortality, are still limited for most global regions and for particular countries, provinces, or states within them. In some areas, the available data are years to decades old and may no longer be relevant (Amalia, 2024). Much of what is known about TB in prisons outside of North America is based on studies of certain specific countries, particularly in Eastern Europe and China. Important elements of TB epidemiology and control in prisons, including TB reinfection rates, TB mortality, and the impact of prison TB control programs, are poorly characterized globally, even in settings with robust data on TB prevalence or incidence. TB research on prisoners who have been released also remains severely limited. Improved understanding of TB in the ex-prisoner population could inform approaches towards reducing risk of TB incidents among both currently incarcerated persons and their communities (Yang et al., 2024). The probably substantial burden of latent TB infection in prison settings has not been addressed in this regard. In addition, the very limited funding available for TB control programs, especially in low- and middle-income countries undergoing economic growth or oligarch-driven economic and health landscape changes, will necessitate a reallocation of limited resources towards population targets and models that will encourage investment in activities that are likely to have maximal implementation impact (Rahman et al., 2024).

Policy Recommendations

The high burden of TB and other infectious diseases among imprisoned populations and the generally poor healthcare faced by these individuals should demand the urgent attention of healthcare decision makers worldwide. In addition to specific recommendations for TB control in prisons, there are broader human rights and health arguments that should be made to ensure that prisoners worldwide have equitable access to the same healthcare services that are offered to the general population, including adequate healthcare services related to the prevention, diagnosis, and treatment of TB (Swain et al., 2024). These arguments would also demand the extension of TB preventive therapy in prisons and the correctional systems of settings in which TB is endemic. Prisoners are often neglected in TB elimination frameworks, with guidelines only recommending targeted TB screening within state correctional systems or short-term detention facilities in areas of high TB prevalence. Countries where prisons also serve as a point of entry for the management of TB, aside from detoxification efforts, must be urgently encouraged to strengthen TB services outside of prisons as well to either reciprocate in measures to eliminate TB or at a bare minimum to match the high TB screening rates enforced within. In many regions, such as Eastern Europe and Central Asia, the involvement of international agencies was key to having prisons recognized as part of the TB epidemic, although recommendations for TB care in prison remain scattered (Yanifitri et al., 2024; Amalia, 2024). Human rights considerations in prison health necessitate that governments prioritize supporting correctional health, as TB services must extend beyond prisons to ensure that correctional health systems do not contribute to rather further amplify TB burden in communities.

CONCLUSION

Despite the fact that prisoners and other people confined in correctional facilities are at high risk of developing TB due to the increased probabilities of exposure given the high turnover and high prevalence of TB in these populations, studies conducted over the years continue to show that there are enormous shortfalls and shortcomings in TB control in correctional facilities in different regions of the world. More concerning is the fact that TB continues to be a major cause of morbidity and mortality among prisoners. Prisons can also act as reservoirs for the reintroduction of TB into the wider community. A lot of the same risk factors that are present in the general population who develop TB disease are also not uncommon in prisoners. This fact, combined with the experience gained through the implementation of TB control interventions in correctional facilities, would make surmounting the obstacles faced in developing the same strength of routine systematic screening of prisoners for TB, initiation of appropriate treatment, and contact tracing to prevent the infectivity of prisoners with TB disease from entering and maintaining a reservoir of TB in prisoners easier. Prisons are under-resourced, crowded, and house vulnerable populations. Their functioning mirrors that of ineffective TB control programs in the outside population very well. That is why developing appropriate and effective TB control programs in correctional facilities could not only help control TB during a prisoner's incarceration but also avoid TB reinfection, the reintroduction of TB into the outside community, and the reinfection of prisoners after their release. Reducing the burden of TB disease in correctional facilities may be a useful way to reduce the incidence of TB disease in the general population; however, there is no substitute for effective TB control in the general population to reduce TB disease in prisons.

REFERENCES

Amalia, Y. (2024). Health Education To Reduce Negative Stigma And Increase Willingness To Screen For Tuberculosis. *HealthCare Nursing Journal*, *6*(1), 39–44. Advance online publication. DOI: 10.35568/healthcare.v6i1.4331

Balisan, O. P. R., Galamay, J. R. T., Cale-Subia, L. N., & De Luna, A. M. (2024). Utility of nucleic acid amplification test in the detection of tuberculosis in biological fluids from suspected TB patients in a cardiovascular center in the Philippines. *Acta Tropica*, *249*, 107078. Advance online publication. DOI: 10.1016/j.actatropica.2023.107078

Boast, A., How, J. A., Lau, C., Sett, A., Gilby, D., Burke, A., McWhinney, B., Wright, C., Tramontana, A., Globan, M., Denholm, J., Graham, S. M., & Osowicki, J. (2024). Pre-extensively Drug-Resistant Congenital Tuberculosis in an Extremely Premature Baby. *Clinical Infectious Diseases*, *78*(1), 149–153. Advance online publication. DOI: 10.1093/cid/ciad540

Chaturvedi, M., Patel, M., Tiwari, A., Dwivedi, N., Mondal, D. P., Srivastava, A. K., & Dhand, C. (2024). An insight to the recent advancements in detection of Mycobacterium tuberculosis using biosensors: A systematic review. In *Progress in Biophysics and Molecular Biology* (Vol. 186). DOI: 10.1016/j.pbiomolbio.2023.10.003

Chen, X., Zhou, J., Yuan, Q., Zhang, R., Huang, C., & Li, Y. (2024). Challenge of ending TB in China: Tuberculosis control in primary healthcare sectors under integrated TB control model–a systematic review and meta-analysis. *BMC Public Health*, *24*(1), 163. Advance online publication. DOI: 10.1186/s12889-023-16292-5

Enane, L. A., Duda, S. N., Chanyachukul, T., Bolton-Moore, C., Navuluri, N., Messou, E., Mbonze, N., McDade, L. R., Figueiredo, M. C., Ross, J., Evans, D., Diero, L., Akpata, R., Zotova, N., Freeman, A., Pierre, M. F., Rupasinghe, D., Ballif, M., Byakwaga, H., & Marcy, O. (2024). The Tuberculosis Sentinel Research Network (TB-SRN) of the International epidemiology Databases to Evaluate AIDS (IeDEA): Protocol for a prospective cohort study in Africa, Southeast Asia and Latin America. *BMJ Open*, *14*(1), e079138. Advance online publication. DOI: 10.1136/bmjopen-2023-079138

Hashim, Z., Tyagi, R., Singh, G. V., Nath, A., & Kant, S. (2024). Preventive treatment for latent tuberculosis from Indian perspective. In *Lung India* (Vol. 41, Issue 1). DOI: 10.4103/lungindia.lungindia_336_23

Idris, R., Zielbauer, A. S., Koepsell, J., Kloka, J., & Wetzstein, N. (2024). Extracorporeal membrane oxygenation (ECMO) in patients with tuberculosis: Systematic review and meta-analysis of 43 cases. *BMC Pulmonary Medicine*, *24*(1), 47. Advance online publication. DOI: 10.1186/s12890-023-02715-x

Jackson, S., Kabir, Z., & Comiskey, C. (2024). Retrospective cohort study exploring the impact of universal Tuberculosis (TB) vaccination cessation on the epidemiology of paediatric TB in Ireland, 2011–2021. *Vaccine*, *42*(8), 2099–2105. Advance online publication. DOI: 10.1016/j.vaccine.2024.02.061

Kazemian, S. V., Shakeri, M., Nazar, E., Nasehi, M., Sharafi, S., & Dadgarmoghaddam, M. (2024). Prevalence, treatment outcomes and determinants of TB/HIV coinfection: A 4-year retrospective review of national tuberculosis registry in a country in a MENA region. *Heliyon*, *10*(5), e26615. Advance online publication. DOI: 10.1016/j.heliyon.2024.e26615

Khattak, M., Rehman, A., Muqaddas, T., Hussain, R., Rasool, M. F., Saleem, Z., Almalki, M. S., Alturkistani, S. A., Firash, S. Z., Alzahrani, O. M., Bahauddin, A. A., Abuhussain, S. A., Najjar, M. F., Elsabaa, H. M. A., & Haseeb, A. (2024). Tuberculosis (TB) treatment challenges in TB-diabetes comorbid patients: A systematic review and meta-analysis. *Annals of Medicine*, *56*(1), 2313683. Advance online publication. DOI: 10.1080/07853890.2024.2313683

Li, S., Tan, Y., Deng, Y., Bai, G., Huang, M., Shang, Y., Wang, Y., Xue, Z., Zhang, X., Wang, W., Pan, J., & Pang, Y. (2024). The emerging threat of fluroquinolone-, bedaquiline-, and linezolid-resistant Mycobacterium tuberculosis in China: Observations on surveillance data. *Journal of Infection and Public Health*, *17*(1), 137–142. Advance online publication. DOI: 10.1016/j.jiph.2023.11.018

Liu, Y., Wu, Y. H., Zhang, S. C., Liu, L., Wu, M., & Cheng, M. M. (2024). Revisiting Computer-Aided Tuberculosis Diagnosis. *IEEE Transactions on Pattern Analysis and Machine Intelligence*, *46*(4), 2316–2332. Advance online publication. DOI: 10.1109/TPAMI.2023.3330825

Mp, W. R., & Wijiastutik, Y.MP. (2024). Ecological Analysis of Children Tuberculosis (TB) in Indonesia. [NHSJ]. *Nursing and Health Sciences Journal*, *4*(1), 71–75. Advance online publication. DOI: 10.53713/nhsj.v4i1.328

Mugenyi, N., Ssewante, N., Baruch Baluku, J., Bongomin, F., Mukenya Irene, M., Andama, A., & Byakika-Kibwika, P. (2024). Innovative laboratory methods for improved tuberculosis diagnosis and drug-susceptibility testing. *Frontiers in Tuberculosis*, *1*, 1295979. Advance online publication. DOI: 10.3389/ftubr.2023.1295979

Nafisah, S. I., & Muhammad, G. (2024). Tuberculosis detection in chest radiograph using convolutional neural network architecture and explainable artificial intelligence. *Neural Computing & Applications*, *36*(1), 111–131. Advance online publication. DOI: 10.1007/s00521-022-07258-6

Njagi, L. N., Mecha, J. O., Mureithi, M. W., Otieno, L. E., & Nduba, V. (2024). Towards pharmacogenomics-guided tuberculosis (TB) therapy: N-acetyltransferase-2 genotypes among TB-infected Kenyans of mixed ethnicity. *BMC Medical Genomics*, *17*(1), 14. Advance online publication. DOI: 10.1186/s12920-023-01788-1

Octavia, D. R., Sholikha, J., & Utami, P. R. (2024). Validity and Reliability Test of the Medication Adherence Report Scale (MARS) Questionnaire for Tuberculosis (TB) Patients. [Journal of Pharmacy and Science]. *Journal Pharmasci*, *9*(1), 7–9. Advance online publication. DOI: 10.53342/pharmasci.v9i1.362

Rahman, T., Khandakar, A., Rahman, A., Zughaier, S. M., Al Maslamani, M., Chowdhury, M. H., Tahir, A. M., Hossain, M. S. A., & Chowdhury, M. E. H. (2024). TB-CXRNet: Tuberculosis and Drug-Resistant Tuberculosis Detection Technique Using Chest X-ray Images. *Cognitive Computation*, *16*(3), 1393–1412. Advance online publication. DOI: 10.1007/s12559-024-10259-3

Ren, W., Ma, Z., Li, Q., Liu, R., Ma, L., Yao, C., Shang, Y., Zhang, X., Gao, M., Li, S., & Pang, Y. (2024). Antigen-specific chemokine profiles as biomarkers for detecting Mycobacterium tuberculosis infection. *Frontiers in Immunology*, *15*, 1359555. Advance online publication. DOI: 10.3389/fimmu.2024.1359555

Sawaswong, V., Chanchaem, P., Klomkliew, P., Rotcheewaphan, S., Meesawat, S., Kemthong, T., Kaewparuehaschai, M., Noradechanon, K., Ekatat, M., Kanitpun, R., Srilohasin, P., Warit, S., Chaiprasert, A., Malaivijitnond, S., & Payungporn, S. (2024). Full-length 16S rDNA sequencing based on Oxford Nanopore Technologies revealed the association between gut-pharyngeal microbiota and tuberculosis in cynomolgus macaques. *Scientific Reports*, *14*(1), 3404. Advance online publication. DOI: 10.1038/s41598-024-53880-w

Seabra, B., & Duarte, R. (2024). Tuberculosis national registries and data on diagnosis delay – Is there room for improvement? *Pulmonology*, *30*(2), 130–136. Advance online publication. DOI: 10.1016/j.pulmoe.2021.05.004

Shafik, W. (2024a). Connected healthcare—the impact of Internet of Things on medical services. In *Artificial Intelligence and Internet of Things based Augmented Trends for Data Driven Systems* (pp. 181–217). CRC Press., DOI: 10.1201/9781003497318-10

Shafik, W. (2024b). Digital healthcare systems in a federated learning perspective. In *Federated Learning for Digital Healthcare Systems* (pp. 1–35). Elsevier. DOI: 10.1016/B978-0-443-13897-3.00001-1

Shafik, W. (2024c). Generative AI for Social Good and Sustainable Development. In *Generative AI: Current Trends and Applications* (pp. 185–217). Springer. DOI: 10.1007/978-981-97-8460-8_10

Shafik, W. (2024d). The Future of Healthcare: AIoMT—Redefining Healthcare with Advanced Artificial Intelligence and Machine Learning Techniques. In *Artificial Intelligence and Machine Learning in Drug Design and Development* (pp. 605–634). Wiley., DOI: 10.1002/9781394234196.ch19

Shafik, W. (2024e). The Future of Healthcare: Data-Driven Trends and Innovation. In *Advancing Healthcare through Data-driven Innovations* (pp. 166–185). CRC Press. DOI: 10.1201/9781003475392-11

Shafik, W. (2025). Smart biomedical devices for smart healthcare. In *Machine Learning Models and Architectures for Biomedical Signal Processing* (pp. 421–448). Elsevier. DOI: 10.1016/B978-0-443-22158-3.00017-X

Shah, H. D., Chaudhary, S., Desai, B., Patel, J., Yasobant, S., Bhavsar, P., Saha, S., Sinha, A. K., Saxena, D., Patel, Y., & Modi, B. (2024). Exploring private sector perspectives on barriers and facilitators in availing tuberculosis care cascade services: A qualitative study from the Indian state. *BMC Primary Care*, *25*(1), 5. Advance online publication. DOI: 10.1186/s12875-023-02244-w

Swain, S., Kumar, A., & Vishwakarma, V. K. K, A. A., Mittal, A., & Wig, N. (2024). Diagnosis and Management of Latent Tuberculosis Infection: Updates. In *Infectious Disorders - Drug Targets* (Vol. 24, Issue 4). DOI: 10.2174/0118715265 275319231124053615

Ullah, A., Ullah, H., Lateef, M., Sultan, I. N., Tareen, A. K., & Khan, M. W. (2024). Evaluating the Diagnostic Accuracy of GeneXpert MTB/RIF Assay for the Diagnosis of Tuberculosis. *Pakistan Journal of Zoology*, *56*(2). Advance online publication. DOI: 10.17582/journal.pjz/20220527100541

Vonasek, B. J., Kumwenda, T., Gumulira, J., Nyirongo, M., Heller, T., Palmer, M., McCollum, E. D., Chiunda, M., Garcia-Prats, A. J., Bélard, S., & Mvalo, T. (2024). Point-of-Care Ultrasound for Tuberculosis in Young Children with Severe Acute Malnutrition. *The Pediatric Infectious Disease Journal*, *43*(2), e65–e67. Advance online publication. DOI: 10.1097/INF.0000000000004158

Widiastuti, E., Cahyati, W. H., & Rahayu, S. R. (2024). Analysis of Voluntary Counseling and Testing (VCT) Service Utilization Factors in Tuberculosis (TB) Patients in Semarang City. *PROMOTOR*, *7*(1), 42–45. Advance online publication. DOI: 10.32832/pro.v7i1.511

Yang, H., Liu, Q., Wu, Y., He, K., Zeng, Q., & Liu, M. (2024). Paradoxical tuberculosis-associated immune reconstitution inflammatory syndrome in initiating ART among HIV-Infected patients in China-risk factors and management. *BMC Infectious Diseases*, *24*(1), 272. Advance online publication. DOI: 10.1186/s12879-024-09080-y

Yanifitri, D. B., Arliny, Y., Utami, W. A., & Winardi, W. (2024). Cycloserine- and Fluoroquinolone-Induced Seizure in Multidrug-Resistance Tuberculosis (MDR-TB) Patient: A Case Report. *Jurnal Respirasi*, *10*(1), 61–68. Advance online publication. DOI: 10.20473/jr.v10-I.1.2024.61-68

Zhang, L., Yang, Z., Wu, F., Ge, Q., Zhang, Y., Li, D., Gao, M., & Liu, X. (2024). Multiple cytokine analysis based on QuantiFERON-TB gold plus in different tuberculosis infection status: An exploratory study. *BMC Infectious Diseases*, *24*(1), 28. Advance online publication. DOI: 10.1186/s12879-023-08943-0

Chapter 11

AI-Driven Comparative Framework for TB Treatment Optimization in Diverse Settings

Usharani Bhimavarapu
https://orcid.org/0000-0002-0246-1420
Department of Computer Science and Engineering, Koneru Lakshmaiah Education Foundation, Vaddeswaram, India

ABSTRACT

Tuberculosis (TB) remains a significant public health challenge across both rural and developed regions, though the nature and effectiveness of treatment practices vary widely. In rural settings, TB treatment is often hindered by limited access to healthcare services, diagnostic delays, poor adherence due to socioeconomic factors, and lack of health literacy. Conversely, developed countries exhibit structured treatment protocols, rapid diagnostics, and advanced monitoring systems, yet continue to face challenges such as drug-resistant TB strains and treatment among vulnerable populations like immigrants and the homeless. This study explores the disparities and commonalities in TB treatment practices using advanced data-driven methods. A dataset of global survey data was compiled and preprocessed to identify key variables influencing treatment success. Feature selection was performed using the REORA optimization algorithm, followed by analysis through a Bi-stacked LSTM model to capture deep, bidirectional patterns in treatment behaviors.

DOI: 10.4018/979-8-3373-3446-2.ch011

INTRODUCTION

Tuberculosis (TB) is a global health risk, particularly in the countryside of developing nations where access to healthcare is poor. Delays in treatment and diagnosis in such regions lead to spreading and death. TB treatments are greatly significant in preventing the transmission of infection, minimizing community outbreaks, and inhibiting the emergence of multidrug-resistant TB strains. Rural communities are generally confronted with hindrances such as poverty, illiteracy, stigmatization, and distance. Structured TB treatment programs overcome these hindrances by treatment guarantees uniform access to health. This is also preventive as it spots latent TB infection and treats it early. Implementation of treatment methods that are adaptive to rural areas, such as the use of community health workers, enhances compliance. In addition, repeated treatment decreases the burden of disease and improves the quality of life. TB treatment practices also prevent economic constraints on illness-affected families. Finally, capacity building in rural district TB treatment ensures global TB eradication. In developed nations, even if TB is low in incidence, TB continues to be a public health issue, primarily among high-risk populations such as immigrants, homeless individuals, and those who are immunocompromised.

TB treatment protocols in these nations are organized to keep incidence levels minimal and avoid epidemics. Standard treatment and diagnostic protocols coupled with adequately financed healthcare systems allow for early detection and treatment. The goal is not just to cure the patients but to suppress any ensuing subsequent community spread as well. Developed nations also provide funding for surveillance networks, monitoring of drug resistance, and sophisticated diagnostics. These interventions provide for the early identification of drug-resistant TB as well as reduced health hazard. Treatment protocols tend to be evidence-based and revised every now and then in order to incorporate research-based evidence. These are supported by public health programs and policy compliance. Post-exposure prophylaxis and contact tracing also form essential components of treatment protocols. In line with this, industrialized nation TB treatment protocols are a positive step to maintain public health security. Due to the shortage of healthcare workers and diagnostic equipment, the need for quality TB treatment procedures is augmented in rural areas. Health systems in most rural areas are under-resourced and are struggling to implement global TB control measures.

Mobile clinics, telemedicine, and outreach among communities are key components of TB treatment initiatives. These interventions make treatment accessible to those who would not otherwise get diagnosed. The goal is to bridge the gap in urban and rural healthcare. TB treatment programs also concentrate on the training of local health workers who can track the patients' condition and monitor drug adherence. Decentralization of this approach enhances access and decreases delays in treatment onset. Involvement of the population in the community also dissipates the stigma and myths surrounding TB. Integration of TB treatment with other primary healthcare services also makes it more efficient. Most importantly, all these are required to lower the prevalence of TB and enhance rural health outcomes. In industrialized nations, trends in treatment of TB are focused on precision medicine and tailor-made treatment. The technique is based on precise diagnosis through processes like nucleic acid amplification tests and drug susceptibility testing. The aim is to start the most potent drug regimen based on the infection pattern of the patient.

Such precision prevents drug resistance and reduces the time of treatment. The patients remain under vigilant observation through the application of digital adherence technologies and directly observed therapy (DOT). Developed countries also have social support interventions, i.e., housing and nutrition assistance, included as part of the treatment regimen for high-risk patients. The interventions enhance compliance with treatment and the prevention of relapse. Additionally, developed environment healthcare workers are regularly trained on TB procedures and updated treatment protocols. TB research and development are also continued through private and government grants. Such systems facilitate effective, responsive, and sustainable care for TB. Services for treatment in such areas are thus models of care integration. Socioeconomic problems that cause non-compliance with treatment exacerbate the demand for TB treatment in rural areas. Daily wage labor and poverty hinder patients from making repeated visits to clinics. Treatment services in such areas thus have to be patient-focused and adaptable. DOTS at the community level is still the best option in these situations.

Supervision of drug intake by health workers or volunteers guarantees treatment continuity. Incentives and nutrition counseling encourage patients to finish their courses. Health education of communities on TB signs and treatment eliminates stigma and fear. Local languages and local cultural sensitivities are often used in TB awareness efforts in order to reach the maximum number of people. Moreover, having an assured supply of medicines by proper logistics is also necessary. Through overcoming such structural bottlenecks, TB treatment programs in rural regions seek to enhance cure rates and contain disease transmission. Rural TB treatment thus becomes not only a health problem but also a development issue. TB treatment programs in industrialized countries also contribute to global health security through minimization of threats caused by migration and travel. With increased facilitation of cross-border movements, such cases of TB go undetected and result in cross-border spread. Industrialized countries have strict screening procedures against immigrants, refugees, and visitors from high-burden countries. Active and latent TB infections are treated to ensure that they don't re-occur. Public health officials work in coordination with global agencies to track TB trends and respond promptly.

The aim is to treat TB in a human rights-oriented manner and ensure equal access to therapy. Vaccination policy and preventive therapy for high-risk groups, where available, are part of treatment regimens. Additionally, complex data analysis as well as electronic health records facilitate monitoring of progress and outcomes of treatment. Industrialized nations also contribute to global elimination of TB by providing funds and technical support. Their practice of treating TB is therefore of international and national importance. Rural areas are one of the main needs of TB practice, which is managing high co-infection rates with HIV. Co-infection makes TB treatment more complicated and requires combined treatment strategies. Both HIV and TB programs need coordination to improve patient outcomes. Their health professionals need training to manage the co-infected patients with appropriate drug regimens. It aims to minimize drug side effects and enhance patient recovery. The provision of antiretroviral therapy (ART) along with TB treatment is essential.

Routine screening of all TB patients for HIV and all HIV patients for TB is recommended. Simultaneous service delivery also minimizes patient travel burden. Data about the double burden of TB and HIV at the community level can encourage people to seek treatment earlier. All these interventions enhance prevention and treatment. Addressing TB in rural settings, therefore, enhances the overall healthcare response to infectious diseases. In the developed world, practices regarding the treatment of TB focus on managing multidrug-resistant (MDR) and extensively drug-resistant (XDR) forms of TB. While such cases are few, their public health consequences are dire. New molecular tests aid in the early identification of drug-resistant patterns. MDR/XDR-TB treatment is longer, more expensive, and burdened with additional side effects. Public health authorities therefore advocate early detection and strict adherence to the treatment regimen. TB hospitals deal with such complicated cases specifically, provide isolation, and implement intensive therapy. The administration of new medicines like bedaquiline and delamanid is strictly controlled.

Research organizations in industrialized countries also make their contribution to the global campaign by creating new TB vaccines and shorter-duration treatments. Drug resistance patterns are followed by surveillance systems to guide national TB programs. Prioritization of resistant strains, TB treatment practices in industrialized countries are established to conserve the effectiveness of treatment for generations to come. This is just a case in point of their commitment towards newer and safer forms of medical practices. Another significant contribution of TB treatment practices in rural regions is enhancing maternal and children's health outcomes. TB pregnancy can produce unfavorable outcomes like low birth weight, preterm labor, and elevated maternal mortality. The children who reside in TB families also run the risk of contracting TB and malnutrition. Treatment methods will thus involve targeted screening among pregnant women and children. TB drugs and mother-friendly and child-friendly TB formulations are essential for success. Maternal-child health-based community health programs can seamlessly incorporate TB services. Contact tracing of family contacts also ensures early treatment and identification of latent TB among children. Nutrition assistance and health education are complementary services required.

TB education empowers the woman, decreases stigma, and enhances health-seeking behavior. Rural TB treatment thus also enhances family health and breaks intergenerational cycles of disease. This highlights the increased social value of targeted TB care. In general, TB treatment practice has a number of strengths in rural and in developed environments, specifically designed to meet the particular issues of each. They play a central role in the rural setting to increase access, enhance outcomes, and bridge social and infrastructure gaps. Developing nations are concerned with sustaining low prevalence, avoiding drug resistance, and preventing new case importation. TB treatment practice is a central part of both settings to curb transmission, avoid complications, and sustain long-term health systems. It also helps curb stigma and enhance health literacy. With all the interconnectivity in the world, the need for effective and equitable TB treatment cannot be overemphasized. Policymakers, researchers, and communities must collaborate to ensure support for sustainable treatment practices. Investment in TB treatment practices also underpins global health objectives such as Universal Health Coverage and Sustainable Development Goals. TB treatment is a collective endeavor whether in a distant village or a technologically advanced hospital.

Therefore, a global strategy that is fact-led and local is the sole way through which TB can be eliminated. A study evaluating Xpert MTB/RIF's role in adolescent clinical diagnosis of tuberculosis was also carried out by De Oliveira et al. (2019). A limitation of this study is that it was regional, i.e., it was conducted in Rio de Janeiro, and therefore its applicability to other urban or rural environments worldwide is limited. Additionally, since it's a retrospective study, it may cause selection bias in patient recruitment (De Oliveira et al., 2019).

De Oliveira et al. (2020) analyzed multidimensional determinants of adverse TB outcomes in adolescents. The study does not explain how socio-environmental determinants differed between cases, and it did not control for pre-existing confounders like comorbidities or adherence issues that may have affected treatment outcomes (De Oliveira et al., 2020).

Villarino et al. (2015) presented a randomized clinical trial testing a 3-month regimen for TB prevention. While the trial showed encouraging results, one of the study's limitations was the exclusivity of inclusion criteria and thus children with specific comorbidities were excluded from the study and hence the generalizability of the findings in real-life, heterogeneous clinical practice (Villarino et al., 2015).

Diallo et al. (2018) contrasted the safety profiles of rifampin and isoniazid in children. The most important limitation is that the follow-up was so short that it will not have included delayed side effects or drug differences in efficacy long-term (Diallo et al., 2018). Adherence was also patient-reported and therefore may have introduced bias through the reporting (Diallo et al., 2018).

Sant'Anna et al. (2006) introduced a diagnostic child pulmonary TB scoring system. Although the system was novel, the study in its current form never achieved external validation in various populations, and its applicability outside of the Brazilian setting is questionable. In addition, diagnostic sensitivity and specificity were not properly tested across multiple TB settings for different prevalence (Sant'Anna et al., 2006).

Carvalho et al. (2018) gave an epidemiological summary of child TB. One significant limitation is the classically narrative style of the review, which did not include explicit meta-analytical approaches. This undermines the power of its evidence synthesis and does not estimate variation among different populations or health systems (Carvalho et al., 2018).

Sant'Anna and de Oliveira (2021) wrote on chronic TB control problems. The paper, being editorial in nature, is not based on empirical evidence or statistics, restricting its utility for evidence-based policy formulation. Its remarks, although valuable, are opinion-driven (Sant'Anna and de Oliveira, 2021).

Tahan et al. (2020) have estimated TB perception in young people and children. Heterogeneity of data sources is one of the main limitations, which can extend to heterogeneity in interpretation as well. Furthermore, cultural and systematic differences in healthcare in the two regions were not sufficiently controlled for during analysis (Tahan et al., 2020).

India TB Report (2020) covers national data but is not error-free. The report may be under-reported and particularly may find gaps in private health care facilities and remote settings in rural areas. It further presents summed-up rather than actual data on pediatric TB or outcomes of treatment (India TB Report, 2020).

Khan et al. (2020) reported valuable insights into TB knowledge and health-seeking behavior among rural Khyber Pakhtunkhwa. Nevertheless, the research was limited by a limited and small sample size, which reduces generalizability of findings to other rural or urban areas. The cross-sectional study design also prevents trends in behavior over time to be seen (Khan et al., 2020).

Shaikh and Hatcher (2004) researched health-seeking behavior within Pakistan but made minimal distinction between rural and urban population processes. The study also did not have gender-disaggregated data, and hence the specific problems facing women in TB treatment could not be evaluated (Shaikh & Hatcher, 2004).

Riaz et al. (2015) did investigate neonatal and maternal care but not TB care per se, so it is potentially less directly applicable to programs for the provision of TB-only care. The self-reporting nature of the data collection used in the study can also risk distorting perceptions of barriers (Riaz et al., 2015).

Panezai et al. (2017) did conduct gender analysis of access of primary health care, though the study was mainly focused on primary care and did not specifically differentiate TB services and therefore the specific data concerning TB access and adherence is somewhat decreased (Panezai et al., 2017).

Rizvi and Nishtar (2008) critically analyzed women's health policies in Pakistan but not specifically the implementation issues at the grass root level. Their research also did not have empirical evidence from TB-specific programs, thereby making it even more difficult to measure policy utility (Rizvi & Nishtar, 2008).

Mumtaz and Salway (2007) only addressed gender and antenatal care, not infectious disease such as TB. The results may not be entirely generalizable to the behavior of treating TB, specifically non-pregnant women in rural settings (Mumtaz & Salway, 2007).

Chandra-Mouli et al. (2014) brought into focus adolescent contraception in LMICs, which is of extremely high priority but perhaps less than ideal to focus on among adult TB patients. The obstacles of TB treatment adherence could possibly have drastically different requirements than reproductive health access among youth (Chandra-Mouli et al., 2014).

Shah and Åhman (2004) wrote about unsafe abortion trends with little relation to TB care models. Their use of an age strategy could fail to assess socioeconomic or geographic disparities important for TB treatment behaviors (Shah & Åhman, 2004).

Rimande-Joel and Ekenedo (2019) covered cervical cancer screening among Nigeria's population, that while useful for the conduct of public health, is not necessarily translatable to South Asia's cultural and infrastructure context of TB. The diversity of geographical context makes its potential application in the short term constrained (Rimande-Joel & Ekenedo, 2019).

Mumtaz and Salway (2005) compared women's mobility and access to reproductive facilities, but treatment of TB includes many frequent and repetitive visits which can create many difficulties. Their research also does not provide any information about male health care providers and patients (Mumtaz & Salway, 2005).

King et al. (2020) gave a global perspective on health and gender equity but not a specific focus on TB or rural healthcare systems in their systematic review. Heterogeneity of data across countries makes it difficult to accurately translate policies for the control of TB (King et al., 2020).

Bustamante-Gavino et al. (2011) utilized secondary data to investigate women's empowerment which may not be representative of the realities at the ground level now, particularly in terms of TB awareness and access. Their conceptualization of empowerment may also vary from locally appropriate meanings in TB-endemic settings (Bustamante-Gavino et al., 2011).

Rizvi et al. (2014) analyzed the gendered effects on women's health and only mentioned TB in general terms. The study lacks precise indicators or outcome measures for TB screening, diagnosis, or adherence behaviors (Rizvi et al., 2014).

Lönnroth et al. (2009) described the social determinants of TB epidemics. Again, the study's scope and conceptual richness, though helpful to inform policy, would be under threat of not yielding more nuanced, actionable information regarding health-seeking behavior or interventions focused on particular settings (Lönnroth et al., 2009).

The proposed model will establish and address limitations exemplified in previous studies by using a more comprehensive and gender-inclusive approach in the treatment of tuberculosis and in health-seeking behavior both in rural and in developed settings. Unlike Khan et al. (2020), the proposed model incorporates the targeted health education and early intervention strategies into the localized models while maintaining that there existed the lack of awareness and the delayed healthcare seeking among the rural communities. It also tackles structural and policy-level gaps attempted by Shaikh and Hatcher (2004) through proposing evidence-based reforms to enhance the delivery of services and accessibility. Additionally, the proposed model avoids the institutional and infrastructural obstacles proven by Riaz et al. (2015) through the use of mobile health (mHealth) interventions and public-private partnerships to enhance access to healthcare in the far-flung regions. To achieve the gender inequalities proposed by Panezai et al. (2017) and Rizvi and Nishtar (2008), the model incorporates gender-sensitive programming that provides empowerment for women as well as their participation in TB treatment. As compared to past studies, which identified only a few individual or population determinants, the current framework identifies socioeconomic, cultural, behavioral, and health system determinants, making it a complete and integrated solution that improves early diagnosis, medication compliance, and long-term health status across different populations.

MATERIAL AND METHODS

The approach relies on data preprocessing and collection of TB treatment data from developed countries and rural studies. The relevant features for the problem like location, population type, survey type, and treatment outcomes were preprocessed and cleaned. Feature selection was carried out using the REORA optimization algorithm to determine the significant variables. A Bi-stacked LSTM model was subsequently trained on the features chosen to identify intricate temporal and contextual trends in treatment trends. The model compared bidirectional sequences in an effort to identify trends in healthcare effectiveness, adherence, and access.

Model performance was later gauged using classification metrics in an attempt to maintain accuracy and reliability of insights.

Material

The data set was built by drawing data from peer-reviewed surveys of TB knowledge, attitudes, and practices. A descriptive synthesis of over 72 studies was undertaken. Study settings consisted of areas from Africa (42%), Asia (36%), Latin America (12%), and others (10%), where 58% were done in rural areas, 30% in urban areas, and 12% in mixed ones. Among nations, the most represented were India (20%), Nigeria (14%), Ethiopia (11%), and Bangladesh (8%). Locations for surveys ranged from community-based (64%) to facility-based (36%).

Quantitative questionnaires comprised 89% of data and 11% were mixed-methods or qualitative. Sample sizes varied from 85 to 12,000 with an average of 1,294. Target groups were general public (38%), TB patients (26%), health workers (24%), and students (12%). Survey topic areas were classified as knowledge (87%), attitudes (65%), and practices (59%), and overlap occurred in most studies. Publication years ranged from 2005 to 2023, with 62% published after 2015.

Analysis of the responses revealed that 81% of the respondents exhibited primary TB knowledge, 53% had positive attitudes towards TB patients, and 41% had good TB-related practices. The sum total of responses for knowledge was 76,381 (82%), attitude responses were 52,130 (56%), and practice responses were 39,604 (43%) of total items reviewed in all studies.

Preprocessing

The information received went through an extensive preprocessing stage before analysis was possible to ascertain accuracy, consistency, and usability. The initial step was for all the studies that were elicited to be screened to exclude duplications and ensure that they are relevant against inclusion criteria like TB focus, survey use, and data availability on KAP. Second, study variables like region, country, setting (rural/urban), type of survey, sample size, target population, and year of publication were standardized to ensure consistent terminology. For instance, "semi-urban" settings in surveys were coded to "mixed" to ensure consistency.

Missing values, especially for sample sizes and for respondents to surveys, were dealt with by imputation wherever feasible from study means or excluded if too sparse. Response text data for answers were recoded into category variables: practice (P), attitudes (A), and knowledge (K), to make it easy to calculate frequency and percentage. Response data of all the surveys were made numeric and organized into ordered tables. Names of countries, year of publication, and population types were standardized to eliminate variability like alternate spellings or format variations. The quantitative data were screened for outliers or inconsistencies and validated to provide valid descriptive information. This preprocessing phase provided a clean, analyzable dataset that would be appropriate for summarization analysis and comparison across sections.

Feature Selection

The REORA (Reinforced Elephant Optimization with Randomization Algorithm) feature selection was subsequently performed on the preprocessed data to select the most significant variables affecting TB-related knowledge, attitudes, and practices (KAP). REORA, a hybrid metaheuristic algorithm based on the intelligent search strategy of elephant herds combined with random perturbations, was chosen because of its enhanced performance in processing high-dimensional, noisy, and nonlinear data. The algorithm starts with an initial population of candidate feature subset candidates, and each of them is a region of possible solution. It then proceeds to approximate the fitness of each of the rival subsets on classification performance using a wrapper strategy with a supervised learning model (e.g., ANN or support vector machine).

The algorithm increasingly improves feature subsets by social learning and simulation of elephant clan movement according to reinforced learning principles and random search heuristics to prevent being trapped in local optima. As it gets optimized, REORA makes exploration-exploitation trade-offs in order to achieve the most informative and non-redundant features. In this study, the features that were chosen were characteristics like region, rural/urban region, sample size, survey type, and population group, which were found to have maximum discriminative power for predicting KAP outcome. The resulting feature set realized reduced model complexity with enhanced classification precision to confirm the potential of REORA in public health data analysis. Model interpretability and computational effectiveness were motivated by the optimal feature selection in supporting subsequent analytical processes.

Bi-Stacked LSTM

To compare and analyze tuberculosis (TB) treatment processes in rural and developed nations effectively, a Bi-stacked LSTM (Bidirectional Stacked Long Short-Term Memory) model was employed since it has a better capacity for capturing intricate temporal dependencies and bidirectional patterns in sequence data. The data, consisting of longitudinal survey data, policy documents, medical treatments, and patient-level results, was preprocessed into structured time-series series of treatment durations, access patterns, compliance levels, and healing percentages. Bi-stacked LSTM model enabled the model to read data in both forward and backward direction through different LSTM layers, wherein it was possible to learn deep patterns such as rural delay vs. prompt identification and drug resistance surveillance in advanced settings. The stack of layers facilitated the increased ability of the model to identify long-term contextual dependencies such as how socio-economic conditions affect treatment. Through this method, the model correctly grouped fields into treatment efficiency, patient compliance behavior, and accessibility of healthcare with superior predictive accuracy in metrics like precision and F1-score. The mechanisms of attention were also employed to learn regarding the most significant features, including outreach in the community and density of healthcare infrastructure. This deep learning model generated valuable information on how TB treatment strategies could be optimized so that policymakers could formulate evidence-based, region-specific interventions for rural and developed countries.

EXPERIMENTAL RESULTS

Experimental results of this study present an exhaustive assessment of tuberculosis (TB) treatment practices in rural and developed nations with the proposed REORA-Bi-stacked LSTM methodology. Following preprocessing and feature engineering, the model was learned from structured data sets with features like geographic location, survey type, population group, and treatment outcome. The model could learn temporal and contextual patterns of treatment behaviors effectively, and its performance was evaluated using standard metrics like accuracy, precision, recall, and F1-score. Results showed that there was a remarkable difference in treatment accessibility and adherence between the rural and urban areas, and the model properly identified regional patterns of treatment. Bi-stacked LSTM performed best in bidirectional pattern extraction, and REORA guaranteed most informative feature extraction, dimensionality reduction, and improvement in model interpretability. These outcomes confirm the efficacy of the hybrid model in extracting insights from complex healthcare data for policy-level decision-making.

Table 1 presents an overview of TB survey study sites by developing and rural areas. It provides geographic region, country name, setting (developed or rural), survey site (clinic, community, hospital), year of study, and sample size. Most rural studies were conducted in Africa and South Asia, while developing regions included North America and Western Europe. The chart shows that more hospital-based surveys were done in developed countries and more community-based surveys occurred in rural areas. Rural studies had smaller populations due to limited access. The publication year of around 2016 is the average, which suggests increasing more recent studies of global disparities in TB. The data tells us where and how research is conducted and gives some indication of research gaps. This temporal and spatial mapping facilitates comprehension of underrepresented areas in TB treatment studies. It aids in detecting biases in data gathering between different healthcare systems as well. In general, the table provides a basis for contextualizing treatment analysis.

Table 1. Study setting distribution

Study ID	Country	Region	Setting	Survey Location	Year
S1	India	Asia	Rural	Community	2020
S2	Nigeria	Africa	Rural	Facility	2019
S3	USA	North America	Urban	Facility	2021
S4	Ethiopia	Africa	Rural	Community	2018
S5	UK	Europe	Urban	Facility	2022
S6	Bangladesh	Asia	Rural	Community	2020
S7	Canada	North America	Urban	Community	2017
S8	Kenya	Africa	Rural	Facility	2019
S9	Germany	Europe	Urban	Facility	2021
S10	Brazil	Latin America	Mixed	Community	2016

Table 2 classifies the surveys into type—quantitative, qualitative, or mixed—and area of focus: knowledge, attitude, or practices (KAP). The majority of the surveys in developed nations were quantitative, while rural surveys utilized mixed methods. Practices-based surveys were common in both settings, reflecting interest in behavioral outcomes. Rural locations reflected a higher percentage of attitude-based studies, perhaps linked to cultural barriers in treatment. Developed settings reflected knowledge assessment interest, consistent with formal health educational programs. Survey types also differed geographically, the table suggests, implying trends in methodology. The distribution of this highlights the need for a balanced approach to handling behavioral, emotional, and informational aspects of TB care. This data is critical in organizing interventions that are appropriate for different populations. Table 2 allows comparison of rigor and specificity of method between the rural and urban areas. It also allows the calibration of future surveys by enabling identification of unemphasized dimensions.

Table 2. Survey type and population

Study ID	Survey Type	Sample Size	Target Population	Knowledge (%)	Attitudes (%)
S1	Quantitative	1300	General Public	78	59
S2	Quantitative	1200	TB Patients	65	52
S3	Mixed	1100	Immigrants	82	70
S4	Quantitative	1450	General Public	71	60
S5	Quantitative	980	Healthcare Workers	89	85
S6	Quantitative	1020	General Public	68	50
S7	Quantitative	950	Homeless	74	55
S8	Mixed	800	TB Patients	60	49
S9	Quantitative	1125	Refugees	77	66
S10	Quantitative	1050	Students	69	58

Table 3 lists the population groups targeted under TB treatment research, such as the general population, health workers, patients, students, immigrants, and children. Rural studies predominantly had patients and the general population, but developed country studies also had health workers and immigrants. Children and adolescents were not represented in either setting. Developed countries had population groups such as prison inmates or refugees based on their risk profiles of TB. Rural studies focused mainly on adults and families living in rural locations. This table describes how different groups are faced with certain challenges in TB care and adherence maintenance. It also suggests a need to extend the studies to capture vulnerable and hard-to-reach groups. Information educates policymakers about how to tailor outreach and education initiatives. Table 3 points out the importance of inclusive study designs in public health interventions. It provides a glimpse of the most frequently studied populations and those that most critically need more attention.

Table 3. Feature importance from REORA

Rank	Feature Name	Importance Score	Selected (Yes/No)	Type	Weight
1	Region	0.912	Yes	Categorical	High
2	Survey Type	0.874	Yes	Categorical	High
3	Setting	0.851	Yes	Categorical	High
4	Knowledge Score	0.832	Yes	Numeric	High
5	Attitudes Score	0.785	Yes	Numeric	Medium
6	Practices Score	0.744	Yes	Numeric	Medium
7	Year of Publication	0.715	No	Numeric	Low

continued on following page

Table 3. Continued

Rank	Feature Name	Importance Score	Selected (Yes/No)	Type	Weight
8	Sample Size	0.689	No	Numeric	Low
9	Country	0.672	No	Categorical	Low
10	Population Category	0.661	No	Categorical	Low

Table 4 displays the responses to knowledge-based questions regarding TB causes, symptoms, transmission, and treatment availability. Developed countries' respondents registered greater percentages of correct responses. Rural dwellers had gaps in their knowledge, particularly regarding the need for completing treatment. A significant proportion of rural respondents falsely believed that TB is hereditary or that it is incurable. Industrialized countries had good knowledge levels about aerial transmission and the need for early diagnosis. However, knowledge about drug resistance was limited even with urban populations. This table indicates the knowledge gaps that are the basis for late diagnosis and treatment failure. Addressing these gaps is essential both for prevention as well as for treatment adherence. Table 4 illustrates the rationale for health education in TB control programs. It also suggests areas of content for potential awareness campaigns on various regions. The information contained in this table provides foundation data for knowledge-based intervention development.

Table 4. Bi-stacked LSTM performance metrics

Model Variant	Accuracy (%)	Precision (%)	Recall (%)	F1-Score (%)	AUC (%)
Rural Model	86.5	84.2	83.7	83.9	89.0
Urban Model	88.9	87.5	85.8	86.6	91.2
Combined Model	90.3	89.0	88.7	88.8	92.5
Baseline LSTM	82.1	80.5	78.6	79.5	85.2
GRU	84.0	82.0	81.5	81.7	87.0
CNN-LSTM	87.0	85.2	83.9	84.5	90.0
RNN	79.2	76.8	75.3	76.0	82.1
RF Classifier	81.6	80.1	79.5	79.8	84.7
SVM	78.9	77.0	76.2	76.6	81.0
Proposed Model	91.5	90.2	89.6	89.9	93.1

Table 5 summarizes participants' attitudes towards TB patients and treatment, including stigma, fear, and trust in health systems. The rural communities experienced more stigma, with most associating TB with social shame. It was also common to fear being isolated and losing jobs as a result of a diagnosis of TB. In industrial settings, the interviewees were kinder but still not willing to closely engage with TB patients. Mistrust in health facilities in rural communities was founded on past negative experiences or cultural beliefs. The table indicates that negative attitudes can indeed affect treatment-seeking behavior. Public awareness and sensitivity to culture are needed to increase social acceptance. Table 5 is a good indicator of emotional and social barriers against TB care. It indicates the need for stigma-reduction interventions in rural settings. The results inform campaigns for changing public attitudes and reducing delay in treatment.

Table 5. Knowledge domain

Country	Mean Knowledge (%)	Rural (%)	Urban (%)	Target Group	Sample Size
India	74.1	70.2	82.3	General Public	1300
Nigeria	66.4	65.7	69.0	TB Patients	1200
USA	82.4	—	82.4	Immigrants	1100
Ethiopia	72.8	72.8	—	General Public	1450
UK	89.2	—	89.2	Healthcare Workers	980
Bangladesh	67.3	67.3	—	General Public	1020
Canada	76.0	—	76.0	Homeless	950
Kenya	60.5	60.5	—	TB Patients	800
Germany	78.7	—	78.7	Refugees	1125
Brazil	70.4	68.2	74.6	Students	1050

Table 6 illustrates self-reported behavior during TB treatment, such as early diagnosis, treatment initiation, adherence, and follow-up. Rural participants reported delayed treatment and irregular consumption of medication, sometimes due to lack of transport or adequate knowledge. Developed countries showed higher rates of treatment initiation but also faced issues of adherence in marginalized groups. Repeat visits were lower in rural areas, resulting in treatment failure. The use of traditional medicine was common in the rural settings, often interfering with regular TB treatment. Information on the use of DOTS (Directly Observed Therapy Short-Course) programs is also included in the table. Healthcare access and trust in modern medicine greatly influenced practices. Table 6 provides valuable information regarding the behavioral nature of treatment success. The results point towards the importance of infrastructural support at the local level and patient education. The results inform interventions towards improved treatment compliance and TB transmission elimination.

Table 6. Attitude scores by region

Region	Mean Score (%)	Positive (%)	Neutral (%)	Negative (%)	Studies
Africa	61.4	54.0	31.2	14.8	18
Asia	64.7	57.5	29.1	13.4	22
Europe	79.3	70.4	21.2	8.4	10
North America	77.6	68.8	23.0	8.2	8
Latin America	67.1	60.0	25.0	15.0	7
Mixed	69.0	63.5	24.5	12.0	7
Global Avg	69.8	62.4	25.7	11.9	—

Table 7 presents the most significant characteristics that were selected according to the REORA optimization approach, listed in order of their importance score. Significant variables included region type, treatment start time, knowledge score, stigma index, survey type, and level of healthcare access. The highest weighted attribute in both contexts was health care access, followed by knowledge and stigma. REORA was able to screen out extraneous or redundant attributes, which improved LSTM model precision. The optimization process allowed the model to focus on influential predictors while streamlining computation. The table supports the use of REORA as a viable instrument for health care analytics. It also identifies the variables with the greatest impacts on treatment outcomes. These findings can be used to guide resource allocation in public health programming. Table 7 illustrates how feature selection improves modeling and interpretation. It maintains the multidimensionality of TB treatment practices and drivers.

Table 7. Practices distribution by setting

Country	Rural (%)	Urban (%)	Practices Score	Sample Size	Year
India	42.0	63.3	53.5	1300	2020
Nigeria	39.1	54.7	46.9	1200	2019
USA	—	71.2	71.2	1100	2021
Ethiopia	48.6	—	48.6	1450	2018
UK	—	77.5	77.5	980	2022
Bangladesh	41.3	—	41.3	1020	2020
Canada	—	65.1	65.1	950	2017
Kenya	36.9	—	36.9	800	2019
Germany	—	69.4	69.4	1125	2021
Brazil	45.2	58.6	52.1	1050	2016

Table 8 displays the classification accuracy of the Bi-stacked LSTM model between rural and developed datasets. Accuracy, precision, recall, F1-score, AUC, and loss rate are the metrics employed. The model performed better in developed settings, perhaps due to having more standardized and organized data. Nevertheless, rural settings achieved higher recall with more sensitivity to positive outcomes of TB treatment. AUC measures were always greater than 0.85 for both data sets and represented correct classification. Loss rate was ever so marginally higher for rural data due to heterogeneity in types of surveys and missing values. The model performed excellently to identify high- and low-risk patterns of treatment adherence. This table presents evidence of the model's generalizability across regions. It confirms the merit of combining REORA and LSTM for health prediction tasks. Table 8 aids in explaining the model's capacity to guide policy and intervention design.

Table 8. Time-series performance on adherence prediction

Epoch	Accuracy (%)	Loss	Precision (%)	Recall (%)	F1-Score (%)
1	72.3	0.63	70.5	69.8	70.1
2	78.4	0.52	76.8	75.5	76.1
3	82.1	0.43	80.5	79.2	79.8
4	85.6	0.35	83.7	82.3	83.0
5	87.2	0.30	85.5	84.1	84.8
6	88.5	0.27	86.9	85.6	86.2
7	89.7	0.24	88.0	87.1	87.5
8	90.2	0.22	88.5	87.8	88.1
9	90.8	0.20	89.0	88.3	88.6
10	91.5	0.18	90.2	89.6	89.9

Table 9 summarizes the most significant treatment barriers noted in studies and across regions as cost, transport, stigma, and quality of care. Cost and transport emerged as the top barriers in rural environments, with developed countries noting system navigation and patient activation. Stigma was a universal barrier in both settings but more pronounced within rural communities. The table demonstrates that logistic issues are the top in underdeveloped countries, yet psychological and bureaucratic issues take center stage within the city environment. Such a contrast provides pattern-based solutions to match regional requirements. Supply of TB drugs was a small issue within developed countries but a main problem within far-off rural communities. The evidence supports decentralized care and mobile clinic introduction within rural communities. Table 9 is a roadmap for resolving and evading treatment barriers. It assigns treatment barriers by levels of health system development. They guide regionally applicable interventions to control TB.

Table 9. KAP summary by population type

Population	Knowledge (%)	Attitude (%)	Practice (%)	Sample Size	Countries
General Public	72.5	60.3	50.6	18470	10
TB Patients	66.7	55.2	44.1	8200	6
Healthcare Workers	88.6	84.3	76.5	4300	4
Students	70.4	58.9	49.7	3200	3
Immigrants	82.4	70.0	71.2	1100	2
Homeless	74.0	55.0	65.1	950	1
Refugees	77.0	66.0	69.4	1125	1
Mixed	71.8	60.5	53.7	3100	3
Community Workers	79.1	67.3	60.4	2450	2
Total/Average	74.7	62.7	54.3	50095	10

Table 10 provides an overview of policy and intervention recommendations based on evidence-based findings. Recommendations are grouped by region and category: infrastructure, education, policy, digital tools, reduction of stigma, and workforce training. For rural environments, priorities that have been recommended are mobile clinics, community health worker programs, and transport support. High-income countries are requested to make a priority of migrant health outreach, electronic adherence instruments, and stigma education. The table aligns each recommendation with the same respective challenge in earlier tables. It highlights the importance of scalable and culturally appropriate policies. Table 10 is an accessible guidebook for policymakers and NGOs involved in TB control. The recommendations are derived from actual data patterns and behavioral insight. They can be tuned in relation to funding, local capacity, and disease load.

Table 10. TB intervention timeliness

Country	Avg. Diagnosis Delay (days)	Avg. Treatment Start (days)	Adherence (%)	Completion (%)	Default Rate (%)
India	21	7	68	62	12
Nigeria	25	10	64	58	16
USA	8	3	82	79	4
Ethiopia	23	9	66	60	14

continued on following page

Table 10. Continued

Country	Avg. Diagnosis Delay (days)	Avg. Treatment Start (days)	Adherence (%)	Completion (%)	Default Rate (%)
UK	6	2	89	85	3
Bangladesh	24	11	63	57	15
Canada	7	4	78	74	5
Kenya	27	12	60	55	18
Germany	5	2	87	84	4
Brazil	19	6	70	65	10

CONCLUSION

The comparative examination of rural and developed country TB treatment practice reveals unique challenges and advantages of each. Rural settings are confronted with systemic issues of low care and treatment default, whereas developed countries have the challenge of maintaining low incidence as well as drug-resistant cases. Application of REORA to feature selection and Bi-stacked LSTM modeling allowed systematic analysis of treatment dynamics to reveal the most critical factors that drive TB management. The results inform the design of context-specific interventions that recognize the differentiated demands of each setting. Building community-driven care in rural settings and ensuring strong surveillance and innovation in high-income settings are key. The research emphasizes the need for region-specific, evidence-based strategies to drive global TB elimination.

REFERENCES

Bustamante-Gavino, M. I., Rattani, S., & Khan, K. (2011). Women's empowerment in Pakistan—Definitions and enabling and disenabling factors: A secondary data analysis. *Journal of Transcultural Nursing*, *22*(2), 174–181. DOI: 10.1177/1043659610395762 PMID: 21467269

Carvalho, A. C. C., Cardoso, C. A. A., Martire, T. M., Migliori, G. B., & Sant'Anna, C. C. (2018). Epidemiological aspects, clinical manifestations and prevention of pediatric tuberculosis from the perspective of the End TB strategy. *Jornal Brasileiro de Pneumologia : Publicaçao Oficial da Sociedade Brasileira de Pneumologia e Tisilogia*, *44*(2), 134–144. DOI: 10.1590/s1806-37562017000000461 PMID: 29791553

Chandra-Mouli, V., McCarraher, D. R., Phillips, S. J., Williamson, N. E., & Hainsworth, G. (2014). Contraception for adolescents in low and middle income countries: Needs, barriers, and access. *Reproductive Health*, *11*(1), 1. Advance online publication. DOI: 10.1186/1742-4755-11-1 PMID: 24383405

de Oliveira, M. C. B., Sant'Anna, C. C., Luiz, R. R., & Kritski, A. L. (2020). Unfavorable outcomes in tuberculosis: Multidimensional factors among adolescents in Rio de Janeiro, Brazil. *The American Journal of Tropical Medicine and Hygiene*, *103*(6), 2492–2500. DOI: 10.4269/ajtmh.20-0209 PMID: 32959763

de Oliveira, M. C. B., Sant'Anna, C. C., Luiz, R. R., Soares, E. C. C., & Kritski, A. L. (2019). Contribution of Xpert MTB/RIF to clinical diagnosis in adolescents with tuberculosis in Rio de Janeiro, Brazil. *The International Journal of Tuberculosis and Lung Disease : the Official Journal of the International Union against Tuberculosis and Lung Disease*, *23*(10), 1115–1121. DOI: 10.5588/ijtld.18.0778 PMID: 31627777

Diallo, T., Adjobimey, M., Ruslami, R., Trajman, A., Sow, O., Obeng Baah, J., Marks, G. B., Long, R., Elwood, K., Zielinski, D., Gninafon, M., Wulandari, D. A., Apriani, L., Valiquette, C., Fregonese, F., Hornby, K., Li, P.-Z., Hill, P. C., Schwartzman, K., & Menzies, D. (2018). Safety and side effects of rifampin versus isoniazid in children. *The New England Journal of Medicine*, *379*(5), 454–463. DOI: 10.1056/NEJMoa1714284 PMID: 30067928

Khan, A., Shaikh, B. T., & Baig, M. A. (2020). Knowledge, awareness, and health-seeking behaviour regarding tuberculosis in a rural district of Khyber Pakhtunkhwa, Pakistan. *BioMed Research International*, *2020*(1), 1852015. Advance online publication. DOI: 10.1155/2020/1850541 PMID: 32382530

King, T. L., Kavanagh, A., Scovelle, A. J., & Milner, A. (2020). Associations between gender equality and health: A systematic review. *Health Promotion International, 35*(1), 27–41. DOI: 10.1093/heapro/day093 PMID: 31916577

Lönnroth, K., Jaramillo, E., Williams, B., Dye, C., & Raviglione, M. (2009). Drivers of tuberculosis epidemics: The role of risk factors and social determinants. *Social Science & Medicine, 68*(12), 2240–2246. DOI: 10.1016/j.socscimed.2009.03.041 PMID: 19394122

Mumtaz, Z., & Salway, S. (2005). 'I never go anywhere': Extricating the links between women's mobility and uptake of reproductive health services in Pakistan. *Social Science & Medicine, 60*(8), 1751–1765. DOI: 10.1016/j.socscimed.2004.08.019 PMID: 15686807

Mumtaz, Z., & Salway, S. M. (2007). Gender, pregnancy and the uptake of antenatal care services in Pakistan. *Sociology of Health & Illness, 29*(1), 1–26. DOI: 10.1111/j.1467-9566.2007.00519.x PMID: 17286703

Panezai, S., Ahmad, M. M., & Saqib, S. E. (2017). Factors affecting access to primary health care services in Pakistan: A gender-based analysis. *Development in Practice, 27*(6), 813–827. DOI: 10.1080/09614524.2017.1344188

Riaz, A., Zaidi, S., & Khowaja, A. R. (2015). Perceived barriers to utilizing maternal and neonatal health services in contracted-out versus government-managed health facilities in the rural districts of Pakistan. *International Journal of Health Policy and Management, 4*(5), 279–284. DOI: 10.15171/ijhpm.2015.50 PMID: 25905478

Rimande-Joel, R., & Ekenedo, G. O. (2019). Knowledge, belief and practice of cervical cancer screening and prevention among women of Taraba, North-East Nigeria. *Asian Pacific Journal of Cancer Prevention : APJCP, 20*(11), 3291–3298. DOI: 10.31557/APJCP.2019.20.11.3291 PMID: 31759351

Rizvi, N., Khan, K. S., & Shaikh, B. T. (2014). Gender: Shaping personality, lives and health of women in Pakistan. *BMC Women's Health, 14*(1), 53. Advance online publication. DOI: 10.1186/1472-6874-14-53 PMID: 24690271

Rizvi, N., & Nishtar, S. (2008). Pakistan's health policy: Appropriateness and relevance to women's health needs. *Health Policy (Amsterdam), 88*(2-3), 269–281. DOI: 10.1016/j.healthpol.2008.03.011 PMID: 18479774

Sant'Anna, C. C., & de Oliveira, M. C. B. (2021). The long-running issues of tuberculosis. *The Lancet. Global Health, 9*(10), e1339–e1340. DOI: 10.1016/S2214-109X(21)00401-0 PMID: 34534470

Sant'Anna, C. C., Orfaliais, C. T., March, M. F., & Conde, M. B. (2006). Evaluation of a proposed diagnostic scoring system for pulmonary tuberculosis in Brazilian children. *The International Journal of Tuberculosis and Lung Disease : the Official Journal of the International Union against Tuberculosis and Lung Disease, 10*(4), 463–465. PMID: 16602415

Shah, I., & Åhman, E. (2004). Age patterns of unsafe abortion in developing country regions. *Reproductive Health Matters, 12*(24, Suppl.), 9–17. DOI: 10.1016/S0968-8080(04)24002-2 PMID: 15938153

Shaikh, B. T., & Hatcher, J. (2004). Health seeking behaviour and health service utilization in Pakistan: Challenging the policy makers. *Journal of Public Health (Oxford, England), 27*(1), 49–54. DOI: 10.1093/pubmed/fdh207 PMID: 15590705

Tahan, T. T., Gabardo, B. M., & Rossoni, A. M. (2020). Tuberculosis in childhood and adolescence: A view from different perspectives. *Jornal de Pediatria, 96*(Suppl. 1), 99–110. DOI: 10.1016/j.jped.2019.11.002 PMID: 31862302

Villarino, M. E., Scott, N. A., Weis, S. E., Weiner, M., Conde, M. B., Jones, B., Nachman, S., Oliveira, R., Moro, R. N., Shang, N., Goldberg, S. V., & Sterling, T. R. (2015). Treatment for preventing tuberculosis in children and adolescents: A randomized clinical trial of a 3-month, 12-dose regimen of a combination of rifapentine and isoniazid. *JAMA Pediatrics, 169*(3), 247–255. DOI: 10.1001/jamapediatrics.2014.3158 PMID: 25580725

Chapter 12
New Drugs, Clinical Trials, and Innovations in Tuberculosis Treatment

Monali Priyadarsini Mishra
https://orcid.org/0000-0002-8548-1784
Centurion University of Technology and Management, Bhubaneswar, India

ABSTRACT

The emergence of drug-resistant tuberculosis and limitations of existing treatment regimens have underscored the urgent need for new therapeutic strategies. This chapter explores recent advancements in TB treatment, focusing on novel and repurposed drugs such as bedaquiline, delamanid, and pretomanid, along with the development of shorter, all-oral regimens. It reviews key clinical trials that have shaped current treatment guidelines and examines innovative drug delivery systems, including nanotechnology and inhaled therapies. The role of host-directed therapies, and supportive diagnostic innovations are also discussed. Challenges such as drug resistance and equitable access to new treatments are critically analysed. By highlighting ongoing research and global initiatives, the chapter emphasizes the potential of a multifaceted approach to transform TB care and contribute to global TB elimination efforts.

INTRODUCTION

The World Health Organisation (WHO) reports that the number of people afflicted with tuberculosis (TB) is at an all-time high, making it the biggest infectious illness cause of mortality worldwide, (Lange et al., 2025). The WHO Global Tuberculosis Report 2024 estimates that 10.8 million people (95% UI: 10.1-11.7 million)

DOI: 10.4018/979-8-3373-3446-2.ch012

contracted tuberculosis in 2023, continuing the upward trend from 10.1 million of 2021 cases, (World Health Organization, 2024). With a combined 56% of all cases, 5 nations have the largest global burden of TB. Among them are India (26%), Indonesia (10%) China (6.8%), the Philippines (6.8%), and Pakistan (6.3%), (World Health Organization, 2024). An estimated 12% of TB cases in 2023- approximately 1.3 million people- occurred in children and young adolescents (ages 0-14 years), a group that is especially susceptible to severe illness and for whom microbiological confirmation is still challenging. In 2023, a projected 1.25 million people died from TB, (World Health Organization, 2024). Even though TB has long been a human scourge, controlling and treating it now presents a number of complex and changing issues. Years of advancements in TB detection and treatment were reversed when the COVID-19 pandemic drastically impacted TB services around the world, (Togun et al., 2020). A decrease in TB case notifications and delays in diagnosis and treatment resulted from many health systems shifting their staff and resources to treating COVID-19. These interruptions exacerbated community transmission and worsened outcomes by generating a backlog of untreated and undetected TB cases, (Togun et al., 2020). Another issue that has surfaced in high-income, low –incidence countries is the increase of non-tuberculous mycobacterial (NTM) infections. NTM cases are now outnumbering TB in absolute terms in areas where TB has been all but eradicated, such as Denmark, Scotland, the United States and Canada. Despite not being spread from person to person like TB, these illnesses present serious diagnostics and treatment difficulties and frequently call for drawn-out and intricate treatment plans, (Dahl, Fløe, & Wejse, 2023). Treatment outcomes are inadequate in many regions due to delayed diagnosis, drug resistance, treatment interruption, and poor patient adherence, even though there are effective first-line anti-TB medications such as isoniazid, rifampicin, ethambutol, and pyrazinamide. Completing the typical six-month program can be challenging, especially in settings with limited resources where patient support may be low and healthcare access is irregular. A growing concern to world health, multidrug-resistant TB (MDR- TB) is a result of these challenges, (Institute of Medicine, Indian National Science Academy, & Indian Council of Medical Research, 2012)

Particularly the clinical concern is MDR-TB, which is characterised as TB resistant to at least isoniazid and rifampicin. Compared to drug susceptible TB, MDR-TB treatment is more costly, time-consuming, and toxic, and the results are typically worse. In 2023, there were about 410,000 new cases of MDR-TB according to WHO forecast, (World Health Organization, 2024). Remarkably, only over half of MDR-TB patients finish their medication. The situation is made more difficult by the introduction of extensively drug-resistant TB (XDR-TB), which is resistant to at least one second line injectable medication in addition to fluoroquinolones and MDR criteria, (Oliveira et al., 2021). Strong public health systems, social support networks, and Medical solutions are all necessary to address these treatment issues. Social determinants like poverty, malnutrition, overcrowding, and stigma are closely linked to TB. Significant socioeconomic obstacles, including as prejudice, transportation issues, and income loss, prevent many people with TB from finishing treatment. For underprivileged groups, including immigrants, criminals, HIV-positive individuals, and those suffering from drug abuse, (Hudson et al., 2025). The WHO's End TB strategy, which aims to cut TB fatalities by 95% and incidence by 90% by 2035 compared to 2015 levels, serves as the cornerstone of international efforts to battle TB. Strengthening health systems, increasing access to rapid diagnostics like GeneXpert MTB/RIF, boosting the availability and affordability of new and repurposed medications like bedaquiline and delamanid, and funding TB vaccine research and development are all necessary to meet these challenging goals, (Gilmour & Alene, 2024). In certain areas, there has been progress. For drug-susceptible and MDR-TB, shorter and more manageable treatment plans are already available and being tested in a number of nations. Digital adherence tools like video DOT and 99DOTS, as well as community-based care models, have demonstrated potential in raising treatment completion rates. Access and continuity of care hurdles may also be lessened by integrating TB treatment into larger primary healthcare systems and universal health coverage programs, (Zary et al., 2024).

However, particularly in high-burden, low-income nations, these developments are not uniformly applied and are frequently constrained by resource shortages. The Global Fund to fight AIDS, Tuberculosis, and Malaria has documented ongoing deficiencies in both domestic and foreign investments for TB, which continues to be a significant barrier. Countries find it difficult to expand vital services like active case detection, contact tracing, preventive therapy and health professional training in the absence of sufficient finance. The emergence and dissemination of drug resistance to more recent medications is another serious concern. MDR-TB treatment results have improved with the use of medications such as bedaquiline and linezolid; nevertheless, resistance to these medications is already being documented. Resistance is accelerated by the improper or uncontrolled administration of anti-TB medications, (Tiberi et al., 2018; Pontali et al., 2018).

The necessity for novel medications and therapeutic advancements is highlighted by the growing threat of drug-resistant TB and the shortcomings of existing treatment plans. Shorter, safer, and more efficient regimens that are also appropriate for usage in children, HIV-positive individuals, and other vulnerable groups are desperately needed. To improve patient outcomes and stop transmission, drug research innovations such host-directed therapy, new antibacterial agents, and fixed-dose combinations are crucial. To improve treatment accuracy, accessibility, and efficacy, new developments in digital adherence technology, diagnostic tools, and personalized medicine must be included into care models concurrently. This book chapter will offer a comprehensive and up-to-date analysis of the evolving landscape of tuberculosis treatment, making it an essential resource for researchers, clinicians and public health professionals. By covering the discovery and developments of new repurposed anti-TB drugs, the chapter will shed light on cutting-edge therapeutic options and their mechanisms of action. Through a detailed discussion of recent landmark clinical trials, it will share insights in to the real-world effectiveness, safety, and applicability of innovative treatment regimens, including for MDR and XDR TB. The inclusion of current challenges and future directions will not only highlight critical gaps in research and policy but also inspire future innovations. By integrating scientific advances with clinical applications, this chapter will uniquely bridge the gap between laboratory research, bedside care, and public health implementation, thereby contributing meaningfully to the global fight against TB.

LIMITATIONS OF CURRENT TB THERAPIES

Drug Resistance: MDR and XDR TB

The development and dissemination of drug-resistant *Mycobacterium tuberculosis* strains is one of the most difficult obstacles in the worldwide battle against TB. XDR-TB and MDR-TB increasingly threaten TB control initiatives and public health in general. TB that is resistant to at least isoniazid and rifampicin, the two most effective first-line anti-TB medications, is known as MDR-TB. In addition to being resistant to any fluoroquinolone and at least one of the second-line medications with second-line injectable drugs (SLID), XDR-TB, a more severe variant, is also resistant to isoniazid and rifampicin, (Oostvogels et al., 2022).

The WHO Global Tuberculosis Report 2024 estimates that 410,000 new cases of MDR-TB were reported in 2023. The global treatment success rate for MDR-TB is still around 50% despite advancements in diagnosis and treatment, which reflects the complexity and frequently inefficiency of existing regimens, (Diriba et al., 2023). MDR-TB treatment usually takes 18-24 months, needs continuous monitoring, and involves several toxic medications, which puts a significant strain on individuals and health systems, (Varshney et al., 2021). Common side effects that result in poor adherence and high default rates include hearing loss, renal impairment and gastrointestinal irritations, (Diriba et al., 2023)

The landscape of treatment is further complicated by the emergence of XDR-TB. Even fewer therapy options, longer treatment periods, and much worse cure rates-typically less than 30%- are faced by patients with XDR-TB. More than 120 nations have recorded cases of XDR-TB spreading, which, if unchecked, could lead to a crisis, (World Health Organization, 2024). Inappropriate prescribing methods, a lack of drug susceptibility testing, inadequate infection control procedures, and irregular drug supply chains are some of the contributing reasons. Uncontrolled use of antibiotics in the private healthcare sector speeds up the emergence of resistance and jeopardises government TB control initiatives in many high-burden nations.

More alarming situation is the emergence and spread of resistance to more recent medications, like linezolid and bedaquiline, which are now essential treatments for MDR-TB and XDR-TB. Particularly, resistance to bedaquiline has been reported in several nations, frequently as a result of the adoption of less-than-ideal regimens or insufficient programmatic assistance. The hard-won progress in treating drug resistant in TB over the last 10 years is in danger of being undermined by this new trend, (Kaniga et al., 2022).

MDR-Tb and XDR-TB represent significant setbacks in global TB control, demanding urgent and coordinated international action. Without innovative strategies and robust implementation, drug-resistant TB will continue to spread, posing a serious threat to global health security.

Treatment Duration and Adherence Issues

The length of therapy and the patient's capacity to follow it regularly are important factors in the efficiency of TB treatment, in addition to the availability of effective medications. The length of the treatment plans, which frequently results in poor adherence, treatment default, and the development of drug resistance, is one of the ongoing problems in TB control. Standard first-line treatment for drug-susceptible TB takes at least six months and consists of a two-month intensive phase with four medications such as isoniazid, rifampicin, pyrazinamide, and ethambutol, followed by a continuation phase with isoniazid and rifampicin for four months, (Rabahi et al., 2017). Even though this regimen is quite effective when followed, it can be challenging to keep patients adhering to it for such a long time, particularly in settings with limited resources.

For patients, the protracted course of treatment presents a lot of difficulties. Among these are the inconveniences of taking pills every day, the adverse effects like hepatotoxicity and gastrointestinal issues, and the disruption of daily routine brought on by frequent clinic appointments. Transportation expenses and lost wages from missing work can be major obstacles to adherence for people with limited access to healthcare. In order to prevent discrimination, patients frequently conceal their diagnosis or stop treatment early due to the social stigma attached to TB, (Johnston, Cooper, & Menzies, 2022).

Poor adherence not only affects individual outcomes but also has broader public health implications. Incomplete treatment contributes to treatment failure, disease relapse, ongoing transmission of *M. tuberculosis*, and the development of drug-resistant strains. These consequences make adherence a central concern in global TB control strategies.

NEW AND REPURPOSED ANTI-TB DRUGS

Bedaquiline

Bedaquiline is the revolutionary anti-TB medication that has significantly changed the landscape of treatment for drug-resistant TB. It is the first new drug with a unique mechanism of action. It was approved by the U.S. Food and Drug Administration (FDA) in 2012 under accelerated approval for treatment in adult with MDR-TB. Bedaquiline functions by blocking mycobacterial ATP synthase, an enzyme necessary for *M. tuberculosis* to produce energy, while other conventional drugs targets cell wall formation and nucleic acid synthesis. Bedaquiline works against both replicating and non-replicating (dormant) bacilli due to its unique mechanism of action, (Fox & Menzies, 2013). When used in combination with other effective drugs, bedaquiline has been shown to increase treatment success rates and reduce mortality. One of the key advantages of this drug is its inclusion in all-oral regimens recommended by WHO, such as the BPal and BPaLM regimens, (Yadav, 2024).

Concerns regarding the emergence of bedaquiline resistance are developing, especially in high-burden settings where monitoring and diagnostic methods may not be sufficient. Mutations in regulatory genes including Rv0678 and the atpE gene, which codes for the ATP synthase target, have been connected to resistance. It ensures that this drug can be a part of an effective combination regimen. Bedaquiline has transformed the management of drug-resistant TB by providing a strong, oral, and shorter duration substitute for conventional treatments. However, its continued effectiveness depends on careful stewardship, routine resistance monitoring, and global access strategies that ensure equitable use in all high-burden settings, (Zimenkov et al., 2025).

Delamanid

In 2014, the European Medicines Agency (EMA) authorised delamanid in addition to bedaquiline for the treatment of adult pulmonary MDR-TB. It is a member of the nitroimidazole class and works by preventing the production of mycolic acids, which are vital parts of the cell wall of *M. tuberculosis*. Delamanid has bactericidal effects by weakening the integrity of the cell wall, especially in the rapidly growing bacilli, (Igarashi, 2017).

In clinical trials, delamanid has shown encouraging outcomes when used with optimised background therapy (OBT) for MDR-TB. When delamanid was used in conjunction with other second-line medicines, studies such as the Phase IIb trial 204 demonstrated improved sputum culture conversion rates at two months, (Szumowski & Lynch, 2015). In longer-term follow-up trials, this effect resulted in lower mortality and higher treatment success rates. Delamanid is currently advised by the WHO as a component of extended MDR-TB therapy regimens for adults and children of 6years or more of age, especially in cases when there are few or no other suitable alternatives is available, (Zhu et al., 2023).

Despite of the potential, delamanid has some limitations also. Similar to bedaquiline, delamanid may result in QT interval prolongation, a cardiac adverse effect that necessitates ECG monitoring, particularly when taken concurrently with other drugs that lengthen the QT. However, if patients are closely monitored, research has indicated that using bedaquiline and delamanid together does not always result in cardiac risks, (Zhu et al., 2023).

In addition to its limited bioavailability, delamanid resistance can arise from mutations in genes associated with the F420-dependent bioactivation pathway, including ddn, fgd1, fbiA, fbiB, and fbiC. These genetic alterations may impair the drug's activation, reducing its efficacy. Consequently, it is crucial for healthcare providers to monitor patients for signs of emerging resistance during delamanid therapy and consider alternative treatment options when necessary to ensure optimal clinical outcomes, (Liu et al., 2022).

The treatment of drug-resistant TB has advanced significantly with delamanid, raising the prospect of more efficient and bearable regimens.

Pretomanid

A relatively new and extremely promising anti-TB medication, pretomanid, was approved by the U.S. FDA in 2019 for use in conjunction with bedaquiline and linezolid (BPaL regimen) to treat adults with treatment-intolerant or non-responsive MDR-TB or pulmonary XDR-TB. It belongs to the antimicrobial class nitroimidazooxazine and has shown strong efficacy against both replicating and non-replicating *M. tuberculosis* bacilli.

Pretomanid exerts its action by multiple mechanisms. Under anaerobic conditions, it releases nitric oxide, which disrupts respiratory processes in non-replicating TB bacilli, while under aerobic conditions, it inhibits mycolic acid synthesis essential for cell wall construction. These dual mechanisms allow pretomanid to act against both actively dividing and dormant bacilli- a major advantage in treating chronic and resistant forms of TB, (Stancil, Mirzayev, & Abdel-Rahman, 2021).

This drug's inclusion in the BPaL regimen (bedaquiline, pretomanid and linezolid), a completely oral, six-month therapy option for XDR-TB and complicated MDR-TB, is among its most noteworthy contributions. Compared to the conventional 18–24-month regimen that mostly depended on toxic and cumbersome injectable medicines, this regimen represented a considerable change. In contrast to the prior success rates for XDR-TB, which were frequently less than 30%, the BPaL regimen produced a favourable outcome in about 90% of patients, according to the historic Nix-TB trial, (Budak et al., 2024).

The utilisation of pharmaceutical resources, treatment length, pill count, and toxicity have all decreased as a result of the introduction of pretomanid into treatment plans. Additionally, it has decreased the risk of injection-related problems like hearing loss and abscess formation and increased patient adherence by doing away with injectable drugs. Concerns regarding resistance also exist. Resistance to pretomanid can emerge through mutations affecting the bacterial genes responsible for drug activation, such as fgd1 and ddn. Thus, pretomanid must always be used in combination with other effective anti-TB drugs to prevent monotherapy-induced resistance, (Rifat et al., 2021).

Linezolid and Clofazimine

Existing antibiotics are repurposed and included in TB treatment regimens due to the worldwide burden of XDR-TB and MDR-TB. Among these, linezolid and clofazimine have emerged as vital components in managing drug-resistant TB due to their potent antimycobacterial activity and compatibility with newer therapeutic strategies. Both drugs, although originally developed for other infections, have proven invaluable in recent years and are endorsed by WHO as part of standardized regimen for MDR and XDR-TB.

Linezolid, an oxazolidinone antibiotic, was originally approved for the treatment of gram-positive infections such as MRSA and VRE. Its mechanism of action is to bind with the 50S ribosomal subunit and inhibit protein synthesis, giving it significant activity against the Tubercle bacilli. Linezolid is bacteriostatic against most TB bacilli but has demonstrated bactericidal activity when used in combination with other drugs, (Garcia-Prats et al., 2019).

This drug's role in TB treatment was solidified with its inclusion in the BPaL regimen, designed for patients with highly resistant forms of TB. Linezolid's excellent oral bioavailability, deep tissue penetration, and effectiveness in both intracellular and extracellular environments make it highly suitable for TB, which often involves granulomatous and poorly vascularized lesions, (Conradie et al., 2022). However, this drug is associated with several dose-dependent adverse effects with its prolonged use. It is associated with Peripheral neuropathy, optic neuritis and myelosuppression. Given its pivotal role linezolid is currently categorized by the WHO as a Group A drug, (Garcia-Prats et al., 2019).

Clofazimine is a riminophenazine dye that has been in medical use since the 1960s, primarily for the treatment of leprosy. Due to its bactericidal and anti-inflammatory activities its repurposing is driven for TB. Unlike most anti-TB drugs, it accumulates in macrophages and fatty tissues, creating a drug reservoir that can sustain activity over extended periods. This drug is known to disrupt bacterial membrane function and generate reactive oxygen species, leading to cell death. Additionally, its anti-inflammatory effects help modulating immune response and reduce tissue damage during infection. It was included in Who recommendations as a Group B drug for MDR-TB and more recently shifted to Group A, (Kengo et al., 2024).

Oral administration, Low toxicity profile, and anti-inflammatory actions are the key advantages of this drug in TB therapy. However, adverse effects like skin discoloration, gastrointestinal disturbances and photosensitivity do occur. Unlike linezolid, clofazimine's toxicity profile is generally more manageable, making it suitable for inclusion in longer regimens for patients.

The integration of linezolid and clofazimine into combination regimens for MDR and XDR –TB has led to transformative changes in treatment outcomes. Both the drugs are recommended by WHO in BPaL and BPaLM regimens. These regimens achieved reduced treatment duration from 18-24 months to 6-9 months, elimination of injectable agents, improving patient compliance and comfort, and higher cure rates and reduced mortality in complicated TB cases. Linezolid contributes strong bacteriostatic and sterilizing activity, while clofazimine enhances bactericidal effects along with anti-inflammatory activity which reduces tissue damage. When used together, they help cover a broad range of bacterial states-from actively growing bacilli to those in persistent or dormant phases, (Shiromwar, Khan, & Chidrawar, 2023).

SHORTER AND ALL-ORAL REGIMENS IN TUBERCULOSIS TREATMENT

Recent years have seen a dramatic change in the management of drug-resistant tuberculosis, with shorter, all-oral, patient-friendly treatments replacing lengthy, toxic, injection-based regimens. Up to 24 months of therapy were previously needed to treat MDR-TB and XDR-TB, frequently involving uncomfortable intramuscular injections and medications with serious adverse effects. However, shorter, entirely oral regimens that are safer and more effective have been made possible by advancements in medication research, clinical trial data, and updated international regulations.

In response to growing evidence and the need to improve patient outcomes, the WHO has recommended new all-oral regimens for MDR-TB and XDR-TB. These include (a) The BPaL regimen- comprising bedaquiline, pretomanid, and linezolid for six months- is specifically recommended for adults with pulmonary MDR-TB that is resistant or intolerant to fluoroquinolones, including XDR-TB (Evans et al., 2024), (b) The BPaLM regimen- BPaL with moxifloxacin-for a broader group of MDR-TB patients, including those with fluoroquinolone-susceptible strains (Silva et al., 2025), and (c) Modified longer regimens- incorporating bedaquiline, linezolid, clofazimine, and fluoroquinolones for 9-12 months, offering alternatives where shorter regimens are not suitable, (Mirzayev et al., 2021).

Compared to conventional treatments, the shorter, all-oral TB regimens have several benefits. The shortened treatment period- from the traditional 18-24 months to just 6-9 months- significantly reduces the load on patients and is one of the biggest advantages. Additionally, these regimens also eliminate the need for injectable drugs such as kanamycin and amikacin, thereby avoiding complications like ototoxicity, painful administration and injection-site abscesses. In contrast to the 50% success rates observed with previous treatments, clinical studies such as Nix TB and Ze-Nix have shown greater efficacy, with cure rates approaching 85-90% in patients with drug-resistant TB. By lowering the dosage and eliminating injections, the all-oral method also enhances patient adherence and quality of life while lowering psychological and physical suffering. Hospitalization can also be reduced when these regimens can be managed in outpatient settings, which relieves the burden on healthcare systems and reduces the risk of hospital-acquired infections. However, their successful implementation requires a concerted global effort to ensure drug access, build health system capacity, and invest in research and surveillance. If these challenges can be addressed, shorter regimens may become the new standard of care, accelerating progress toward ending the global TB epidemic, (Dookie et al., 2022).

ONGOING AND RECENT CLINICAL TRIALS IN TUBERCULOSIS TREATMENT

Phase I – III Trials in Tuberculosis Drug Development

The pathway for developing new TB treatments involves a structured series of clinical trial phases- Phase I, II, III. Each phase plays a vital role in ensuring that candidate drugs are safe, effective, and appropriate for use in diverse populations. Given the complexity and chronicity of TB infection, especially in drug-resistant

TB, clinical trials design in TB often face unique scientific and logistical challenges. Below in Table 1 is an overview of each clinical trial phase emphasizing recent advancements and examples specific to TB research.

Table 1. Overview of phase I-III trials in tuberculosis drug development

Trials	Objectives	Participants	Sub-Phases	Examples in TB	Importance
Phase I Trials: First-in-Human Safety Studies	To assess safety, tolerability, and pharmacokinetics of new anti-TB compounds in humans	Small group (20-100) of healthy volunteers or, TB patients		1. Pretomanid, a nitroimidazole drug, underwent Phase I trials to establish oral dosing and basic safety before it advanced to the Nix-TB study [37]. 2. OPC-167832, a novel DprE1 inhibitor, completed Phase I trials demonstrating promising safety and pharmacokinetics for further study [38].	Phase I ensures that a compound does not pose unacceptable risks, forming the foundations for later trials that assess efficacy.
Phase II Trials: Efficacy and Dose Optimization	To evaluate the efficacy of the drug, determine optimal dosing, and further examine safety.	Several hundred patients with active TB	1. Phase IIa: Focuses on EBA over 14 days 2. Phase IIb: Evaluates different doses or drug combinations over 8 weeks	1. The BPaZ and BPaMZ regimens underwent Phase II trials showing super EBA compared to standard treatment [39]. 2. Delamanid went through Phase II trials demonstrating its utility in MDR-TB, particularly in combination regimens, (Rodriguez et al., 2019).	This phase is critical for narrowing down the best drug combinations and treatment durations while refining risk benefit profiles.
Phase III Trials: Large Scale efficacy and Safety studies	To confirm the effectiveness, monitor adverse reactions, and compare the new regimen with the current standard of care in real-world, diverse populations	Several hundreds to several thousand TB patients from multiple geographic and demographic backgrounds.		1. Nix-TB Trial (Phase III): tested the BPaL regimen in XDR- TB and demonstrated > 90% cure rates, (Li et al., 2019). 2. ZeNix Trial: Evaluated linezolid dose reduction in the BPaL regimen to improve safety while maintain efficacy, (Phillips et al., 2019). 3. STREAM Stage 2: Assessed bedaquiline-based, all-oral regimens in place of injectables for MDR-TB, (Moodley, Godec, & STREAM Trial Team, 2016). 4. TB-PRACTECAL Trial: A multi-country Phase III trial that confirmed BPaLM as a superior regimen over conventional MDR-TB therapy, (Gotham et al., 2025)	Phase III trials are the final step before regulatory approval and Who guideline recommendations. They generate the high-quality evidence needed for national TB programs to adopt new regimens at scale.

The global TB community has witnessed remarkable progress through well-conducted trials, particularly in the shift towards shorter, all-oral, and less toxic regimens. However, sustained investment in trial infrastructure, participant diversity, and post-approval surveillance is critical to ensure that innovations reach and benefit all patients- especially in high burden, resource limited settings.

Key Clinical Trials and their Impact

The rise of MDR/XDR-TB and the challenges posed by prolonged, conventional TB treatment regimens have driven global initiatives to develop shorter, more effective, and safer therapeutic alternatives. In this context, clinical trials-both completed and ongoing – play a pivotal role in shaping the future of TB management. These trials focus on optimizing drug combinations, shortening treatment duration, evaluating novel therapeutic agents, and expanding treatment accessibility for high-risk groups, including children, individuals living with HIV, and patients with extra-pulmonary TB, (Aguilar Diaz et al., 2023).

Nix-TB Trial

The Nix-TB trial was a landmark Phase III study conducted in south Africa, evaluating a novel three-drug combination: bedaquiline, pretomanid, and linezolid (BPaL). This all-oral, 6-month regimen targeted patients with XDR-TB or treatment-intolerant MDR-TB. The results published in 2020, showed a 90% favourable outcome, far exceeding historical success rates in this patient population. Importantly, the regimen eliminated the need for injectable agents, improving tolerability and patient adherence, (Gomez et al., 2021).

ZeNix Trial

The ZeNix trial followed Nix-TB, specifically assessing linezolid dose and duration within the BPaL regimen. The goal was to reduce linezolid-associated toxicity like peripheral neuropathy, myelosuppression, without compromising efficacy. Results confirmed that lower doses (600 mg/day) and shorter duration (2 months instead of 6) maintained high cure rates while significantly reducing adverse effects. These findings are shaping WHO guidance and Programmatic implementation worldwide, (Conradie, 2021).

TB PRACTECAL Trial

TB PRACTECAL, led by Medecins Sans Frontieres (MSF), evaluated multiple short, all-oral regimens for MDR-TB, including combinations like bedaquiline, pretomanid, linezolid, and moxifloxacin (BPaLM). The trial demonstrated that the 6-month BPaLM regimen was superior to standard 18–24-month treatment in terms of efficacy, safety, and adherence. These results prompted WHO in 2022 to recommend BPaLM as a preferred regimen for most patients with MDR-TB, including those with fluoroquinolone-sensitive disease, (Nyang'wa et al., 2021).

STREAM Trial (Stage 1 and 2)

STREAM is one of the largest multi-country clinical trials focusing on MDR-TB. Stage 1 compared a shorter 9-11 month injectable –based regimen with the conventional 20–24-month regimen. Although the shorter regimen was non-inferior, toxicities and the continued reliance on injectables limited its appeal. Stage 2 examined all-oral regimens that include bedaquiline and avoided injectables. Early results indicate good tolerability and efficacy, contributing to the growing shift toward injectable-free TB treatment, (Hughes et al., 2022).

Ongoing and Emerging Clinical Trials

SimpliciTB Trial

The SimpliciTB trial is testing a 4-month BPaMZ regimen (bedaquiline, pretomanid, moxifloxacin, pyrazinamide) in both drug-sensitive and drug-resistant TB. If successful, this regimen could potentially unify TB treatment under a single, shorter protocol for all patients, simplifying programmatic implementation and improving outcomes across the board, (Timm et al., 2023).

BEAT-TB and BEAT-Tuberculosis Trials (India)

The BEAT-TB trial, coordinated by the Indian Council of Medical Research (ICMR), is testing shorter, all-oral regimens including bedaquiline and delamanid, in combination with other agents. These trials are pain India and similar countries-rticularly relevant for high-burden settings and are expected to inform national TB policy in India and similar countries, (Muniyandi et al., 2023).

endTB and endTB-Q Trials

These large, multi-country Phase III trials led by Partners in Health and MSF are evaluating five novel, all-oral regimens for MDR and pre-XDR TB using combinations of bedaquiline, delamanid, linezolid, moxifloxacin, and clofazimine. The endTB-Q trial specifically focuses on patients with highly resistant TB. Interim results are promising, and final data are anticipated in the coming years, (Masini et al., 2023)

TRUNCATE-TB Trial

This innovative trial is investigating whether a "response-guided" short-course therapy could be used for drug-sensitive TB. Patients receive a 2-month intensive regimen followed by close monitoring, with extended treatment only if needed. This individualized treatment approach could reduce unnecessary drug exposure and improve patient experience, (Paton et al., 2023).

The recent ongoing clinical trials in tuberculosis mark a pivotal shift in global TB control, offering broader implications beyond the development of new treatments. These studies are enhancing treatment precision by enabling clinicians to tailor regimens according to individual resistance profiles and patient characteristics. They are also reducing treatment-related morbidity through the elimination of toxic injectable drugs, thereby improving patient safety and comfort. Importantly, these trials are promoting greater treatment access and equity, particularly in low- and middle-income countries, where the burden of TB is highest. Additionally, the outcomes of these trials are influencing regulatory approvals and driving policy changes, ensuring that scientific advancements are swiftly translated in to public health interventions. The inclusion of previously underrepresented groups- such as children, HIV patients, and those with extra pulmonary TB- is also helping to close critical evidence gaps and support more inclusive, effective TB care.

INNOVATIVE DRUG DELIVERY SYSTEMS IN TB TREATMENT

To address the limitations associated with TB, innovative drug delivery systems are being developed and investigated to enhance the therapeutic efficacy, reduce treatment duration, and improve patient compliance. Among the most promising technologies are nanoparticle –based drug delivery systems, inhaled drug formulations, and long-acting injectable therapies. These strategies offer targeted drug delivery, controlled release, and potentially simplified dosing regimens- all critical steps toward more effective TB management, especially in the era of drug –resistant TB, (Omoteso et al., 2025).

Nanoparticle-Based Drug Delivery Systems

Nanoparticles (NPs) are tiny carriers, usually ranging from 1 to 1000 nanometers in size, designed to deliver drugs directly to target tissues or cells. In TB, nanoparticle–based formulations are being investigated for their ability to enhance drug delivery to macrophages, the primary host cells for *M. tuberculosis*, (Suman, Chandrasekaran, & Priya Doss, 2023).

NPs offer several advantages in the treatment of TB, particularly by enhancing the efficacy and precision of drug delivery. One key benefit is targeted drug delivery, as NPs can be engineered to selectively release drugs within infected macrophages or granulomas, thereby increasing local drug concentrations while minimizing systemic toxicity. Additionally, nanoparticles improve the solubility and bioavailability of poorly water-soluble TB drugs such as Rifampicin and isoniazid through lipid-or polymer – based formulations. They also enable sustained drug release, allowing for a controlled, gradual release of medication over time, which reduces the frequency of dosing and enhances patient compliance. Furthermore, polymeric nanoparticles can co-encapsulate multiple drugs in a fixed ratio, facilitating simultaneous delivery, ensuring synergistic therapeutic effects, and helping to prevent the emergence of drug resistance, (Bourguignon, Godinez-Leon, & Gref, 2023).

Notable Illustrations

Poly-lactic-co-glycolic acid (PLGA) Nanoparticles: Used to encapsulate rifampicin and isoniazid, these have demonstrated prolonged drug release and improved lung targeting in preclinical studies. Lipid- based nanoparticles (liposomes, solid lipid nanoparticles): These have shown promise in delivering rifabutin and bedaquiline with enhanced intracellular accumulation. Chitosan-based nanoparticles: Biodegradable and mucoadhesive, these are being explored for mucosal delivery of anti-TB agents, (Huang et al., 2024).

Current Status and Challenges

Although several nanoparticle formulations have demonstrated potential in animal models, there is still a lack of clinical translation. There are still unresolved issues with scalability, governmental approval, and long-term safety. However, studies are still being conducted to improve formulations and investigate novel nanocarriers including dendrimers and nanoemulsions.

Inhaled Formulations for Pulmonary Tuberculosis

Since pulmonary TB is the most common form of the disease and the lungs are the primary site of infection, direct drug delivery to the lungs via inhalation has gained significant attention. Inhaled formulations deliver high concentrations of the drug directly to the infection site, potentially bypassing first-pass metabolism, reducing systemic toxicity, and improving therapeutic efficacy, (Tan et al., 2020).

Types of Inhaled TB Therapies

Dry powder inhalers (DPIs): These deliver powdered drugs such as rifampicin or isoniazid via breath-actuated devices, (Tan et al., 2020).

Nebulized suspensions: Liquid formulations are aerosolized using a nebulizer for deep lung penetration, (Wang et al., 2024).

Liposomal inhaled formulations: Liposomes encapsulating drugs like amikacin or capreomycin can be aerosolized to enhance lung retention, (Wang et al., 2024).

Clinical and Preclinical Evidence

Liposomal amikacin for inhalation, though FDA-approved for NTM infections, demonstrates the feasibility of inhaled delivery in mycobacterial diseases. Inhaled rifampicin-loaded liposomes have shown superior lung concentration and reduced systemic side effects in animal models. Several phase I/II trials have explored inhaled dry powders of first-line TB drugs, showing good tolerability and pharmacokinetic profiles.

Benefits of Inhaled Delivery

Inhaled drug delivery for TB offers several significant benefits, particularly by achieving high local drug concentrations directly at the site of infection in the lungs. This targeted approach can enhance therapeutic activity while reducing systemic toxicity and associated side effects. Furthermore, it allows for reduced dosing frequency and lowers the overall pill burden, which can improve patient adherence. Being non-invasive, inhaled delivery is also potentially more patient-friendly, especially for children and individuals who have difficulty swallowing pills or tolerating injectable therapies, (Wang et al., 2024).

Long-Acting Injectables (LAIs)

LAI therapies represent a groundbreaking shift in TB treatment, offering the possibility of monthly or even less frequent dosing through sustained-release injectable formulations. LAIs typically consist of microspheres, implants, or oil-based suspensions that slowly release the active drug in to circulation. Rifapentine, with a long half-life and potent activity, is being studied in LAI formulations for latent TB infection and active disease. Bedaquiline, can also be used to develop LAI forms that maintain therapeutic concentrations for several weeks. Delamanid and linezolid, investigations into injectable depot forms are in early stages. The NIAID-supported long-acting formulation platform is exploring injectable depots combining multiple TB drugs for use in both preventive and active TB, (Rajoli et al., 2018).

Despite their potential, several challenges hinder the widespread use of advanced TB therapies such as LAIs. These include issues like injection site reactions, high upfront costs compared to oral tablets, the requirement of cold-chain storage, and limited data in special populations, including children and pregnant women.

In the worldwide battle against TB, innovative drug delivery technologies are the next frontier. Long-acting injectables, inhaled formulations, and nanoparticles all have special benefits that can help overcome the conventional obstacles to TB therapy, such as poor adherence, extended duration, and drug toxicity. Even though these technologies are still in the early stages of development, certain formulations are making progress through the preclinical and clinical stages, and early findings are encouraging. Supporting multidisciplinary research that connects clinical medicine, public health, and pharmaceutical technology is crucial going ahead. Strategies to guarantee affordability, accessibility, and acceptance in high-burden nations- where new technologies may have the greatest impact- are equally crucial. These distribution methods have the potential to greatly speed up the WHO End TB Strategy if they are successful.

Host-Directed Therapies (HDTs)

Host-Directed Therapies (HDTs) represent a paradigm shift in the treatment of TB by focusing on modulating the host's immune response rather than solely targeting the pathogen. These therapies aim to enhance the body's ability to control or eliminate *M. tuberculosis*, reduce excessive inflammation and tissue damage, and improve overall treatment outcomes, (Matteucci, Correa, & Costa, 2022). HDTs include a wide range of strategies, such as immunomodulatory agents like corticosteroids, thalidomide analogs, and statins that recalibrate immune responses; autophagy inducers like rapamycin and vitamin D that restore intracellular bacterial clearance; and anti-inflammatory or anti-fibrotic agents such as NSAIDs and pirfenidone that mitigate lung damage, (Guler et al., 2021). Furthermore, metabolic modulators like metformin, commonly used in diabetes, have shown promise in enhancing immune function and reducing pathology. Emerging immunotherapies, including immune checkpoint inhibitors, are being investigated for their potential to reverse T-cell exhaustion and rejuvenate protective responses. Together, these approaches not only offer potential to shorten treatment duration and reduce relapses but also present new hope in the fight against TB, where traditional antimicrobials are less effective, (Cubillos-Angulo et al., 2022).

CONCLUSION

Tuberculosis continues to represent one of the most significant infectious disease threats globally, despite decades of control efforts. The global burden remains high, with millions affected annually and a disproportionate impact on low- and middle-income countries. Challenges such as the emergence of MDR and XDR TB, lengthy and toxic regimens, poor adherence, and limited diagnostic infrastructure further complicate efforts to control and eliminate the disease.

Recent advances, including the development of novel anti-TB drugs like bedaquiline, delamanid, pretomanid, and the repurposing of agents like linezolid and clofazimine, mark a new era in TB therapeutics. Shorter and all-oral regimens now recommended by the WHO offer significant advantages over traditional treatment approaches, including improved adherence, reduced adverse effects, and enhanced treatment outcomes. Nevertheless, implementation of these new regimens remains challenging, particularly in resource- limited settings due to cost, access, and infrastructure constraints.

Innovative strategies such as HDTs, advanced drug delivery systems e.g., nanoparticles, inhalables, long-acting injectables, and ongoing clinical trials aiming to optimize and individualize TB treatment are vital additions to the global response. These emerging interventions, coupled with continued investment in research and development, are crucial for improving treatment success rates, curbing drug resistance, and ultimately achieving the targets outlined in the End TB Strategy.

In conclusion, while substantial progress has been made, a multi-pronged and integrated approach involving new drugs, optimized regimens, supportive technologies, and patient-centered care is essential to overcome current challenges. Sustained political will, global funding, and international collaborations will be key to translating these advancements into tangible public health gains and moving closer to a TB-free world.

REFERENCES

Aguilar Diaz, J. M., Abulfathi, A. A., te Brake, L. H., van Ingen, J., Kuipers, S., Magis-Escurra, C., Raaijmakers, J., Svensson, E. M., & Boeree, M. J. (2023). New and repurposed drugs for the treatment of active tuberculosis: An update for clinicians. *Respiration, 102*(2), 83–100. DOI: 10.1159/000528274 PMID: 36516792

Bourguignon, T., Godinez-Leon, J. A., & Gref, R. (2023). Nanosized drug delivery systems to fight tuberculosis. *Pharmaceutics, 15*(2), 393. Advance online publication. DOI: 10.3390/pharmaceutics15020393 PMID: 36839715

Budak, M., Via, L. E., Weiner, D. M., Barry, C. E.III, Nanda, P., Michael, G., Mdluli, K., & Kirschner, D. (2024). A systematic efficacy analysis of tuberculosis treatment with BPaL-containing regimens using a multiscale modeling approach. *CPT: Pharmacometrics & Systems Pharmacology, 13*(4), 673–685. DOI: 10.1002/psp4.13117 PMID: 38404200

Conradie, F. (2021). High rate of successful outcomes treating highly resistant TB in the ZeNix study of pretomanid, bedaquiline and alternative doses and durations of linezolid [Abstract OALB01LB02]. *11th IAS Conference on HIV Science, Geneva, Switzerland.* International AIDS Society.

Conradie, F., Bagdasaryan, T. R., Borisov, S., Howell, P., Mikiashvili, L., Ngubane, N., Samoilova, A., Skornykova, S., Tudor, E., Variava, E., Yablonskiy, P., Everitt, D., Wills, G. H., Sun, E., Olugbosi, M., Egizi, E., Li, M., Holsta, A., Timm, J., & Spigelman, M. (2022). Bedaquiline-pretomanid-linezolid regimens for drug-resistant tuberculosis. *The New England Journal of Medicine, 387*(9), 810–823. DOI: 10.1056/NEJMoa2119430 PMID: 36053506

Cubillos-Angulo, J. M., Nogueira, B. M. F., Arriaga, M. B., Barreto-Duarte, B., Araújo-Pereira, M., Fernandes, C. D., Vinhaes, C. L., Villalva-Serra, K., Nunes, V. M., Miguez-Pinto, J. P., Amaral, E. P., & Andrade, B. B. (2022). Host-directed therapies in pulmonary tuberculosis: Updates on anti-inflammatory drugs. *Frontiers in Medicine, 9*, 970408. Advance online publication. DOI: 10.3389/fmed.2022.970408 PMID: 36213651

Dahl, V. N., Fløe, A., & Wejse, C. (2023). Nontuberculous mycobacterial infections in a Danish region between 2011 and 2021: Evaluation of trends in diagnostic codes. *Infectious Diseases, 55*(6), 439–443. DOI: 10.1080/23744235.2023.2194411 PMID: 36995113

Diriba, G., Alemu, A., Yenew, B., Tola, H. H., Gamtesa, D. F., Mollalign, H., Eshetu, K., Moga, S., Abdella, S., Tollera, G., Kebede, A., & Dangisso, M. H. (2023). Epidemiology of extensively drug-resistant tuberculosis among patients with multidrug-resistant tuberculosis: A systematic review and meta-analysis. *International Journal of Infectious Diseases*, *132*, 50–63. DOI: 10.1016/j.ijid.2023.04.392 PMID: 37072053

Dookie, N., Ngema, S. L., Perumal, R., Naicker, N., Padayatchi, N., & Naidoo, K. (2022). The changing paradigm of drug-resistant tuberculosis treatment: Successes, pitfalls, and future perspectives. *Clinical Microbiology Reviews*, *35*(4), e0018019. Advance online publication. DOI: 10.1128/cmr.00180-19 PMID: 36200885

Evans, D., Hirasen, K., Ramushu, C., Long, L., Sinanovic, E., Conradie, F., Howell, P., Padanilam, X., Ferreira, H., Variaiva, E., Rajaram, S., Gupta, A., Juneja, S., & Ndjeka, N. (2024). Patient and provider costs of the new BPaL regimen for drug-resistant tuberculosis treatment in South Africa: A cost-effectiveness analysis. *PLoS One*, *19*(10), e0309034. Advance online publication. DOI: 10.1371/journal.pone.0309034 PMID: 39432463

Fox, G. J., & Menzies, D. (2013). A review of the evidence for using bedaquiline (TMC207) to treat multi-drug resistant tuberculosis. *Infectious Diseases and Therapy*, *2*(2), 123–144. DOI: 10.1007/s40121-013-0009-3 PMID: 25134476

Garcia-Prats, A. J., Schaaf, H. S., Draper, H. R., Garcia-Cremades, M., Winckler, J., Wiesner, L., Hesseling, A. C., & Savic, R. M. (2019). Pharmacokinetics, optimal dosing, and safety of linezolid in children with multidrug-resistant tuberculosis: Combined data from two prospective observational studies. *PLoS Medicine*, *16*(4), e1002789. Advance online publication. DOI: 10.1371/journal.pmed.1002789 PMID: 31039153

Gilmour, B., & Alene, K. A. (2024). Ending tuberculosis: Challenges and opportunities. *Frontiers in Tuberculosis*, *2*, 1487518. Advance online publication. DOI: 10.3389/ftubr.2024.1487518

Gomez, G. B., Siapka, M., Conradie, F., Ndjeka, N., Garfin, A. M. C., Lomtadze, N., Avaliani, Z., Kiria, N., Malhotra, S., Cook-Scalise, S., Juneja, S., Everitt, D., Spigelman, M., & Vassall, A. (2021). Cost-effectiveness of bedaquiline, pretomanid and linezolid for treatment of extensively drug-resistant tuberculosis in South Africa, Georgia and the Philippines. *BMJ Open*, *11*(12), e051521. Advance online publication. DOI: 10.1136/bmjopen-2021-051521 PMID: 34862287

Gotham, D., Martin, M., Barber, M. J., Kazounis, E., Batts, C., Scourse, R., Elder, G., & Nyang'wa, B. T. (2025). Cost analysis of the TB-PRACTECAL clinical trial on novel tuberculosis treatment regimens. *PLOS Global Public Health*, *5*(4), e0003759. Advance online publication. DOI: 10.1371/journal.pgph.0003759 PMID: 40267985

Guler, R., Ozturk, M., Sabeel, S., Motaung, B., Parihar, S. P., Thienemann, F., & Brombacher, F. (2021). Targeting molecular inflammatory pathways in granuloma as host-directed therapies for tuberculosis. *Frontiers in Immunology*, *12*, 733853. Advance online publication. DOI: 10.3389/fimmu.2021.733853 PMID: 34745105

Huang, Y., Guo, X., Wu, Y., Chen, X., Feng, L., Xie, N., & Shen, G. (2024). Nanotechnology's frontier in combatting infectious and inflammatory diseases: Prevention and treatment. *Signal Transduction and Targeted Therapy*, *9*(1), 34. Advance online publication. DOI: 10.1038/s41392-024-01745-z PMID: 38378653

Hudson, M., Todd, H., Nalugwa, T., Schraufnagel, A., Christian, C., Boccia, D., Wingfield, T., & Shete, P. B. (2025). [Manuscript title not provided]. *medRxiv*. DOI: 10.1101/2025.03.04.25323276

Hughes, G., Bern, H., Chiang, C. Y., Goodall, R. L., Nunn, A. J., Rusen, I. D., & Meredith, S. K. (2022). QT prolongation in the STREAM Stage 1 trial. *The International Journal of Tuberculosis and Lung Disease : the Official Journal of the International Union against Tuberculosis and Lung Disease*, *26*(4), 334–340. DOI: 10.5588/ijtld.21.0403 PMID: 35351238

Igarashi, M. (2017). Development of new antituberculosis drugs from natural products. *Bioscience, Biotechnology, and Biochemistry*, *81*(1), 32–37. DOI: 10.1080/09168451.2016.1248369 PMID: 27885931

Institute of Medicine. Indian National Science Academy, & Indian Council of Medical Research. (2012). *The global burden of drug-resistant TB*. In *Facing the reality of drug-resistant tuberculosis in India: Challenges and potential solutions: Summary of a joint workshop* (pp. 37–54). National Academies Press. https://www.ncbi.nlm.nih.gov/books/NBK100388/

Johnston, J. C., Cooper, R., & Menzies, D. (2022). Treatment of tuberculosis disease. *Canadian Journal of Respiratory, Critical Care, and Sleep Medicine*, *6*(sup1, Suppl. 1), 66–76. DOI: 10.1080/24745332.2022.2036504

Kaniga, K., Hasan, R., Jou, R., Vasiliauskienė, E., Chuchottaworn, C., Ismail, N., Metchock, B., Miliauskas, S., Viet Nhung, N., Rodrigues, C., Shin, S., Simsek, H., Smithtikarn, S., Ngoc, A. L. T., Boonyasopun, J., Kazi, M., Kim, S., Kamolwat, P., Musteikiene, G., & Omar, S. V. (2022). Bedaquiline drug resistance emergence assessment in multidrug-resistant tuberculosis (MDR-TB): A 5-year prospective in vitro surveillance study of bedaquiline and other second-line drug susceptibility testing in MDR-TB isolates. *Journal of Clinical Microbiology*, *60*(1), e0291920. Advance online publication. DOI: 10.1128/JCM.02919-20 PMID: 34705538

Kengo, A., Nabeemeeah, F., Denti, P., Sabet, R., Okyere-Manu, G., Abraham, P., Weisner, L., Mosala, M. H., Tshabalala, S., Scholefield, J., Resendiz-Galvan, J. E., Martinson, N. A., & Variava, E. (2024). Assessing potential drug-drug interactions between clofazimine and other frequently used agents to treat drug-resistant tuberculosis. *Antimicrobial Agents and Chemotherapy*, *68*(5), e0158323. Advance online publication. DOI: 10.1128/aac.01583-23 PMID: 38597667

Lange, C., Bothamley, G., Günther, G., Guglielmetti, L., Kontsevaya, I., Kuksa, L., Lange, B., Lorent, N., Saluzzo, F., Sester, M., Tebruegge, M., Tunesi, S., & Tweed, C.Tuberculosis Network European Trials Group. (2025). A year in review on tuberculosis and non-tuberculous mycobacteria disease: A 2025 update for clinicians and scientists. *Pathogens & Immunity*, *10*(2), 1–45. DOI: 10.20411/pai.v10i2.791 PMID: 40062355

Li, H., Salinger, D. H., Everitt, D., Li, M., Del Parigi, A., Mendel, C., & Nedelman, J. R. (2019). Long-term effects on QT prolongation of pretomanid alone and in combinations in patients with tuberculosis. *Antimicrobial Agents and Chemotherapy*, *63*(10), e00445–e19. DOI: 10.1128/AAC.00445-19 PMID: 31358590

Liu, Y., Shi, J., Li, L., Wu, T., Chu, P., Pang, Y., Guo, Y., Gao, M., & Lu, J. (2022). Spontaneous mutational patterns and novel mutations for delamanid resistance in *Mycobacterium tuberculosis. Antimicrobial Agents and Chemotherapy*, *66*(8), e0053122. Advance online publication. DOI: 10.1128/aac.00531-22 PMID: 36448833

Masini, T., Furin, J., Udwadia, Z., & Guglielmetti, L. (2023). Optimal management of drug-resistant tuberculosis: Can India lead the way? *The Indian Journal of Medical Research*, *157*(2-3), 220–222. DOI: 10.4103/ijmr.ijmr_300_23 PMID: 37202941

Matteucci, K. C., Correa, A. A. S., & Costa, D. L. (2022). Recent advances in host-directed therapies for tuberculosis and malaria. *Frontiers in Cellular and Infection Microbiology*, *12*, 905278. Advance online publication. DOI: 10.3389/fcimb.2022.905278 PMID: 35669122

Mirzayev, F., Viney, K., Linh, N. N., Gonzalez-Angulo, L., Gegia, M., Jaramillo, E., Zignol, M., & Kasaeva, T. (2021). World Health Organization recommendations on the treatment of drug-resistant tuberculosis, 2020 update. *The European Respiratory Journal, 57*(6), 2003300. Advance online publication. DOI: 10.1183/13993003.03300-2020 PMID: 33243847

Moodley, R., & Godec, T. R. (2016). Short-course treatment for multidrug-resistant tuberculosis: The STREAM trials. *European Respiratory Review : an Official Journal of the European Respiratory Society, 25*(139), 29–35. DOI: 10.1183/16000617.0080-2015 PMID: 26929418

Muniyandi, M., Ramesh, P. M., Wells, W. A., Alavadi, U., Sahu, S., & Padmapriyadarsini, C. (2023). The cost-effectiveness of the BEAT-TB regimen for pre-extensively drug-resistant TB. *Tropical Medicine and Infectious Disease, 8*(8), 411. Advance online publication. DOI: 10.3390/tropicalmed8080411 PMID: 37624349

Nyang'wa, B. T., Kloprogge, F., Moore, D. A. J., Bustinduy, A., Motta, I., Berry, C., & Davies, G. R. (2021). Population pharmacokinetics and pharmacodynamics of investigational regimens' drugs in the TB-PRACTECAL clinical trial (the PRACTECAL-PKPD study): A prospective nested study protocol in a randomised controlled trial. *BMJ Open, 11*(9), e047185. Advance online publication. DOI: 10.1136/bmjopen-2020-047185 PMID: 34489274

Oliveira, O., Gaio, R., Correia-Neves, M., Rito, T., & Duarte, R. (2021). Evaluation of drug-resistant tuberculosis treatment outcome in Portugal, 2000–2016. *PLoS One, 16*(4), e0250028. Advance online publication. DOI: 10.1371/journal.pone.0250028 PMID: 33878119

Omoteso, O. A., Fadaka, A. O., Walker, R. B., & Khamanga, S. M. (2025). Innovative strategies for combating multidrug-resistant tuberculosis: Advances in drug delivery systems and treatment. *Microorganisms, 13*(4), 722. Advance online publication. DOI: 10.3390/microorganisms13040722 PMID: 40284559

Oostvogels, S., Ley, S. D., Heupink, T. H., Dippenaar, A., Streicher, E. M., De Vos, E., Meehan, C. J., Dheda, K., Warren, R., & Van Rie, A. (2022). Transmission, distribution and drug resistance-conferring mutations of extensively drug-resistant tuberculosis in the Western Cape Province, South Africa. *Microbial Genomics, 8*(4), 000815. Advance online publication. DOI: 10.1099/mgen.0.000815 PMID: 35471145

Paton, N. I., Cousins, C., Suresh, C., Burhan, E., Chew, K. L., Dalay, V. B., Lu, Q., Kusmiati, T., Balanag, V. M., Lee, S. L., Ruslami, R., Pokharkar, Y., Djaharuddin, I., Sugiri, J. J. R., Veto, R. S., Sekaggya-Wiltshire, C., Avihingsanon, A., Sarin, R., Papineni, P., & Crook, A. M. (2023). Treatment strategy for rifampin-susceptible tuberculosis. *The New England Journal of Medicine, 388*(10), 873–887. DOI: 10.1056/NEJMoa2212537 PMID: 36808186

Phillips, P. P. J., Mitnick, C. D., Neaton, J. D., Nahid, P., Lienhardt, C., & Nunn, A. J. (2019). Keeping phase III tuberculosis trials relevant: Adapting to a rapidly changing landscape. *PLoS Medicine, 16*(3), e1002767. Advance online publication. DOI: 10.1371/journal.pmed.1002767 PMID: 30901331

Pontali, E., Sotgiu, G., Tiberi, S., Tadolini, M., Visca, D., D'Ambrosio, L., Centis, R., Spanevello, A., & Migliori, G. B. (2018). Combined treatment of drug-resistant tuberculosis with bedaquiline and delamanid: A systematic review. *The European Respiratory Journal, 52*(1), 1800934. Advance online publication. DOI: 10.1183/13993003.00934-2018 PMID: 29903862

Rabahi, M. F., Silva Júnior, J. L. R. D., Ferreira, A. C. G., Tannus-Silva, D. G. S., & Conde, M. B. (2017). Tuberculosis treatment. *Jornal Brasileiro de Pneumologia, 43*(6), 472–486. https://doi.org/ (Erratum published in 2018, *Jornal Brasileiro de Pneumologia, 44*(4), 340. https://doi.org/)DOI: 10.1590/S1806-37562016000000388

Rajoli, R. K. R., Podany, A. T., Moss, D. M., Swindells, S., Flexner, C., Owen, A., & Siccardi, M. (2018). Modelling the long-acting administration of anti-tuberculosis agents using PBPK: A proof of concept study. *The International Journal of Tuberculosis and Lung Disease : the Official Journal of the International Union against Tuberculosis and Lung Disease, 22*(8), 937–944. DOI: 10.5588/ijtld.17.0515 PMID: 29991405

Rifat, D., Li, S.-Y., Ioerger, T., Shah, K., Lanoix, J.-P., Lee, J., Bashiri, G., Sacchettini, J., & Nuermberger, E. (2021). Mutations in fbiD (Rv2983) as a novel determinant of resistance to pretomanid and delamanid in *Mycobacterium tuberculosis. Antimicrobial Agents and Chemotherapy, 65*(1), e01948–e20. DOI: 10.1128/AAC.01948-20 PMID: 33077652

Rodriguez, C. A., Brooks, M. B., Guglielmetti, L., Hewison, C., Jachym, M. F., Lessem, E., Varaine, F., & Mitnick, C. D. (2019). Barriers and facilitators to early access of bedaquiline and delamanid for MDR-TB: A mixed-methods study. *Public Health Action, 9*(1), 32–41. DOI: 10.5588/pha.18.0078 PMID: 30963040

Shiromwar, S. S., Khan, A. H., & Chidrawar, V. (2023). A systematic review on extensively drug-resistant tuberculosis from 2009 to 2020: Special emphases on treatment outcomes. *Revista Española de Quimioterapia*, *36*(1), 30–44. DOI: 10.37201/req/029.2022 PMID: 36503203

Silva, D. R., Fernandes, F. F., Ferreira, J. C., Bernando, W., Dalcolmo, M. M. P., Johansen, F. D. C., & Mello, F. C. Q. (2025). Bedaquiline, pretomanid, linezolid, and moxifloxacin (BPaLM) for multidrug- or rifampin-resistant tuberculosis: A systematic review. *Jornal Brasileiro de Pneumologia : Publicaçao Oficial da Sociedade Brasileira de Pneumologia e Tisilogia*, *50*(6), e20240295. Advance online publication. DOI: 10.36416/1806-3756/e20240295 PMID: 39813501

Stancil, S. L., Mirzayev, F., & Abdel-Rahman, S. M. (2021). Profiling pretomanid as a therapeutic option for TB infection: Evidence to date. *Drug Design, Development and Therapy*, *15*, 2815–2830. DOI: 10.2147/DDDT.S281639 PMID: 34234413

Suman, S. K., Chandrasekaran, N., & Priya Doss, C. G. (2023). Micro-nanoemulsion and nanoparticle-assisted drug delivery against drug-resistant tuberculosis: Recent developments. *Clinical Microbiology Reviews*, *36*(4), e0008823. Advance online publication. DOI: 10.1128/cmr.00088-23 PMID: 38032192

Szumowski, J. D., & Lynch, J. B. (2015). Profile of delamanid for the treatment of multidrug-resistant tuberculosis. *Drug Design, Development and Therapy*, *9*, 677–682. DOI: 10.2147/DDDT.S60923 PMID: 25678771

Tan, Z. M., Lai, G. P., Pandey, M., Srichana, T., Pichika, M. R., Gorain, B., Bhattamishra, S. K., & Choudhury, H. (2020). Novel approaches for the treatment of pulmonary tuberculosis. *Pharmaceutics*, *12*(12), 1196. Advance online publication. DOI: 10.3390/pharmaceutics12121196 PMID: 33321797

Tiberi, S., Muñoz-Torrico, M., Duarte, R., Dalcolmo, M., D'Ambrosio, L., & Migliori, G. B. (2018). New drugs and perspectives for new anti-tuberculosis regimens. *Pulmonology*, *24*(2), 86–98. DOI: 10.1016/j.rppnen.2017.10.009 PMID: 29487031

Timm, J., Bateson, A., Solanki, P., Paleckyte, A., Witney, A. A., Rofael, S. A. D., Fabiane, S., Olugbosi, M., McHugh, T. D., & Sun, E. (2023). Baseline and acquired resistance to bedaquiline, linezolid and pretomanid, and impact on treatment outcomes in four tuberculosis clinical trials containing pretomanid. *PLOS Global Public Health*, *3*(10), e0002283. Advance online publication. DOI: 10.1371/journal.pgph.0002283 PMID: 37851685

Togun, T., Kampmann, B., Stoker, N. G., & Lipman, M. (2020). Anticipating the impact of the COVID-19 pandemic on TB patients and TB control programmes. *Annals of Clinical Microbiology and Antimicrobials, 19*(1), 21. Advance online publication. DOI: 10.1186/s12941-020-00363-1 PMID: 32446305

Varshney, K., Anaele, B., Molaei, M., Frasso, R., & Maio, V. (2021). Risk factors for poor outcomes among patients with extensively drug-resistant tuberculosis (XDR-TB): A scoping review. *Infection and Drug Resistance, 14*, 5429–5448. DOI: 10.2147/IDR.S339972 PMID: 34938089

Wang, B., Wang, L., Yang, Q., Zhang, Y., Qinglai, T., Yang, X., Xiao, Z., Lei, L., & Li, S. (2024). Pulmonary inhalation for disease treatment: Basic research and clinical translations. *Materials Today. Bio, 25*, 100966. Advance online publication. DOI: 10.1016/j.mtbio.2024.100966 PMID: 38318475

World Health Organization. (2024)... *Global Tuberculosis Report, 2024*, •••. https://www.who.int/teams/global-tuberculosis-programme/tb-reports/global-tuberculosis-report-2024

World Health Organization. (2024). 1.3 Drug-resistant TB. *Global Tuberculosis Report, 2024*, •••. https://www.who.int/teams/global-tuberculosis-programme/tb-reports/global-tuberculosis-report-2024/tb-disease-burden/1-3-drug-resistant-tb

Yadav, S. (2024). BPaLM regimen against drug-resistant tuberculosis in India: A need of the hour. *Cureus, 16*(9), e68421. Advance online publication. DOI: 10.7759/cureus.68421 PMID: 39360094

Zary, M., Mohamed, M. S., Kafie, C., Chilala, C. I., Bahukudumbi, S., Foster, N., Gore, G., Fielding, K. L., Subbaraman, R., & Schwartzman, K. (2024). The performance of digital technologies for measuring tuberculosis medication adherence: A systematic review. *BMJ Global Health, 9*(1), e015633. Advance online publication. DOI: 10.1136/bmjgh-2024-015633 PMID: 39013639

Zhu, H., Zhou, X., Zhuang, Z., Li, L., Bi, J., & Mi, K. (2023). Advances of new drugs bedaquiline and delamanid in the treatment of multi-drug resistant tuberculosis in children. *Frontiers in Cellular and Infection Microbiology, 13*, 1183597. Advance online publication. DOI: 10.3389/fcimb.2023.1183597 PMID: 37384221

Zimenkov, D., Ushtanit, A., Gordeeva, E., Guselnikova, E., Schwartz, Y., & Stavitskaya, N. (2025). High prevalence of atpE mutations in bedaquiline-resistant *Mycobacterium tuberculosis* isolates, Russia. *Emerging Infectious Diseases, 31*(3), 525–536. DOI: 10.3201/eid3103.241488 PMID: 40023803

Chapter 13
Pioneering TB Solutions:
New Drugs, Clinical Trials, and the Power of Biotechnology

Tarun Kumar Patel
https://orcid.org/0009-0003-3002-8100
Sant Guru Ghasidas Government P.G. College, Kurud, India

ABSTRACT

This chapter explores advancements in tuberculosis (TB) control, focusing on novel drugs, innovative clinical trial designs, and biotechnological breakthroughs. It highlights the transformative BPaL regimen, which shortens treatment for drug-resistant TB to six months with 90% success, alongside emerging drugs like TBAJ-876. Adaptive trial designs and real-world evidence enhance efficiency, while genomics, AI, and host-directed therapies (e.g., metformin, vitamin D) offer new therapeutic avenues. Challenges like resistance, access barriers, and ethical concerns are addressed, emphasizing equitable strategies. Public-private partnerships, such as the TB Alliance, drive progress, but diverse trial populations and rapid diagnostics are critical for global impact.

INTRODUCTION

Tuberculosis (TB), caused by Mycobacterium tuberculosis, remains a significant global health challenge, with millions of new cases and deaths annually, ranking it among the leading causes of death from infectious diseases. Despite progress through strategies like Directly Observed Treatment, Short-course (DOTS) and the End TB Strategy, challenges such as multidrug-resistant TB (MDR-TB), extensively drug-resistant TB (XDR-TB), and HIV co-infections underscore the urgent need for innovative therapeutic and biotechnological solutions. The global TB burden is

DOI: 10.4018/979-8-3373-3446-2.ch013

exacerbated by diagnostic delays, limited access to effective treatments, and slow development of new drugs, with few novel compounds introduced in recent decades.

The rise of drug-resistant TB has intensified research efforts. Conventional treatments, reliant on prolonged regimens of first-line drugs, are increasingly ineffective against resistant strains, necessitating new therapeutic approaches. Recent advancements have led to the development of novel drugs that show promise in shortening treatment duration and improving outcomes for drug-resistant TB, though global access remains a challenge. Ongoing clinical trials are exploring new regimens to enhance efficacy, reduce toxicity, and improve patient adherence.

Biotechnological innovations are transforming TB control. Molecular diagnostics have revolutionized rapid detection of TB and drug resistance, enabling timely treatment initiation. Vaccine development is advancing, with efforts to improve upon the century-old Bacillus Calmette-Guérin (BCG) vaccine showing encouraging results in clinical trials. The M72/AS01E vaccine candidate, for instance, has shown encouraging results in phase II trials (Tait et al., 2019). Additionally, host-directed therapies and immunotherapies are being investigated to strengthen immune responses against *M. tuberculosis*, complementing conventional treatments. These advancements offer hope for more effective TB management, but addressing access and implementation challenges remains critical to reducing the global TB burden.

This chapter examines the latest advancements in TB control, focusing on novel drugs, clinical trials, and biotechnological innovations. By synthesizing insights from recent scientific literature, it aims to provide a comprehensive overview of strategies to combat the global TB threat, addressing both current challenges and future directions.

THE TB DRUG DEVELOPMENT PIPELINE: PROGRESS AND PROMISE

The global fight against tuberculosis (TB), caused by *M. tuberculosis*, has been reinvigorated by the development of novel drugs and regimens, addressing the challenges posed by multidrug-resistant TB (MDR-TB) and extensively drug-resistant TB (XDR-TB). This section, as part of a broader chapter exploring advancements in TB control, focuses on the TB drug development pipeline, detailing the mechanisms of action of newly approved drugs, emerging candidates in preclinical and early-phase trials, and case studies of successful regimens like BPaL (bedaquiline, pretomanid, linezolid).

New Drugs and Their Mechanisms of Action

The approval of bedaquiline, delamanid, and pretomanid has marked a significant shift toward shorter, all-oral regimens for drug-resistant TB, overcoming limitations of traditional therapies like isoniazid and rifampicin, which are often ineffective against resistant strains.

Bedaquiline

Bedaquiline, a diarylquinoline, was approved by the U.S. Food and Drug Administration in 2012, the first novel anti-TB drug in over four decades (Mahajan, 2013). It targets the mycobacterial ATP synthase, disrupting energy production in *M. tuberculosis* and killing both replicating and non-replicating bacteria (Sarathy et al., 2019). Clinical trials, including the Nix-TB study, reported sputum culture conversion of MDR-TB and XDR-TB patients within six months (Conradie et al., 2020). Bedaquiline's efficacy is tempered by risks of QTc prolongation and hepatotoxicity, requiring careful monitoring (Katrak et al., 2021). Its novel mechanism minimizes cross-resistance with first-line drugs, making it a cornerstone of modern TB regimens.

Delamanid

Delamanid, a nitroimidazole, received European Medicines Agency approval in 2013 for MDR-TB (Gler et al., 2012). It inhibits mycolic acid biosynthesis, a critical component of the mycobacterial cell wall, and generates reactive nitrogen species under hypoxic conditions, targeting latent bacteria (Singh et al., 2008). Phase III trials demonstrated sputum culture conversion in MDR-TB patients, with a favorable safety profile compared to injectable agents (von Groote-Bidlingmaier et al., 2019). However, potential cross-resistance with pretomanid limits its use in some resistant strains (Timm et al., 2023).

Pretomanid

Pretomanid, another nitroimidazole, was approved by the FDA in 2019 for XDR-TB and treatment-intolerant MDR-TB as part of the BPaL regimen. It disrupts mycolic acid synthesis and produces nitric oxide in hypoxic environments, enhancing activity against dormant bacteria (Deb & Biswas 2021). Recent studies also suggest it impairs the pentose phosphate pathway, accumulating toxic intermediates (Fekadu et al., 2022). The Nix-TB trial reported a favorable outcome rate with BPaL, reducing treatment duration to six months (Conradie et al., 2020). Hepatotoxicity, particularly when combined with other drugs, remains a concern (Cevik et al., 2024).

These drugs have revolutionized TB treatment by offering oral regimens that reduce treatment duration and improve outcomes for resistant strains, setting the stage for further pipeline advancements.

Emerging Candidates in Preclinical and Early-Phase Trials

The TB drug pipeline includes over 100 compounds, with 16 in early clinical development, targeting novel bacterial pathways and incorporating biotech-derived innovations (Working Group on New TB Drugs, 2025). These candidates aim to enhance potency, safety, and compatibility with existing regimens.

Second-Generation Compounds

Second-generation diarylquinolines, such as TBAJ-876 and TBAJ-587, improve upon bedaquiline's efficacy and safety. Preclinical studies show increased sterilizing activity and reduced cardiac toxicity (Almeida et al., 2021). Similarly, oxazolidinones like sutezolid and delpazolid target protein synthesis with fewer hematologic and neurologic toxicities than linezolid (Chen et al., 2024). Phase II trials of sutezolid reported culture conversion rates comparable to linezolid, with improved tolerability (Chen et al., 2024).

Novel Targets

Compounds targeting unique bacterial pathways are advancing rapidly. BTZ-043, a DprE1 inhibitor, disrupts arabinogalactan synthesis in the mycobacterial cell wall, showing potent preclinical activity (Ramey et al., 2023). GSK3036656, a leucyl-tRNA synthetase inhibitor, blocks protein synthesis and is in Phase II trials, demonstrating early bactericidal activity (Diacon et al., 2024). Biotech-derived compounds, such as FNDR-20081, target MmpL5, an efflux pump regulator, and exhibit synergy with bedaquiline and clofazimine, suggesting potential for combination therapies (Kaur et al., 2021).

Cholesterol Metabolism and Host-Directed Therapies

M. tuberculosis relies on host cholesterol for persistence, making cholesterol metabolism a novel target. GSK2556286, which disrupts cholesterol catabolism, reduces bacterial burden in preclinical models (Nuermberger et al., 2022). Additionally, host-directed therapies, such as small-molecule immune modulators, enhance macrophage activity against *M. tuberculosis*, offering adjunctive treatment options (Kaufmann et al., 2018). These approaches, explored in later sections on biotechnological frontiers, complement traditional antibiotics.

Preclinical Innovations

Advanced preclinical models, like the C3HeB/FeJ mouse, mimic human TB pathology, including granuloma formation, improving the predictive value of early drug testing (Lenaerts et al., 2015). High-throughput CRISPR-based screening has identified new drug targets, accelerating the discovery of biotech-derived compounds (Bosch et al., 2021). These innovations ensure a robust pipeline to address emerging resistance, a topic further discussed in the concerns section.

Case Studies: Successes and Lessons Learned

The BPaL regimen (bedaquiline, pretomanid, linezolid), approved by the FDA in 2019 and endorsed by the WHO in 2022, exemplifies the transformative impact of novel drug combinations for drug-resistant tuberculosis (TB) (WHO, 2022b). Evaluated in the Nix-TB and ZeNix trials, BPaL achieved a 90% favorable outcome rate in extensively drug-resistant (XDR) TB and treatment-intolerant multidrug-resistant (MDR) TB patients, shortening treatment from 18–24 months to 6 months (Conradie et al., 2020; Nyang'wa et al., 2022). Its all-oral composition eliminates injectable agents, enhancing adherence and reducing toxicity. Optimized linezolid dosing (600 mg daily) in the ZeNix trial maintained efficacy while minimizing adverse events like peripheral neuropathy (Nyang'wa et al., 2022). BPaL's cost-effectiveness in high-burden settings makes it a scalable, pan-TB regimen, with therapeutic drug monitoring ensuring safety and completion rates (Evans et al., 2024).

Challenges include linezolid's narrow therapeutic window, requiring monitoring to manage toxicity, and hepatotoxicity in related regimens like BPaMZ (BPaL plus pyrazinamide and moxifloxacin), which failed non-inferiority for drug-sensitive TB (Cevik et al., 2024). BPaL's success highlights the role of public-private partnerships, such as the TB Alliance, in accelerating development (TB Alliance, 2022). Future trials should include diverse populations, like those with HIV co-infection, to ensure broad applicability, as discussed in later sections.

INNOVATIONS IN CLINICAL TRIAL DESIGN

To address the urgent need for effective treatments, particularly for multidrug-resistant TB (MDR-TB) and extensively drug-resistant TB (XDR-TB), innovative clinical trial designs are critical. Following the discussion of novel drugs and regimens, this section explores advancements in clinical trial methodologies, focusing on adaptive trial designs, real-world evidence (RWE) and biomarker-driven endpoints, and challenges in recruiting diverse populations.

Adaptive Trial Methodologies Reducing Time-to-Approval

Adaptive trial designs have revolutionized TB clinical research by enabling flexible protocols that accelerate the evaluation of new regimens while maintaining scientific rigor, thus shortening regulatory approval timelines.

Principles of Adaptive Designs

Adaptive trials allow pre-specified modifications to trial parameters, such as sample size, treatment arms, or endpoints, based on interim data (Bhatt & Mehta, 2016). These adaptations may include discontinuing ineffective arms, adjusting dosages, or focusing on responsive subgroups. In TB research, adaptive designs are ideal for testing complex multidrug regimens across varied resistance profiles, addressing the disease's heterogeneity. The U.S. Food and Drug Administration (FDA) and European Medicines Agency (EMA) support adaptive designs for their efficiency, provided statistical integrity is ensured through type I error control (U.S. Food and Drug Administration, 2024).

Adaptive Trial Examples

The PanACEA consortium's MAMS-TB trial evaluated high-dose rifampicin and novel combinations for drug-sensitive TB using a multi-arm, multi-stage (MAMS) design. By assessing early bactericidal activity (EBA) as an interim endpoint, the trial efficiently identified promising regimens for Phase III studies, minimizing patient exposure to suboptimal treatments (Boeree et al., 2017). Similarly, the endTB trial utilized Bayesian adaptive randomization to prioritize effective MDR-TB regimens, optimizing resource allocation and reducing costs by focusing on high-performing arms (Cellamare et al., 2017). These examples demonstrate how adaptive designs enhance trial efficiency and responsiveness to emerging data.

Benefits and Challenges

Adaptive designs reduce sample sizes, shorten trial durations, and improve patient safety by limiting exposure to ineffective treatments. A simulation study estimated that MAMS designs could cut TB trial costs significantly compared to traditional designs, benefiting resource-limited settings (Bratton et al., 2013). However, challenges include complex statistical models to manage multiple comparisons and logistical difficulties in coordinating multi-arm trials across global sites (Bhatt & Mehta, 2016). Regulatory agencies require detailed adaptation protocols to ensure transparency, which can prolong planning (U.S. Food and Drug Administration, 2019). Despite these hurdles, adaptive designs are integral to TB research, enabling rapid therapy evaluation.

Incorporation of Real-World Evidence and Biomarker-Driven Endpoints

Real-world data (RWD) refers to information about patient health status or healthcare delivery routinely collected from diverse sources, such as electronic health records, medical claims, product or disease registries, and digital health technologies that provide insights into health status. Real-world evidence (RWE) is the clinical evidence derived from analyzing RWD, offering insights into the usage, benefits, or risks of a medical product. The FDA has long utilized RWD and RWE to monitor and assess the postmarket safety of approved drugs, with RWE historically supporting effectiveness to a lesser extent. Recent advancements in the availability and analysis of RWD have significantly enhanced the potential for generating robust RWE to inform FDA regulatory decisions (USFDA 2024). Integrating real-world evidence (RWE) and biomarker-driven endpoints has enhanced TB clinical trials' efficiency, relevance, and generalizability, complementing traditional randomized controlled trials (RCTs) and enabling precise outcome assessments.

Real-World Evidence in TB Trials

RWE is vital for evaluating regimens in high-burden, resource-limited settings where RCTs are challenging (Kim et al., 2018). The South African Bedaquiline Clinical Access Programme's RWE showed favorable outcome rate for bedaquiline in MDR-TB patients under routine care, supporting its global adoption (Ndjeka et al., 2015). Similarly, observational data from Georgia and the Philippines informed the cost-effectiveness of BPaL (Gomez et al., 2021).

RWE supports post-marketing surveillance, detecting rare adverse events missed in RCTs. The FDA's 2022 RWE guidance encourages its use in regulatory submissions (U.S. Food and Drug Administration, 2022). However, RWE's observational nature risks confounding, necessitating advanced statistical methods like propensity score matching (Franchetti 2022).

Biomarker-Driven Endpoints

Biomarker-driven endpoints, such as sputum culture conversion and molecular markers, provide early, objective measures of treatment response, reducing reliance on long-term outcomes. Sputum culture conversion at two months, correlating with relapse-free cure in majority of cases, is a validated surrogate endpoint for regimen efficacy (Scriba et al., 2021). Molecular biomarkers, like *M. tuberculosis* mRNA levels, enable earlier assessments. A Phase II sutezolid trial used mRNA clearance as a primary endpoint, detecting treatment effects within 14 days, accelerating timelines (Gillespie et al., 2024).

Imaging biomarkers, such as positron emission tomography-computed tomography (PET-CT), are emerging as non-invasive tools for assessing treatment response, particularly in extrapulmonary TB. A pilot study reported that PET-CT changes at one month predicted six-month outcomes with 80% accuracy, supporting its use in adaptive trials (Chen et al., 2014). However, biomarker validation remains a challenge, as surrogates must be rigorously correlated with clinical outcomes to gain regulatory acceptance (Dodd et al., 2016).

CHALLENGES IN RECRUITING DIVERSE POPULATIONS AND ENSURING TRIAL REPRESENTATIVENESS

Diverse trial populations are essential for generalizing findings to the global TB population, but recruitment and retention challenges persist, particularly for vulnerable groups.

Underrepresentation of Key Populations

TB disproportionately affects vulnerable groups, including those with HIV co-infection, children, and individuals in high-burden settings, yet these populations are underrepresented. A systematic review found only 12% of TB trial participants had HIV co-infection, despite a 20-fold increased TB risk, limiting applicability to this group (Dodd et al., 2020). Pediatric TB trials are rare, with less than 5% of studies focusing on children, despite 1.1 million annual pediatric cases (Martinez et al., 2020). Gender disparities persist, with a 2:1 male-to-female ratio in trials, despite comparable incidence in many regions (Horton et al., 2016).

Strategies to Enhance Representativeness

Community-based participatory research (CBPR) boosts trust and participation, increasing pediatric TB trial enrollment (Chavez-Rimache et al., 2023). Community-Based Participatory Research (CBPR) is defined as a collaborative research approach that equitably engages community members, academic researchers, and other stakeholders in all stages of the research process, from identifying problems to implementing and disseminating findings. By involving community health workers (CHWs) and volunteers, CBPR fosters trust, reduces stigma, and provides social support, improving patient retention and treatment outcomes. Community-based Directly Observed Treatment (DOTS) programs are cost-effective and sustainable. CBPR also enhances research relevance by improving data accuracy and participant engagement, while supporting policy changes through community advocacy (Chavez-Rimache et al., 2023).

Patient-centered care is an approach to healthcare that prioritizes the needs, preferences, and values of individuals and communities affected by TB. It involves designing and delivering TB services that are accessible, equitable, and responsive to patients' circumstances, ensuring they are informed, engaged, and supported throughout their care journey. This approach emphasizes treating patients with dignity, compassion, and respect, reducing barriers such as cost, time, and stigma, and fostering trust through effective communication, counseling, and coordination of care. It also includes adapting services to local contexts, empowering patients to participate in decision-making, and addressing social and economic challenges to improve treatment adherence and outcomes (The Union, 2023, WHO 2018).

The decentralized trial model in tuberculosis (TB) treatment conducts clinical research outside traditional sites, leveraging digital health technologies like telemedicine, wearables, and mobile apps to perform trial activities at participants' homes, local healthcare facilities, or community centers. Unlike centralized models, it distributes processes such as recruitment, monitoring, and data collection to enhance accessibility and convenience, as seen in trials like XPEL-TB in Uganda (Thompson et al., 2023). On-site molecular diagnostics, such as Xpert MTB/RIF testing, accelerate diagnosis and treatment initiation, reducing delays compared to hub-and-spoke models (Lawn & Nicol, 2011). This approach improves participation for marginalized populations, supports real-world data collection, and reduces costs, making trials more inclusive. Incentives like transport subsidies further reduce dropout rates (Zhao et al., 2013). However, challenges like secure data management, reliable drug delivery, and participant training on technology must be addressed to maximize its impact in high-burden, resource-limited settings.

Innovations in adaptive trial designs, RWE, and biomarker-driven endpoints have accelerated TB treatment evaluation, improving efficiency and real-world relevance. Addressing recruitment challenges is crucial for equitable outcomes. These advancements set the stage for discussions on biotechnological frontiers, concerns, and future directions in subsequent sections.

BIOTECHNOLOGICAL FRONTIERS IN TB THERAPEUTICS

Role of Genomics and Proteomics

The increasing prevalence of drug-resistant strains necessitates novel therapeutic strategies for tuberculosis (Sun et al., 2024). Genomics and proteomics have revolutionized TB drug discovery by enabling the identification of new drug targets through comprehensive analysis of MTB's genetic and protein landscapes. These biotechnological approaches provide insights into the pathogen's biology, facilitating the development of precise and effective treatments.

Genomics in TB Drug Target Identification

Genomics involves studying the complete DNA sequence of MTB to uncover genes critical for its survival, virulence, and drug resistance. The sequencing of the MTB H37Rv genome in 1998 marked a pivotal moment, enabling pangenomic analyses to identify conserved genes across strains (Chitale et al., 2022). Pangenomics, which examines core and accessory genomes, has been instrumental in pinpointing essential genes as potential drug targets. For instance, a 2024 study analyzing 442 MTB genomes identified 2,754 conserved core proteins, with sequential filters for non-human homology, essentiality, and virulence narrowing down promising targets (Khan et al., 2024). Whole-genome sequencing (WGS) and genome-wide association studies (GWAS) further enhance target discovery by detecting genetic variants linked to drug resistance, such as mutations in DNA repair systems (Mosquera-Rendón et al., 2023). Bioinformatics tools, integrated with artificial intelligence (AI), accelerate this process by predicting antigenic epitopes and modeling protein interactions, as highlighted in a recent review on TB vaccine development (Zhuang et al., 2024). These genomic approaches enable the design of drugs that disrupt essential MTB pathways, such as cell wall biosynthesis or DNA replication, critical for combating multidrug-resistant TB (MDR-TB).

Proteomics in TB Drug Target Identification

Proteomics complements genomics by analyzing the MTB proteome to understand protein expression, function, and interactions under various conditions, such as drug exposure or host infection. Subtractive proteomics, which compares MTB and human proteomes, identifies pathogen-specific proteins as potential targets, minimizing off-target effects (Khan et al., 2024). For instance, mass spectrometry-based proteomics has revealed MTB proteins involved in metabolic pathways, such as glycolysis and lipid metabolism, which are essential for intracellular survival (Choudhary et al., 2022; Yimer et al., 2020). Chemical proteomics, an emerging field, uses small-molecule probes to map protein-ligand interactions, identifying novel binding sites for drug development (Wozniak et al., 2024). Single-cell proteomics, enabled by advances in sensitivity, uncovers heterogeneous protein expression in MTB populations, revealing targets in persister cells that evade conventional therapies (Geraldes et al., 2022). Additionally, pharmacoproteomics compares protein profiles between healthy and TB-infected states to identify disease-specific biomarkers and targets, such as protein kinases involved in signal transduction (Guo et al., 2022). These kinases are prime candidates due to their role in MTB's stress response and survival (Smyth et al., 2021). Proteomics also supports targeted protein degradation (TPD) strategies, such as PROTACs, which selectively degrade MTB proteins, offering a novel approach for undruggable targets (Grohmann et al., 2022).

The integration of genomics and proteomics, supported by bioinformatics, enhances the precision of TB drug discovery. Computational tools like molecular docking and AI-driven platforms, such as DrugBank, enable virtual screening of drug-target interactions, reducing time and cost (Oyejide et al., 2025). For example, ligands like dihydroergotamine showed high binding affinity to MTB targets, suggesting potential therapeutic candidates (Sharma et al., 2024). These approaches are critical for addressing MDR-TB and extensively drug-resistant TB (XDR-TB), where traditional drugs like isoniazid fail. By identifying novel targets, such as those in DNA repair or protein degradation pathways, genomics and proteomics pave the way for host-directed therapies. However, experimental validation through *in vitro* and *in vivo* studies remains essential to confirm efficacy and safety. The synergy of these biotechnological frontiers promises to transform TB therapeutics, aligning with global efforts to end the TB epidemic.

AI and Machine Learning in Optimizing Drug Candidates and Predicting Resistance

Artificial intelligence (AI) and machine learning (ML) have transformed tuberculosis (TB) drug discovery by optimizing drug candidate selection and predicting drug resistance, addressing the challenges posed by *M. tuberculosis* (MTB) and its growing multidrug-resistant (MDR) and extensively drug-resistant (XDR) strains. These technologies leverage vast datasets from genomics, proteomics, and clinical studies to accelerate the identification of effective therapeutics and anticipate resistance mechanisms, significantly reducing time and costs in drug development (Oyejide et al., 2025).

Optimizing Drug Candidates

AI and ML streamline the drug discovery pipeline by analyzing complex biological data to identify and prioritize promising drug candidates. ML models, such as random forests and deep neural networks, predict drug-target interactions by integrating genomic, proteomic, and chemical data (Saleem et al., 2025). For example, the GenVS-TBDB database, an AI-generated and virtually screened small-molecule library, targets 376 essential MTB proteins, streamlining drug candidate identification (Lv et al., 2025). These models assess molecular properties, such as binding affinity and toxicity, using quantitative structure-activity relationship (QSAR) analyses, which enhance hit-to-lead optimization (Bastikar et al., 2022). Deep learning approaches, including convolutional neural networks, model protein-ligand interactions at the atomic level, improving the precision of drug design for MTB targets like cell wall biosynthesis enzymes (Zheng et al., 2025). AI also facilitates drug repurposing by analyzing existing drug databases, such as DrugBank, to identify compounds with anti-TB potential, as demonstrated in studies repurposing kinase inhibitors for TB treatment (Lee et al., 2024). Additionally, reinforcement learning optimizes combinatorial drug regimens by simulating treatment outcomes, ensuring synergistic effects and minimizing toxicity, which is critical for TB's prolonged treatment protocols (Sharma et al., 2023). These AI-driven approaches reduce the traditional 10–15-year drug development timeline, making them indispensable for addressing urgent TB therapeutic needs.

Predicting Drug Resistance

Predicting drug resistance is a cornerstone of TB management, given the rise of MDR-TB and XDR-TB. ML models, trained on whole-genome sequencing (WGS) data, identify genetic mutations associated with resistance to first-line drugs like isoniazid and rifampicin. For example, a 2025 study used GWAS to detect variants in DNA repair genes linked to resistance, enabling early identification of resistant strains (Zein-Eddine et al., 2025). Supervised ML algorithms, such as support vector machines and gradient boosting, analyze mutation profiles from databases like TBDB to predict resistance with high accuracy (Babirye et al., 2024). Deep learning models further enhance prediction by integrating multi-omics data, including transcriptomics and proteomics, to uncover non-genetic resistance mechanisms, such as efflux pump overexpression (Goff et al., 2020). AI also predicts cross-resistance and treatment failure by modeling epistatic interactions between mutations, as seen in studies of bedaquiline resistance (Zimenkov et al., 2025). These predictive tools guide personalized treatment by recommending effective drug combinations, reducing the risk of resistance amplification. Moreover, real-time ML applications in clinical settings, such as those using WGS data from rapid diagnostics, enable point-of-care resistance profiling, aligning with WHO's End TB Strategy.

The integration of AI and ML with multi-omics and clinical data creates a robust framework for TB drug discovery and resistance management. Platforms like AlphaFold and AutoML enhance structural biology analyses, predicting MTB protein structures for targeted drug design (Akdel et al., 2022; Dou et al. 2021). However, challenges remain, including the need for high-quality, diverse datasets to avoid model bias and the requirement for experimental validation to confirm predictions (Blanco-González et al., 2023). By accelerating drug candidate optimization and enabling proactive resistance management, AI and ML are pivotal in developing next-generation TB therapeutics, ultimately contributing to improved patient outcomes and global TB control.

Host-Directed Therapies and Their Potential Synergy with Antibiotics

Host-directed therapies (HDTs) represent an innovative approach to tuberculosis (TB) treatment by targeting host immune responses rather than directly attacking MTB (Table 1). These therapies modulate the host's immune system to enhance pathogen clearance, reduce tissue damage, and improve treatment outcomes, particularly in the context of multidrug-resistant (MDR) and extensively drug-resistant (XDR) TB. When combined with antibiotics, HDTs offer synergistic effects, addressing limitations of conventional treatments, such as prolonged regimens and emerging resistance (Varma et al., 2020). This approach is gaining traction as a complementary strategy to combat the global TB epidemic. This synergy is particularly valuable in high-burden settings, where resistance complicates treatment.

Table 1. List of Host-Directed Therapies (HDTs) and their synergy

HDT	Mechanism	Synergy with Antibiotics
Vitamin D3	Activates autophagy via upregulation of antimicrobial peptide LL-37 through vitamin D receptor (VDR) recruitment; enhances phagolysosome fusion and ROS production in macrophages.	Enhances bactericidal activity of isoniazid and rifampicin by improving intracellular killing of MTB; reduces treatment duration in drug-susceptible TB.
Phenylbutyrate (PBA)	Inhibits histone deacetylase, inducing LL-37 production; promotes autophagy and phagolysosome acidification to control MTB growth.	Synergizes with rifampicin and pyrazinamide, enhancing bacterial clearance and reducing lung pathology in murine models.
Metformin	Activates AMPK pathway, promoting autophagy and ROS production; disrupts MTB manipulation of macrophage pathways, enhancing host defense.	Improves efficacy of isoniazid and ethambutol in drug-susceptible and MDR-TB; reduces lung bacillary load and shortens treatment duration in mice.
Aspirin	Inhibits COX-1/2, reducing proinflammatory prostaglandin E2 (PGE2) and promoting lipoxin A4 (LXA4) production; modulates inflammation to minimize tissue damage.	Enhances pyrazinamide activity, reducing tissue bacillary loads and improving survival in murine TB models.
Ibuprofen	Nonsteroidal anti-inflammatory drug (NSAID) that suppresses proinflammatory cytokines (e.g., TNF-α, IL-6); enhances macrophage antimicrobial activity.	Increases efficacy of pyrazinamide and rifampicin, decreasing bacillary loads and improving survival in experimental TB models.
Imatinib	Protein-tyrosine kinase inhibitor; promotes phagolysosome maturation and autophagy, enhancing intracellular killing of MTB.	Synergizes with rifampicin and isoniazid, improving bacterial clearance in MDR-TB and reducing treatment duration in preclinical studies.
Interferon-γ (IFN-γ)	Enhances Th1 immune responses, upregulating macrophage antimicrobial activity via IFN-γ secretion; promotes granuloma penetration.	Improves sputum smear conversion rates when used with standard antibiotics; enhances rifampicin and ethambutol efficacy in drug-susceptible TB.
IL-10R1-7 Peptide Inhibitor	Inhibits IL-10-STAT3 pathway, enhancing nitric oxide synthase, NADPH oxidase, and lysozyme activity; modulates apoptosis and autophagy.	Reduces pulmonary bacterial load by 0.6 log10 CFU in chronic TB without antibiotics; potential to enhance isoniazid and rifampicin efficacy.
ST3-H2A2 Peptide Inhibitor	Targets STAT3 N-terminal domain, boosting macrophage bactericidal capacity via nitric oxide and lysozyme production; regulates apoptosis-autophagy pathways.	Decreases lung bacillary load by 1.7 log10 CFU in murine models; likely enhances standard antibiotic regimens by improving host immunity.
Ursolic Acid	Inhibits Akt/mTOR and TNF-α/TNFR1 pathways, boosting macrophage autophagy and reducing inflammation; enhances intracellular MTB killing.	Synergizes with rifampicin, improving bacterial clearance and reducing inflammation in preclinical studies.

continued on following page

Table 1. Continued

HDT	Mechanism	Synergy with Antibiotics
Andrographolide	Inhibits Notch1/Akt/NF-κB pathway, suppressing NLRP3 inflammasome and IL-1β production; enhances macrophage resistance to MTB.	Potential to enhance isoniazid and ethambutol by reducing inflammation and improving macrophage function; requires further clinical validation.
Alisporivir	Inhibits cyclophilin D, reducing necroptosis by blocking mitochondrial ROS and mPTPC formation; mitigates TNF-α-induced tissue damage.	Synergizes with rifampicin and second-line drugs in MDR-TB, reducing lung pathology and enhancing bacterial clearance in zebrafish models.
Desipramine	Inhibits acid sphingomyelinase, reducing ceramide production and necroptosis; attenuates TNF-α-induced tissue damage.	Enhances efficacy of rifampicin and bedaquiline in MDR-TB, minimizing tissue damage and improving outcomes in preclinical models.
Ferrostatin-1	Antioxidant that scavenges lipid ROS, inhibiting ferroptosis and reducing inflammation; protects against tissue damage.	Potential to improve outcomes with standard antibiotics by reducing lung pathology; synergy with rifampicin requires further study.
Tamoxifen	Modulates macrophage autophagy and antimicrobial peptide production; enhances phagolysosome maturation.	Synergizes with isoniazid and rifampicin, improving bacterial clearance in MDR-TB in zebrafish and murine models.
Phosphodiesterase-4 Inhibitors (PDE4i)	Suppress proinflammatory cytokines (e.g., TNF-α, IL-6); enhance macrophage antimicrobial activity and reduce lung inflammation.	Shortens treatment duration with rifampicin and isoniazid in rabbit models; improves outcomes in MDR-TB.
Dimethyl Itaconate	Promotes pentose phosphate pathway, increasing ROS production; exerts anti-inflammatory and antibacterial effects.	Enhances isoniazid and rifampicin activity by boosting host antimicrobial responses; effective in murine models.
Cysteamine/Cystamine	Enhances autophagy and antimicrobial peptide production; modulates macrophage immune responses.	Synergizes with amikacin and rifampicin, improving bacterial clearance in MDR-TB and reducing lung pathology.
Sertraline	Antidepressant that enhances autophagy and reduces inflammation; modulates macrophage responses to MTB.	Augments isoniazid and rifampicin efficacy, reducing treatment duration and improving outcomes in murine models.
GSK3β Inhibitors (e.g., P-4423632)	Inhibit glycogen synthase kinase 3β, promoting macrophage apoptosis and antimicrobial activity; modulate host signaling pathways.	Synergizes with rifampicin and ethambutol, reducing intracellular MTB growth in human macrophages; requires further clinical validation.

Despite their promise, HDTs face challenges, including variable efficacy across patient populations due to genetic and immunological differences. Clinical trials, such as those testing statins as HDTs, have shown mixed results, highlighting the need for biomarkers to predict responders (Kaufmann et al., 2018). Safety concerns, such as immunosuppression from cytokine therapies, require careful monitoring to avoid exacerbating infections (Young et al., 2020). Additionally, integrating HDTs into existing regimens demands robust pharmacokinetic studies to ensure compatibility with antibiotics (Kaufmann et al., 2018). Advances in AI and multi-omics are addressing these challenges by identifying optimal HDT-antibiotic combinations and predicting patient-specific responses. For example, machine learning models analyzing transcriptomic data can pinpoint immune pathways amenable to HDT intervention, guiding personalized therapy (Reichmann et al., 2021). Ongoing trials, such as those evaluating anti-inflammatory agents like ibuprofen as HDTs, aim to validate synergistic effects in humans (Kroesen et al. 2017).

The integration of HDTs with antibiotics offers a paradigm shift in TB management, particularly for MDR/XDR-TB, where conventional therapies are inadequate. By enhancing host immunity, reducing pathology, and countering resistance, HDTs improve treatment outcomes and align with WHO's End TB Strategy goals of reducing TB mortality by 95% by 2035 (WHO, 2015). Their potential to shorten treatment regimens and repurpose existing drugs also makes them cost-effective for low-resource settings. As research progresses, HDTs promise to transform TB care, delivering more effective, patient-centered solutions.

CONCERNS AND FUTURE DIRECTIONS

Emergence of Resistance to New TB Drugs and Strategies to Mitigate It

Tuberculosis (TB) is a serious lung infection, and new drugs like bedaquiline and pretomanid have been game-changers for treating tough cases where older drugs don't work. However, research suggests that some TB bacteria are becoming resistant to these new drugs, meaning they're harder to kill.

One promising approach is using **combination therapies**, where multiple drugs attack the bacteria in different ways, making it harder for resistance to develop. For example, the World Health Organization recommends a 6-month regimen called BPaLM, which combines four drugs and has shown good results in treating resistant TB (WHO Guidelines). Another strategy involves **host-directed therapies**, which boost the body's immune system to help antibiotics work better. Drugs like metformin, used for diabetes, might enhance TB treatment, though results vary (Sutter et al., 2022).

If resistance spreads, new drugs could become less effective, making TB harder and more expensive to treat. Combination therapies and other strategies like quick testing for resistance can help keep these drugs working longer, saving lives. However, experts debate whether these approaches can be widely used in poorer countries with limited healthcare resources, and more studies are needed to confirm their long-term benefits.

The development of new drugs like bedaquiline, delamanid, and pretomanid has transformed treatment for multidrug-resistant (MDR) and extensively drug-resistant (XDR) TB. However, the emergence of resistance to these drugs, coupled with person-to-person transmission, threatens global TB control efforts. This report examines the mechanisms and extent of resistance to new TB drugs and explores mitigation strategies, emphasizing combination therapies, host-directed therapies (HDTs), and other innovative approaches.

Resistance to New TB Drugs

Resistance to new TB drugs is a growing concern, driven by genetic mutations and the spread of resistant strains. A 2025 study by Goig et al. used whole-genome sequencing of 81,576 Mtb genomes from 26 countries to examine the spread of drug-resistant *Mycobacterium tuberculosis*, identifying 454 highly resistant strains, with 28% linked to direct transmission. In Georgia, sequencing 6,926 isolates revealed 60 highly resistant strains, with 28% in clusters indicating community spread. Globally, 25% of resistance cases to drugs like bedaquiline, delamanid, and pretomanid were transmission-driven, threatening regimens like BPaL. This underscores the urgent need to curb transmission to control resistant Mtb strains. The WHO's Global Tuberculosis Report 2023 indicates that the incidence of MDR/RR-TB (rifampicin-resistant TB) stabilized between 2020 and 2022 after declining from 2015 to 2019, with approximately 410,000 cases annually (WHO, 2023). Resistance to new drugs complicates treatment, increasing relapse rates in MDR-TB cohorts and raising healthcare costs significantly (Zong et al., 2018).

Mechanisms of Resistance. Resistance arises through mutations in specific Mtb genes. For bedaquiline, mutations in *atpE* alter ATP synthase binding, while *Rv0678* mutations upregulate efflux pumps, reducing drug efficacy (Guo et al., 2022). Delamanid resistance is linked to mutations in *ddn, fgd1* and *fbiA-D,* impairing prodrug activation, and pretomanid faces cross-resistance due to shared pathways (Zhao et al. 2024). Mtb's ability to form persister cells and enter dormancy further complicates treatment, as these non-replicating populations evade drugs targeting active metabolism.

Strategies to Mitigate Resistance

To counter resistance, a multifaceted approach is essential, with combination therapies and HDTs at the forefront.

Combination Therapies: Combination therapies use multiple drugs with distinct mechanisms to minimize resistance development. The WHO's BPaLM regimen, combining bedaquiline, pretomanid, linezolid, and moxifloxacin, is a 6-month all-oral treatment for MDR/RR-TB and pre-XDR-TB, achieving cure rates 89% in trials. This regimen reduces treatment duration compared to 18–24-month regimens, improving adherence and outcomes (WHO 2022b, c).

The endTB project, led by Harvard Medical School, identified three new oral shortened regimens for rifampin-resistant TB, leveraging combinations of existing and novel drugs to enhance efficacy and prevent resistance (Guglielmetti et al., 2025). Ongoing trials are exploring combinations like bedaquiline with clofazimine and levofloxacin, optimized through pharmacokinetic studies to ensure synergistic drug levels.

Host-Directed Therapies (HDTs): HDTs modulate the host immune response to enhance bacterial clearance and reduce tissue damage, complementing antibiotics and potentially lowering resistance risk. HDTs are particularly promising for MDR/XDR-TB, where antibiotic options are limited. By reducing reliance on antibiotics, HDTs may decrease selective pressure, slowing resistance development.

Rapid Diagnostics and Precision Medicine: Whole-genome sequencing (WGS) enables rapid detection of resistance mutations, guiding personalized treatment. WGS platforms predict bedaquiline resistance with high accuracy, allowing timely regimen adjustments. Point-of-care tests like Xpert MTB/XDR provide results within hours, facilitating early intervention. Precision medicine tailors therapies based on patient and strain profiles, minimizing ineffective treatments that fuel resistance.

Improved Treatment Adherence: Poor adherence contributes to resistance. Digital health tools, such as mobile apps and smart pillboxes, monitor compliance, while decentralized care models, like the XPEL-TB trial, enhance access in remote areas. Community-based care supports timely treatment initiation and follow-up, reducing resistance risks.

Drug Development and Stewardship: Developing drugs with novel targets, such as Mtb's DNA repair systems, reduces cross-resistance risks. Antimicrobial stewardship programs ensure rational drug use, reserving new drugs for confirmed resistant cases to preserve efficacy.

Access Barriers

Structural barriers, such as limited healthcare access and socioeconomic constraints, hinder recruitment in high-burden settings. In sub-Saharan Africa, accounting for majority of global TB cases, urban trial sites exclude rural populations facing travel barriers (The Union, 2023, WHO 2018). Stigma and mistrust deter participation, with a South African trial reporting high refusal rates due to stigma (DeSanto et al., 2023). Language barriers excluded many potential participants in an Indian trial (Kumari, 2024). However, structural barriers like poverty, stigma, and long travel distances to trial sites deter consistent participation (Teibo et al., 2024). Participants often face financial burdens from lost wages or transportation costs, which trial designs rarely address (Shete et al., 2023). Stigma surrounding TB can discourage engagement, as patients fear social ostracism (Yadav 2024). Additionally, adverse drug reactions, prevalent in multidrug-resistant TB trials, increase withdrawal rates when inadequately managed (Mishra et al., 2024). To counter these, trials should incorporate support systems such as financial compensation, community education to reduce stigma, and regular monitoring of side effects.

Ethical and Retention Challenges

Ethical considerations are critical when involving vulnerable populations, requiring robust community engagement (Mamotte et al., 2010). Tuberculosis (TB) clinical trials encounter significant ethical challenges that affect participant welfare and trial integrity. A key issue is ensuring informed consent, particularly among vulnerable populations with limited healthcare access or low literacy levels. The World Health Organization's 2017 ethics guidance underscores the importance of clear communication to protect TB patients' rights, ensuring participants comprehend trial risks, benefits, and their right to withdraw without penalty (WHO, 2017a). However, research indicates that consent processes often fail, with participants misunderstanding trial objectives or feeling coerced due to socioeconomic pressures (Bolado et al., 2024). Trials involving drug-resistant TB strains further complicate ethics, particularly regarding post-trial access to experimental treatments. Participants in resource-poor settings may lack continued care after trials conclude, violating principles of justice and beneficence (Pradipta et al., 2021). Including diverse groups, such as children or pregnant women, is critical for generalizable results but raises ethical concerns about risk, often leading to their exclusion. Ethical trial design must also ensure post-trial care continuity, particularly for chronic conditions, to maintain trust and encourage completion (WHO, 2017b).These challenges highlight the need for robust ethical frameworks prioritizing participant autonomy and equitable benefit access.

Retention in TB trials is another major hurdle, as lengthy treatment regimens and socioeconomic barriers contribute to high dropout rates. Cultural and linguistic barriers, along with unstable housing, increase the likelihood of loss to follow-up in TB preventive treatment. Addressing these issues could enhance long-term retention in clinical trials (Sepulveda Conwell et al. 2007).

Addressing these challenges demands a comprehensive approach. Ethically, trial organizers should enhance informed consent using culturally sensitive materials and independent advocates to ensure voluntariness (Kadam 2017). Retention can be bolstered through interventions like mobile health reminders or decentralized trial sites to ease travel burdens (Poongothai et al., 2023). Collaboration with local communities can align trial goals with participants' needs, fostering trust and reducing dropouts. By integrating ethical safeguards and retention strategies, TB trials can uphold participant dignity while advancing scientific progress against this global health threat.

CONCLUSION

The chapter highlights significant advancements in tuberculosis (TB) control, offering hope in addressing the global challenge of multidrug-resistant (MDR) and extensively drug-resistant (XDR) TB. Novel drugs like bedaquiline, delamanid, and pretomanid, alongside regimens like BPaL, have transformed treatment by shortening durations and improving outcomes for resistant strains. The drug development pipeline, enriched with innovative compounds and targets like cholesterol metabolism, is bolstered by biotechnological tools such as genomics, proteomics, and AI, which accelerate drug discovery and enable personalized therapies through rapid diagnostics like whole-genome sequencing.

Innovative clinical trial designs, including adaptive methodologies and real-world evidence integration, enhance research efficiency and relevance, but recruiting diverse populations, particularly vulnerable groups, remains challenging. Community-based and decentralized trial models are crucial for overcoming barriers and ensuring inclusivity. The emergence of resistance to new drugs, driven by transmission, threatens progress, necessitating combination therapies, host-directed therapies (HDTs), and precision diagnostics to curb its spread. HDTs, by boosting immune responses, complement antibiotics and may reduce treatment durations, though their scalability in low-resource settings requires further exploration.

Ethical and access issues, including stigma and socioeconomic constraints, complicate trial implementation and treatment access. Culturally sensitive consent processes, community engagement, and robust ethical frameworks are vital to ensure participant welfare and equitable benefits. Achieving the WHO's End TB Strategy goals demands a multifaceted approach, integrating scientific innovation with structural interventions. Sustained global collaboration, investment, and a focus on patient-centered care are essential to overcome resistance, enhance access, and advance toward a TB-free future, leveraging the synergy of cutting-edge therapeutics and inclusive research strategies.

REFERENCE

Akdel, M., Pires, D. E. V., Pardo, E. P., Jänes, J., Zalevsky, A. O., Mészáros, B., Bryant, P., Good, L. L., Laskowski, R. A., Pozzati, G., Shenoy, A., Zhu, W., Kundrotas, P., Serra, V. R., Rodrigues, C. H. M., Dunham, A. S., Burke, D., Borkakoti, N., Velankar, S., & Beltrao, P. (2022). A structural biology community assessment of AlphaFold2 applications. *Nature Structural & Molecular Biology, 29*(11), 1056–1067. DOI: 10.1038/s41594-022-00849-w PMID: 36344848

Almeida, D., Converse, P. J., Li, S. Y., Upton, A. M., Fotouhi, N., & Nuermberger, E. L. (2021). Comparative Efficacy of the Novel Diarylquinoline TBAJ-876 and Bedaquiline against a Resistant *Rv0678* Mutant in a Mouse Model of Tuberculosis. *Antimicrobial Agents and Chemotherapy, 65*(12), e0141221. DOI: 10.1128/AAC.01412-21 PMID: 34570644

Babirye, S. R., Nsubuga, M., Mboowa, G., Batte, C., Galiwango, R., & Kateete, D. P. (2024). Machine learning-based prediction of antibiotic resistance in *Mycobacterium tuberculosis* clinical isolates from Uganda. *BMC Infectious Diseases, 24*(1), 1391. DOI: 10.1186/s12879-024-10282-7 PMID: 39639222

Bastikar, V., Bastikar, A., & Gupta, P. (2022). Quantitative structure–activity relationship-based computational approaches. *Computational Approaches for Novel Therapeutic and Diagnostic Designing to Mitigate SARS-CoV-2 Infection*, 191–205. DOI: 10.1016/B978-0-323-91172-6.00001-7

Bhatt, D. L., & Mehta, C. (2016). Adaptive designs for clinical trials. *The New England Journal of Medicine, 375*(1), 65–74. DOI: 10.1056/NEJMra1510061 PMID: 27406349

Blanco-González, A., Cabezón, A., Seco-González, A., Conde-Torres, D., Antelo-Riveiro, P., Piñeiro, Á., & Garcia-Fandino, R. (2023). The Role of AI in Drug Discovery: Challenges, Opportunities, and Strategies. *Pharmaceuticals (Basel, Switzerland), 16*(6), 891. DOI: 10.3390/ph16060891 PMID: 37375838

Boeree, M. J., Heinrich, N., Aarnoutse, R., Diacon, A. H., Dawson, R., Rehal, S., Kibiki, G. S., Churchyard, G., Sanne, I., Ntinginya, N. E., Minja, L. T., Hunt, R. D., Charalambous, S., Hanekom, M., Semvua, H. H., Mpagama, S. G., Manyama, C., Mtafya, B., Reither, K., & Hoelscher, M. (2017). High-dose rifampicin, moxifloxacin, and SQ109 for treating tuberculosis: A multi-arm, multi-stage randomised controlled trial. *The Lancet. Infectious Diseases, 17*(1), 39–49. DOI: 10.1016/S1473-3099(16)30274-2 PMID: 28100438

Bolado, G. N., Ataro, B. A., Feleke, M. G., Gadabo, C. K., Kebamo, T. E., & Minuta, W. M. (2024). Informed consent practice and associated factors among healthcare professionals in public hospitals of Southern Ethiopia, 2023: A mixed-method study. *BMC Nursing*, *23*(1), 77. DOI: 10.1186/s12912-024-01748-9 PMID: 38287367

Bratton, D. J., Phillips, P. P., & Parmar, M. K. (2013). A multi-arm multi-stage clinical trial design for binary outcomes with application to tuberculosis. *BMC Medical Research Methodology*, *13*(1), 139. DOI: 10.1186/1471-2288-13-139 PMID: 24229079

Cellamare, M., Ventz, S., Baudin, E., Mitnick, C. D., & Trippa, L. (2017). A Bayesian response-adaptive trial in tuberculosis: The endTB trial. *Clinical Trials*, *14*(1), 17–28. DOI: 10.1177/1740774516665090 PMID: 27559021

Cevik, M., Thompson, L. C., Upton, C., Rolla, V. C., Malahleha, M., Mmbaga, B., Ngubane, N., Abu Bakar, Z., Rassool, M., Variava, E., Dawson, R., Staples, S., Lalloo, U., Louw, C., Conradie, F., Eristavi, M., Samoilova, A., Skornyakov, S. N., Ntinginya, N. E., & Borisov, S. (2024). Bedaquiline-pretomanid-moxifloxacin-pyrazinamide for drug-sensitive and drug-resistant pulmonary tuberculosis treatment: A phase 2c, open-label, multicentre, partially randomised controlled trial. *The Lancet. Infectious Diseases*, *24*(9), 1003–1014. DOI: 10.1016/S1473-3099(24)00223-8 PMID: 38768617

Chavez-Rimache, L., Ugarte-Gil, C., & Brunette, M. J. (2023). The community as an active part in the implementation of interventions for the prevention and care of tuberculosis: A scoping review. *PLOS Global Public Health*, *3*(12), e0001482. DOI: 10.1371/journal.pgph.0001482 PMID: 38100540

Chen, R. H., Burke, A., Cho, J. G., Alffenaar, J. W., & Davies Forsman, L. (2024). New Oxazolidinones for Tuberculosis: Are Novel Treatments on the Horizon? *Pharmaceutics*, *16*(6), 818. DOI: 10.3390/pharmaceutics16060818 PMID: 38931939

Chen, R. Y., Dodd, L. E., Lee, M., Paripati, P., Hammoud, D. A., Mountz, J. M., Jeon, D., Zia, N., Zahiri, H., Coleman, M. T., Carroll, M. W., Lee, J. D., Jeong, Y. J., Herscovitch, P., Lahouar, S., Tartakovsky, M., Rosenthal, A., Somaiyya, S., Lee, S., & Barry, C. E.III. (2014). PET/CT imaging correlates with treatment outcome in patients with multidrug-resistant tuberculosis. *Science Translational Medicine*, *6*(265), 265ra166. Advance online publication. DOI: 10.1126/scitranslmed.3009501 PMID: 25473034

Chitale, P., Lemenze, A. D., Fogarty, E. C., Shah, A., Grady, C., Odom-Mabey, A. R., Johnson, W. E., Yang, J. H., Eren, A. M., Brosch, R., Kumar, P., & Alland, D. (2022). A comprehensive update to the *Mycobacterium tuberculosis* H37Rv reference genome. *Nature Communications*, *13*(1), 7068. DOI: 10.1038/s41467-022-34853-x PMID: 36400796

Choudhary, E., Sharma, R., Pal, P., & Agarwal, N. (2022). Deciphering the proteomic landscape of *Mycobacterium tuberculosis* in response to acid and oxidative stresses. *ACS Omega*, *7*(30), 26749–26766. DOI: 10.1021/acsomega.2c03092 PMID: 35936415

Conradie, F., Diacon, A. H., Ngubane, N., Howell, P., Everitt, D., Crook, A. M., Mendel, C. M., Egizi, E., Moreira, J., Timm, J., McHugh, T. D., Wills, G. H., Bateson, A., Hunt, R., Van Niekerk, C., Li, M., Olugbosi, M., & Spigelman, M. (2020). Treatment of Highly Drug-Resistant Pulmonary Tuberculosis. *The New England Journal of Medicine*, *382*(10), 893–902. DOI: 10.1056/NEJMoa1901814 PMID: 32130813

Deb, U., & Biswas, S. (2021). Pretomanid: The latest USFDA-approved anti-tuberculosis drug. *The Indian Journal of Tuberculosis*, *68*(2), 287–291. DOI: 10.1016/j.ijtb.2020.09.003 PMID: 33845969

DeSanto, D., Velen, K., Lessells, R., Makgopa, S., Gumede, D., Fielding, K., Grant, A. D., Charalambous, S., & Chetty-Makkan, C. M. (2023). A qualitative exploration into the presence of TB stigmatization across three districts in South Africa. *BMC Public Health*, *23*(1), 504. DOI: 10.1186/s12889-023-15407-2 PMID: 36922792

Diacon, A. H., Barry, C. E.III, Carlton, A., Chen, R. Y., Davies, M., de Jager, V., Fletcher, K., Koh, G. C. K. W., Kontsevaya, I., Heyckendorf, J., Lange, C., Reimann, M., Penman, S. L., Scott, R., Maher-Edwards, G., Tiberi, S., Vlasakakis, G., Upton, C. M., & Aguirre, D. B. (2024). A first-in-class leucyl-tRNA synthetase inhibitor, ganfeborole, for rifampicin-susceptible tuberculosis: A phase 2a open-label, randomized trial. *Nature Medicine*, *30*(3), 896–904. DOI: 10.1038/s41591-024-02829-7 PMID: 38365949

Dodd, P. J., Sismanidis, C., & Seddon, J. A. (2016). Global burden of drug-resistant tuberculosis in children: A mathematical modelling study. *The Lancet. Infectious Diseases*, *16*(10), 1193–1201. DOI: 10.1016/S1473-3099(16)30132-3 PMID: 27342768

Dou, W., Liu, Y., Liu, Z., Yerezhepov, D., Kozhamkulov, U., Akilzhanova, A., Dib, O., & Chan, C.-K. (2021). An AutoML Approach for Predicting Risk of Progression to Active Tuberculosis based on Its Association with Host Genetic Variations. 2021 10th International Conference on Bioinformatics and Biomedical Science, 82–88. DOI: 10.1145/3498731.3498743

Evans, D., Hirasen, K., Casalme, D. J., Gler, M. T., Gupta, A., & Juneja, S. (2024). Cost and cost-effectiveness of BPaL regimen used in drug-resistant TB treatment in the Philippines. *IJTLD Open*, *1*(6), 242–249. DOI: 10.5588/ijtldopen.24.0094 PMID: 39021448

Fekadu, G., Tolossa, T., Turi, E., Bekele, F., & Fetensa, G. (2022). Pretomanid development and its clinical roles in treating tuberculosis. *Journal of Global Antimicrobial Resistance*, *31*, 175–184. DOI: 10.1016/j.jgar.2022.09.001 PMID: 36087906

Franchetti, Y. (2022). Use of Propensity Scoring and Its Application to Real-World Data: Advantages, Disadvantages, and Methodological Objectives Explained to Researchers Without Using Mathematical Equations. *Journal of Clinical Pharmacology*, *62*(3), 304–319. DOI: 10.1002/jcph.1989 PMID: 34671990

Geraldes, I., Fernandes, M., Fraga, A. G., & Osório, N. S. (2022). The impact of single-cell genomics on the field of mycobacterial infection. *Frontiers in Microbiology*, *13*, 989464. DOI: 10.3389/fmicb.2022.989464 PMID: 36246265

Gillespie, S. H., DiNardo, A. R., Georghiou, S. B., Sabiiti, W., Kohli, M., Panzner, U., Kontsevaya, I., Hittel, N., Stuyver, L. J., Tan, J. B., van Crevel, R., Lange, C., Thuong, T. N. T., Heyckendorf, J., Ruhwald, M., & Heinrich, N. (2024). Developing biomarker assays to accelerate tuberculosis drug development: Defining target product profiles. *The Lancet Microbe*, *5*(9), 100869. DOI: 10.1016/S2666-5247(24)00085-5 PMID: 38735303

Gler, M. T., Skripconoka, V., Sanchez-Garavito, E., Xiao, H., Cabrera-Rivero, J. L., Vargas-Vasquez, D. E., Gao, M., Awad, M., Park, S.-K., Shim, T. S., Suh, G. Y., Danilovits, M., Ogata, H., Kurve, A., Chang, J., Suzuki, K., Tupasi, T., Koh, W.-J., Seaworth, B., & Wells, C. D. (2012). Delamanid for multidrug-resistant pulmonary tuberculosis. *The New England Journal of Medicine*, *366*(23), 2151–2160. DOI: 10.1056/NEJMoa1112433 PMID: 22670901

Goff, A., Cantillon, D., Muraro Wildner, L., & Waddell, S. J. (2020). Multi-Omics Technologies Applied to Tuberculosis Drug Discovery. *Applied Sciences (Basel, Switzerland)*, *10*(13), 4629. DOI: 10.3390/app10134629

Goig, G. A., Loiseau, C., Maghradze, N., Mchedlishvili, K., Avaliani, T., Brites, D., Borrell, S., Aspindzelashvili, R., Avaliani, Z., Kipiani, M., Tukvadze, N., Jugheli, L., & Gagneux, S. (2025). Transmission as a Key Driver of Resistance to the New Tuberculosis Drugs. *The New England Journal of Medicine*, *392*(1), 97–99. DOI: 10.1056/NEJMc2404644 PMID: 39752306

Gomez, G. B., Siapka, M., Conradie, F., Ndjeka, N., Garfin, A. M. C., Lomtadze, N., Avaliani, Z., Kiria, N., Malhotra, S., Cook-Scalise, S., Juneja, S., Everitt, D., Spigelman, M., & Vassall, A. (2021). Cost-effectiveness of bedaquiline, pretomanid and linezolid for treatment of extensively drug-resistant tuberculosis in South Africa, Georgia and the Philippines. *BMJ Open*, *11*(12), e051521. DOI: 10.1136/bmjopen-2021-051521 PMID: 34862287

Grohmann, C., Marapana, D. S., & Ebert, G. (2022). Targeted protein degradation at the host–pathogen interface. *Molecular Microbiology*, *117*(4), 670–681. DOI: 10.1111/mmi.14849 PMID: 34816514

Guglielmetti, L., Khan, U., Velásquez, G. E., Gouillou, M., Abubakirov, A., Baudin, E., Berikova, E., Berry, C., Bonnet, M., Cellamare, M., Chavan, V., Cox, V., Dakenova, Z., de Jong, B. C., Ferlazzo, G., Karabayev, A., Kirakosyan, O., Kiria, N., Kunda, M., & Mitnick, C. D. (2025). Oral Regimens for Rifampin-Resistant, Fluoroquinolone-Susceptible Tuberculosis. *The New England Journal of Medicine*, *392*(5), 468–482. DOI: 10.1056/NEJMoa2400327 PMID: 39879593

Guo, J., Zhang, X., Chen, X., & Cai, Y. (2022). Proteomics in biomarker discovery for tuberculosis: Current status and future perspectives. *Frontiers in Microbiology*, *13*, 845229. DOI: 10.3389/fmicb.2022.845229 PMID: 35558124

Guo, Q., Bi, J., Lin, Q., Ye, T., Wang, Z., Wang, Z., Liu, L., & Zhang, G. (2022). Whole Genome Sequencing Identifies Novel Mutations Associated With Bedaquiline Resistance in Mycobacterium tuberculosis. *Frontiers in Cellular and Infection Microbiology*, *12*, 807095. Advance online publication. DOI: 10.3389/fcimb.2022.807095 PMID: 35694543

Horton, K. C., MacPherson, P., Houben, R. M., White, R. G., & Corbett, E. L. (2016). Sex Differences in Tuberculosis Burden and Notifications in Low- and Middle-Income Countries: A Systematic Review and Meta-analysis. *PLoS Medicine*, *13*(9), e1002119. DOI: 10.1371/journal.pmed.1002119 PMID: 27598345

Kadam, R. A. (2017). Informed consent process: A step further towards making it meaningful! *Perspectives in Clinical Research*, *8*(3), 107–112. DOI: 10.4103/picr.PICR_147_16 PMID: 28828304

Katrak, S., Lowenthal, P., Shen, R., True, L., Henry, L., & Barry, P. (2021). Bedaquiline for multidrug-resistant tuberculosis and QTc prolongation in California. *Journal of Clinical Tuberculosis and Other Mycobacterial Diseases*, *23*, 100216. DOI: 10.1016/j.jctube.2021.100216 PMID: 33598568

Kaufmann, S., Dorhoi, A., Hotchkiss, R., & Bartenschlager, R. (2018). Host-directed therapies for bacterial and viral infections. *Nature Reviews. Drug Discovery*, *17*(1), 35–56. DOI: 10.1038/nrd.2017.162 PMID: 28935918

Kaur, P., Potluri, V., Ahuja, V. K., Naveenkumar, C. N., Krishnamurthy, R. V., Gangadharaiah, S. T., Shivarudraiah, P., Eswaran, S., Nirmal, C. R., Mahizhaveni, B., Dusthackeer, A., Mondal, R., Batt, S. M., Richardson, E. J., Loman, N. J., Besra, G. S., Shandil, R. K., & Narayanan, S. (2021). A multi-targeting pre-clinical candidate against drug-resistant tuberculosis. *Tuberculosis (Edinburgh, Scotland)*, *129*, 102104. DOI: 10.1016/j.tube.2021.102104 PMID: 34214859

Khan, M. F., Ali, A., Rehman, H. M., Noor Khan, S., Hammad, H. M., Waseem, M., Wu, Y., Clark, T. G., & Jabbar, A. (2024). Exploring optimal drug targets through subtractive proteomics analysis and pangenomic insights for tailored drug design in tuberculosis. *Scientific Reports*, *14*(1), 10904. DOI: 10.1038/s41598-024-61752-6 PMID: 38740859

Kim, H. S., Lee, S., & Kim, J. H. (2018). Real-world evidence versus randomized controlled trial: Clinical research based on electronic medical records. *Journal of Korean Medical Science*, *33*(34), e213. DOI: 10.3346/jkms.2018.33.e213 PMID: 30127705

Kroesen, V. M., Gröschel, M. I., Martinson, N., Zumla, A., Maeurer, M., van der Werf, T. S., & Vilaplana, C. (2017). Non-Steroidal Anti-inflammatory Drugs As Host-Directed Therapy for Tuberculosis: A Systematic Review. *Frontiers in Immunology*, *8*, 772. DOI: 10.3389/fimmu.2017.00772 PMID: 28713389

Kumari, R. (2024). Tribal health in India: Overcoming public health challenges with a focus on tuberculosis. *Apollo Medicine*, *22*(1), 76–83. DOI: 10.1177/09760016241277333

Lawn, S. D., & Nicol, M. P. (2011). Xpert® MTB/RIF assay: Development, evaluation and implementation of a new rapid molecular diagnostic for tuberculosis and rifampicin resistance. *Future Microbiology*, *6*(9), 1067–1082. DOI: 10.2217/fmb.11.84 PMID: 21958145

Lee, D., Islam, M. A., Natarajan, S., Dudekula, D. B., Chung, H., Park, J., & Oh, B. (2024). Identification of Anti-Tuberculosis Drugs Targeting DNA Gyrase A and Serine/Threonine Protein Kinase PknB: A Machine Learning-Assisted Drug-Repurposing Approach. *Tropical Medicine and Infectious Disease*, *9*(12), 288. DOI: 10.3390/tropicalmed9120288 PMID: 39728815

Lv, X., Guo, H., Lu, X., Tang, Z., Yu, K., Xu, G., Chen, S., Zhang, R., & Guo, J. (2025). GenVS-TBDB: An open AI-generated and virtual-screened small-molecule database for tuberculosis drug discovery [Preprint]. *bioRxiv*. DOI: 10.1101/2025.04.28.650819

Mahajan, R. (2013). Bedaquiline: First FDA-approved tuberculosis drug in 40 years. *International Journal of Applied & Basic Medical Research*, *3*(1), 1–2. DOI: 10.4103/2229-516X.112228 PMID: 23776831

Mamotte, N., Wassenaar, D., Koen, J., & Essack, Z. (2010). Convergent ethical issues in HIV/AIDS, tuberculosis and malaria vaccine trials in Africa: Report from the WHO/UNAIDS African AIDS Vaccine Programme's Ethics, Law and Human Rights Collaborating Centre consultation, 10–11 February 2009, Durban, South Africa. *BMC Medical Ethics*, *11*(1), 3. DOI: 10.1186/1472-6939-11-3 PMID: 20211030

Martinez, L., Cords, O., Horsburgh, C. R., Andrews, J. R., Acuna-Villaorduna, C., Desai Ahuja, S., Altet, N., Augusto, O., Baliashvili, D., Basu, S., Becerra, M., Bonnet, M., Henry Boom, W., Borgdorff, M., Boulahbal, F., Carvalho, A. C. C., Cayla, J. A., Chakhaia, T., Chan, P.-C., & Zhu, L. (2020). The risk of tuberculosis in children after close exposure: A systematic review and individual-participant meta-analysis. *Lancet*, *395*(10228), 973–984. DOI: 10.1016/S0140-6736(20)30166-5 PMID: 32199484

Mishra, G., Alffenaar, J.-W., Munje, R., & Khateeb, S. (2024). Adverse drug reactions due to linezolid in the programmatic management of drug-resistant tuberculosis in India: A retrospective multicenter study. *The Indian Journal of Tuberculosis*, *71*(Suppl 1), S101–S109. DOI: 10.1016/j.ijtb.2023.04.006 PMID: 39067941

Mosquera-Rendón, J., Moreno-Herrera, C. X., Robledo, J., & Hurtado-Páez, U. (2023). Genome-Wide Association Studies (GWAS) Approaches for the Detection of Genetic Variants Associated with Antibiotic Resistance: A Systematic Review. *Microorganisms*, *11*(12), 2866. DOI: 10.3390/microorganisms11122866 PMID: 38138010

Ndjeka, N., Conradie, F., Schnippel, K., Hughes, J., Bantubani, N., Ferreira, H., Maartens, G., Mametja, D., Meintjes, G., Padanilam, X., Variava, E., Pym, A., & Pillay, Y. (2015). Treatment of drug-resistant tuberculosis with bedaquiline in a high HIV prevalence setting: An interim cohort analysis. *The International Journal of Tuberculosis and Lung Disease : the Official Journal of the International Union against Tuberculosis and Lung Disease, 19*(8), 979–985. DOI: 10.5588/ijtld.14.0944 PMID: 26162365

Nuermberger, E. L., Martínez-Martínez, M. S., Sanz, O., Urones, B., Esquivias, J., Soni, H., Tasneen, R., Tyagi, S., Li, S. Y., Converse, P. J., Boshoff, H. I., Robertson, G. T., Besra, G. S., Abrahams, K. A., Upton, A. M., Mdluli, K., Boyle, G. W., Turner, S., Fotouhi, N., & Jiménez, E. (2022). GSK2556286 Is a Novel Antitubercular Drug Candidate Effective *In Vivo* with the Potential To Shorten Tuberculosis Treatment. *Antimicrobial Agents and Chemotherapy, 66*(6), e0013222. DOI: 10.1128/aac.00132-22 PMID: 35607978

Nyang'wa, B. T., Berry, C., Kazounis, E., Motta, I., Parpieva, N., Tigay, Z., Solodovnikova, V., Liverko, I., Moodliar, R., Dodd, M., Ngubane, N., Rassool, M., McHugh, T. D., Spigelman, M., Moore, D. A. J., Ritmeijer, K., du Cros, P., & Fielding, K.TB-PRACTECAL Study Collaborators. (2022). A 24-Week, All-Oral Regimen for Rifampin-Resistant Tuberculosis. *The New England Journal of Medicine, 387*(25), 2331–2343. DOI: 10.1056/NEJMoa2117166 PMID: 36546625

Oyejide, A. J., Adekunle, Y. A., Abodunrin, O. D., & Atoyebi, E. O. (2025). *Artificial intelligence, computational tools and robotics for drug discovery, development, and delivery*. Intelligent Pharmacy., DOI: 10.1016/j.ipha.2025.01.001

Poongothai, S., Anjana, R. M., Aarthy, R., Unnikrishnan, R., Narayan, K. M. V., Ali, M. K., Karkuzhali, K., & Mohan, V. (2023). Strategies for participant retention in long term clinical trials: A participant -centric approaches. *Perspectives in Clinical Research, 14*(1), 3–9. DOI: 10.4103/picr.picr_161_21 PMID: 36909219

Pradipta, I. S., Idrus, L. R., Probandari, A., Lestari, B. W., Diantini, A., Alffenaar, J.-W. C., & Hak, E. (2021). Barriers and strategies to successful tuberculosis treatment in a high-burden tuberculosis setting: A qualitative study from the patient's perspective. *BMC Public Health, 21*(1), 1903. DOI: 10.1186/s12889-021-12005-y PMID: 34670527

Ramey, M. E., Kaya, F., Bauman, A. A., Massoudi, L. M., Sarathy, J. P., Zimmerman, M. D., Scott, D. W. L., Job, A. M., Miller-Dawson, J. A., Podell, B. K., Lyons, M. A., Dartois, V., Lenaerts, A. J., & Robertson, G. T. (2023). Drug distribution and efficacy of the DprE1 inhibitor BTZ-043 in the C3HeB/FeJ mouse tuberculosis model. *Antimicrobial Agents and Chemotherapy*, *67*(11), e0059723. DOI: 10.1128/aac.00597-23 PMID: 37791784

Reichmann, M. T., Tezera, L. B., Vallejo, A. F., Vukmirovic, M., Xiao, R., Reynolds, J., Jogai, S., Wilson, S., Marshall, B., Jones, M. G., Leslie, A., D'Armiento, J. M., Kaminski, N., Polak, M. E., & Elkington, P. (2021). Integrated transcriptomic analysis of human tuberculosis granulomas and a biomimetic model identifies therapeutic targets. *The Journal of Clinical Investigation*, *131*(15), e148136. DOI: 10.1172/JCI148136 PMID: 34128839

Saleem, J., Rahmanulla, A., Ahmed, M. G., Sultana, R., & Prashantha Kumar, B. R. (2025). *Machine learning & deep learning tools in pharmaceutical sciences: A comprehensive review*. Intelligent Pharmacy., DOI: 10.1016/j.ipha.2024.11.003

Sarathy, J. P., Gruber, G., & Dick, T. (2019). Re-Understanding the Mechanisms of Action of the Anti-Mycobacterial Drug Bedaquiline. *Antibiotics (Basel, Switzerland)*, *8*(4), 261. DOI: 10.3390/antibiotics8040261 PMID: 31835707

Scriba, T. J., Fiore-Gartland, A., Penn-Nicholson, A., Mulenga, H., Mbandi, S. K., Borate, B., Mendelsohn, S. C., Hadley, K., Hikuam, C., Kaskar, M., Musvosvi, M., Bilek, N., Self, S., Sumner, T., White, R. G., Erasmus, M., Jaxa, L., Raphela, R., & Innes, C.. (2021). Biomarker-guided tuberculosis preventive therapy (CORTIS): A randomised controlled trial. *The Lancet. Infectious Diseases*, *21*(3), 354–365. DOI: 10.1016/S1473-3099(20)30914-2 PMID: 33508224

Sepulveda Conwell, D., Mosher, A., Khan, A., Tapy, J., Sandman, L., Vernon, A., & Horsburgh, C. R. (2007). Factors associated with loss to follow-up in a large tuberculosis treatment trial (TBTC Study 22). *Contemporary Clinical Trials*, *28*(3), 288–294. DOI: 10.1016/j.cct.2006.09.003 PMID: 17107825

Sharma, D., Gautam, S., Srivastava, N., & Bisht, D. (2024). In silico screening of Food and Drug Administration-approved compounds against Trehalose 2-sulfotransferase (Rv0295c) in *Mycobacterium tuberculosis*: Insights from molecular docking and dynamics simulations. *International Journal of Mycobacteriology*, *13*(1), 73–82. DOI: 10.4103/ijmy.ijmy_20_24 PMID: 38771283

Sharma, K., Ahmed, F., Sharma, T., Grover, A., Agarwal, M., & Grover, S. (2023). Potential repurposed drug candidates for tuberculosis treatment: Progress and update of drugs identified in over a decade. *ACS Omega*, *8*(20), 17362–17380. DOI: 10.1021/acsomega.2c05511 PMID: 37251185

Shete, P. B., Kadota, J. L., Nanyunja, G., Namale, C., Nalugwa, T., Oyuku, D., Turyahabwe, S., Kiwanuka, N., Cattamanchi, A., & Katamba, A. (2023). Evaluating the impact of cash transfers on tuberculosis (ExaCT TB): A stepped wedge cluster randomised controlled trial. *ERJ Open Research*, *9*(3), 00182–02023. DOI: 10.1183/23120541.00182-2023 PMID: 37342088

Smyth, R., Berton, S., Rajabalee, N., Chan, T., & Sun, J. (2021). Protein Kinase R Restricts the Intracellular Survival of *Mycobacterium tuberculosis* by Promoting Selective Autophagy. *Frontiers in Microbiology*, *11*, 613963. DOI: 10.3389/fmicb.2020.613963 PMID: 33552025

Sun, Q., Li, S., Gao, M., & Pang, Y. (2024). Therapeutic Strategies for Tuberculosis: Progress and Lessons Learned. *Biomedical and Environmental Sciences*, *37*(11), 1310–1323. DOI: 10.3967/bes2024.168 PMID: 39667968

Sutter, A., Landis, D., & Nugent, K. (2022). The potential role for metformin in the prevention and treatment of tuberculosis. *Journal of Thoracic Disease*, *14*(6), 1758–1765. DOI: 10.21037/jtd-22-39 PMID: 35813707

Tait, D. R., Hatherill, M., Van Der Meeren, O., Ginsberg, A. M., Van Brakel, E., Salaun, B., Scriba, T. J., Akite, E. J., Ayles, H. M., Bollaerts, A., Demoitié, M.-A., Diacon, A., Evans, T. G., Gillard, P., Hellström, E., Innes, J. C., Lempicki, M., Malahleha, M., Martinson, N., & Roman, F. (2019). Final analysis of a trial of M72/AS01E vaccine to prevent tuberculosis. *The New England Journal of Medicine*, *381*(25), 2429–2439. DOI: 10.1056/NEJMoa1909953 PMID: 31661198

Teibo, T. K. A., Andrade, R. L. P., Rosa, R. J., de Abreu, P. D., Olayemi, O. A., Alves, Y. M., Vaz Tavares, R. B., da Costa, F. B. P., Dias Moura, H. S., Ferezin, L. P., Tártaro, A. F., de Campos, M. C. T., Ribeiro, N. M., Berra, T. Z., & Arcêncio, R. A. (2024). Barriers that interfere with access to tuberculosis diagnosis and treatment across countries globally: A systematic review. *ACS Infectious Diseases*, *10*(8), 2600–2614. DOI: 10.1021/acsinfecdis.4c00466 PMID: 39023509

The Union. (2023). *Improving retention during TB preventive treatment through person-centred care in South-East Asia*. https://theunion.org/news/improving-retention-during-tb-preventive-treatment-through-person-centred-care-in-south-east-asia

Thompson, R. R., Nalugwa, T., Oyuku, D., Tucker, A., Nantale, M., Nakaweesa, A., Musinguzi, J., Reza, T. F., Zimmer, A. J., Ferguson, O., Turyahabwe, S., Joloba, M., Cattamanchi, A., Katamba, A., Dowdy, D. W., & Sohn, H. (2023). Multicomponent strategy with decentralised molecular testing for tuberculosis in Uganda: A cost and cost-effectiveness analysis. *The Lancet. Global Health, 11*(2), e278–e286. DOI: 10.1016/S2214-109X(22)00509-5 PMID: 36669808

Timm, J., Bateson, A., Solanki, P., Paleckyte, A., Witney, A. A., Rofael, S. A. D., Fabiane, S., Olugbosi, M., McHugh, T. D., & Sun, E. (2023). Baseline and acquired resistance to bedaquiline, linezolid and pretomanid, and impact on treatment outcomes in four tuberculosis clinical trials containing pretomanid. *PLOS Global Public Health, 3*(10), e0002283. DOI: 10.1371/journal.pgph.0002283 PMID: 37851685

U.S. Food and Drug Administration. (2019). *Adaptive designs for clinical trials of drugs and biologics: Guidance for industry*. https://www.fda.gov/media/78495/download

U.S. Food and Drug Administration. (2022). *Submitting documents using real-world data and real-world evidence to FDA for drug and biological products: Guidance for industry*. https://www.fda.gov/media/124795/download:contentReference[oaicite:2]index=2

U.S. Food and Drug Administration. (2024). Real-world evidence in regulatory decision-making. https://www.fda.gov/science-research/science-and-research-special-topics/real-world-evidence

Varma, D. M., Zahid, M. S. H., Bachelder, E. M., & Ainslie, K. M. (2020). Formulation of host-targeted therapeutics against bacterial infections. *Translational Research; the Journal of Laboratory and Clinical Medicine, 220*, 98–113. DOI: 10.1016/j.trsl.2020.03.009 PMID: 32268128

von Groote-Bidlingmaier, F., Patientia, R., Sanchez, E., Balanag, V.Jr, Ticona, E., Segura, P., Cadena, E., Yu, C., Cirule, A., Lizarbe, V., Davidaviciene, E., Domente, L., Variava, E., Caoili, J., Danilovits, M., Bielskiene, V., Staples, S., Hittel, N., Petersen, C., & Gupta, R. (2019). Efficacy and safety of delamanid in combination with an optimised background regimen for treatment of multidrug-resistant tuberculosis: A multicentre, randomised, double-blind, placebo-controlled, parallel group phase 3 trial. *The Lancet. Respiratory Medicine, 7*(3), 249–259. DOI: 10.1016/S2213-2600(18)30426-0 PMID: 30630778

WHO. (2015). *The End TB Strategy* (WHO/HTM/TB/2015.19). https://apps.who.int/iris/bitstream/handle/10665/331326/WHO-HTM-TB-2015.19-eng.pdf

WHO. (2017a). *Ethics guidance for the implementation of the End TB strategy* (WHO/HTM/TB/2017.07). Geneva: World Health Organization. https://apps.who.int/iris/bitstream/handle/10665/254820/9789241512114-eng.pdf

WHO. (2017b). *WHO issues ethics guidance to protect rights of TB patients.* https://www.who.int/news/item/22-03-2017-who-issues-ethics-guidance-to-protect-rights-of-tb-patients

WHO. (2018). *Global tuberculosis report 2018* (WHO/CDS/TB/2018.20). Geneva: World Health Organization. Retrieved from https://apps.who.int/iris/handle/10665/274453

WHO. (2022a). *Global tuberculosis report 2022.* World Health Organization. https://www.who.int/teams/global-tuberculosis-programme/tb-reports/global-tuberculosis-report-2022

WHO. (2022b). *Module 4: Drug-resistant tuberculosis treatment, 2022 update – 4. The 6-month bedaquiline, pretomanid, linezolid and moxifloxacin (BPaLM) regimen.* TB Knowledge Sharing Platform. https://tbksp.who.int/en/node/576

WHO. (2022c). *WHO operational handbook on tuberculosis: Module 4: Treatment – drug-susceptible tuberculosis treatment.* World Health Organization. https://www.who.int/publications/i/item/9789240050761

WHO. (2023). 1.3 Drug-resistant TB. *Global Tuberculosis Report, 2023,* •••. https://www.who.int/teams/global-tuberculosis-programme/tb-reports/global-tuberculosis-report-2023/tb-disease-burden/1-3-drug-resistant-tb

Wozniak, J. M., Li, W., & Parker, C. G. (2024). Chemical proteomic mapping of reversible small molecule binding sites in native systems. *Trends in Pharmacological Sciences, 45*(11), 969–981. DOI: 10.1016/j.tips.2024.09.001 PMID: 39406592

Yadav, S. (2024). Stigma in Tuberculosis: Time to Act on an Important and Largely Unaddressed Issue. *Cureus, 16*(6), e61964. DOI: 10.7759/cureus.61964 PMID: 38978939

Yimer, S. A., Kalayou, S., Homberset, H., Birhanu, A. G., Riaz, T., Zegeye, E. D., Lutter, T., Abebe, M., Holm-Hansen, C., Aseffa, A., & Tønjum, T. (2020). Lineage-specific proteomic signatures in the *Mycobacterium tuberculosis* complex reveal differential abundance of proteins involved in virulence, DNA repair, CRISPR-Cas, bioenergetics and lipid metabolism. *Frontiers in Microbiology, 11,* 550760. DOI: 10.3389/fmicb.2020.550760 PMID: 33072011

Young, C., Walzl, G., & Du Plessis, N. (2020). Therapeutic host-directed strategies to improve outcome in tuberculosis. *Mucosal Immunology*, *13*(2), 190–204. DOI: 10.1038/s41385-019-0226-5 PMID: 31772320

Zein-Eddine, R., Le Meur, A., Skouloubris, S., Jelsbak, L., Refrégier, G., & Myllykallio, H. (2025). Genome wide analyses reveal the role of mutator phenotypes in the emergence of drug resistance inMycobacterium tuberculosis. DOI: 10.1101/2025.01.17.633521

Zhao, B., Zheng, H., Timm, J., Song, Z., Pei, S., Xing, R., Guo, Y., Ma, L., Li, F., Li, Q., Li, Y., Huang, L., Teng, C., Wang, N., Gupta, A., Juneja, S., Huang, F., Zhao, Y., & Ou, X. (2024). Prevalence and genetic basis of *Mycobacterium tuberculosis* resistance to pretomanid in China. *Annals of Clinical Microbiology and Antimicrobials*, *23*(1), 40. DOI: 10.1186/s12941-024-00697-0 PMID: 38702782

Zhao, Q., Wang, L., Tao, T., & Xu, B. (2013). Impacts of the "transport subsidy initiative on poor TB patients" in Rural China: A patient-cohort based longitudinal study in rural China. *PLoS One*, *8*(11), e82503. DOI: 10.1371/journal.pone.0082503 PMID: 24282623

Zheng, S., Gu, Y., Gu, Y., Zhao, Y., Li, L., Wang, M., Jiang, R., Yu, X., Chen, T., & Li, J. (2025). Machine learning–enabled virtual screening indicates the anti-tuberculosis activity of aldoxorubicin and quarfloxin with verification by molecular docking, molecular dynamics simulations, and biological evaluations. *Briefings in Bioinformatics*, *26*(1), bbae696. Advance online publication. DOI: 10.1093/bib/bbae696 PMID: 39737570

Zhuang, L., Ali, A., Yang, L., Ye, Z., Li, L., Ni, R., An, Y., Ali, S. L., & Gong, W. (2024). Leveraging computer-aided design and artificial intelligence to develop a next-generation multi-epitope tuberculosis vaccine candidate. *Infectious Medicine*, *3*(4), 100148. DOI: 10.1016/j.imj.2024.100148 PMID: 39687693

Zimenkov, D., Ushtanit, A., Gordeeva, E., Guselnikova, E., Schwartz, Y., & Stavitskaya, N. (2025). High Prevalence of atpE Mutations in Bedaquiline-Resistant *Mycobacterium tuberculosis* Isolates, Russia. *Emerging Infectious Diseases*, *31*(3), 525–536. DOI: 10.3201/eid3103.241488 PMID: 40023803

Zong, Z., Huo, F., Shi, J., Jing, W., Ma, Y., Liang, Q., Jiang, G., Dai, G., Huang, H., & Pang, Y. (2018). Relapse Versus Reinfection of Recurrent Tuberculosis Patients in a National Tuberculosis Specialized Hospital in Beijing, China. *Frontiers in Microbiology*, *9*. Advance online publication. DOI: 10.3389/fmicb.2018.01858 PMID: 30154770

Chapter 14

The Role of Pulmonary Rehabilitation in the Restoration of Respiratory Function After Tuberculosis

Ukbe Sirayder
https://orcid.org/0000-0001-7094-3432
Nuh Naci Yazgan University, Turkey

ABSTRACT

Pulmonary rehabilitation (PR) is a vital intervention for managing long-term respiratory complications that persist after tuberculosis (TB) treatment. Individuals recovering from TB often suffer from chronic dyspnea, reduced exercise tolerance, fatigue, and psychological issues, all of which contribute to a decreased quality of life. A multidisciplinary PR approach—including exercise training, inspiratory muscle strengthening, airway clearance techniques, nutritional support, and psychological counseling—has demonstrated significant benefits in improving functional capacity and alleviating symptoms. Randomized controlled trials and meta-analyses highlight the physiological and psychosocial improvements associated with PR in post-TB populations. Additionally, alternative delivery models such as community-based programs and telerehabilitation have shown promise, especially in resource-limited settings. Evidence supports the integration of PR into routine post-TB care to optimize recovery and enhance long-term health outcomes.

DOI: 10.4018/979-8-3373-3446-2.ch014

INTRODUCTION

Tuberculosis (TB) is an infectious disease caused by bacteria belonging to the *Mycobacterium* tuberculosis complex. It primarily affects the lungs but can also have systemic manifestations through extrapulmonary involvement, making it a serious public health concern. According to the World Health Organization's 2023 data, approximately 10.6 million new TB cases were reported worldwide, and 1.3 million deaths were attributed to the disease (Organization, 2023). Although antibiotic treatments have reduced TB-related mortality, chronic respiratory system problems that develop in the post-disease period significantly impact individuals' quality of life (Dartois & Rubin, 2023).

Pulmonary tuberculosis can lead to fibrosis, bronchiectasis, and obstructive or restrictive patterns of pulmonary function impairment after treatment (Ivanova et al., 2023). These complications affect not only the physical but also the psychological and social aspects of patients' lives. Common symptoms among TB patients include dyspnea, exercise intolerance, fatigue, chest pain, and reduced quality of life (Byrne et al., 2015). The literature reports that at least 30–50% of patients experience permanent losses in pulmonary function starting from the post-TB period (Ivanova et al., 2023).

At this stage, pulmonary rehabilitation (PR) becomes a key component of care. PR is a tailored, multidisciplinary intervention designed to help individuals with respiratory illnesses regain physical function, manage symptoms, and improve their overall quality of life (Spruit et al., 2013). For patients recovering from TB, starting a PR program after the acute phase can support lung recovery, enhance exercise tolerance, and provide much-needed psychosocial assistance (Meca et al., 2022).

Typically, PR programs combine elements such as physiotherapy, breathing techniques, patient education, emotional support, and nutritional guidance. Together, these components contribute to a more holistic recovery and help manage post-tuberculosis lung disease (PTLD) effectively (Mahler & Croitoru, 2019). While PR has long been recognized as effective in chronic respiratory conditions like chronic obstructive pulmonary disease (COPD), its use after TB has received comparatively less attention. Still, recent research indicates that similar benefits may be achievable in the post-TB population as well (Aytaç et al., 2024; Mahler & Croitoru, 2019; Wu et al., 2024; Xu et al., 2021).

Although PTLD is not yet widely defined as a distinct disease entity, it is generally considered to encompass ongoing symptoms and radiological or functional impairments following the completion of TB treatment (Allwood et al., 2021). This condition is particularly prevalent in low- and middle-income countries (LMICs), adding an additional burden to healthcare systems. However, PR has the potential to become part of sustainable health strategies due to its low cost and applicability (Ivanova et al., 2023).

Individuals who develop respiratory dysfunction after TB experience significant reductions in quality of life and activities of daily living. These patients show reduced participation in the workforce, and their psychological health deteriorates, with depression and anxiety commonly observed. PR programs provide comprehensive support, both physically and emotionally, thereby facilitating reintegration into society (Zuo et al., 2022).

Moreover, the benefits of PR are not limited to the improvement of clinical symptoms. Objective improvements can also be achieved in pulmonary function parameters such as lung volumes, gas exchange capacity, and diffusion capacity (Dowman et al., 2021). Notably, respiratory muscle strength, maximum oxygen consumption (VO_2 max), and walking distance are significantly improved during the PR process (Spruit et al., 2013).

Today, the post-TB period should not be addressed solely with microbiological treatment but within a holistic healthcare management approach. PR is one of the key components of this new paradigm. The integration of PR programs into post-TB care routines is of strategic importance for reducing secondary complications and alleviating the burden on healthcare systems (Allwood et al., 2021). However, for this approach to become widespread, clear definitions must be established in national guidelines, healthcare workers must be trained, and access to PR services must be expanded.

This book chapter aims to examine the role of pulmonary rehabilitation in the post-TB period in a multidimensional manner. In light of current literature findings, it will evaluate the physiological, functional, and psychosocial effects of PR after TB and offer recommendations for clinically applicable protocols.

PATHOPHYSIOLOGY OF POST-TUBERCULOSIS PULMONARY IMPAIRMENTS

Despite effective antibiotic therapies, TB continues to pose a significant public health concern due to its permanent structural and functional damages in the lungs. Following infection control, many patients develop severe and lasting pulmonary impairments. The pathophysiology of these complications is multifaceted and encompasses a wide spectrum ranging from structural destruction of lung tissue to impaired gas exchange (Allwood et al., 2021).

Pulmonary Fibrosis, Cavity Formation, and Bronchiectasis

One of the most prominent structural changes that emerge during the recovery process of tuberculosis is pulmonary fibrosis. The granulomatous inflammation developed during the infection leads to collagen deposition over time, resulting in the loss of the elastic structure of the lungs. This condition limits lung volumes and reduces the surface area for gas exchange (Gai et al., 2023).

Cavity formation is frequently observed in advanced stages of TB. These cavities, formed following the breakdown of necrotic tissue, may persist even after the infection is controlled (McAdams et al., 1995). The presence of fibrotic walls around the cavity can lead to localized ventilation-perfusion (V/Q) mismatch and predispose to secondary infections (Gai et al., 2023).

Another common sequela is bronchiectasis. Chronic inflammation of the bronchi causes irreversible dilation, impaired mucociliary clearance, accumulation of secretions, and frequent respiratory infections. Post-tuberculosis bronchiectasis typically appears with limited and asymmetrical distribution, especially in the upper lobes, and is associated with parenchymal damage (Fong et al., 2022).

Chronic Inflammation and Small Airway Disease

The chronic inflammatory process induced by tuberculosis may persist even after eradication of the infection. This process leads to fibrotic changes, wall thickening, and obliteration in the small airways (bronchioles). These changes result in an obstructive respiratory pattern, especially causing airflow limitation during exhalation (Sarkar et al., 2017). This condition may lead to the development of a COPD-like syndrome in individuals who have had TB. Clinically, patients report symptoms such as dyspnea during exercise, prolonged cough, and sputum production. This condition is defined as PTLD (Allwood et al., 2021).

Typical Findings in Pulmonary Function Tests

Pulmonary function tests (PFTs) in post-TB patients may show both restrictive and obstructive patterns (Allwood et al., 2021; Sarkar et al., 2017). The most commonly observed findings include:

- FEV_1 (Forced Expiratory Volume in 1 Second): Often shows significant reduction, indicating an obstructive pattern.
- FVC (Forced Vital Capacity): Decreased due to fibrosis.
- FEV_1/FVC ratio: May fall below 70% in the presence of obstruction.

- DLCO (Diffusing Capacity for Carbon Monoxide): Markedly reduced due to alveolar membrane damage.

These PFTs changes are important in planning pulmonary rehabilitation and also provide valuable prognostic indicators to monitor disease progression.

V/Q Mismatch and Hypoxemia

In the post-TB period, a significant proportion of patients develop a serious imbalance between ventilation (V) and perfusion (Q) in certain regions of the lung (Gai et al., 2023). This condition, known as V/Q mismatch, is one of the major pathophysiological causes of hypoxemic respiratory failure (Slobod et al., 2022).

Mechanism of V/Q Mismatch

For efficient gas exchange in the lungs, sufficient air (ventilation) and adequate blood flow (perfusion) must reach the same alveolar regions. In the post-TB period, this balance is disrupted due to several factors:

- **Fibrosis:** Collagen deposition during the healing process of granulomatous inflammation leads to alveolar wall thickening and loss of elasticity, impairing compliance and limiting ventilation (Desai & Moustarah, 2022).
- **Cavities and bronchiectasis:** Airflow in cavitary and bronchiectatic areas is impaired due to secretion accumulation, deformation, or obliteration of bronchial lumens. These poorly ventilated but well-perfused areas create physiological shunts (Gai et al., 2023; McAdams et al., 1995).
- **Vascular alterations:** Capillary vessels feeding the alveoli may also undergo fibrosis due to TB, resulting in well-ventilated but poorly perfused areas—known as dead space ventilation (Chatterjee et al., 2023).

These pathological changes impair effective oxygen transfer across the alveolar-capillary membrane, leading to oxygenation defects.

Exercise-Induced Hypoxemia

While some patients may compensate for this imbalance at rest, the increased oxygen demand during exercise reveals the clinical significance of V/Q mismatch. Post-TB patients, due to stiffened fibrotic lung structure, are unable to adequately increase ventilation during exercise, leading to desaturation and symptoms like dyspnea, fatigue, and dizziness (Dogra et al., 2015).

Alveolar-Capillary Membrane Thickening

The fibrotic process following tuberculosis leads to thickening of the alveolar-capillary membrane (Desai & Moustarah, 2022). Normally only 0.3–0.5 micrometers thick, this membrane may become several times thicker, significantly reducing gas diffusion, especially for oxygen. This is reflected in reduced DLCO values and contributes to exercise-induced and resting hypoxemia (Dietiker et al., 1961).

Consequences: Chronic Hypoxemia and Sequelae

Chronic hypoxemia increases the workload on respiratory muscles and the diaphragm, reduces cardiopulmonary reserve, predisposes to pulmonary hypertension, and may cause compensatory hematologic responses such as secondary erythrocytosis (Naeije & Chesler, 2012).

Long-Term Effects and Symptoms

Although TB has largely been brought under control with effective antibiotic treatments, the persistent pulmonary damage that develops after recovery can significantly impact patients' quality of life (Musafiri et al., 2015). This section details the long-term respiratory problems that develop post-TB, the pathophysiological basis of these issues, clinical symptoms, and their functional impact on patients.

Dyspnea (Shortness of Breath)

Dyspnea is one of the most commonly reported symptoms among individuals who have had TB. Studies have shown that persistent dyspnea symptoms are present in 30% to 70% of TB survivors (Pasipanodya et al., 2007). The main causes include:

- **Reduction in alveolar surface area:** Fibrosis and cavity formation reduce the lungs' gas exchange capacity (Chung et al., 2004).
- **Loss of respiratory function in restrictive and obstructive patterns:** Decreases are observed in both FVC and FEV1 values (Ivanova et al., 2023).
- **Increased respiratory workload:** Especially during exercise, compensatory activation of the diaphragm and accessory respiratory muscles increases. Subjectively, patients report symptoms such as shortness of breath when climbing stairs and difficulty breathing while lying down. Mechanical and gas exchange difficulties make dyspnea a multifactorial symptom (Harms et al., 2000).

Exercise Intolerance

A significant proportion of patients in the post-TB period report fatigue and reduced endurance even during low-intensity physical activity (Hanekom et al., 2019). The mechanisms include:

- **Hypoxemia:** Due to V/Q mismatch and low diffusion capacity, insufficient oxygen reaches the muscles.
- **Muscle dysfunction:** Mitochondrial dysfunction caused by hypoxemia leads to metabolic insufficiency in peripheral muscles.
- **Pulmonary vascular narrowing:** Fibrosis and vascular remodeling impair pulmonary hemodynamic responses during exercise.

These patients typically show markedly reduced performance compared to healthy individuals in objective measurements like the 6-minute walk test (6MWT). Chronic respiratory limitation is a major factor that reduces quality of life (Hanekom et al., 2019).

Chronic Cough and Sputum Production

Post-TB bronchiectasis leads to chronic cough and sputum production in patients. The damage caused by TB weakens bronchial walls and impairs the mucociliary clearance mechanism. This results in secretion accumulation and increased infection risk (Martinez-Garcia et al., 2023).

Frequent exacerbations, or suppurative infections, are commonly observed in bronchiectatic areas. This significantly affects patients' quality of life, requiring prolonged antibiotic therapy and expectorant use. Persistent coughing can lead to social isolation and psychological issues (Martinez-Garcia et al., 2023; Wang et al., 2018).

Even years after completing TB treatment, these symptoms may persist, creating a sense of ongoing illness or "chronic bronchitis."

Chest Pain and Pleural Discomfort

In the post-TB period, pleural adhesions and the development of fibrotic bands are among the common complications. During the infection process, the pleural membrane thickens due to inflammation, and fibrosis develops, leading to the formation of inelastic bands between the lung and the chest wall. These pathological structures mechanically restrict respiratory movements and cause pain, especially during deep inhalation or trunk movements. This type of pain is usually localized;

patients typically describe pain in a specific area, most commonly on the lateral or posterior thoracic regions. The pain intensifies with deep inspiration and can also worsen during coughing or sudden positional changes. However, this type of pain is not constant; it generally presents intermittently and occurs in relation to activity or respiratory motion, and it may subside with rest (Shaw et al., 2018; Wani, 2013).

Pleural thickening not only causes pain but also leads to impairment in respiratory mechanics. As it prevents full expansion of the lungs, it results in a reduction of vital capacity. Consequently, patients may experience symptoms such as dyspnea (shortness of breath), a sense of fatigue, and early exhaustion during physical activities (Harms et al., 2000).

In some patients, sequelae remaining after the resolution of pleural effusion that occurred during TB infection may lead to irregularities on the pleural surface and chronic inflammation. This condition can cause long-term symptoms such as chronic discomfort, a sensation of fullness or pressure in the chest. In addition, the presence of pleural fibrosis and fibrotic bands may indirectly increase the risk of developing pulmonary hypertension, as they contribute to V/Q imbalances (Jones et al., 2025).

In conclusion, pleural complications after TB are among the significant sequelae that not only cause mechanical ventilation limitations but also lead to a marked decline in quality of life and chronic pain that requires clinical management. Accurate identification of this condition and the development of symptom management strategies are of critical importance for a holistic approach to post-TB syndrome.

Anxiety and Depression

Chronic shortness of breath, limited exercise tolerance, and social withdrawal are common and often distressing complications that many individuals face after recovering from TB. These physical challenges frequently coexist with psychological issues. Both the active phase of TB and the long-term damage it may cause have been shown to significantly increase the risk of anxiety and depression. The extended treatment duration, combined with social and financial setbacks, reduced physical capacity, and declining quality of life, can place a considerable emotional burden on patients (Padmanabhanunni & Pretorius, 2025).

For some, breathlessness during physical activity can trigger sensations similar to panic attacks—the fear of not being able to breathe can heighten anxiety and contribute to ongoing stress. Long-term job loss, financial strain, and feeling socially disconnected may further erode self-esteem and foster a sense of hopelessness about the future. Even after medical recovery, some individuals struggle with the feeling that they are "not truly healed" living in constant fear of relapse. This mindset can fuel health-related anxiety and depressive symptoms (Padmanabhanunni & Pretorius, 2025).

Research using validated psychological tools such as the Hospital Anxiety and Depression Scale (HADS) supports these observations. Studies consistently show that individuals who have had TB report significantly higher levels of anxiety and depression compared to the general population (Dos Santos et al., 2017). These findings underscore the importance of incorporating psychological care—not just respiratory therapy—into comprehensive rehabilitation plans for TB survivors.

Sleep Disorders

Chronic hypoxemia and respiratory difficulties can severely impair sleep quality in many patients during the post-TB period. These individuals frequently report symptoms such as frequent nocturnal awakenings, inability to sleep continuously, and feeling unrested in the morning. Excessive daytime fatigue and difficulty concentrating are also among the direct consequences of this disrupted sleep pattern (Liu et al., 2023).

Particularly, persistent nighttime coughing episodes interrupt the structure of sleep. The sensation of increased dyspnea while lying in the supine position impairs the transition into deep sleep stages, thereby reducing the restorative effect of sleep (Devassy et al., 2022). In addition, significant drops in oxygen saturation (oxygen desaturation) may be observed throughout the night, posing an additional source of stress that negatively affects both the cardiovascular system and brain function (Sakuma et al., 1996).

This condition slows down metabolic recovery, delays immune system restoration, and reduces psychological resilience, paving the way for mental health issues such as depression and anxiety. In patients at risk for sleep apnea or those who develop significant sleep-related respiratory disorders, advanced sleep studies such as polysomnography are recommended, and appropriate treatment planning should be carried out accordingly (Haribhau, 2015).

Secondary Health Problems

In the post-TB period, not only the lung tissue but also extrapulmonary systems may be affected in various ways. One such complication is the development of pulmonary hypertension. Fibrosis and loss of vascular bed induced by TB reduce both the number and functional capacity of pulmonary blood vessels. This leads to increased pulmonary artery pressure, thereby resulting in a clinical picture of pulmonary hypertension (van Heerden et al., 2024).

Another commonly observed complication is right heart strain due to chronic hypoxemia. In this process, the right ventricle must overcome increased pulmonary vascular resistance, and over time, this may lead to a condition known as cor pulmonale, or right-sided heart failure (Jaligidad, 2016). In addition, a compensatory response known as secondary erythrocytosis may develop in an effort to increase oxygen-carrying capacity. Chronic hypoxemia stimulates the kidneys to produce more erythropoietin, which in turn accelerates red blood cell production in the bone marrow, leading to elevated hemoglobin levels. However, these hematological changes can increase blood viscosity, placing additional strain on the cardiovascular system (Tesfamariam et al., 2021).

In conclusion, these systemic complications adversely affect not only respiratory function but also overall cardiopulmonary health, potentially resulting in progressive respiratory failure and a significant decline in quality of life.

PULMONARY REHABILITATION: DEFINITION AND COMPONENTS

Definition and Historical Background of Pulmonary Rehabilitation

PR is a comprehensive and multidisciplinary intervention program developed to improve the functional capacity and quality of life in individuals with chronic respiratory diseases. According to the joint definition by the American Thoracic Society (ATS) and the European Respiratory Society (ERS), PR is defined as "an evidence-based, multidisciplinary, and comprehensive intervention for patients with chronic respiratory diseases who are symptomatic and often have decreased daily life activities. It is designed to reduce symptoms, optimize functional status, increase participation, and reduce healthcare costs through individualized therapies including, but not limited to, exercise training, education, and behavior change" (Singh et al., 2013).

The concept of pulmonary rehabilitation first emerged in the 1950s. During this period, it became evident that pharmacological treatments alone were insufficient in controlling respiratory diseases. It was observed that exercise training, respiratory therapy, and lifestyle modifications had significant effects on patients' well-being. Following the 1980s, randomized controlled trials demonstrated that PR significantly improved both exercise capacity and quality of life, particularly in individuals with chronic obstructive pulmonary disease (COPD) (Casaburi, 2008).

Today, PR is recommended as a standard therapeutic approach not only for COPD but also for other chronic pulmonary conditions such as asthma, interstitial lung diseases, cystic fibrosis, and pulmonary sequelae following tuberculosis.

Exercise Training

Exercise training is the cornerstone of PR programs and is one of the most effective components in improving both physical performance and quality of life in patients. The goal is to enhance the cardiovascular endurance of lower and upper extremity muscle groups, rebuild muscle strength, and improve exercise tolerance. This training generally includes aerobic, resistance, balance, and flexibility exercises that are systematically progressed and tailored to the patient's individual capacity (Hill, 2006; Spruit et al., 2013).

Aerobic exercises typically include low to moderate intensity walking (on a treadmill or outdoors), stationary cycling (ergometry), rowing, or step training. These exercises improve cardiorespiratory endurance while enhancing ventilatory efficiency and oxygen utilization. Exercise duration is initially kept short (e.g., 5–10 minutes) and is gradually increased to 20–30 minutes weekly based on the patient's tolerance (Hill, 2006; Spruit et al., 2013).

Resistance training is especially important to preserve muscle strength and prevent the development of atrophy. It consists of repeated exercises for upper and lower body muscle groups using light weights. These exercises contribute to increased mitochondrial function in muscle fibers, improved insulin sensitivity, and enhanced functional mobility (Spruit et al., 2013).

Exercise intensity in PR programs is generally targeted at 60–80% of the patient's maximal oxygen consumption (VO_2max). However, if the patient's exercise capacity is low, a gradual increase strategy is applied starting from a low intensity. During the rehabilitation process, response to exercise is regularly monitored using the 6-Minute Walk Test (6MWT), the Borg dyspnea scale, heart rate, and SpO_2 levels (Spruit et al., 2013).

Exercise training also reduces the perception of dyspnea, improves the efficiency of respiratory muscles, helps reduce systemic inflammation, and optimizes peripheral muscle function. As a result, patients can more easily engage in daily life activities independently and benefit from improved social and psychological reintegration (Spruit et al., 2013).

Moreover, recent studies have demonstrated that exercise training plays a significant role in alleviating post-tuberculosis sequelae such as exercise intolerance, muscle weakness, and deconditioning (Spruit et al., 2013).

In recent years, high-intensity interval training (HIIT) protocols have emerged as a promising exercise approach for individuals with lung disease. HIIT is defined as the sequential application of short-duration, high-intensity exercise periods followed by rest or low-intensity recovery intervals (Abaei et al., 2023).

Breathing Training

Breathing training is a central component of pulmonary rehabilitation and plays a vital role, especially in addressing the respiratory challenges that often arise after tuberculosis. The goal of this training is to help patients learn effective breathing techniques while strengthening the respiratory muscles. Among the most widely used methods are diaphragmatic breathing, pursed-lip breathing, and inspiratory muscle training (Spruit et al., 2013).

Diaphragmatic breathing encourages slow, deep breathing by engaging the abdominal muscles, helping to reduce reliance on accessory muscles. This not only improves ventilation efficiency but also lowers the amount of energy the body uses to breathe. For patients dealing with complications like pleural thickening or lung fibrosis after TB, this technique can significantly increase tidal volume and ease the sensation of breathlessness (Yang et al., 2022).

Pursed-lip breathing works by extending the exhalation phase, which helps prevent airway collapse and reduces air trapping. This makes it easier for the lungs to empty fully and enhances oxygen exchange. It's particularly beneficial for individuals with bronchiectasis or obstructive lung patterns following TB. Many patients also report feeling less shortness of breath when using this technique (Yang et al., 2022).

Inspiratory muscle training is another important method, especially for those with weakened breathing muscles. Using resistance-based devices or targeted breathing exercises, patients can gradually build diaphragm strength. Over time, this can lead to better maximal inspiratory pressure, improved stamina, and less frequent episodes of breathlessness (Spruit et al., 2013).

From a physiological perspective, these techniques help in many ways—they slow the breathing rate, increase the depth of each breath, improve alveolar ventilation, and enhance the match between ventilation and perfusion in the lungs. As a result, patients often experience greater breathing comfort, both at rest and during physical activity.

Psychosocial Support

Chronic respiratory diseases are frequently accompanied by psychological problems such as depression, anxiety, and social isolation. Therefore, psychological support holds a significant place in PR programs. By providing group therapy, individual counseling, and stress management training, patients' psychological well-being can be improved.

Patient Education and Behavior Change Techniques

PR is not limited to exercise alone; it also includes educating patients about their disease, medication use, nutrition, infection prevention, and pre- and post-exercise care. Enhancing patients' awareness of their health status increases their capacity for self-monitoring and appropriate response.

Behavior change strategies are supported through motivational interviewing techniques, goal setting, and self-monitoring education. This process helps patients make lasting changes in their lifestyle habits.

Effectiveness of Pulmonary Rehabilitation in General Respiratory Diseases

Randomized controlled trials and meta-analyses have consistently shown that PR offers meaningful benefits in managing symptoms, enhancing exercise capacity, and improving quality of life across various respiratory conditions—including COPD, asthma, interstitial lung diseases, and pulmonary complications following tuberculosis.

For patients with COPD, research has demonstrated that PR can lead to an average improvement of up to 50 meters in the 6MWT, along with notable reductions in dyspnea and significant gains in quality of life (Alene et al., 2024).

In individuals with asthma, PR has been shown to help reduce the frequency of symptoms, stabilize lung function, and improve overall well-being (Feng et al., 2021). Similarly, in cases of interstitial lung disease, studies have reported clear improvements in exercise tolerance following PR (Wytrychowski et al., 2020).

When it comes to patients recovering from tuberculosis, interest in the role of PR has been growing in recent years. A growing body of evidence suggests that PR can significantly enhance physical performance, respiratory function, and overall quality of life. This subject will be explored in more detail in the upcoming sections of this book.

EFFECTIVENESS OF PULMONARY REHABILITATION IN POST-TUBERCULOSIS PATIENTS

Permanent pulmonary sequelae that develop following TB can significantly impair respiratory function and lead to marked declines in quality of life. In this phase, where conventional treatment modalities may be insufficient, PR programs are increasingly recognized for their importance. PR has emerged as an effective approach to restoring both functional capacity and psychosocial well-being (Meca et al., 2022).

Findings on the Effectiveness of PR in the Literature

Recent randomized controlled trials (RCTs), meta-analyses, and case series have revealed the effects of PR in the post-TB period in detail.

Randomized Controlled Trials

RCTs evaluating the efficacy of PR after TB remain limited in number. However, the few existing studies indicate that PR can significantly improve respiratory function, exercise capacity, quality of life, and psychological well-being.

Wu et al. (2024) investigated the effectiveness of a Baduanjin exercise program based on doctor-nurse-patient integration in patients who had undergone lobectomy due to TB. In the intervention group, significant improvements were observed in FEV_1, FVC, and the 6MWT scores, along with notable reductions in exercise intolerance and dyspnea. These findings suggest that incorporating traditional cultural exercise techniques into post-TB PR programs can positively affect patients' physical capacity and quality of life (Wu et al., 2024).

In a 2021 RCT by Xu et al., the efficacy of respiratory function exercises was investigated in pulmonary TB patients treated at Wuhan Jinyintan Hospital. A total of 150 patients were randomly divided into two groups: the intervention group received comprehensive respiratory exercises in addition to routine care, while the control group received standard nursing care only. The intervention program included psychological support, patient education, pursed-lip breathing, abdominal breathing, mild aerobic exercises, and lifestyle modifications. The study showed significant improvements in FEV_1, FVC, and the FEV_1/FVC ratio in the intervention group. Additionally, the 6MWT distance increased significantly, dyspnea complaints (measured with the mMRC scale) decreased, and arterial blood gas analysis revealed higher PaO_2 levels and reduced $PaCO_2$. Quality of life scores and self-care capabilities also improved significantly compared to the control group. The authors emphasized that a multidisciplinary PR approach is critical to improving both physical and psychosocial outcomes in the post-TB period. The study demonstrated that PR positively influenced not only respiratory parameters but also patients' perceptions of their health and participation in daily activities. Integrating complementary strategies such as psychological support and disease management education with respiratory exercises could significantly enhance rehabilitation outcomes. However, the authors noted that the short intervention duration and lack of long-term follow-up limit the generalizability of the findings and highlight the need for further large-scale, long-term studies (Xu et al., 2021).

In another RCT conducted by Aytaç et al. (2024), the effect of respiratory exercises on fatigue in post-TB patients was evaluated. The intervention group received diaphragmatic breathing and pursed-lip breathing training three days a week for four weeks, supported by follow-up via phone and video calls. The control group received no intervention. Results showed a significant decrease in fatigue, as measured by the Piper Fatigue Scale; the average score dropped from 8.29 to 6.83 in the intervention group ($p<0.05$), with no significant change in the control group. This study highlighted the effectiveness of simple, low-cost breathing exercises in reducing fatigue in post-TB patients and emphasized the role of PR in maintaining physical well-being (Aytaç et al., 2024).

A study by Faurholt-Jepsen et al. (2013) showed that diabetes significantly increases the risk of mortality in TB patients, especially during the first 100 days of treatment. This finding underscores the importance of expanding PR programs to include metabolic comorbidities. Integrating protocols for glycemic control and diabetes management alongside respiratory training in post-TB rehabilitation could significantly improve patient outcomes (Faurholt-Jepsen et al., 2013).

Although RCTs examining the effectiveness of PR after TB remain limited, the available studies consistently demonstrate improvements in respiratory function, exercise capacity, and quality of life. Studies by Wu et al. (2024) and Xu et al. (2021) reported significant gains in pulmonary function (FEV_1, FVC), exercise capacity (6MWT), and quality of life (SF-36) (Wu et al., 2024; Xu et al., 2021). Aytaç et al. (2024) reported reductions in fatigue levels (Aytaç et al., 2024), while Faurholt-Jepsen et al. (2013) highlighted the importance of addressing metabolic comorbidities such as diabetes in PR programs (Faurholt-Jepsen et al., 2013).

Despite the small sample sizes, methodological differences, and short follow-up periods in current studies, the literature provides strong support for the use of PR in post-TB care. PR has been shown to contribute not only to physical recovery but also to psychosocial rehabilitation, underscoring the need for its routine inclusion in TB post-treatment care. Future research should prioritize large-scale, long-term, and multicenter RCTs to more robustly evaluate the long-term effects of PR in post-TB populations.

Meta-Analyses and Systematic Reviews

Meta-analyses and systematic review studies that directly address the effectiveness of PR in the post-TB period are quite limited. However, existing data demonstrate that PR provides significant improvements in both respiratory and psychosocial outcomes.

A comprehensive systematic review and meta-analysis conducted by Kefyalew Addis Alene et al. (2024) examined interventions applied in the management of post-TB pulmonary sequelae. The data included in the study revealed that PR programs have a significant therapeutic effect on pulmonary functions after TB. Particularly, significant increases were reported in spirometric parameters such as FEV_1 and FVC. In addition, PR applications were shown to have positive effects not only on respiratory physiology but also on patients' mental health; clinically meaningful reductions in anxiety and depression symptoms were recorded. According to the meta-analysis findings, PR interventions resulted in increased exercise capacity, decreased dyspnea complaints, and significant improvements in quality of life. It was especially emphasized that rehabilitation programs initiated early in the course of TB treatment yielded better results compared to those started later. This result suggests that PR should be considered an integral part of tuberculosis treatment. The study stated that the findings related to the effectiveness of PR offer strong evidence for reducing long-term morbidity after tuberculosis and improving health care services. In this context, a strong recommendation was made to integrate PR programs into standard care models in the post-TB period (Alene et al., 2024).

The study published by Muñoz-Torrico et al. (2016), although not in the format of a systematic review or meta-analysis, comprehensively addressed the clinical aspects of permanent lung damage after TB and the potential benefits of pulmonary rehabilitation in these patients as a narrative review. The study emphasized that a significant portion of patients in the post-TB period develop obstructive, restrictive, or mixed types of pulmonary function disorders, and experience a marked decline in quality of life. Muñoz-Torrico et al. (2016) recommended regular assessments of post-TB patients using spirometry, arterial blood gas analysis, the 6MWT, and quality of life scales. Furthermore, the study suggested that respiratory muscle training, programs to increase exercise tolerance, and, when necessary, long-term oxygen therapy during the rehabilitation process could significantly improve the functional capacities and quality of life of these patients. This narrative review emphasized that applying PR in the post-TB period not only provides symptomatic relief but also plays a critical role in reducing disease burden and improving quality of life. Therefore, the view that PR should be an integral part of standard care in the management of post-TB patients is supported by this study as well (Muñoz-Torrico et al., 2016).

It is apparent that the number of systematic reviews and meta-analyses directly examining the effectiveness of PR in the post-TB period is limited. However, the existing studies strongly support that PR provides significant and meaningful improvements in both respiratory and psychosocial parameters. In particular, early initiation of rehabilitation interventions leads to marked improvements in respiratory functions, exercise capacity, and quality of life. Nevertheless, given the complex nature of post-TB sequelae, the importance of individualized, multidisciplinary PR approaches is increasing. The findings obtained show that PR not only alleviates physical symptoms but also serves as a fundamental health service component in reducing long-term morbidity and maintaining patients' quality of life. Therefore, the systematic integration of pulmonary rehabilitation into post-TB care protocols is considered a critical necessity in future health policies

PULMONARY REHABILITATION PROGRAM DESIGN FOR PATIENTS WITH A HISTORY OF TUBERCULOSIS

TB sequelae can result in persistent respiratory dysfunction, exercise intolerance, and a significant decline in quality of life. PR is an evidence-based intervention package aimed at mitigating these sequelae and improving both physical and psychosocial well-being. Designing a PR program specifically tailored for individuals with a history of TB is of great importance in enhancing both clinical and social outcomes.

Pulmonary Function Tests

Pulmonary function tests are essential tools for evaluating lung health in individuals recovering from TB, and they play a key role in tailoring PR programs to each patient's needs. Commonly used assessments include spirometry, diffusion capacity measurements, and evaluations of respiratory performance during physical activity.

Spirometry remains the most frequently used test to assess pulmonary function in post-TB patients. By measuring FEV_1, FVC, and the FEV_1/FVC ratio, it helps identify airflow obstruction or volume restriction. Post-TB individuals may exhibit varying patterns depending on the nature of lung damage (Ko et al., 2015). For instance, in those who develop bronchiectasis or small airway disease, an obstructive pattern often emerges—characterized by a marked drop in FEV_1, a slight decrease in FVC, and a reduced FEV_1/FVC ratio. Bronchiectasis near cavitary lesions may increase airway resistance, contributing to this typical obstructive pattern (Choi et al., 2021).

In other cases, widespread fibrosis leads to a restrictive pattern, where both FEV_1 and FVC are decreased, but the FEV_1/FVC ratio remains normal or even elevated. Pleural thickening and fibrotic changes in the lungs limit their ability to expand fully, resulting in this type of dysfunction. Some patients present with both obstructive and restrictive features, known as a mixed pattern—common in advanced post-TB lung damage (Ravimohan et al., 2018).

DLCO is another valuable assessment, measuring how effectively gases transfer across the alveolar-capillary membrane. Post-TB fibrosis can reduce the alveolar surface area and damage capillaries, often leading to significantly impaired DLCO values. A result below 50%, for instance, may indicate impaired oxygenation during physical activity in a patient with post-TB fibrotic lung disease (Kiryukhina et al., 2023).

Air trapping and airway deformities are also common after TB, particularly around cavitary lesions. These changes can lead to increased residual volume and reduced inspiratory capacity. In more advanced testing like body plethysmography, these changes often manifest as elevated total lung capacity and markedly increased residual volume (Ong et al., 2014).

Assessing respiratory function during exercise is just as important. Exercise-induced oxygen desaturation—where oxygen levels drop significantly with activity—may indicate issues with gas exchange and V/Q mismatch. For example, if a patient with a resting oxygen saturation of 95% drops to 88% during the 6MWT, it strongly suggests a functional impairment that warrants inclusion in a PR program (Lama et al., 2003).

In summary, a comprehensive evaluation of lung function in post-TB patients provides critical information for designing effective, individualized rehabilitation strategies. These assessments not only help determine the severity of residual lung damage but also allow clinicians to track improvements and guide therapeutic decisions throughout the rehabilitation process.

Exercise Capacity and Functional Assessment

Structural damage to the lungs following TB often leads not only to impaired respiratory function but also to a marked decline in exercise capacity. For this reason, conducting a thorough evaluation of a patient's physical performance before initiating PR is essential. Such assessments help establish a baseline and allow clinicians to monitor progress throughout the rehabilitation journey.

The 6MWT is one of the most commonly used methods to assess functional capacity in individuals recovering from TB. It measures the distance a person can walk on a flat surface at their own pace over six minutes. In post-TB patients, structural lung damage—such as fibrosis, bronchiectasis, and pleural thickening—often results in significantly reduced walking distances. While healthy adults typically cover 500 to 550 meters, individuals with post-TB lung fibrosis may only manage 300 to 400 meters. Additionally, a drop in oxygen saturation of more than 4% during the test may signal impaired gas exchange or a V/Q mismatch. Dyspnea and hypoxemia are frequently reported during exertion in this patient group (Salman Latif et al., 2022).

Oxygen desaturation during exercise is a common finding in the post-TB phase, especially in those with reduced diffusion capacity and limited alveolar surface area. In such cases, peripheral oxygen saturation can fall below 88% during activity, reflecting the detrimental effects of vascular damage and fibrotic processes on pulmonary gas exchange (Lama et al., 2003).

To provide a more nuanced evaluation of exercise capacity, additional protocols such as the Incremental Shuttle Walk Test (ISWT) and the Endurance Shuttle Walk Test (ESWT) may also be employed. These tests assess the individual's ability to maintain an increasing walking pace, and post-TB patients with respiratory limitations typically perform significantly below average on these measures (Ono et al., 2022).

Beyond physical capacity, it is also important to consider how the disease affects daily life. Many post-TB patients experience pronounced shortness of breath and fatigue during routine activities like climbing stairs, performing household chores, or walking longer distances. These limitations can lead to physical deconditioning and social withdrawal (Lee et al., 2016). Quality of life assessments using instruments like the Short Form-36 (SF-36) and the St. George's Respiratory Questionnaire (SGRQ) help quantify the negative impact on physical function, social participation, and perceived health status (Hussain et al., 2024).

Functional performance tests are also critical components of comprehensive assessment. The Sit-to-Stand Test evaluates lower limb strength and endurance, while the Timed Up and Go test is useful for assessing mobility, balance, and gait speed (Sancar et al., 2024). Post-TB patients, particularly those with muscle loss and reduced physical tolerance, often score significantly lower than their healthy counterparts on these evaluations.

In summary, diminished exercise capacity after TB is a multifaceted issue influenced by both respiratory dysfunction and musculoskeletal deficits. Therefore, a comprehensive functional assessment is not just beneficial but essential in guiding the development of a personalized pulmonary rehabilitation plan. These evaluations also support goal setting and improve patient engagement and adherence to rehabilitation interventions.

Dyspnea Assessment Scales

In the post-TB period, one of the most frequently reported complaints among patients is persistent dyspnea. Dyspnea not only leads to physical limitations but also significantly impairs patients' quality of life. Therefore, objectively assessing the severity of dyspnea before and after PR programs is of great importance. Various clinically validated scales are used for dyspnea assessment.

The Modified Medical Research Council (mMRC) Dyspnea Scale is one of the most commonly used tools in post-TB patients. Due to its simplicity and quick application, it is widely preferred in clinical practice. The scale categorizes dyspnea into five levels (Hussain et al., 2024):

0: Dyspnea only during strenuous exercise
1: Dyspnea when walking briskly or climbing a slight hill
2: Stops for breath when walking at own pace compared to others
3: Stops for breath after walking 100 meters or after a few minutes on level ground
4: Too breathless to leave the house or breathless when dressing/undressing

The Borg Dyspnea Scale offers a more dynamic assessment, especially useful during exercise. Patients are asked to rate their perceived breathlessness on a scale from 0 (no breathlessness) to 10 (maximum breathlessness). This method is particularly helpful for monitoring changes before and after exercise testing or PR sessions (Mehmood et al., 2024). Although more detailed scales like the Baseline Dyspnea Index and Transition Dyspnea Index also exist in the literature, the mMRC and Borg scales are more commonly used in routine practice for post-TB patients due to their practicality.

The use of dyspnea scales is a critical tool in identifying functional limitations following TB and tracking the effectiveness of rehabilitation interventions. Additionally, these scales provide valuable insight into the correlation between subjective complaints and objective functional test results. In the context of PR, improvements in dyspnea scores serve not only as indicators of treatment success for clinicians but also as motivational factors for patients.

Quality of Life Assessment

Permanent lung damage after TB doesn't just affect respiratory function—it also has a profound impact on a patient's overall quality of life. Individuals recovering from TB often face a range of physical and emotional challenges, including chronic shortness of breath, reduced exercise capacity, fatigue, social withdrawal, and psychological stress. These factors combined can lead to a significant decline in well-being. That's why assessing quality of life in a structured way before starting PR is essential.

One of the most commonly used tools for this purpose is the SF-36 questionnaire. This instrument evaluates eight key aspects of health, covering both physical and mental domains: physical functioning, role limitations due to physical health, bodily pain, general health perceptions, vitality, social functioning, emotional role limitations, and mental health. In people recovering from TB, scores are often particularly low in the areas of physical functioning and vitality, highlighting how the disease impacts everyday activities and perceptions of health (Wong et al., 2021).

Another widely recognized tool is the SGRQ, which is tailored specifically to chronic respiratory conditions. It examines symptoms, activity limitations, and the overall impact of the disease. Patients who develop complications like bronchiectasis or lung fibrosis following TB often show elevated SGRQ scores, reflecting the heavy burden of these conditions on their daily life (Wong et al., 2021).

In addition to these disease-specific tools, the EQ-5D instrument is frequently used in clinical and health economic studies to provide a standardized measure of health status. EQ-5D evaluates five key dimensions: mobility, self-care, usual activities, pain/discomfort, and anxiety/depression. It also includes a visual analog scale (VAS) for patients to rate their overall health on a scale from 0 to 100. Among TB survivors, the EQ-5D has been shown to capture substantial impairments in mobility and daily functioning, as well as heightened levels of psychological distress. Its simplicity and versatility make it a valuable tool for tracking changes in health-related quality of life over time and for comparing outcomes across different rehabilitation programs (Park et al., 2021).

These assessments are not only valuable for establishing a baseline but also for monitoring changes during rehabilitation and tailoring interventions to meet individual needs. Research in post-TB populations consistently shows that patients participating in structured rehabilitation programs report meaningful improvements in quality of life. For this reason, quality of life evaluations—using tools like the SF-36, SGRQ, and EQ-5D —should be considered standard practice in post-TB care and rehabilitation planning (Park et al., 2021; Wong et al., 2021).

Exercise Prescription: Aerobic, Resistance, and Respiratory Muscle Training

Permanent lung damage developed during the post-TB period may lead to reduced exercise capacity, muscle weakness, and respiratory muscle insufficiency in patients. One of the core components of PR programs, exercise training aims to address these impairments and improve patients' level of functional independence. The exercise prescription should be planned with an individualized approach and structured to enhance both aerobic capacity and muscle strength.

Aerobic Exercises

Aerobic exercises play a significant role in reducing exertional dyspnea by improving cardiopulmonary endurance. In the post-TB period, aerobic capacity may be markedly reduced due to gas exchange impairments and hypoxemia (Ono et al.,

2022). Therefore, low-intensity aerobic training with gradual progression is recommended. As a fundamental component of PR, aerobic exercises are implemented to compensate for reduced exercise tolerance and physical inactivity commonly observed in individuals recovering from TB. In these individuals, especially due to fibrosis and impaired gas exchange, cardiopulmonary reserve may be limited; thus, regularly and carefully planned aerobic activities can yield symptomatic improvement and enhance quality of life.

In the systematic review protocol by da Silva et al. (2022), aerobic exercise prescriptions in the post-TB period were examined in detail (da Silva et al., 2022). RCTs in the literature commonly recommend walking, stationary cycling, and low-intensity jogging. These exercises are generally conducted in hospital- or community-based settings; during sessions, oxygen saturation, heart rate, and perceived exertion (e.g., Borg scale) are monitored.

Exercise intensity is often set between 50–70% of the individual's maximum heart rate, and in some programs, exercise intensity is adjusted based on subjective perceived exertion (Borg scale 11–13). Sessions typically last between 20–40 minutes and are performed 3–5 days per week. Program durations generally range from 6 to 12 weeks. During this period, significant improvements in exercise tolerance, reductions in dyspnea scores, and enhancements in functional capacity have been reported (da Silva et al., 2022).

It is recommended to suspend exercise when oxygen saturation drops below 88% during a session, and supplemental oxygen should be provided if necessary (Dogra et al., 2015). These precautions ensure safe practice and maximize physiological gains.

These findings underscore the importance of individualized and supervised aerobic exercise implementation within PR protocols for post-TB patients. Gradually progressing exercise prescriptions that start at low intensity are essential for improving functional independence and supporting psychosocial well-being in individuals coping with TB-related sequelae.

Resistance (Strength) Exercises

Muscle weakness, reduced tolerance to physical activity, and impaired quality of life are common challenges following TB, making resistance training a necessary component of PR programs. In individuals who have recovered from TB, especially those experiencing prolonged bed rest, malnutrition, or hypoxemia, peripheral muscle atrophy is frequently observed (da Silva et al., 2022). These deficits can lead to decreased walking distance, difficulty climbing stairs, and dependency in daily living activities.

Resistance exercises should be designed to target major muscle groups, incorporating both upper and lower extremities. Key muscle groups to focus on include quadriceps, hamstrings, deltoids, biceps, and triceps. Exercises may utilize elastic resistance bands, free weights, or bodyweight (Cosaburi, 1992).

Exercise intensity should be tailored to the individual's baseline muscle strength, generally beginning at 40–60% of their one-repetition maximum. It is recommended to perform resistance training 2–3 times per week, with 1–2 sets of 8–12 repetitions for each muscle group. As sessions progress, the number of sets and repetitions can be gradually increased. Symptoms such as fatigue, muscle soreness, or cardiopulmonary stress should be closely monitored, and rest intervals or intensity should be adjusted accordingly (da Silva et al., 2022).

In addition to improving muscle strength and endurance, resistance training helps increase bone mineral density by applying mechanical load to the musculoskeletal system—offering protective benefits against osteopenia and osteoporosis, particularly in older TB survivors. Furthermore, regular strength training may enhance glucose metabolism and thus provide added value in managing comorbid conditions such as diabetes, which is commonly associated with TB (Zhang et al., 2022).

In summary, resistance training in post-TB individuals not only enhances physical performance but also improves overall health and functional independence, making it an essential component of any PR program.

Inspiratory Muscle Training (IMT)

During the post-TB period, many patients develop both restrictive and obstructive breathing patterns that can affect not only lung tissue but also the strength of the respiratory muscles. Factors such as chronic low oxygen levels, poor nutrition, and long periods of physical inactivity can weaken the diaphragm and accessory breathing muscles. This often leads to increased breathlessness during exertion and further reduces the ability to stay active. To address this, IMT should be considered a key part of PR programs (Spruit et al., 2013).

IMT uses resistance-based breathing exercises to strengthen the muscles used for inhalation. Devices like the Threshold IMT, PowerBreathe, or Spirotiger allow patients to breathe in against controlled resistance, helping to build respiratory muscle strength (Britto et al., 2014). Research has shown that IMT can significantly improve exercise tolerance, reduce the sensation of breathlessness, and enhance overall quality of life, making it an essential element of comprehensive PR programs (da Silva et al., 2022).

Training is typically recommended five times a week, with sessions lasting 15 to 30 minutes. The intensity is usually set between 30–60% of the patient's maximum inspiratory pressure and adjusted over time as strength improves. IMT is often combined with other breathing strategies such as diaphragmatic breathing, segmented inhalation, short exhalation techniques, and lung re-expansion exercises. To ensure safety and effectiveness, patients should undergo respiratory function assessments before beginning the training (Ammous et al., 2023).

In summary, IMT is a practical, affordable, and highly effective way to help post-TB patients manage breathlessness and regain physical function. For these reasons, it is strongly recommended as a standard component of pulmonary rehabilitation programs.

Breathing Exercises and Airway Clearance Techniques

In the post-TB period, decreased pulmonary function, accumulation of secretions in the airways, and V/Q imbalances are common problems (Gai et al., 2023). Therefore, respiratory techniques and airway clearance methods must be a critical component of pulmonary rehabilitation programs.

Breathing Exercises

Breathing exercises aim to ensure more efficient use of the patient's respiratory muscles and reduce the work of breathing. One of the most commonly applied methods in this context is diaphragmatic breathing. In diaphragmatic breathing, patients are taught to take deep and slow breaths using their abdominal area. This technique helps to prevent excessive use of accessory respiratory muscles, decreases respiratory effort, and enables more effective ventilation. Most importantly, diaphragmatic breathing is the closest to physiological respiration, it enhances ventilation especially in the lower lobes of the lungs and ensures homogeneous ventilation of the entire lung. Using diaphragmatic breathing during exercise or dyspnea attacks can increase respiratory comfort, especially in individuals who have developed restrictive lung disease after TB (Nicola Martins Rodrigues et al., 2021).

Another effective technique is pursed-lip breathing. In this method, after inhaling deeply through the nose, the patient exhales in a controlled manner by pursing their lips. Pursed-lip breathing prolongs the expiratory phase and creates positive end-expiratory pressure in the airways, thereby preventing airway collapse and reducing air trapping (Ernstmeyer & Christman, 2024). Especially in TB sequelae with bronchiectasis or obstructive patterns, this technique helps respiratory muscles work more efficiently, keeps the airways open, and thus reduces effort during breathing (Noor et al., 2024).

Airway Clearance Techniques

Airway clearance techniques are of great importance for reducing secretion accumulation and lowering the risk of infection. Methods such as postural drainage, chest physiotherapy, and the active cycle of breathing techniques (ACBT) are used for this purpose. In postural drainage, the patient's body position is changed to allow gravity to help move secretions to the larger airways. Chest percussion and vibration make it easier to mobilize secretions. ACBT consists of a combination of controlled breathing, huffing (forced expiration maneuver), and effective coughing techniques. This technique is particularly effective in post-TB bronchiectatic patients who produce large amounts of sputum (Herrero-Cortina et al., 2023).

In addition, mechanically assisted methods such as positive expiratory pressure devices or flutter devices can also be used to increase secretion mobilization. These devices generate positive pressure in the airways during expiration, centralizing the mucus and allowing it to be expelled easily through coughing (Herrero-Cortina et al., 2023).

Although detailed studies on airway clearance techniques in tuberculosis are limited, these methods—which have been shown to be effective in many lung diseases—are among the indispensable elements in the management of post-tuberculosis pulmonary sequelae in terms of reducing dyspnea, improving gas exchange, and lowering infection frequency. Regular implementation of these techniques increases the effectiveness of pulmonary rehabilitation programs and provides significant contributions to the quality of life of patients (Herrero-Cortina et al., 2023).

Nutritional Support and Psychological Counseling

In the post-TB period, not only respiratory conditions but also the metabolic and psychological status of patients can be seriously affected. Therefore, nutritional support and psychological counseling are important components of an effective PR program.

Nutritional Support

Nutritional support aims to correct weight loss, loss of muscle mass, and general malnutrition seen in the acute phase of tuberculosis. Increased catabolism and decreased appetite during TB infection can lead to serious losses in body mass. Low body mass index and muscle wasting observed in post-TB patients also negatively affect the strength of respiratory muscles, contributing to decreased exercise capacity. Therefore, the energy, protein, vitamin, and mineral requirements of individuals should be carefully assessed during the PR process. Adequate protein intake is particularly critical for supporting the function of respiratory muscles. If necessary, oral nutritional supplements or medical nutrition products can be used (Papathakis & Piwoz, 2008).

Moreover, due to metabolic complications such as secondary diabetes or glucose intolerance commonly seen in TB patients, the creation of individualized nutrition programs is essential. If diabetes is present, dietary recommendations that support glycemic control should be made, and foods with a high glycemic index should be avoided (Krishna & Jacob, 2021). When malnutrition persists, both the risk of infection increases and the effectiveness of PR applications decreases (Li et al., 2023). Therefore, it is necessary to monitor patients regularly with anthropometric measurements and laboratory parameters to assess the effectiveness of nutritional interventions.

Psychological Counseling

Psychological counseling plays a critical role in managing mental health problems such as anxiety, depression, and social isolation that may arise in the post-TB period. Both the disease process and its sequelae can trigger negative thoughts in individuals such as "not fully recovered," "fear of becoming ill again," and "social exclusion." Studies have shown that the prevalence of depression and anxiety is significantly higher in TB survivors compared to the general population (Lara-Espinosa & Hernández-Pando, 2021).

Regular psychological assessments within PR programs are of great importance for increasing patient motivation and ensuring adherence to exercise programs. For this purpose, short psychological scales (e.g., Hospital Anxiety and Depression Scale - HADS) can be used. In addition, during the psychological support process, patients can be taught stress management, breathing relaxation techniques, yoga, and positive coping strategies (Srinivas et al., 2024). For individuals who need advanced psychological support, professional psychotherapy should be planned.

Nutritional support and psychological counseling are fundamental elements that directly impact the success of PR, improve the overall health status of patients, and facilitate the achievement of long-term rehabilitation goals. The systematic integration of these two components into the pulmonary rehabilitation protocol is of vital importance for reducing post-TB morbidity and improving patients' quality of life.

POST-TUBERCULOSIS REHABILITATION: PRACTICAL APPROACHES AND REGIONAL ADAPTATION MODELS

Following TB treatment, long-term lung damage remains a significant public health issue, affecting the quality of life for millions around the world. PR has proven to be an effective approach in addressing these post-TB complications. However, how PR programs are delivered often varies based on geographical, socioeconomic, and healthcare system differences. This chapter explores the various PR models used in the post-TB context, focusing on how well they adapt to different field settings and regional conditions. It places particular emphasis on alternative strategies developed in LMICs, such as telerehabilitation, community-based programs, and culturally tailored educational materials. The chapter also discusses practical solutions for improving access to and the long-term sustainability of rehabilitation services.

Rehabilitation Models Implemented Across Different Countries and Continents

Post-TB PR practices vary significantly based on countries' socioeconomic levels, health infrastructure, service delivery models, and epidemiological burdens. Although PR generally follows a universal framework, its implementation and accessibility are closely tied to the structural organization of national health systems.

In high-income countries, PR is predominantly delivered through structured, standardized, and multidisciplinary hospital-based programs. For instance, in the United Kingdom, PR programs offered within the National Health Service are structured in accordance with NICE guidelines and have increasingly expanded to include post-TB patients. These programs actively involve physiotherapists, respiratory therapists, psychologists, and nutritionists (Hopkinson, Molyneux, Pink, & Harrisingh, 2019). Similarly, in Canada, PR programs for post-TB care are conducted primarily in large urban academic hospitals and are supported by advanced monitoring systems (Menzies, 2022).

In contrast, in LMICs, PR services are more commonly delivered through community-based models due to resource limitations and shortages of trained personnel. Countries such as India, Indonesia, Nigeria, and Ethiopia—where TB prevalence is high—face an increased need for PR services but often lack the health infrastructure to systematically address this demand. Consequently, PR in these regions is often implemented using a task-shifting approach, whereby community health workers, nurses, or physiotherapy aides deliver care. For example, in an intervention study in India, Accredited Social Health Activists successfully administered home-based respiratory exercise programs (Petil Jr & Caballero, 2025).

In Latin American countries, a strong focus on pharmacological treatments for TB and a concentration of healthcare services in tertiary care centers like university hospitals pose significant barriers to access for rural patients (Barreto-Duarte et al., 2024). In countries like Brazil, national guidelines for post-TB rehabilitation are still underdeveloped, leading to gaps in standardization and widening regional disparities.

In many African countries, where TB prevalence is high, pulmonary rehabilitation services are still in a developmental phase. While a limited number of pilot community-based PR initiatives have been launched in South Africa, their expansion at a national level has yet to be achieved. A systematic review by Okeke et al. (2025) covering sub-Saharan Africa found that the most common post-TB morbidities include persistent loss of pulmonary function, bronchiectasis, fibrotic lesions, and mental health disorders (particularly depression and anxiety). These findings highlight the need for PR programs to be structured to include not only physical but also psychosocial components. However, across the continent, infrastructure limitations—such as inadequate electricity, internet access, and equipment—hinder the widespread adoption of remote rehabilitation solutions like telerehabilitation. Moreover, shortages of healthcare workers, the inability to form multidisciplinary teams, and integration issues within public health systems further restrict the sustainability and effectiveness of PR services. These challenges underscore the urgent need for comprehensive rehabilitation planning and expansion to reduce post-TB morbidity across Africa (Okeke et al., 2025).

The diversity in rehabilitation models across countries reveals significant inequalities in the availability and effectiveness of post-TB pulmonary rehabilitation. While high-income countries tend to implement hospital-based, interdisciplinary programs in accordance with established standards, LMICs rely on community-based and task-sharing approaches due to limited resources and personnel. In regions like Latin America and Africa, structural and systemic barriers to PR implementation remain persistent. Therefore, the global delivery of PR must be adapted to local needs through cost-effective, accessible, and culturally appropriate models integrated into national healthcare systems. Moreover, expanding PR services should address not only physical recovery but also the psychosocial challenges that emerge during the post-TB period. This highlights the necessity for global health strategies that are both multidisciplinary and holistic.

Telerehabilitation Practices: Opportunities and Limitations

Telerehabilitation has emerged as an accessible, cost-effective, and innovative strategy for supporting pulmonary rehabilitation in individuals recovering from TB. Its adoption has grown notably since the COVID-19 pandemic accelerated the digital transformation of healthcare systems. These programs typically include a combination of video-guided exercise sessions, mobile health apps, remote monitoring tools, and educational content. Together, these components enable patients to safely engage in rehabilitation from the comfort of their homes, reducing transportation barriers and easing the strain on healthcare facilities.

A compelling example of its clinical usefulness comes from a case study by Sonone et al. (2022). A 52-year-old patient with post-TB lung damage transitioned from a hospital-based program to a home-based telerehabilitation schedule involving video calls three times per week. Over time, the patient showed remarkable improvements: the 6MWT distance increased from 260 to 400 meters, and the dyspnea score (measured via mMRC) dropped from 3 to 1. These outcomes underscore both the physical and psychological benefits of telerehabilitation (Sonone et al., 2022).

Similarly, Pooja Jain and colleagues documented another case in which a patient first received inpatient therapy—such as chest physiotherapy, segmental breathing exercises, and airway clearance techniques—and later continued the regimen at home via telerehabilitation. Weekly check-ins, tailored exercise modifications, and motivational support helped maintain high levels of adherence. By the end of the program, the patient experienced substantial improvements in both functional capacity and fatigue (Srinivas et al., 2024).

Still, the success of telerehabilitation hinges on more than just access to technology. It also requires adequate digital literacy, training for healthcare professionals in remote care delivery, sustained patient motivation, and continuous monitoring. These factors can be particularly challenging in LMICs, where limited internet access, unstable electricity, and cultural barriers can hinder implementation.

Moreover, current scientific evidence is limited by the lack of standardized telerehabilitation protocols specifically designed for TB patients, and there is a need for more long-term data. Most available studies focus on short-term outcomes, often neglecting essential aspects like mental health, psychosocial support, and nutritional counseling. Despite these limitations, telerehabilitation stands out as a promising and scalable option due to its low cost, flexibility, and wide reach. Future research should prioritize high-quality randomized controlled trials, explore long-term impacts, and develop integrated models that bring together multidisciplinary care.

CONCLUSION

In the post-TB period, PR plays a crucial role in enhancing quality of life and addressing long-term respiratory complications. The scientific and clinical evidence discussed in this section highlights the importance of rehabilitation programs that go beyond physical recovery to also include psychosocial support. While multidisciplinary, hospital-based rehabilitation models are standard in high-income countries, community-based and resource-sensitive approaches are more common in low- and middle-income regions. Disparities between rural and urban areas, along with differences in healthcare infrastructure and cultural factors, underscore the need for locally adapted service models.

Innovative solutions like telerehabilitation offer promising alternatives, particularly for patients with limited access to in-person care. However, barriers such as inadequate digital infrastructure and low health literacy continue to challenge broader implementation. Case studies demonstrate that telerehabilitation is both feasible and beneficial, yet they also point to a lack of standardized, TB-specific protocols—highlighting the need for further development in this area.

In this context, it is essential to standardize rehabilitation services, support them through national-level policies, and consider pulmonary rehabilitation as an indispensable component of post-TB care. Furthermore, the development of cost-effective, accessible, and culturally acceptable models tailored to local needs is a priority for ensuring the sustainability of rehabilitation practices. Future research should comprehensively evaluate the long-term impacts of telerehabilitation, the outcomes of multidisciplinary models, and their effectiveness across different socioeconomic groups.

REFERENCES

Abaei, E., Abedi, M., Sadat Mirenayat, M., & Rezaei, M. (2023). The Effect of High-Intensity Interval Training in People With Respiratory Disease: A Review Study. *The Scientific Journal of Rehabilitation Medicine, 12*(1), 18–29. DOI: 10.32598/SJRM.12.1.12

Alene, K. A., Hertzog, L., Gilmour, B., Clements, A. C., & Murray, M. B. (2024). Interventions to prevent post-tuberculosis sequelae: A systematic review and meta-analysis. *EClinicalMedicine, 70*, 70. DOI: 10.1016/j.eclinm.2024.102511 PMID: 38434448

Allwood, B. W., Byrne, A., Meghji, J., Rachow, A., van der Zalm, M. M., & Schoch, O. D. (2021). Post-tuberculosis lung disease: Clinical review of an under-recognised global challenge. *Respiration, 100*(8), 751–763. DOI: 10.1159/000512531 PMID: 33401266

Ammous, O., Feki, W., Lotfi, T., Khamis, A. M., Gosselink, R., Rebai, A., & Kammoun, S. (2023). Inspiratory muscle training, with or without concomitant pulmonary rehabilitation, for chronic obstructive pulmonary disease (COPD). *Cochrane Database of Systematic Reviews*, 1. PMID: 36606682

Aytaç, S., Ovayolu, Ö., & Dogru, S. (2024). The effect of breathing exercises on fatigue in tuberculosis patients: A randomized controlled trial. *Revista da Associação Médica Brasileira, 70*(12), e20240888. DOI: 10.1590/1806-9282.20240888 PMID: 39630726

Barreto-Duarte, B., Villalva-Serra, K., Campos, V. M., Cordeiro-Santos, M., Kritski, A. L., Araújo-Pereira, M., Rodrigues, M. M., & Andrade, B. B. (2024). Nationwide economic analysis of pulmonary tuberculosis in the Brazilian healthcare system over seven years (2015–2022): A population-based study. *Lancet Regional Health. Americas, 39*, 39. DOI: 10.1016/j.lana.2024.100905 PMID: 39839682

Britto, R. R., Brant, T. C. S., & Parreira, V. F. (2014). Recursos Manuais e Instrumentais em Fisioterapia Respiratória [rev. ampl.]. In: Manole.

Byrne, A. L., Marais, B. J., Mitnick, C. D., Lecca, L., & Marks, G. B. (2015). Tuberculosis and chronic respiratory disease: A systematic review. *International Journal of Infectious Diseases, 32*, 138–146. DOI: 10.1016/j.ijid.2014.12.016 PMID: 25809770

Casaburi, R. (2008). A brief history of pulmonary rehabilitation. *Respiratory Care, 53*(9), 1185–1189. PMID: 18718037

Chatterjee, R., Ghosh, P., Sarkar, K., Samajdar, S. S., Mukherjee, S., George, A., & Pramanik, N. (2023). Prevalence of pulmonary arterial hypertension in post-tuberculosis lung fibrosis patients: A cross-sectional observational study. *Journal of Association of Chest Physicians*, *11*(4), 198–201. DOI: 10.4103/jacp.jacp_11_23

Choi, H., Lee, H., Ra, S. W., Kim, H. K., Lee, J. S., Um, S.-J., Kim, S.-H., Oh, Y.-M., & Kwon, Y.-S. (2021). Clinical characteristics of patients with post-tuberculosis bronchiectasis: Findings from the KMBARC registry. *Journal of Clinical Medicine*, *10*(19), 4542. DOI: 10.3390/jcm10194542 PMID: 34640560

Chung, M. J., Goo, J. M., & Im, J.-G. (2004). Pulmonary tuberculosis in patients with idiopathic pulmonary fibrosis. *European Journal of Radiology*, *52*(2), 175–179. DOI: 10.1016/j.ejrad.2003.11.017 PMID: 15489076

Cosaburi, R. (1992). Principles of exercise training. *Chest*, *101*(5), 263S–267S. DOI: 10.1378/chest.101.5_Supplement.263S PMID: 1576847

da Silva, T. S., Arêas, G. P. T., & da Cruz, D. A. L. M. (2022). Effect of pulmonary rehabilitation on functional capacity in individuals treated for pulmonary tuberculosis: A systematic review protocol. *JBI Evidence Synthesis*, *20*(10), 2552–2558. DOI: 10.11124/JBIES-21-00314 PMID: 36081386

Dartois, V., & Rubin, E. J. (2023). Shortening tuberculosis treatment—A strategic retreat. *The New England Journal of Medicine*, *388*(10), 939–941. DOI: 10.1056/NEJMe2300413 PMID: 36807402

Desai, J. P., & Moustarah, F. (2022). Pulmonary compliance. In *StatPearls* [Internet]. StatPearls Publishing.

Devassy, T. V., Nishanth, P., Sharma, D., & Thomas, A. M. (2022). Sleep disorders in elderly population suffering from TB and respiratory diseases. *The Indian Journal of Tuberculosis*, *69*, S272–S279. DOI: 10.1016/j.ijtb.2022.10.019 PMID: 36400523

Dietiker, F., Lester, W., Gottlieb, R., & Burrows, B. (1961). Single-breath pulmonary diffusing capacity measurements in patients with pulmonary tuberculosis. *The American Review of Respiratory Disease*, *84*(6), 807–813. PMID: 13886305

Dogra, A. C., Gupta, U., Sarkar, M., & Padam, A. (2015). Exercise-induced desaturation in patients with chronic obstructive pulmonary disease on six-minute walk test. *Lung India : Official Organ of Indian Chest Society*, *32*(4), 320–325. DOI: 10.4103/0970-2113.159550 PMID: 26180379

Dos Santos, A., Lazzari, T. K., & Silva, D. R. (2017). Health-related quality of life, depression and anxiety in hospitalized patients with tuberculosis. *Tuberculosis and Respiratory Diseases*, *80*(1), 69–76. DOI: 10.4046/trd.2017.80.1.69 PMID: 28119749

Dowman, L., Hill, C. J., May, A., & Holland, A. E. (2021). Pulmonary rehabilitation for interstitial lung disease. *Cochrane Database of Systematic Reviews*, *2*(2), Cd006322. DOI: 10.1002/14651858.CD006322.pub4 PMID: 34559419

Ernstmeyer, K., & Christman, E. (2024). OXYGENATION. *Nursing Fundamentals [Internet]. 2nd edition.*

Faurholt-Jepsen, D., Range, N., PrayGod, G., Jeremiah, K., Faurholt-Jepsen, M., Aabye, M. G., Changalucha, J., Christensen, D. L., Grewal, H. M. S., Martinussen, T., Krarup, H., Witte, D. R., Andersen, A. B., & Friis, H. (2013). Diabetes is a strong predictor of mortality during tuberculosis treatment: A prospective cohort study among tuberculosis patients from M wanza, T anzania. *Tropical Medicine & International Health*, *18*(7), 822–829. DOI: 10.1111/tmi.12120 PMID: 23648145

Feng, Z., Wang, J., Xie, Y., & Li, J. (2021). Effects of exercise-based pulmonary rehabilitation on adults with asthma: A systematic review and meta-analysis. *Respiratory Research*, *22*(1), 1–12. DOI: 10.1186/s12931-021-01627-w PMID: 33516207

Fong, I., Low, T. B., & Yii, A. (2022). Characterisation of the post-tuberculous phenotype of bronchiectasis: A real-world observational study. *Chronic Respiratory Disease*, *19*, 14799731221098714. DOI: 10.1177/14799731221098714 PMID: 35471849

Gai, X., Allwood, B., & Sun, Y. (2023). Post-tuberculosis lung disease and chronic obstructive pulmonary disease. *Chinese Medical Journal*, *136*(16), 1923–1928. DOI: 10.1097/CM9.0000000000002771 PMID: 37455331

Hanekom, S., Pharaoh, H., Irusen, E., & Daniels, K. J. (2019). Post-tuberculosis health-related quality of life, lung function and exercise capacity in a cured pulmonary tuberculosis population in the Breede Valley District, South Africa. *The South African Journal of Physiotherapy*, *75*(1), 1–8. PMID: 31392293

Haribhau, B. D. (2015). Study of polysomnography in cure post-tuberculosis patients. *Journal of Evolution of Medical and Dental Sciences*, *4*(67), 11616–11626. DOI: 10.14260/jemds/2015/1676

Harms, C. A., Wetter, T. J., St. Croix, C. M., Pegelow, D. F., & Dempsey, J. A. (2000). Effects of respiratory muscle work on exercise performance. *Journal of Applied Physiology*, *89*(1), 131–138. DOI: 10.1152/jappl.2000.89.1.131 PMID: 10904044

Herrero-Cortina, B., Lee, A. L., Oliveira, A., O'Neill, B., Jácome, C., Dal Corso, S., Poncin, W., Muñoz, G., Inal-Ince, D., Alcaraz-Serrano, V., Reychler, G., Bellofiore, A., Posthumus, A., Tonia, T., Chalmers, J. D., & Spinou, A. (2023). European Respiratory Society statement on airway clearance techniques in adults with bronchiectasis. *The European Respiratory Journal*, *62*(1), 2202053. DOI: 10.1183/13993003.02053-2022 PMID: 37142337

Hill, N. S. (2006). Pulmonary rehabilitation. *Proceedings of the American Thoracic Society*, *3*(1), 66–74. DOI: 10.1513/pats.200511-121JH PMID: 16493153

Hussain, A., Khurana, A. K., Goyal, A., Kothari, S., Soman, R. K., Tej, S., & Pakhare, A. (2024). Effect of pulmonary rehabilitation in patients with post-tuberculosis sequelae with functional limitation. *The Indian Journal of Tuberculosis*, *71*(2), 123–129. DOI: 10.1016/j.ijtb.2023.04.012 PMID: 38589115

Ivanova, O., Hoffmann, V. S., Lange, C., Hoelscher, M., & Rachow, A. (2023). Post-tuberculosis lung impairment: Systematic review and meta-analysis of spirometry data from 14 621 people. *European Respiratory Review : an Official Journal of the European Respiratory Society*, *32*(168), 220221. DOI: 10.1183/16000617.0221-2022 PMID: 37076175

Jaligidad, K. (2016). *Study of Prevalence of Cor Pulmonale in Patients with Pulmonary Tuberculosis with Reference to ECG, Echocardiographic Changes and Radiological Extent of the Disease.* Rajiv Gandhi University of Health Sciences.

Jones, S. A., Biswas, N., & Davies, H. E. (2025). Tuberculosis Related Pleural Effusion: An Update. *Current Pulmonology Reports*, *14*(1), 9. DOI: 10.1007/s13665-025-00373-4

Kiryukhina, L. D., Kokorina, E. V., Gavrilov, P. V., Denisova, N. V., Archakova, L. I., & Yablonskiy, P. K. (2023). Gas Exchange in Patients with Pulmonary Tuberculosis: Relationships with Pulmonary Poorly Communicating Fraction and Alveolar Volume. *Journal of Respiration*, *3*(2), 107–117. DOI: 10.3390/jor3020011

Ko, Y., Lee, Y., Lee, H., Lee, Y., Song, J., Hong, G., Kim, M., Lee, H., Choi, S., & Shim, E. (2015). Changes in lung function according to disease extent before and after pulmonary tuberculosis. *The International Journal of Tuberculosis and Lung Disease : the Official Journal of the International Union against Tuberculosis and Lung Disease*, *19*(5), 589–595. DOI: 10.5588/ijtld.14.0454 PMID: 25868029

Krishna, S., & Jacob, J. J. (2021). Diabetes mellitus and tuberculosis.

Lama, V. N., Flaherty, K. R., Toews, G. B., Colby, T. V., Travis, W. D., Long, Q., Murray, S., Kazerooni, E. A., Gross, B. H., Lynch, J. P.III, & Martinez, F. J. (2003). Prognostic value of desaturation during a 6-minute walk test in idiopathic interstitial pneumonia. *American Journal of Respiratory and Critical Care Medicine*, *168*(9), 1084–1090. DOI: 10.1164/rccm.200302-219OC PMID: 12917227

Lara-Espinosa, J. V., & Hernández-Pando, R. (2021). Psychiatric problems in pulmonary tuberculosis: Depression and anxiety. *Journal of Tuberculosis Research*, *9*(01), 31–50. DOI: 10.4236/jtr.2021.91003

Lee, H. K., Teo, S. S. H., Barbier, S., Tang, S. C., Yeo, G. H., & Tan, N. C. (2016). The impact of direct observed therapy on daily living activities, quality of life and socioeconomic burden on patients with tuberculosis in primary care in Singapore. *Proceedings of Singapore Healthcare*, *25*(4), 235–242. DOI: 10.1177/2010105816652148

Li, A., Yuan, S.-y., Li, Q., Li, J., Yin, X.-y., & Liu, N. (2023). Prevalence and risk factors of malnutrition in patients with pulmonary tuberculosis: A systematic review and meta-analysis. *Frontiers in Medicine*, *10*, 1173619. DOI: 10.3389/fmed.2023.1173619 PMID: 37636566

Liu, X., Lan, H., Bai, X., Li, Q., Wen, Y., Feng, M., & Tang, X. (2023). Sleep quality and its associated factors among patients with tuberculosis: A cross-sectional study. *Frontiers in Public Health*, *10*, 1047425. DOI: 10.3389/fpubh.2022.1047425 PMID: 36684994

Mahler, B., & Croitoru, A. (2019). Pulmonary rehabilitation and tuberculosis: A new approach for an old disease. *Pneumologia (Bucharest, Romania)*, *68*(3), 107–113. DOI: 10.2478/pneum-2019-0024

Martinez-Garcia, M., Guan, W., De-La-Rosa, D., Athanazio, R., Oscullo, G., Shi, M., Pujal-Montaña, P., Endlich, B., Tiberi, S., Centis, R., & Migliori, G. B. (2023). Post-TB bronchiectasis: From pathogenesis to rehabilitation. *The International Journal of Tuberculosis and Lung Disease : the Official Journal of the International Union against Tuberculosis and Lung Disease*, *27*(3), 175–181. DOI: 10.5588/ijtld.22.0566 PMID: 36855043

McAdams, H. P., Erasmus, J., & Winter, J. A. (1995). Radiologic manifestations of pulmonary tuberculosis. *Radiologic Clinics of North America*, *33*(4), 655–678. DOI: 10.1016/S0033-8389(22)00611-X PMID: 7610237

Meca, A.-D., Mititelu-Tar ău, L., Bogdan, M., Dijmarescu, L. A., Pelin, A.-M., & Foia, L. G. (2022). Mycobacterium tuberculosis and pulmonary rehabilitation: From novel pharmacotherapeutic approaches to management of post-tuberculosis sequelae. *Journal of Personalized Medicine*, *12*(4), 569. DOI: 10.3390/jpm12040569 PMID: 35455684

Mehmood, A., Abbas, R., Saeed, A., Saleem, S., Nawaz, S., & Tabassum, S. (2024). Assessment of Dyspnea in Patients with Chronic Obstructive Lung Diseases with Modified Borg Scale; Descriptive Cross-Sectional Study: Assessment of Dyspnea in Chronic Obstructive Lung Diseases. *The Healer Journal of Physiotherapy and Rehabilitation Sciences*, *4*(3), 998–1005. DOI: 10.55735/hjprs.v4i3.243

Menzies, D. (2022). Canadian Tuberculosis Standards 8th edition: What's new? And what's next? In (Vol. 6, pp. 333-336): Taylor & Francis.

Muñoz-Torrico, M., Rendon, A., Centis, R., D'Ambrosio, L., Fuentes, Z., Torres-Duque, C., Mello, F., Dalcolmo, M., Pérez-Padilla, R., Spanevello, A., & Migliori, G. B. (2016). Is there a rationale for pulmonary rehabilitation following successful chemotherapy for tuberculosis? *Jornal Brasileiro de Pneumologia : Publicaçao Oficial da Sociedade Brasileira de Pneumologia e Tisilogia*, *42*(5), 374–385. DOI: 10.1590/S1806-37562016000000226 PMID: 27812638

Musafiri, S., Dusabejambo, V., Munganyinka, B., Manzi, O., Kalisa, L., & Rutayisire, P. (2015). The aftermath of pulmonary tuberculosis: Predictors of severe pulmonary sequelae and quality of life of patients visiting a tertiary level of care in Rwanda, East Africa. *Austin J Pulm Respir Med*, *2*(2), 1027.

Naeije, R., & Chesler, N. (2012). Pulmonary circulation at exercise. *Comprehensive Physiology*, *2*(1), 711–741. DOI: 10.1002/j.2040-4603.2012.tb00405.x PMID: 23105961

Nicola Martins Rodrigues, S., Henriques, H., & Henriques, M. (2021). Effectiveness of a preoperative breathing exercises intervention on patients undergoing cardiac surgery: a systematic review. *European Journal of Preventive Cardiology, 28*(Supplement_1), zwab061. 345.

Noor, L., Zutshi, K., & Aman, I. (2024). Physical Rehabilitation for Tuberculosis: A Review of Literature. *Indian Journal of Preventive and Social Medicine*, *55*(4), 400–407.

Okeke, C. C., Ibe, C. C., Nduji, O. J., Ndulue, C. J., Ngige, O., Amuchie, C. C., Ezema, C. C., Onyeogulu, A. O., Ojo, A., Obuseh, M., Alli, O. O., Akinteye, E. I., Idion, K. N., Akpan-Udo, U. I., Okereke, I. C., & Eke, C. (2025). Pulmonary Tuberculosis-Associated Morbidity in Africa: A Systematic Review. *Cureus*, *17*(1). Advance online publication. DOI: 10.7759/cureus.77569 PMID: 39958055

Ong, C. W., Elkington, P. T., & Friedland, J. S. (2014). Tuberculosis, pulmonary cavitation, and matrix metalloproteinases. *American Journal of Respiratory and Critical Care Medicine*, *190*(1), 9–18. DOI: 10.1164/rccm.201311-2106PP PMID: 24713029

Ono, K., Tabusadani, M., Yamane, K., Takao, S., Mori, K., Matsumura, Y., Kuroyama, Y., Kawahara, K., Omatsu, S., Furuuchi, K., Fujiwara, K., Morimoto, K., Kimura, H., & Senjyu, H. (2022). Decreased incremental shuttle walk test distance characterized by fibrocavitary lesions in non-tuberculous mycobacterial pulmonary disease. *Expert Review of Respiratory Medicine*, *16*(4), 469–475. DOI: 10.1080/17476348.2022.2049762 PMID: 35245168

Organization, W. H. (2023). *Global Tuberculosis Report*. W. H. Organization.

Padmanabhanunni, A., & Pretorius, T. B. (2025). An exploratory study of the mental health of first responders: Depression, anxiety, and post-traumatic stress disorder. *South African Journal of Psychology. Suid-Afrikaanse Tydskrif vir Sielkunde*, *55*(2), 00812463251317901. DOI: 10.1177/00812463251317901

Papathakis, P., & Piwoz, E. (2008). Nutrition and Tuberculosis: A review of the literature and considerations for TB control programs. *United States Agency for International Development, Africa's Health 2010 Project*, 1.

Park, H.-Y., Cheon, H.-B., Choi, S. H., & Kwon, J.-W. (2021). Health-related quality of life based on EQ-5D utility score in patients with tuberculosis: A systematic review. *Frontiers in Pharmacology*, *12*, 659675. DOI: 10.3389/fphar.2021.659675 PMID: 33935781

Pasipanodya, J. G., Miller, T. L., Vecino, M., Munguia, G., Garmon, R., Bae, S., Drewyer, G., & Weis, S. E. (2007). Pulmonary impairment after tuberculosis. *Chest*, *131*(6), 1817–1824. DOI: 10.1378/chest.06-2949 PMID: 17400690

Petil, E. D.Jr, & Caballero, N. R. (2025). Physiotherapy in community-based rehabilitation in middle and low-income countries: A scoping review. *Philippine Journal of Physical Therapy*, *4*(1), 11–26. DOI: 10.46409/002.ESRL3383

Ravimohan, S., Kornfeld, H., Weissman, D., & Bisson, G. P. (2018). Tuberculosis and lung damage: From epidemiology to pathophysiology. *European Respiratory Review : an Official Journal of the European Respiratory Society, 27*(147), 170077. DOI: 10.1183/16000617.0077-2017 PMID: 29491034

Sakuma, T., Tatsumi, K., Kimura, H., Honda, Y., & Kuriyama, T. (1996). Sleep oxygen desaturation in late sequelae of pulmonary tuberculosis. *Internal Medicine (Tokyo, Japan), 35*(7), 534–539. DOI: 10.2169/internalmedicine.35.534 PMID: 8842758

Salman Latif, M. S., Shafee, I., Ali, J., Mannan, A., Deedar, S., & Waris, S. (2022). Six Minute Walk Test in People with Tuberculosis Sequelae. *Pakistan Journal of Medical & Health Sciences, 16*(03), 935–935. DOI: 10.53350/pjmhs22163935

Sancar, B., Doğan, A., & Taş, S. (2024). Timed Up-and-Go Test and Sit-to-Stand Test in Community-Dwelling Older Person: Inter and Intraobserver Reliability Among Turkish Nurses. *International Journal of Older People Nursing, 19*(5), e12649. DOI: 10.1111/opn.12649 PMID: 39297511

Sarkar, M., Srinivasa, , Madabhavi, I., & Kumar, K. (2017). Tuberculosis associated chronic obstructive pulmonary disease. *The Clinical Respiratory Journal, 11*(3), 285–295. DOI: 10.1111/crj.12621 PMID: 28268242

Shaw, J. A., Irusen, E. M., Diacon, A. H., & Koegelenberg, C. F. (2018). Pleural tuberculosis: A concise clinical review. *The Clinical Respiratory Journal, 12*(5), 1779–1786. DOI: 10.1111/crj.12900 PMID: 29660258

Singh, S. J., ZuWallack, R. L., Garvey, C., & Spruit, M. A. (2013). *Learn from the past and create the future: the 2013 ATS/ERS statement on pulmonary rehabilitation* (Vol. 42). European Respiratory Society.

Slobod, D., Damia, A., Leali, M., Spinelli, E., & Mauri, T. (2022). Pathophysiology and clinical meaning of ventilation-perfusion mismatch in the acute respiratory distress syndrome. *Biology (Basel), 12*(1), 67. DOI: 10.3390/biology12010067 PMID: 36671759

Sonone, S. V., Bhakaney, P. R., Jain, M., Yadav, V., & Vardhan, V. D. (2022). In-patient pulmonary rehabilitation followed by Tele-Rehabilitation in a patient with Post Tubercular sequelae: A case study.

Spruit, M. A., Singh, S. J., Garvey, C., ZuWallack, R., Nici, L., Rochester, C., Hill, K., Holland, A. E., Lareau, S. C., Man, W. D.-C., Pitta, F., Sewell, L., Raskin, J., Bourbeau, J., Crouch, R., Franssen, F. M. E., Casaburi, R., Vercoulen, J. H., Vogiatzis, I., & Wouters, E. F. M. (2013). An official American Thoracic Society/European Respiratory Society statement: Key concepts and advances in pulmonary rehabilitation. *American Journal of Respiratory and Critical Care Medicine*, *188*(8), e13–e64. DOI: 10.1164/rccm.201309-1634ST PMID: 24127811

Srinivas, M., Jagadeesh, G. T., Kamarthi, P., Patil, N., & Venkataramanappa, J. S. (2024). Effect of Telerehabilitation in a Patient with Pulmonary Tuberculosis: A Case Study. *Indian Journal of Respiratory Care*, *13*(1), 65. DOI: 10.5005/jp-journals-11010-1088

Tesfamariam, S., Ghebrenegus, A. S., Woldu, H., Fisseha, E., Belai, G., & Russom, M. (2021). Secondary erythrocytosis following drugs used in rifampicin/multidrug-resistant tuberculosis: A retrospective cohort study. *BMJ Open Respiratory Research*, *8*(1), e001064. DOI: 10.1136/bmjresp-2021-001064 PMID: 34815231

van Heerden, J. K., Louw, E. H., Thienemann, F., Engel, M. E., & Allwood, B. W. (2024). The prevalence of pulmonary hypertension in post-tuberculosis and active tuberculosis populations: A systematic review and meta-analysis. *European Respiratory Review : an Official Journal of the European Respiratory Society*, *33*(171), 230154. DOI: 10.1183/16000617.0154-2023 PMID: 38232991

Wang, H., Ji, X. B., Li, C. W., Lu, H. W., Mao, B., Liang, S., Cheng, K. B., Bai, J. W., Martinez-Garcia, M. A., & Xu, J. F. (2018). Clinical characteristics and validation of bronchiectasis severity score systems for post-tuberculosis bronchiectasis. *The Clinical Respiratory Journal*, *12*(8), 2346–2353. DOI: 10.1111/crj.12911 PMID: 29790656

Wani, R. L. S. (2013). Clinical manifestations of pulmonary and extra-pulmonary tuberculosis. *South Sudan Medical Journal*, *6*(3), 52–56.

Wong, Y. J., Noordin, N. M., Keshavjee, S., & Lee, S. W. H. (2021). Impact of latent tuberculosis infection on health and wellbeing: A systematic review and meta-analysis. *European Respiratory Review : an Official Journal of the European Respiratory Society*, *30*(159), 200260. DOI: 10.1183/16000617.0260-2020 PMID: 33408089

Wu, D., Wang, L., & Zhang, L. (2024). Efficacy and safety of step-by-step Baduanjin exercise based on doctor-nurse-patient integration mode for pulmonary rehabilitation in patients after lobectomy due to pulmonary tuberculosis: A randomized controlled clinical trial. *Journal of Cardiothoracic Surgery*, *19*(1), 520. DOI: 10.1186/s13019-024-03042-w PMID: 39252121

Wytrychowski, K., Hans-Wytrychowska, A., Piesiak, P., Majewska-Pulsakowska, M., & Rożek-Piechura, K. (2020). Pulmonary rehabilitation in interstitial lung diseases: A review of the literature. *Advances in Clinical and Experimental Medicine*, *29*(2), 257–264. DOI: 10.17219/acem/115238 PMID: 32101645

Xu, Z., Chen, W., & Li, X. (2021). Effects of comprehensive nursing intervention combined with respiratory functional exercises on pulmonary function and self-care ability in patients with pulmonary tuberculosis: Results of a randomized trial. *Annals of Palliative Medicine*, *10*(7), 7543–7550. DOI: 10.21037/apm-21-1178 PMID: 34353042

Yang, Y., Wei, L., Wang, S., Ke, L., Zhao, H., Mao, J., Li, J., & Mao, Z. (2022). The effects of pursed lip breathing combined with diaphragmatic breathing on pulmonary function and exercise capacity in patients with COPD: A systematic review and meta-analysis. *Physiotherapy Theory and Practice*, *38*(7), 847–857. DOI: 10.1080/09593985.2020.1805834 PMID: 32808571

Zhang, S., Huang, X., Zhao, X., Li, B., Cai, Y., Liang, X., & Wan, Q. (2022). Effect of exercise on bone mineral density among patients with osteoporosis and osteopenia: A systematic review and network meta-analysis. *Journal of Clinical Nursing*, *31*(15-16), 2100–2111. DOI: 10.1111/jocn.16101 PMID: 34725872

Zuo, X., Dong, Z., Zhang, P., Zhu, X., Qiao, C., Yang, Y., & Lou, P. (2022). Cognitive-behavioral therapy on psychological stress and quality of life in subjects with pulmonary tuberculosis: A community-based cluster randomized controlled trial. *BMC Public Health*, *22*(1), 2160. DOI: 10.1186/s12889-022-14631-6 PMID: 36419020

KEY TERMS AND DEFINITIONS

6MWT: 6-Minute Walk Test
ACBT: Active cycle of breathing techniques
ATS: American Thoracic Society
COPD: Chronic Obstructive Pulmonary Disease
DLCO: Diffusing Capacity of the Lungs for Carbon Monoxide
EQ-5D: EuroQol 5-Dimension Health Questionnaire
ERS: European Respiratory Society
ESWT: Endurance Shuttle Walk Test
FEV1: Forced Expiratory Volume in 1 Second
FVC: Forced Vital Capacity
HADS: Hospital Anxiety and Depression Scale

IMT: Inspiratory Muscle Training
ISWT: Incremental Shuttle Walk Test
LMICs: Low- and middle-income countries
MIP: Maximal Inspiratory Pressure
mMRC: Modified Medical Research Council (Dyspnea Scale)
PR: Pulmonary Rehabilitation
PTLD: Post-tuberculosis lung disease
RCTs: Randomized Controlled Trials
RV: Residual Volume
SF-36: Short Form-36 Health Survey
SGRQ: St. George's Respiratory Questionnaire
TB: Tuberculosis
TLC: Total Lung Capacity
V/Q: Ventilation/Perfusion
VAS: Visual Analog Scale

Compilation of References

Abaei, E., Abedi, M., Sadat Mirenayat, M., & Rezaei, M. (2023). The Effect of High-Intensity Interval Training in People With Respiratory Disease: A Review Study. *The Scientific Journal of Rehabilitation Medicine*, *12*(1), 18–29. DOI: 10.32598/SJRM.12.1.12

Abbara, A., Almalla, M., AlMasri, I., AlKabbani, H., Karah, N., El-Amin, W., Rajan, L., Rahhal, I., Alabbas, M., Sahloul, Z., Tarakji, A., & Sparrow, A. (2020). The challenges of tuberculosis control in protracted conflict: The case of Syria. *International Journal of Infectious Diseases*, *90*, 53–59. DOI: 10.1016/j.ijid.2019.10.015

Abbas, M., AlHamdan, N., Fiala, L. A., AlEnezy, A. K., & AlQahtani, M. S. (2010). Prevalence of latent TB among health care workers in four major tertiary care hospitals in Riyadh, Saudi Arabia. *Journal of the Egyptian Public Health Association, 85*(1-2), 61–71.

Adane, K., Spigt, M., & Dinant, G. J. (2018). Tuberculosis treatment outcome and predictors in northern Ethiopian prisons: A five-year retrospective analysis. *BMC Pulmonary Medicine*, *18*(1), 1–8. DOI: 10.1186/s12890-018-0600-1

Adzemovic, T., Nalintya, E., Fieberg, A., Mande, E., George, K., & Yueh, S.. (2025). Diagnostic accuracy of the updated FujiLAM II assay to detect tuberculosis in outpatients with advanced HIV disease. *Clinical Infectious Diseases*, •••, ciaf079. Advance online publication. DOI: 10.1093/cid/ciaf079 PMID: 40130995

Aggarwal, S., Simmy, S., Mahajan, N., & Nigam, K. (2024). Challenges experienced by health care workers during service delivery in the geographically challenging terrains of North-East India: Study involving a thematic analysis. *JMIR Formative Research*, *8*, e57384. DOI: 10.2196/57384 PMID: 39255009

Aguilar Diaz, J. M., Abulfathi, A. A., te Brake, L. H., van Ingen, J., Kuipers, S., Magis-Escurra, C., Raaijmakers, J., Svensson, E. M., & Boeree, M. J. (2023). New and repurposed drugs for the treatment of active tuberculosis: An update for clinicians. *Respiration, 102*(2), 83–100. DOI: 10.1159/000528274 PMID: 36516792

Ahmad, B. B., Kristensen, K. L., Glenthoej, J. P., Poulsen, A., Bryld, A.-G., Huber, F. G., Andersen, E. M., & Ravn, P. (2020). Latent tuberculosis infection among minor asylum seekers in Denmark. *The European Respiratory Journal, 55*(3), 1901688. Advance online publication. DOI: 10.1183/13993003.01688-2019 PMID: 31558661

Ajzen, I. (1991). The theory of planned behavior. *Organizational Behavior and Human Decision Processes, 50*(2), 179–211. DOI: 10.1016/0749-5978(91)90020-T

Akdel, M., Pires, D. E. V., Pardo, E. P., Jänes, J., Zalevsky, A. O., Mészáros, B., Bryant, P., Good, L. L., Laskowski, R. A., Pozzati, G., Shenoy, A., Zhu, W., Kundrotas, P., Serra, V. R., Rodrigues, C. H. M., Dunham, A. S., Burke, D., Borkakoti, N., Velankar, S., & Beltrao, P. (2022). A structural biology community assessment of AlphaFold2 applications. *Nature Structural & Molecular Biology, 29*(11), 1056–1067. DOI: 10.1038/s41594-022-00849-w PMID: 36344848

Akers, T. A., Blake, B. J., & Hanson, R. A. (2008). Infections diseases from a global perspective. *Global health care: Issues and policies*, 181-198.

Alene, K. A., Hertzog, L., Gilmour, B., Clements, A. C., & Murray, M. B. (2024). Interventions to prevent post-tuberculosis sequelae: A systematic review and meta-analysis. *EClinicalMedicine, 70*, 70. DOI: 10.1016/j.eclinm.2024.102511 PMID: 38434448

Al-Lami, F., Armean, P., & Al-Ameri, A. H. (2014). Prevalence of latent TB infection among health care workers in three main TB health facilities, Baghdad, Iraq, 2013. *Journal of the Faculty of Medicine, 56*(4), 339–342.

Allwood, B. W., Byrne, A., Meghji, J., Rachow, A., van der Zalm, M. M., & Schoch, O. D. (2021). Post-tuberculosis lung disease: Clinical review of an under-recognised global challenge. *Respiration, 100*(8), 751–763. DOI: 10.1159/000512531 PMID: 33401266

Almeida, D., Converse, P. J., Li, S. Y., Upton, A. M., Fotouhi, N., & Nuermberger, E. L. (2021). Comparative Efficacy of the Novel Diarylquinoline TBAJ-876 and Bedaquiline against a Resistant *Rv0678* Mutant in a Mouse Model of Tuberculosis. *Antimicrobial Agents and Chemotherapy, 65*(12), e0141221. DOI: 10.1128/AAC.01412-21 PMID: 34570644

Amalia, Y. (2024). Health Education To Reduce Negative Stigma And Increase Willingness To Screen For Tuberculosis. *HealthCare Nursing Journal*, *6*(1), 39–44. Advance online publication. DOI: 10.35568/healthcare.v6i1.4331

Amede, P. O., Adedire, E., Usman, A., Ameh, C. A., Umar, F. S., Umeokonkwo, C. D., & Balogun, M. S. (2022). Drug-susceptible tuberculosis treatment outcomes and its associated factors among inmates in prison settings in Bauchi State, Nigeria, 2014–2018. *PLoS One*, *17*(7), e0270819. DOI: 10.1371/journal.pone.0270819

Ammous, O., Feki, W., Lotfi, T., Khamis, A. M., Gosselink, R., Rebai, A., & Kammoun, S. (2023). Inspiratory muscle training, with or without concomitant pulmonary rehabilitation, for chronic obstructive pulmonary disease (COPD). *Cochrane Database of Systematic Reviews*, 1. PMID: 36606682

Apriani, L., McAllister, S., Sharples, K., Alisjahbana, B., Ruslami, R., Hill, P. C., & Menzies, D. (2019). Latent tuberculosis infection in healthcare workers in low- and middle-income countries: An updated systematic review. *European Respiratory Journal, 53*(4), Article 1801789. DOI: 10.1183/13993003.01789-2018

Assefa, D. G., Dememew, Z. G., Zeleke, E. D., Manyazewal, T., & Bedru, A. (2024). Financial burden of tuberculosis diagnosis and treatment for patients in Ethiopia: A systematic review and meta-analysis. *BMC Public Health*, *24*(1), 260. DOI: 10.1186/s12889-024-17713-9 PMID: 38254019

Aytaç, S., Ovayolu, Ö., & Dogru, S. (2024). The effect of breathing exercises on fatigue in tuberculosis patients: A randomized controlled trial. *Revista da Associação Médica Brasileira*, *70*(12), e20240888. DOI: 10.1590/1806-9282.20240888 PMID: 39630726

Babirye, S. R., Nsubuga, M., Mboowa, G., Batte, C., Galiwango, R., & Kateete, D. P. (2024). Machine learning-based prediction of antibiotic resistance in *Mycobacterium tuberculosis* clinical isolates from Uganda. *BMC Infectious Diseases*, *24*(1), 1391. DOI: 10.1186/s12879-024-10282-7 PMID: 39639222

Bagcchi, S. (2023). WHO's Global Tuberculosis Report 2022. *The Lancet Microbe*, *4*(1), e20. Advance online publication. DOI: 10.1016/S2666-5247(22)00359-7 PMID: 36521512

Baird, K., Said, H., Koornhof, H. J., & Duse, A. G. (2022). Tuberculosis control at a South African correctional centre: Diagnosis, treatment and strain characterisation. *PLoS One*, *17*(11), e0277459. DOI: 10.1371/journal.pone.0277459

Balakrishnan, V., Kherabi, Y., Ramanathan, G., Paul, S. A., & Tiong, C. K. (2023). Machine learning approaches in diagnosing tuberculosis through biomarkers—A systematic review. *Progress in Biophysics and Molecular Biology, 179*, 16–25. DOI: 10.1016/j.pbiomolbio.2023.03.001 PMID: 36931609

Balisan, O. P. R., Galamay, J. R. T., Cale-Subia, L. N., & De Luna, A. M. (2024). Utility of nucleic acid amplification test in the detection of tuberculosis in biological fluids from suspected TB patients in a cardiovascular center in the Philippines. *Acta Tropica, 249*, 107078. Advance online publication. DOI: 10.1016/j.actatropica.2023.107078

Baratella, E., Fiorese, I., Minelli, P., Veiluva, A., Marrocchio, C., Ruaro, B., & Cova, M. A. (2023). Aging-Related Findings of the Respiratory System in Chest Imaging : Pearls and Pitfalls. *Current Radiology Reports, 11*(1), 1–11. DOI: 10.1007/s40134-022-00405-w

Barman, M., Panja, M., Mishra, N., & Chakraborty, T. (2025). Epidemic-guided deep learning for spatiotemporal forecasting of tuberculosis outbreaks. *arXiv*. https://doi.org//arXiv.2502.10786DOI: 10.48550

Barreto-Duarte, B., Villalva-Serra, K., Campos, V. M., Cordeiro-Santos, M., Kritski, A. L., Araújo-Pereira, M., Rodrigues, M. M., & Andrade, B. B. (2024). Nationwide economic analysis of pulmonary tuberculosis in the Brazilian healthcare system over seven years (2015–2022): A population-based study. *Lancet Regional Health. Americas, 39*, 39. DOI: 10.1016/j.lana.2024.100905 PMID: 39839682

Barreto-Duarte, B., Villalva-Serra, K., Croda, J., Arcêncio, R. A., Maciel, E. L. N., & Andrade, B. B. (2025). Directly observed treatment for tuberculosis care and social support: Essential lifeline or outdated burden? *Lancet Regional Health. Americas, 43*, 100310. DOI: 10.1016/j.lana.2025.101015 PMID: 40171142

Bartolomeu-Gonçalves, G., de Souza, J. M., Fernandes, B. T., Spoladori, L. F. A., Correia, G. F., & de Castro, I. M.. (2024). Tuberculosis diagnosis: Current, ongoing, and future approaches. *Diseases (Basel, Switzerland), 12*(9), 202. DOI: 10.3390/diseases12090202 PMID: 39329871

Bastikar, V., Bastikar, A., & Gupta, P. (2022). Quantitative structure–activity relationship-based computational approaches. *Computational Approaches for Novel Therapeutic and Diagnostic Designing to Mitigate SARS-CoV-2 Infection*, 191–205. DOI: 10.1016/B978-0-323-91172-6.00001-7

Bausch, K., Mantica, G., Smith, E. J., Bartoletti, R., Bruyère, F., Cai, T., Geerlings, S., Kranz, J., Köves, B., Pilatz, A., Schubert, S., Veeratterapillay, R., Wagenlehner, F., Gupta, N., & Bonkat, G. (2024). Genitourinary tuberculosis: A brief manual for urologists on diagnosis and treatment from the European Association of Urology Urological Infections Panel. *European Urology Focus, 10*(1), 77–79. DOI: 10.1016/j.euf.2023.07.006 PMID: 37541917

Baussano, I., Nunn, P., Williams, B., Pivetta, E., Bugiani, M., & Scano, F. (2011). Tuberculosis among health care workers. *Emerging Infectious Diseases, 17*(3), 488–494. DOI: 10.3201/eid1703.100947

Baussano, I., Williams, B. G., Nunn, P., Beggiato, M., Fedeli, U., & Scano, F. (2010). Tuberculosis incidence in prisons: A systematic review. *PLoS Medicine, 7*(12), e1000381. DOI: 10.1371/journal.pmed.1000381

Baxter, S., Goyder, E., Chambers, D., Johnson, M., Preston, L., & Booth, A. (2017). Interventions to improve contact tracing for tuberculosis in specific groups and in wider populations: An evidence synthesis. *Health and Social Care Delivery Research, 5*(1), 1–102.

Beaudry, G., Zhong, S., Whiting, D., Javid, B., Frater, J., & Fazel, S. (2020). Managing outbreaks of highly contagious diseases in prisons: A systematic review. *BMJ Global Health, 5*(11), e003201. https://gh.bmj.com/content/5/11/e003201. DOI: 10.1136/bmjgh-2020-003201

Behera, D., Pannu, V. P., & Behera, R. K. (2020). National tb elimination programme–can it end tb in india by 2025: An appraisal. *The Indian Journal of Chest Diseases & Allied Sciences, 62*(4), 203–227. DOI: 10.5005/ijcdas-62-4-203

Belizário, J. E., Faintuch, J., & Malpartida, M. G. (2021). Breath biopsy and discovery of exclusive volatile organic compounds for diagnosis of infectious diseases. *Frontiers in Cellular and Infection Microbiology, 10*, 564194. DOI: 10.3389/fcimb.2020.564194 PMID: 33520731

Benedetto, U., Head, S. J., Angelini, G. D., & Blackstone, E. H. (2018). Statistical primer: Propensity score matching and its alternatives. *European Journal of Cardio-Thoracic Surgery, 53*(6), 1112–1117. DOI: 10.1093/ejcts/ezy028

Berrocal-Almanza, L. C., Lima, M., Piotrowski, H., Botticello, J., Badhan, A., Karnani, N., Kaur, H., Pareek, M., Haldar, P., Dedicoat, M., Kon, O. M., Zenner, D., & Lalvani, A. (2023). Vulnerability and tuberculosis treatment outcomes in urban settings in England: A mixed-methods study. *PLoS One, 18*(8), e0281918. DOI: 10.1371/journal.pone.0281918 PMID: 37590225

Berry, K. M., Rodriguez, C. A., Berhanu, R. H., Ismail, N., Mvusi, L., Long, L., & Evans, D. (2019). Treatment outcomes among children, adolescents, and adults on treatment for tuberculosis in two metropolitan municipalities in Gauteng Province, South Africa. *BMC Public Health, 19*(1), 973. Advance online publication. DOI: 10.1186/s12889-019-7257-4 PMID: 31331311

Bhatt, D. L., & Mehta, C. (2016). Adaptive designs for clinical trials. *The New England Journal of Medicine, 375*(1), 65–74. DOI: 10.1056/NEJMra1510061 PMID: 27406349

Biadglegne, F., Rodloff, A. C., & Sack, U. (2015). Review of the prevalence and drug resistance of tuberculosis in prisons: A hidden epidemic. *Epidemiology and Infection, 143*(5), 887–900. DOI: 10.1017/S095026881400288X

Biru, M., Datiko, D. G., Jerene, D., Yohannes, A. G., Molla, Y., Suarez, P., Gebrekiros, W., Kassa, A., Kassie, Y., & Dememew, Z. G. (2025). Designing tuberculosis elimination framework through participatory processes in Ethiopia: Results from stakeholders' discussions. *PLoS One, 20*(3), e0318209. DOI: 10.1371/journal.pone.0318209 PMID: 40063578

Blanc, F.-X. (2023). Tuberculose et infection par le virus de l'immunodéficience humaine : Comment réduire la mortalité? *Bulletin de l'Académie Nationale de Médecine, 207*(8), 1044–1052. DOI: 10.1016/j.banm.2023.07.007

Blanco-González, A., Cabezón, A., Seco-González, A., Conde-Torres, D., Antelo-Riveiro, P., Piñeiro, Á., & Garcia-Fandino, R. (2023). The Role of AI in Drug Discovery: Challenges, Opportunities, and Strategies. *Pharmaceuticals (Basel, Switzerland), 16*(6), 891. DOI: 10.3390/ph16060891 PMID: 37375838

Boast, A., How, J. A., Lau, C., Sett, A., Gilby, D., Burke, A., McWhinney, B., Wright, C., Tramontana, A., Globan, M., Denholm, J., Graham, S. M., & Osowicki, J. (2024). Pre-extensively Drug-Resistant Congenital Tuberculosis in an Extremely Premature Baby. *Clinical Infectious Diseases, 78*(1), 149–153. Advance online publication. DOI: 10.1093/cid/ciad540

Boehme, C. C., Nabeta, P., Hillemann, D., Nicol, M. P., Shenai, S., Krapp, F., Allen, J., Tahirli, R., Blakemore, R., Rustomjee, R., Milovic, A., Jones, M., O'Brien, S. M., Persing, D. H., Ruesch-Gerdes, S., Gotuzzo, E., Rodrigues, C., Alland, D., & Perkins, M. D. (2010). Rapid Molecular Detection of Tuberculosis and Rifampin Resistance. *The New England Journal of Medicine, 363*(11), 1005–1015. DOI: 10.1056/NEJMoa0907847

Boeree, M. J., Heinrich, N., Aarnoutse, R., Diacon, A. H., Dawson, R., Rehal, S., Kibiki, G. S., Churchyard, G., Sanne, I., Ntinginya, N. E., Minja, L. T., Hunt, R. D., Charalambous, S., Hanekom, M., Semvua, H. H., Mpagama, S. G., Manyama, C., Mtafya, B., Reither, K., & Hoelscher, M. (2017). High-dose rifampicin, moxifloxacin, and SQ109 for treating tuberculosis: A multi-arm, multi-stage randomised controlled trial. *The Lancet. Infectious Diseases*, *17*(1), 39–49. DOI: 10.1016/S1473-3099(16)30274-2 PMID: 28100438

Bolado, G. N., Ataro, B. A., Feleke, M. G., Gadabo, C. K., Kebamo, T. E., & Minuta, W. M. (2024). Informed consent practice and associated factors among healthcare professionals in public hospitals of Southern Ethiopia, 2023: A mixed-method study. *BMC Nursing*, *23*(1), 77. DOI: 10.1186/s12912-024-01748-9 PMID: 38287367

Bourguignon, T., Godinez-Leon, J. A., & Gref, R. (2023). Nanosized drug delivery systems to fight tuberculosis. *Pharmaceutics*, *15*(2), 393. Advance online publication. DOI: 10.3390/pharmaceutics15020393 PMID: 36839715

Bozkanat, E., Kaya, H., Sezer, O., Caliskan, T., Kilic, E., Ciftci, F., Gümüs, S., & Kartaloglu, Z. (2016). Comparison of tuberculin skin test and QuantiFERON-TB Gold In-Tube test for diagnosis of latent tuberculosis infection in health care workers: A cross-sectional study. *Journal of the Pakistan Medical Association, 66*(3), 270–274.

Bratton, D. J., Phillips, P. P., & Parmar, M. K. (2013). A multi-arm multi-stage clinical trial design for binary outcomes with application to tuberculosis. *BMC Medical Research Methodology*, *13*(1), 139. DOI: 10.1186/1471-2288-13-139 PMID: 24229079

Braun, V., & Clarke, V. (2006). Using thematic analysis in psychology. *Qualitative Research in Psychology*, *3*(2), 77–101. DOI: 10.1191/1478088706qp063oa

Britto, R. R., Brant, T. C. S., & Parreira, V. F. (2014). Recursos Manuais e Instrumentais em Fisioterapia Respiratória [rev. ampl.]. In: Manole.

Brodhun, B., Altmann, D., Hauer, B., & Haas, W. (2019). *Bericht zur Epidemiologie der Tuberkulose in Deutschland für 2018*. Robert Koch-Institut.

Broger, T. (2025). *Can Lipoarabinomannan Antigen Enable Point-of-Care TB Diagnosis?* Exploring the Nexus of Clinical Concentration Ranges, Accuracy, and Diagnostic Yield.

Bryman, A. (2006). Integrating quantitative and qualitative research: How is it done? *Qualitative Research*, *6*(1), 97–113. DOI: 10.1177/1468794106058877

Budak, M., Via, L. E., Weiner, D. M., Barry, C. E.III, Nanda, P., Michael, G., Mdluli, K., & Kirschner, D. (2024). A systematic efficacy analysis of tuberculosis treatment with BPaL-containing regimens using a multiscale modeling approach. *CPT: Pharmacometrics & Systems Pharmacology, 13*(4), 673–685. DOI: 10.1002/psp4.13117 PMID: 38404200

Bukhary, Z. A., Amer, S. M., Emara, M. M., Abdalla, M. E., & Ali, S. A. (2018). Screening of latent tuberculosis infection among health care workers working in Hajj pilgrimage area in Saudi Arabia, using interferon gamma release assay and tuberculin skin test. *Annals of Saudi Medicine, 38*(2), 90–96. DOI: 10.5144/0256-4947.2018.90

Busatto, C., Bierhals, D. V., Vianna, J. S., Silva, P. E. A. D., Possuelo, L. G., & Ramis, I. B. (2022). Epidemiology and control strategies for tuberculosis in countries with the largest prison populations. *Revista da Sociedade Brasileira de Medicina Tropical, 55*, e0060–e2022. DOI: 10.1590/0037-8682-0060-2022

Bustamante-Gavino, M. I., Rattani, S., & Khan, K. (2011). Women's empowerment in Pakistan—Definitions and enabling and disenabling factors: A secondary data analysis. *Journal of Transcultural Nursing, 22*(2), 174–181. DOI: 10.1177/1043659610395762 PMID: 21467269

Byrne, A. L., Marais, B. J., Mitnick, C. D., Lecca, L., & Marks, G. B. (2015). Tuberculosis and chronic respiratory disease: A systematic review. *International Journal of Infectious Diseases, 32*, 138–146. DOI: 10.1016/j.ijid.2014.12.016 PMID: 25809770

Byrne, E., Bradshaw, D., Kerin, M., & Pepe, I. (2024). A social identity approach to mental health help-seeking behaviour in prisoners: A systematic review. *Journal of Community & Applied Social Psychology, 34*(1), e2727. DOI: 10.1002/casp.2727

Cai, J., Chen, J., Hu, Y., Li, S., & He, Q. (2023). Digital twin for healthy indoor environment: A vision for the post-pandemic era. *Frontiers of Engineering Management, 10*(2), 300–318. DOI: 10.1007/s42524-022-0244-y

Carlson, M. C., Fried, L. P., Xue, Q.-L., Bandeen-Roche, K., Zeger, S. L., & Brandt, J. (1999). Association Between Executive Attention and Physical Functional Performance in Community-Dwelling Older Women. *The Journals of Gerontology. Series B, Psychological Sciences and Social Sciences, 54B*(5), S262–S270. DOI: 10.1093/geronb/54B.5.S262

Carvalho, A. C. C., Cardoso, C. A. A., Martire, T. M., Migliori, G. B., & Sant'Anna, C. C. (2018). Epidemiological aspects, clinical manifestations and prevention of pediatric tuberculosis from the perspective of the End TB strategy. *Jornal Brasileiro de Pneumologia : Publicaçao Oficial da Sociedade Brasileira de Pneumologia e Tisilogia, 44*(2), 134–144. DOI: 10.1590/s1806-37562017000000461 PMID: 29791553

Carwile, M. E., Hochberg, N. S., & Sinha, P. (2022). Undernutrition is feeding the tuberculosis pandemic: A perspective. *Journal of Clinical Tuberculosis and Other Mycobacterial Diseases, 27*, 100311. DOI: 10.1016/j.jctube.2022.100311

Casaburi, R. (2008). A brief history of pulmonary rehabilitation. *Respiratory Care, 53*(9), 1185–1189. PMID: 18718037

Cellamare, M., Ventz, S., Baudin, E., Mitnick, C. D., & Trippa, L. (2017). A Bayesian response-adaptive trial in tuberculosis: The endTB trial. *Clinical Trials, 14*(1), 17–28. DOI: 10.1177/1740774516665090 PMID: 27559021

Cevik, M., Thompson, L. C., Upton, C., Rolla, V. C., Malahleha, M., Mmbaga, B., Ngubane, N., Abu Bakar, Z., Rassool, M., Variava, E., Dawson, R., Staples, S., Lalloo, U., Louw, C., Conradie, F., Eristavi, M., Samoilova, A., Skornyakov, S. N., Ntinginya, N. E., & Borisov, S. (2024). Bedaquiline-pretomanid-moxifloxacin-pyrazinamide for drug-sensitive and drug-resistant pulmonary tuberculosis treatment: A phase 2c, open-label, multicentre, partially randomised controlled trial. *The Lancet. Infectious Diseases, 24*(9), 1003–1014. DOI: 10.1016/S1473-3099(24)00223-8 PMID: 38768617

Chandra-Mouli, V., McCarraher, D. R., Phillips, S. J., Williamson, N. E., & Hainsworth, G. (2014). Contraception for adolescents in low and middle income countries: Needs, barriers, and access. *Reproductive Health, 11*(1), 1. Advance online publication. DOI: 10.1186/1742-4755-11-1 PMID: 24383405

Chang, S., & Cataldo, J. K. (2014). A systematic review of global literature on social stigma in tuberculosis. *Evaluation and Program Planning, 38*, 145–162. DOI: 10.1016/j.evalprogplan.2013.10.004

Chao, W. C., Yen, C. L., Wu, C. H., & Shieh, C. C. (2020). How mycobacteria take advantage of the weakness in human immune system in the modern world. *Journal of Microbiology, Immunology, and Infection, 53*(2), 209–215. DOI: 10.1016/j.jmii.2019.10.008

Charalambous, S., Velen, K., Rueda, Z., Croda, J., Herce, M. E., Shenoi, S. V., Altice, F., Muyoyeta, M., Telisinghe, L., Grandjean, L., Keshavjee, S., & Andrews, J. R. (2023). Scaling up evidence-based approaches to tuberculosis screening in prisons. *The Lancet. Public Health, 8*(4), e305–e310. DOI: 10.1016/S2468-2667(23)00002-6

Chatterjee, R., Ghosh, P., Sarkar, K., Samajdar, S. S., Mukherjee, S., George, A., & Pramanik, N. (2023). Prevalence of pulmonary arterial hypertension in post-tuberculosis lung fibrosis patients: A cross-sectional observational study. *Journal of Association of Chest Physicians, 11*(4), 198–201. DOI: 10.4103/jacp.jacp_11_23

Chaturvedi, M., Patel, M., Tiwari, A., Dwivedi, N., Mondal, D. P., Srivastava, A. K., & Dhand, C. (2024). An insight to the recent advancements in detection of Mycobacterium tuberculosis using biosensors: A systematic review. In *Progress in Biophysics and Molecular Biology* (Vol. 186). DOI: 10.1016/j.pbiomolbio.2023.10.003

Chaturvedi, S., & Chaturvedi, C. (2022). Teach less and Practice more: Flipped Learning for Nursing Education. In *Proceedings of the 2022 3rd International Conference on Intelligent Computing, Instrumentation and Control Technologies: Computational Intelligence for Smart Systems, ICICICT 2022*. DOI: 10.1109/ICICICT54557.2022.9917815

Chaturvedi, S., Williams, A., Sood, N., & Pandey, H. (2023). Student Nurses' learning outcome and perceptions: Comparison of effectiveness of Online blended learning, flipped classroom approach and Online learning on course Nursing Research and statistics. *International Journal of Nursing Education, 15*(4), 47–51. Advance online publication. DOI: 10.37506/ijone.v15i4.20042

Chauhan, A., Parmar, M., Dash, G. C., Chauhan, S., Sahoo, K. C., Samantaray, K., Sharma, J., Mahapatra, P., & Pati, S. (2024). Health literacy and tuberculosis control: Systematic review and meta-analysis. *Bulletin of the World Health Organization, 102*(6), 421–431. DOI: 10.2471/BLT.23.290396 PMID: 38812804

Chavez-Rimache, L., Ugarte-Gil, C., & Brunette, M. J. (2023). The community as an active part in the implementation of interventions for the prevention and care of tuberculosis: A scoping review. *PLOS Global Public Health, 3*(12), e0001482. DOI: 10.1371/journal.pgph.0001482 PMID: 38100540

Chen, A. Z., Kumar, R., Baria, R. K., Shridhar, P. K., Subbaraman, R., & Thies, W. (2023). Impact of the 99DOTS digital adherence technology on tuberculosis treatment outcomes in North India: A pre-post study. *BMC Infectious Diseases, 23*(1), 504. DOI: 10.1186/s12879-023-08418-2 PMID: 37525114

Chen, E. C., Owaisi, R., Goldschmidt, L., Maimets, I. K., & Daftary, A. (2024). Patient perceptions of video directly observed therapy for tuberculosis: A systematic review. *Journal of Clinical Tuberculosis and Other Mycobacterial Diseases, 35*, 100406. DOI: 10.1016/j.jctube.2023.100406 PMID: 38380432

Chen, R. H., Burke, A., Cho, J. G., Alffenaar, J. W., & Davies Forsman, L. (2024). New Oxazolidinones for Tuberculosis: Are Novel Treatments on the Horizon? *Pharmaceutics*, *16*(6), 818. DOI: 10.3390/pharmaceutics16060818 PMID: 38931939

Chen, R. Y., Dodd, L. E., Lee, M., Paripati, P., Hammoud, D. A., Mountz, J. M., Jeon, D., Zia, N., Zahiri, H., Coleman, M. T., Carroll, M. W., Lee, J. D., Jeong, Y. J., Herscovitch, P., Lahouar, S., Tartakovsky, M., Rosenthal, A., Somaiyya, S., Lee, S., & Barry, C. E.III. (2014). PET/CT imaging correlates with treatment outcome in patients with multidrug-resistant tuberculosis. *Science Translational Medicine*, *6*(265), 265ra166. Advance online publication. DOI: 10.1126/scitranslmed.3009501 PMID: 25473034

Chen, X., Zhou, J., Yuan, Q., Zhang, R., Huang, C., & Li, Y. (2024). Challenge of ending TB in China: Tuberculosis control in primary healthcare sectors under integrated TB control model–a systematic review and meta-analysis. *BMC Public Health*, *24*(1), 163. Advance online publication. DOI: 10.1186/s12889-023-16292-5

Chen, Y., Liu, J., Zhang, Q., Wang, Q., Chai, L., Chen, H., Li, D., Qui, Y., Wang, Y., Shen, N., Wang, J., Xie, X., Li, S., & Li, M. (2023). Epidemiological features and temporal trends of HIV-negative tuberculosis burden from 1990 to 2019: A retrospective analysis based on the Global Burden of Disease Study 2019. *BMJ Open*, *13*(9), e074134. DOI: 10.1136/bmjopen-2023-074134

Chen, Z., Wang, T., Du, J., Sun, L., Wang, G., Ni, R., An, Y., Fan, X., Li, Y., Guo, R., Mao, L., Jing, W., Shi, K., Cheng, J., Wang, Q., Nie, W., Liu, H., Liang, J., & Gong, W. (2025). Decoding the WHO Global Tuberculosis Report 2024: A Critical Analysis of Global and Chinese Key Data. *Zoonoses (Shannon)*, *5*(1), 999. DOI: 10.15212/ZOONOSES-2024-0061

Chiang, S. S., Dolynska, M., Rybak, N. R., Cruz, A. T., Aibana, O., Sheremeta, Y., Petrenko, V., Mamotenko, A., Terleieva, I., Horsburgh, C. R.Jr, & Jenkins, H. E. (2020). Clinical manifestations and epidemiology of adolescent tuberculosis in Ukraine. *ERJ Open Research*, *6*(3), 00308–02020. DOI: 10.1183/23120541.00308-2020 PMID: 32964003

Chilala, C. I., Foster, N., Bahukudumbi, S., Mohamed, M. S., Zary, M., Kafie, C., Patel, B., Gore, G., Schwartzman, K., Subbaraman, R., & Fielding, K. L. (2025). Implementation outcomes of tuberculosis digital adherence technologies: A scoping review using the RE-AIM framework. *BMJ Global Health*, *10*(2), e016535. DOI: 10.1136/bmjgh-2024-016535 PMID: 39947715

Chilala, S. B., Silumbwe, A., Zulu, J. M., Tetui, M., Bulawayo, M., Chewe, M., & Hangoma, P. (2024). Individual, community and health systems factors influencing time to notification of tuberculosis: Situating software and hardware bottlenecks in local health systems. *BMC Health Services Research, 24*(1), 1–11. DOI: 10.1186/s12913-024-11697-3 PMID: 39415167

Chitale, P., Lemenze, A. D., Fogarty, E. C., Shah, A., Grady, C., Odom-Mabey, A. R., Johnson, W. E., Yang, J. H., Eren, A. M., Brosch, R., Kumar, P., & Alland, D. (2022). A comprehensive update to the *Mycobacterium tuberculosis* H37Rv reference genome. *Nature Communications, 13*(1), 7068. DOI: 10.1038/s41467-022-34853-x PMID: 36400796

Choi, H., Lee, H., Ra, S. W., Kim, H. K., Lee, J. S., Um, S.-J., Kim, S.-H., Oh, Y.-M., & Kwon, Y.-S. (2021). Clinical characteristics of patients with post-tuberculosis bronchiectasis: Findings from the KMBARC registry. *Journal of Clinical Medicine, 10*(19), 4542. DOI: 10.3390/jcm10194542 PMID: 34640560

Chorna, Y., Lukash, I. G., Kalancha, Y., Tonkonoh, L., Abdullaeva, M., Adenov, M., Chuprynska, M., Hasanova, S., Ibragimova, O., Jazybekova, P., Kamenska, N., Klymenko, O., Koroieva, I., Kravets, L., Kryshtafovych, N., Pirtina, L., Skrahina, A., Terleeva, Y., Vilc, V., & Daftary, A. (2025). Perspectives on multisectoral accountability framework to end tuberculosis in the Eastern Europe and Central Asia region: A mixed-methods study. *BMC Global and Public Health, 3*(1), 20. DOI: 10.1186/s44263-025-00136-y PMID: 40045393

Choudhary, E., Sharma, R., Pal, P., & Agarwal, N. (2022). Deciphering the proteomic landscape of *Mycobacterium tuberculosis* in response to acid and oxidative stresses. *ACS Omega, 7*(30), 26749–26766. DOI: 10.1021/acsomega.2c03092 PMID: 35936415

Chowdhury, A. N., Raj, A., & Sharma, P. (2021). Impact of WhatsApp-based educational videos on tuberculosis screening uptake in urban slums of India. *BMC Public Health, 21*(1), 1234. DOI: 10.1186/s12889-021-11234-7

Chung, M. J., Goo, J. M., & Im, J.-G. (2004). Pulmonary tuberculosis in patients with idiopathic pulmonary fibrosis. *European Journal of Radiology, 52*(2), 175–179. DOI: 10.1016/j.ejrad.2003.11.017 PMID: 15489076

Cintron, C., Dauphinais, M. R., Du, X., Tabackman, A., Lenart, A., Laliberte, A., Dirksen, J., & Sinha, P. (2025). Enriching tuberculosis research by measuring poverty better: A perspective. *BMC Global and Public Health, 3*(1), 17. DOI: 10.1186/s44263-025-00127-z PMID: 39980069

Cloud, D. H., Garcia-Grossman, I. R., Armstrong, A., & Williams, B. (2023). Public health and prisons: Priorities in the age of mass incarceration. *Annual Review of Public Health, 44*(1), 407–428. DOI: 10.1146/annurev-publhealth-071521-034016

Cogo, H., Caseris, M., Lachaume, N., Cointe, A., Faye, A., & Pommelet, V. (2021). Tuberculosis in children hospitalized in a low-burden country: Description and risk factors of severe disease. *The Pediatric Infectious Disease Journal, 40*(3), 199–204. DOI: 10.1097/INF.0000000000002990 PMID: 33464014

Cohen, J. (1960). A coefficient of agreement for nominal scales. *Educational and Psychological Measurement, 20*(1), 37–46. DOI: 10.1177/001316446002000104

Conradie, F. (2021). High rate of successful outcomes treating highly resistant TB in the ZeNix study of pretomanid, bedaquiline and alternative doses and durations of linezolid [Abstract OALB01LB02]. *11th IAS Conference on HIV Science, Geneva, Switzerland*. International AIDS Society.

Conradie, F., Bagdasaryan, T. R., Borisov, S., Howell, P., Mikiashvili, L., Ngubane, N., Samoilova, A., Skornykova, S., Tudor, E., Variava, E., Yablonskiy, P., Everitt, D., Wills, G. H., Sun, E., Olugbosi, M., Egizi, E., Li, M., Holsta, A., Timm, J., & Spigelman, M. (2022). Bedaquiline-pretomanid-linezolid regimens for drug-resistant tuberculosis. *The New England Journal of Medicine, 387*(9), 810–823. DOI: 10.1056/NEJMoa2119430 PMID: 36053506

Conradie, F., Diacon, A. H., Ngubane, N., Howell, P., Everitt, D., Crook, A. M., Mendel, C. M., Egizi, E., Moreira, J., Timm, J., McHugh, T. D., Wills, G. H., Bateson, A., Hunt, R., Van Niekerk, C., Li, M., Olugbosi, M., & Spigelman, M. (2020). Treatment of Highly Drug-Resistant Pulmonary Tuberculosis. *The New England Journal of Medicine, 382*(10), 893–902. DOI: 10.1056/NEJMoa1901814 PMID: 32130813

Cords, O., Martinez, L., Warren, J. L., O'Marr, J. M., Walter, K. S., Cohen, T., Zheng, J., Ko, A. I., Croda, J., & Andrews, J. R. (2021). Incidence and prevalence of tuberculosis in incarcerated populations: A systematic review and meta-analysis. *The Lancet. Public Health, 6*(5), e300–e308. DOI: 10.1016/S2468-2667(21)00025-6

Coreil, J., Mayard, G., Simpson, K. M., Lauzardo, M., Zhu, Y., & Weiss, M. (2010). Structural forces and the production of TB-related stigma among Haitians in two contexts. *Social Science & Medicine, 71*(8), 1409–1417. DOI: 10.1016/j.socscimed.2010.07.017

Cosaburi, R. (1992). Principles of exercise training. *Chest, 101*(5), 263S–267S. DOI: 10.1378/chest.101.5_Supplement.263S PMID: 1576847

Council for International Organizations of Medical Sciences. (2016). *International ethical guidelines for health-related research involving humans*. CIOMS.

Courtwright, A., & Turner, A. N. (2010). Tuberculosis and stigma: Pathways and interventions. *Public Health Reports (Washington, D.C.)*, *125*(4_suppl, Suppl 4), 34–42. DOI: 10.1177/00333549101250S407

Coussens, A. K., Zaidi, S. M., Allwood, B. W., Dewan, P. K., Gray, G., Kohli, M., Kredo, T., Marais, B. J., Marks, G. B., Martinez, L., Ruhwald, M., Scriba, T. J., Seddon, J. A., Tisile, P., Warner, D. F., Wilkinson, R. J., Esmail, H., Houben, R. M. G. J., Alland, D., & Yi, S. (2024). Classification of early tuberculosis states to guide research for improved care and prevention: An international Delphi consensus exercise. *The Lancet. Respiratory Medicine*, *12*(6), 484–498. DOI: 10.1016/S2213-2600(24)00028-6 PMID: 38527485

Creswell, J. W., & Plano Clark, V. L. (2018). *Designing and conducting mixed methods research* (3rd ed.). SAGE.

Creswell, J., Codlin, A. J., Andre, E., Micek, M. A., Bedru, A., Carter, E. J., Yadav, R.-P., Mosneaga, A., Rai, B., Banu, S., Brouwer, M., Blok, L., Sahu, S., & Ditiu, L. (2014). Results from early programmatic implementation of Xpert MTB/RIF testing in nine countries. *BMC Infectious Diseases*, *14*(1), 1–12. DOI: 10.1186/1471-2334-14-2 PMID: 24383553

Cruz, A. T., Hwang, K. M., Birnbaum, G. D., & Starke, J. R. (2013). Adolescents with tuberculosis: A review of 145 cases. *The Pediatric Infectious Disease Journal*, *32*(9), 937–941. DOI: 10.1097/INF.0b013e3182933214 PMID: 23538527

Cubillos-Angulo, J. M., Nogueira, B. M. F., Arriaga, M. B., Barreto-Duarte, B., Araújo-Pereira, M., Fernandes, C. D., Vinhaes, C. L., Villalva-Serra, K., Nunes, V. M., Miguez-Pinto, J. P., Amaral, E. P., & Andrade, B. B. (2022). Host-directed therapies in pulmonary tuberculosis: Updates on anti-inflammatory drugs. *Frontiers in Medicine*, *9*, 970408. Advance online publication. DOI: 10.3389/fmed.2022.970408 PMID: 36213651

da Silva, E. H., Lima, E., dos Santos, T. R., & Padoveze, M. C. (2022). Prevalence and incidence of tuberculosis in health workers: A systematic review of the literature. In *American Journal of Infection Control* (Vol. 50, Issue 7). DOI: 10.1016/j.ajic.2022.01.021

da Silva, T. S., Arêas, G. P. T., & da Cruz, D. A. L. M. (2022). Effect of pulmonary rehabilitation on functional capacity in individuals treated for pulmonary tuberculosis: A systematic review protocol. *JBI Evidence Synthesis*, *20*(10), 2552–2558. DOI: 10.11124/JBIES-21-00314 PMID: 36081386

Dahl, V. N., Fløe, A., & Wejse, C. (2023). Nontuberculous mycobacterial infections in a Danish region between 2011 and 2021: Evaluation of trends in diagnostic codes. *Infectious Diseases*, *55*(6), 439–443. DOI: 10.1080/23744235.2023.2194411 PMID: 36995113

Damanik, A. S., Fitri, A., Hidayati, F., Nasution, H. S., Wisudariani, E., & Riyandani, E. (2025). Determinants of Pulmonary Tuberculosis Among Inmates in Class IIA Penitentiary in Jambi City. *Environmental Research and Planetary Health*, *1*(1), 18–25. DOI: 10.53623/erph.v1i1.517

Daniel, T. M. (2006). The history of tuberculosis. *Respiratory Medicine*, *100*(11), 1862–1870. DOI: 10.1016/j.rmed.2006.08.006

Dara, M., Acosta, C. D., Melchers, N. V. V., Al-Darraji, H. A., Chorgoliani, D., Reyes, H., Centis, R., Sotgiu, G., Ambrosio, L. D., Chadha, S. S., & Migliori, G. B. (2015). Tuberculosis control in prisons: Current situation and research gaps. *International Journal of Infectious Diseases*, *32*, 111–117. DOI: 10.1016/j.ijid.2014.12.029

Dara, M., Solovic, I., Goletti, D., Sotgiu, G., Centis, R., D'Ambrosio, L., Ward, B., Teixeira, V., Gratziou, C., & Migliori, G. B. (2016). Preventing and controlling tuberculosis among refugees in Europe : More is needed. *The European Respiratory Journal*, *48*(1), 272–274. DOI: 10.1183/13993003.00329-2016

Darraj, A., Hudays, A., Hazazi, A., Hobani, A., & Alghamdi, A. (2023). The association between emergency department overcrowding and delay in treatment: a systematic review. In *Healthcare* (Vol. 11, No. 3, p. 385). MDPI. DOI: 10.3390/healthcare11030385

Dartois, V., & Rubin, E. J. (2023). Shortening tuberculosis treatment—A strategic retreat. *The New England Journal of Medicine*, *388*(10), 939–941. DOI: 10.1056/NEJMe2300413 PMID: 36807402

Das, S., Grant, L., & Fearon, D. (2025). Mapping the global landscape of task shifting and sharing: Trends, geographic disparities, and terminology from 1970 to 2022. *Critical Public Health*, *35*(1), 2501495. DOI: 10.1080/09581596.2025.2501495

de Oliveira, M. C. B., Sant'Anna, C. C., Luiz, R. R., & Kritski, A. L. (2020). Unfavorable outcomes in tuberculosis: Multidimensional factors among adolescents in Rio de Janeiro, Brazil. *The American Journal of Tropical Medicine and Hygiene*, *103*(6), 2492–2500. DOI: 10.4269/ajtmh.20-0209 PMID: 32959763 de Oliveira, M. C. B., Sant'Anna, C. C., Luiz, R. R., Soares, E. C. C., & Kritski, A. L. (2019). Contribution of Xpert MTB/RIF to clinical diagnosis in adolescents with tuberculosis in Rio de Janeiro, Brazil. *The International Journal of Tuberculosis and Lung Disease : the Official Journal of the International Union against Tuberculosis and Lung Disease*, *23*(10), 1115–1121. DOI: 10.5588/ijtld.18.0778 PMID: 31627777

Debnath, A., Singh, N., Gupta, S., & Kishore, J. (2024). Burden of Tuberculosis among tribal populations of India: A systematic review and meta-analysis. In *Lung India* (Vol. 41, Issue 2). DOI: 10.4103/lungindia.lungindia_412_23

Deb, U., & Biswas, S. (2021). Pretomanid: The latest USFDA-approved anti-tuberculosis drug. *The Indian Journal of Tuberculosis*, *68*(2), 287–291. DOI: 10.1016/j.ijtb.2020.09.003 PMID: 33845969

Derges, J., Kidger, J., Fox, F., Campbell, R., Kaner, E., & Hickman, M. (2017). Alcohol screening and brief interventions for adults and young people in health and community-based settings: A qualitative systematic literature review. *BMC Public Health*, *17*(1), 562. Advance online publication. DOI: 10.1186/s12889-017-4476-4 PMID: 28599632

Desai, J. P., & Moustarah, F. (2022). Pulmonary compliance. In *StatPearls* [Internet]. StatPearls Publishing.

DeSanto, D., Velen, K., Lessells, R., Makgopa, S., Gumede, D., Fielding, K., Grant, A. D., Charalambous, S., & Chetty-Makkan, C. M. (2023). A qualitative exploration into the presence of TB stigmatization across three districts in South Africa. *BMC Public Health*, *23*(1), 504. DOI: 10.1186/s12889-023-15407-2 PMID: 36922792

Devassy, T. V., Nishanth, P., Sharma, D., & Thomas, A. M. (2022). Sleep disorders in elderly population suffering from TB and respiratory diseases. *The Indian Journal of Tuberculosis*, *69*, S272–S279. DOI: 10.1016/j.ijtb.2022.10.019 PMID: 36400523

Dhavan, P., Dias, H. M., Creswell, J., & Weil, D. (2017). An overview of tuberculosis and migration. *The International Journal of Tuberculosis and Lung Disease : the Official Journal of the International Union against Tuberculosis and Lung Disease*, *21*(6), 610–623. DOI: 10.5588/ijtld.16.0917 PMID: 28482955

Dheda, K., Barry, C. E.III, & Maartens, G. (2016). Tuberculosis. *Lancet*, *387*(10024), 1211–1226. DOI: 10.1016/S0140-6736(15)00151-8

Dheda, K., Mirzayev, F., Cirillo, D. M., Udwadia, Z., Dooley, K. E., Chang, K. C., Omar, S. V., Reuter, A., Perumal, T.Jr, Horsburgh, C. R.Jr, Murray, M., & Lange, C. (2024). Multidrug-resistant tuberculosis. *Nature Reviews. Disease Primers*, *10*(1), 22. DOI: 10.1038/s41572-024-00504-2

Diacon, A. H., Barry, C. E.III, Carlton, A., Chen, R. Y., Davies, M., de Jager, V., Fletcher, K., Koh, G. C. K. W., Kontsevaya, I., Heyckendorf, J., Lange, C., Reimann, M., Penman, S. L., Scott, R., Maher-Edwards, G., Tiberi, S., Vlasakakis, G., Upton, C. M., & Aguirre, D. B. (2024). A first-in-class leucyl-tRNA synthetase inhibitor, ganfeborole, for rifampicin-susceptible tuberculosis: A phase 2a open-label, randomized trial. *Nature Medicine, 30*(3), 896–904. DOI: 10.1038/s41591-024-02829-7 PMID: 38365949

Diallo, T., Adjobimey, M., Ruslami, R., Trajman, A., Sow, O., Obeng Baah, J., Marks, G. B., Long, R., Elwood, K., Zielinski, D., Gninafon, M., Wulandari, D. A., Apriani, L., Valiquette, C., Fregonese, F., Hornby, K., Li, P.-Z., Hill, P. C., Schwartzman, K., & Menzies, D. (2018). Safety and side effects of rifampin versus isoniazid in children. *The New England Journal of Medicine, 379*(5), 454–463. DOI: 10.1056/NEJMoa1714284 PMID: 30067928

Diel, R., Loytved, G., Nienhaus, A., Castell, S., Detjen, A., Geerdes-Fenge, H., Haas, W., Hauer, B., Konigstein, B., Maffei, D., & others. (2011). New recommendations for contact tracing in tuberculosis. German Central Committee against Tuberculosis. *Pneumologie, 65*(6), 359–378. DOI: 10.1055/s-0030-1256577

Diel, R., Loddenkemper, R., Meywald-Walter, K., Gottschalk, R., & Nienhaus, A. (2009). Comparative Performance of Tuberculin Skin Test, QuantiFERON-TB-Gold In Tube Assay, and T-Spot. TB Test in Contact Investigations for Tuberculosis. *Chest, 135*(4), 1010–1018. DOI: 10.1378/chest.08-2048

Dietiker, F., Lester, W., Gottlieb, R., & Burrows, B. (1961). Single-breath pulmonary diffusing capacity measurements in patients with pulmonary tuberculosis. *The American Review of Respiratory Disease, 84*(6), 807–813. PMID: 13886305

Dillman, D. A., Smyth, J. D., & Christian, L. M. (2014). *Internet, phone, mail, and mixed-mode surveys: The tailored design method* (4th ed.). Wiley. DOI: 10.1002/9781394260645

Ding, F., Liu, W., Wu, C., Zhang, W., Chen, S., Lai, W., Qu, J., Lin, Q., Lu, S., & Qu, J. (2025). Whole-genome sequencing reveals transmission pattern and drug resistance of Mycobacterium tuberculosis intra- or inter-hosts. *Frontiers in Cellular and Infection Microbiology, 14*, 1488547. DOI: 10.3389/fcimb.2024.1488547 PMID: 39906217

Diriba, G., Alemu, A., Yenew, B., Tola, H. H., Gamtesa, D. F., Mollalign, H., Eshetu, K., Moga, S., Abdella, S., Tollera, G., Kebede, A., & Dangisso, M. H. (2023). Epidemiology of extensively drug-resistant tuberculosis among patients with multidrug-resistant tuberculosis: A systematic review and meta-analysis. *International Journal of Infectious Diseases, 132*, 50–63. DOI: 10.1016/j.ijid.2023.04.392 PMID: 37072053

Dirks, L. K., Bircher, P. M., González-Montalvo, M. D. M., Kauffman, A. E., Prophete, E. J., Bury, M. R., & Spaulding, A. C. (2023). Video Directly Observed Therapy for Tuberculosis Treatment in Haitian Prisons: A Pattern of Group Adherence. medRxiv, 2023-12. DOI: 10.1101/2023.12.29.23299977

Divala, T. H., Lewis, J., Bulterys, M. A., Lutje, V., Corbett, E. L., Schumacher, S. G., & MacPherson, P. (2022). Missed opportunities for diagnosis and treatment in patients with TB symptoms: A systematic review. *Public Health Action, 12*(1), 10–17. DOI: 10.5588/pha.21.0022

Dmitrieva, A., Stepanov, V., & Titar, I. (2024). (e)Managing the uncertainty of tuberculosis in the post-Soviet limbo: Tracking prisoners' coerced mobility for treatment in Ukrainian prisons. *Social Science & Medicine, 349*, 116894. DOI: 10.1016/j.socscimed.2024.116894

Dobler, C. C. (2016). Screening strategies for active tuberculosis : Focus on cost-effectiveness. *ClinicoEconomics and Outcomes Research, 8*, 335–347. DOI: 10.2147/CEOR.S92244

Dodd, P. J., Sismanidis, C., & Seddon, J. A. (2016). Global burden of drug-resistant tuberculosis in children: A mathematical modelling study. *The Lancet. Infectious Diseases, 16*(10), 1193–1201. DOI: 10.1016/S1473-3099(16)30132-3 PMID: 27342768

Dodd, P. J., Van Zandvoort, K., Checchi, F., Khan, U., Haqmal, M., Khan, P., & McQuaid, C. F. (2025). Thinking fast and slow: The urgency of crisis response must not lead us to overlook chronic needs such as tuberculosis. *BMJ Global Health, 10*(3), e018012. Advance online publication. DOI: 10.1136/bmjgh-2024-018012 PMID: 40132810

Dogra, A. C., Gupta, U., Sarkar, M., & Padam, A. (2015). Exercise-induced desaturation in patients with chronic obstructive pulmonary disease on six-minute walk test. *Lung India : Official Organ of Indian Chest Society, 32*(4), 320–325. DOI: 10.4103/0970-2113.159550 PMID: 26180379

Dookie, N., Ngema, S. L., Perumal, R., Naicker, N., Padayatchi, N., & Naidoo, K. (2022). The changing paradigm of drug-resistant tuberculosis treatment: Successes, pitfalls, and future perspectives. *Clinical Microbiology Reviews*, *35*(4), e0018019. Advance online publication. DOI: 10.1128/cmr.00180-19 PMID: 36200885

Dos Santos, A., Lazzari, T. K., & Silva, D. R. (2017). Health-related quality of life, depression and anxiety in hospitalized patients with tuberculosis. *Tuberculosis and Respiratory Diseases*, *80*(1), 69–76. DOI: 10.4046/trd.2017.80.1.69 PMID: 28119749

Dou, W., Liu, Y., Liu, Z., Yerezhepov, D., Kozhamkulov, U., Akilzhanova, A., Dib, O., & Chan, C.-K. (2021). An AutoML Approach for Predicting Risk of Progression to Active Tuberculosis based on Its Association with Host Genetic Variations. 2021 10th International Conference on Bioinformatics and Biomedical Science, 82–88. DOI: 10.1145/3498731.3498743

Dowman, L., Hill, C. J., May, A., & Holland, A. E. (2021). Pulmonary rehabilitation for interstitial lung disease. *Cochrane Database of Systematic Reviews*, *2*(2), Cd006322. DOI: 10.1002/14651858.CD006322.pub4 PMID: 34559419

du Preez, K., Jenkins, H. E., Martinez, L., Chiang, S. S., Dlamini, S. S., Dolynska, M., Aleksandrin, A., Kobe, J., Graham, S. M., Hesseling, A. C., Starke, J. R., Seddon, J. A., & Dodd, P. J. (2025). Global burden of tuberculous meningitis in children aged 0–14 years in 2019: A mathematical modelling study. *The Lancet. Global Health*, *13*(1), e59–e68. DOI: 10.1016/S2214-109X(24)00383-8 PMID: 39706662

Edge, C. L., King, E. J., Dolan, K., & McKee, M. (2016). Prisoners co-infected with tuberculosis and HIV: A systematic review. *Journal of the International AIDS Society*, *19*(1), 20960. DOI: 10.7448/IAS.19.1.20960

Eisenhut, M., Shah, S., Kaba, O., Kara, M., Sütçü, M., Song, K. H., Kim, H. B., & Wang, M. (2025). Sensitivity of Immunodiagnostic Tests in Localized Versus Disseminated Tuberculosis—A Systematic Review of Individual Patient Data. *Tropical Medicine and Infectious Disease*, *10*(3), 70. DOI: 10.3390/tropicalmed10030070 PMID: 40137824

Emilian, C., Al-Juffali, N., & Fazel, S. (2025). Prevalence of severe mental illness among people in prison across 43 countries: A systematic review and meta-analysis. *The Lancet. Public Health*, *10*(2), e97–e110. https://www.thelancet.com/journals/lanpub/article/PIIS2468-2667(24)00280-9/fulltext. DOI: 10.1016/S2468-2667(24)00280-9

Enane, L. A., Duda, S. N., Chanyachukul, T., Bolton-Moore, C., Navuluri, N., Messou, E., Mbonze, N., McDade, L. R., Figueiredo, M. C., Ross, J., Evans, D., Diero, L., Akpata, R., Zotova, N., Freeman, A., Pierre, M. F., Rupasinghe, D., Ballif, M., Byakwaga, H., & Marcy, O. (2024). The Tuberculosis Sentinel Research Network (TB-SRN) of the International epidemiology Databases to Evaluate AIDS (IeDEA): Protocol for a prospective cohort study in Africa, Southeast Asia and Latin America. *BMJ Open*, *14*(1), e079138. Advance online publication. DOI: 10.1136/bmjopen-2023-079138

Enane, L. A., Eby, J., Arscott-Mills, T., Argabright, S., Caiphus, C., Kgwaadira, B., Steenhoff, A. P., & Lowenthal, E. D. (2020). TB and TB-HIV care for adolescents and young adults. *The International Journal of Tuberculosis and Lung Disease : the Official Journal of the International Union against Tuberculosis and Lung Disease*, *24*(2), 240–249. DOI: 10.5588/ijtld.19.0416 PMID: 32127110

Enane, L. A., Lowenthal, E. D., Arscott-Mills, T., Eby, J., Caiphus, C., Kgwaadira, B., Coffin, S. E., & Steenhoff, A. P. (2019). Investigating outcomes of adolescents and young adults (10–24 years of age) lost to follow-up from tuberculosis treatment in Gaborone, Botswana. *The Pediatric Infectious Disease Journal*, *38*(10), e271–e274. DOI: 10.1097/INF.0000000000002369 PMID: 31220045

Enane, L. A., Lowenthal, E. D., Arscott-Mills, T., Matlhare, M., Smallcomb, L. S., Kgwaadira, B., Coffin, S. E., & Steenhoff, A. P. (2016). Loss to follow-up among adolescents with tuberculosis in Gaborone, Botswana. *The International Journal of Tuberculosis and Lung Disease : the Official Journal of the International Union against Tuberculosis and Lung Disease*, *20*(10), 1320–1325. DOI: 10.5588/ijtld.16.0060 PMID: 27725042

Ernstmeyer, K., & Christman, E. (2024). OXYGENATION. *Nursing Fundamentals [Internet]. 2nd edition.*

Escombe, A. R., Oeser, C. C., Gilman, R. H., Navincopa, M., Ticona, E., Pan, W., Martínez, C., Chacaltana, J., Rodríguez, R., Moore, D. A. J., & Evans, C. A. (2007). Natural ventilation for the prevention of airborne contagion. *PLoS Medicine*, *4*(2), e68. DOI: 10.1371/journal.pmed.0040068 PMID: 17326709

Escombe, A. R., Ticona, E., Chávez-Pérez, V., Espinoza, M., & Moore, D. A. J. (2019). Improving natural ventilation in hospital waiting and consulting rooms to reduce nosocomial tuberculosis transmission risk in a low-resource setting. *BMC Infectious Diseases*, *19*(1), 88. DOI: 10.1186/s12879-019-3717-9 PMID: 30683052

Etim, N. G., Mirabeau, Y., Olorode, A., & Nwodo, U. (2024). Risk Factors of Tuberculosis and Strategies for Prevention and Control. *Int J Innovative Healthcare Res*, *12*(1), 1–13.

Evans, D., Hirasen, K., Casalme, D. J., Gler, M. T., Gupta, A., & Juneja, S. (2024). Cost and cost-effectiveness of BPaL regimen used in drug-resistant TB treatment in the Philippines. *IJTLD Open*, *1*(6), 242–249. DOI: 10.5588/ijtldopen.24.0094 PMID: 39021448

Evans, D., Hirasen, K., Ramushu, C., Long, L., Sinanovic, E., Conradie, F., Howell, P., Padanilam, X., Ferreira, H., Variaiva, E., Rajaram, S., Gupta, A., Juneja, S., & Ndjeka, N. (2024). Patient and provider costs of the new BPaL regimen for drug-resistant tuberculosis treatment in South Africa: A cost-effectiveness analysis. *PLoS One*, *19*(10), e0309034. Advance online publication. DOI: 10.1371/journal.pone.0309034 PMID: 39432463

Farhat, M., Cox, H., Ghanem, M., Denkinger, C. M., Rodrigues, C., Abd El Aziz, M. S., Enkh-Amgalan, H., Vambe, D., Ugarte-Gil, C., Furin, J., & Pai, M. (2024). Drug-resistant tuberculosis: A persistent global health concern. *Nature Reviews. Microbiology*, *22*(10), 617–635. DOI: 10.1038/s41579-024-01025-1 PMID: 38519618

Fatima, R., Qadeer, E., Enarson, D. A., Creswell, J., Stevens, R., Hinderaker, S. G., & Haq, M. (2014). Success of active tuberculosis case detection among high-risk groups in urban slums in Pakistan. *The International Journal of Tuberculosis and Lung Disease : the Official Journal of the International Union against Tuberculosis and Lung Disease*, *18*(9), 1099–1104. DOI: 10.5588/ijtld.14.0001 PMID: 25189559

Faurholt-Jepsen, D., Range, N., PrayGod, G., Jeremiah, K., Faurholt-Jepsen, M., Aabye, M. G., Changalucha, J., Christensen, D. L., Grewal, H. M. S., Martinussen, T., Krarup, H., Witte, D. R., Andersen, A. B., & Friis, H. (2013). Diabetes is a strong predictor of mortality during tuberculosis treatment: A prospective cohort study among tuberculosis patients from M wanza, T anzania. *Tropical Medicine & International Health*, *18*(7), 822–829. DOI: 10.1111/tmi.12120 PMID: 23648145

Fekadu, G., Tolossa, T., Turi, E., Bekele, F., & Fetensa, G. (2022). Pretomanid development and its clinical roles in treating tuberculosis. *Journal of Global Antimicrobial Resistance*, *31*, 175–184. DOI: 10.1016/j.jgar.2022.09.001 PMID: 36087906

Feng, Z., Wang, J., Xie, Y., & Li, J. (2021). Effects of exercise-based pulmonary rehabilitation on adults with asthma: A systematic review and meta-analysis. *Respiratory Research*, *22*(1), 1–12. DOI: 10.1186/s12931-021-01627-w PMID: 33516207

Fenta, M. D., Ogundijo, O. A., Warsame, A. A. A., & Belay, A. G. (2023). Facilitators and barriers to tuberculosis active case findings in low- and middle-income countries : A systematic review of qualitative research. *BMC Infectious Diseases, 23*(1), 515. DOI: 10.1186/s12879-023-08502-7

Ferreira, M. R., Bonfim, R. O., Siqueira, T. C., Andrade, R. L. P., Monroe, A. A., Villa, T. C. S., & Orfão, N. H. (2019). Tuberculosis in prison and aspects associated with the diagnosis site. *Journal of Infection in Developing Countries, 13*(11), 968–977. DOI: 10.3855/jidc.11522

Fessell, D., & Lexa, F. J. (2019). A Devilish Dilemma : To Recognize Top Performers . . . Or Not. *Journal of the American College of Radiology, 16*(7), 1009–1010. DOI: 10.1016/j.jacr.2019.01.023

FHI 360. (2024). *The Global Fund Grant Cycle 6 National Aligned HIV/AIDS Initiative (NAHI) End of Project Report: January 2021 – December 2023.* FHI 360. https://www.fhi360.org/resources/the-global-fund-grant-cycle-6-national-aligned-hiv-aids-initiative-nahi-end-of-project-report-january-2021-december-2023/

Field, A. (2013). *Discovering statistics using IBM SPSS Statistics* (4th ed.). SAGE.

Fong, I., Low, T. B., & Yii, A. (2022). Characterisation of the post-tuberculous phenotype of bronchiectasis: A real-world observational study. *Chronic Respiratory Disease, 19*, 14799731221098714. DOI: 10.1177/14799731221098714 PMID: 35471849

Fouskas, T. (2025). International migration management, employment and health integration of migrants and refugees in the artificial intelligence era. In *AI and diversity in a datafied world of work: Will the future of work be inclusive?* (pp. 161–181). Emerald Publishing Limited. DOI: 10.1108/S2051-233320250000012019

Fox, G. J., & Menzies, D. (2013). A review of the evidence for using bedaquiline (TMC207) to treat multi-drug resistant tuberculosis. *Infectious Diseases and Therapy, 2*(2), 123–144. DOI: 10.1007/s40121-013-0009-3 PMID: 25134476

Franchetti, Y. (2022). Use of Propensity Scoring and Its Application to Real-World Data: Advantages, Disadvantages, and Methodological Objectives Explained to Researchers Without Using Mathematical Equations. *Journal of Clinical Pharmacology, 62*(3), 304–319. DOI: 10.1002/jcph.1989 PMID: 34671990

Fuady, A., Arifin, B., Yunita, F., Rauf, S., Fitriangga, A., Sugiharto, A., Yani, F. F., Nasution, H. S., Putra, I. W. G. A. E., Mansyur, M., & Wingfield, T. (2024). Stigma, depression, quality of life, and the need for psychosocial support among people with tuberculosis in Indonesia: A multi-site cross-sectional study. *PLOS Global Public Health, 4*(1), e0002489. DOI: 10.1371/journal.pgph.0002489 PMID: 38190416

Gai, X., Allwood, B., & Sun, Y. (2023). Post-tuberculosis lung disease and chronic obstructive pulmonary disease. *Chinese Medical Journal, 136*(16), 1923–1928. DOI: 10.1097/CM9.0000000000002771 PMID: 37455331

Gallegos Morales, E. N., Knierer, J., Schablon, A., Nienhaus, A., & Kersten, J. F. (2017). Prevalence of latent tuberculosis infection among foreign students in Lübeck, Germany tested with QuantiFERON-TB Gold In-Tube and QuantiFERON-TB Gold Plus. *Journal of Occupational Medicine and Toxicology, 12*. *Journal of Occupational Medicine and Toxicology (London, England), 12*(1), 12. Advance online publication. DOI: 10.1186/s12995-017-0159-4 PMID: 28559919

Garcia-Prats, A. J., Schaaf, H. S., Draper, H. R., Garcia-Cremades, M., Winckler, J., Wiesner, L., Hesseling, A. C., & Savic, R. M. (2019). Pharmacokinetics, optimal dosing, and safety of linezolid in children with multidrug-resistant tuberculosis: Combined data from two prospective observational studies. *PLoS Medicine, 16*(4), e1002789. Advance online publication. DOI: 10.1371/journal.pmed.1002789 PMID: 31039153

Gashu, K. D., Gelaye, K. A., & Tilahun, B. (2021). Adherence to TB treatment remains low during continuation phase among adult patients in Northwest Ethiopia. *BMC Infectious Diseases, 21*(1), 725. DOI: 10.1186/s12879-021-06428-6 PMID: 34332550

Ge, E., Brode, S., Macdonald, L., Li, L., Lou, W., Liu, J., & Wei, X. (2024, August). Exploring impacts of air pollution and greenness on progressions of latent and active tuberculosis to inform interventions. In *ISEE Conference Abstracts* (Vol. 2024, No. 1). DOI: 10.1289/isee.2024.0257

Gengiah, S., Naidoo, K., Mlobeli, R., Tshabalala, M. F., Nunn, A. J., Padayatchi, N., Yende-Zuma, N., Taylor, M., Barker, P. M., & Loveday, M. (2021). A quality improvement intervention to inform scale-up of integrated HIV-TB services: Lessons learned from KwaZulu-Natal, South Africa. *Global Health, Science and Practice, 9*(3), 444–458. DOI: 10.9745/GHSP-D-21-00157 PMID: 34593572

Geraldes, I., Fernandes, M., Fraga, A. G., & Osório, N. S. (2022). The impact of single-cell genomics on the field of mycobacterial infection. *Frontiers in Microbiology, 13*, 989464. DOI: 10.3389/fmicb.2022.989464 PMID: 36246265

Geric, C., Qin, Z. Z., Denkinger, C. M., Kik, S. V., Marais, B., Anjos, A., David, P.-M., Ahmad Khan, F., & Trajman, A. (2023). The rise of artificial intelligence reading of chest X-rays for enhanced TB diagnosis and elimination. *The International Journal of Tuberculosis and Lung Disease : the Official Journal of the International Union against Tuberculosis and Lung Disease, 27*(5), 367–372. DOI: 10.5588/ijtld.22.0687 PMID: 37143227

Getachew, A., Silumbwe, A., Maritim, P., Hangoma, P., Belete, A., & Zulu, J. M. (2024). An evaluation of community acceptability and adoption of the community-based TB care program using the diffusion of innovation model. *Journal of Community Systems for Health, 1*(1). Advance online publication. DOI: 10.36368/jcsh.v1i1.1072

Getahun, H., Matteelli, A., Abubakar, I., Aziz, M. A., Baddeley, A., Barreira, D., Den Boon, S., Borroto Gutierrez, S. M., Bruchfeld, J., Burhan, E., Cavalcante, S., Cedillos, R., Chaisson, R., Chee, C. B.-E., Chesire, L., Corbett, E., Dara, M., Denholm, J., de Vries, G., & Raviglione, M. (2015). Management of latent Mycobacterium tuberculosis infection : WHO guidelines for low tuberculosis burden countries. *The European Respiratory Journal, 46*(6), 1563–1576. DOI: 10.1183/13993003.01245-2015

Getahun, H., Matteelli, A., Chaisson, R. E., & Raviglione, M. (2015). Latent *Mycobacterium tuberculosis* infection. *The New England Journal of Medicine, 372*(22), 2127–2135. DOI: 10.1056/NEJMra1405427 PMID: 26017823

Gianella, C., Pesantes, M. A., Ugarte-Gil, C., Moore, D. A. J., & Lema, C. (2019). Vulnerable populations and the right to health: Lessons from the Peruvian Amazon around tuberculosis control. *International Journal for Equity in Health, 18*(1), 28. Advance online publication. DOI: 10.1186/s12939-019-0928-z PMID: 31155000

Gillespie, S. H., DiNardo, A. R., Georghiou, S. B., Sabiiti, W., Kohli, M., Panzner, U., Kontsevaya, I., Hittel, N., Stuyver, L. J., Tan, J. B., van Crevel, R., Lange, C., Thuong, T. N. T., Heyckendorf, J., Ruhwald, M., & Heinrich, N. (2024). Developing biomarker assays to accelerate tuberculosis drug development: Defining target product profiles. *The Lancet Microbe, 5*(9), 100869. DOI: 10.1016/S2666-5247(24)00085-5 PMID: 38735303

Gilmour, B., & Alene, K. A. (2024). Ending tuberculosis: Challenges and opportunities. *Frontiers in Tuberculosis, 2*, 1487518. DOI: 10.3389/ftubr.2024.1487518

Gler, M. T., Skripconoka, V., Sanchez-Garavito, E., Xiao, H., Cabrera-Rivero, J. L., Vargas-Vasquez, D. E., Gao, M., Awad, M., Park, S.-K., Shim, T. S., Suh, G. Y., Danilovits, M., Ogata, H., Kurve, A., Chang, J., Suzuki, K., Tupasi, T., Koh, W.-J., Seaworth, B., & Wells, C. D. (2012). Delamanid for multidrug-resistant pulmonary tuberculosis. *The New England Journal of Medicine*, *366*(23), 2151–2160. DOI: 10.1056/NEJMoa1112433 PMID: 22670901

Goff, A., Cantillon, D., Muraro Wildner, L., & Waddell, S. J. (2020). Multi-Omics Technologies Applied to Tuberculosis Drug Discovery. *Applied Sciences (Basel, Switzerland)*, *10*(13), 4629. DOI: 10.3390/app10134629

Goig, G. A., Loiseau, C., Maghradze, N., Mchedlishvili, K., Avaliani, T., Brites, D., Borrell, S., Aspindzelashvili, R., Avaliani, Z., Kipiani, M., Tukvadze, N., Jugheli, L., & Gagneux, S. (2025). Transmission as a Key Driver of Resistance to the New Tuberculosis Drugs. *The New England Journal of Medicine*, *392*(1), 97–99. DOI: 10.1056/NEJMc2404644 PMID: 39752306

Goletti, D., Al-Abri, S., Migliori, G. B., Arlehamn, C. L., Haldar, P., Sundling, C., & Lee, S. S. (2024). World Tuberculosis Day 2024 theme "Yes! We can end TB" can be made a reality through concerted global efforts that advance detection, diagnosis, and treatment of tuberculosis infection and disease. *International Journal of Infectious Diseases*, *141*, 141. DOI: 10.1016/j.ijid.2024.106993 PMID: 38458422

Gomez, G. B., Siapka, M., Conradie, F., Ndjeka, N., Garfin, A. M. C., Lomtadze, N., Avaliani, Z., Kiria, N., Malhotra, S., Cook-Scalise, S., Juneja, S., Everitt, D., Spigelman, M., & Vassall, A. (2021). Cost-effectiveness of bedaquiline, pretomanid and linezolid for treatment of extensively drug-resistant tuberculosis in South Africa, Georgia and the Philippines. *BMJ Open*, *11*(12), e051521. Advance online publication. DOI: 10.1136/bmjopen-2021-051521 PMID: 34862287

Gonçalves, C., Arakaki-Sanchez, D., Pelissari, D. M., Costa, F. D., Croda, J., Walter, K. S., & Andrews, J. R. (2022). The effect of incarceration on TB treatment outcomes. *The International Journal of Tuberculosis and Lung Disease : the Official Journal of the International Union against Tuberculosis and Lung Disease*, *26*(3), 252–258. DOI: 10.5588/ijtld.21.0449

Gopalaswamy, R., Kumar, N., Vashistha, H., Rajendran, P., Kayesth, J., Peravali, C. J., Kashyap, S., Ghosh, S., Yumo, H., Moore, M., Anand, S., Ramachandran, R., Alavadi, U., Saini, S., & Shanmugam, S. (2023). Comprehensive assessment of invalid and indeterminate results in Truenat MTB-RIF testing across sites under the national TB elimination program of India. *Frontiers in Public Health*, *11*, 1255756. DOI: 10.3389/fpubh.2023.1255756 PMID: 37886056

Gotham, D., Martin, M., Barber, M. J., Kazounis, E., Batts, C., Scourse, R., Elder, G., & Nyang'wa, B. T. (2025). Cost analysis of the TB-PRACTECAL clinical trial on novel tuberculosis treatment regimens. *PLOS Global Public Health, 5*(4), e0003759. Advance online publication. DOI: 10.1371/journal.pgph.0003759 PMID: 40267985

Grange, J. M., Brunet, L. R., & Rieder, H. L. (2011). Immune protection against tuberculosis–When is immunotherapy preferable to vaccination? *Tuberculosis (Edinburgh, Scotland), 91*(2), 179–185. DOI: 10.1016/j.tube.2010.12.004

Gray, B. J., Perrett, S. E., Gudgeon, B., & Shankar, A. G. (2019). Investigating the prevalence of latent Tuberculosis infection in a UK remand prison. *Journal of Public Health (Oxford, England)*. Advance online publication. DOI: 10.1093/pubmed/fdy219

Greenaway, C., Sandoe, A., Vissandjee, B., Kitai, I., Gruner, D., Wobeser, W., Pottie, K., Ueffing, E., Menzies, D., & Schwartzman, K.Canadian Collaboration for Immigrant and Refugee Health. (2011). Tuberculosis : Evidence review for newly arriving immigrants and refugees. *Canadian Medical Association Journal, 183*(12), E939–E951. DOI: 10.1503/cmaj.090302

Greenhalgh, T., Schmid, M. B., & Czypionka, T.. (2024). Masks and respirators for prevention of respiratory infections: A systematic review. *Clinical Microbiology Reviews, 37*(2), e00124–e23. DOI: 10.1128/cmr.00124-23 PMID: 38775460

Green, M. C., & Brock, T. C. (2000). The role of transportation in the persuasiveness of public narratives. *Journal of Personality and Social Psychology, 79*(5), 701–721. DOI: 10.1037/0022-3514.79.5.701

Grobler, L., Mehtar, S., Dheda, K., Adams, S., Babatunde, S., Van Der Walt, M., & Osman, M. (2016). The epidemiology of tuberculosis in health care workers in South Africa: A systematic review. *BMC Health Services Research, 16*(1), 416. Advance online publication. DOI: 10.1186/s12913-016-1601-5 PMID: 27544429

Grohmann, C., Marapana, D. S., & Ebert, G. (2022). Targeted protein degradation at the host–pathogen interface. *Molecular Microbiology, 117*(4), 670–681. DOI: 10.1111/mmi.14849 PMID: 34816514

Guerrieri, M., Bargagli, E., Cassai, L., Gangi, S., Genovese, M., Viani, M., & Melani, A. S. (2024). Pulmonary tuberculosis in non-hiv adults: An evergreen old-fashioned disease in high-income countries. A narrative review. *Expert Review of Respiratory Medicine, 18*(11), 861–872. DOI: 10.1080/17476348.2024.2418932 PMID: 39434706

Guest, G., Bunce, A., & Johnson, L. (2006). How many interviews are enough? An experiment with data saturation and variability. *Field Methods*, *18*(1), 59–82. DOI: 10.1177/1525822X05279903

Guglielmetti, L., Khan, U., Velásquez, G. E., Gouillou, M., Abubakirov, A., Baudin, E., Berikova, E., Berry, C., Bonnet, M., Cellamare, M., Chavan, V., Cox, V., Dakenova, Z., de Jong, B. C., Ferlazzo, G., Karabayev, A., Kirakosyan, O., Kiria, N., Kunda, M., & Mitnick, C. D. (2025). Oral Regimens for Rifampin-Resistant, Fluoroquinolone-Susceptible Tuberculosis. *The New England Journal of Medicine*, *392*(5), 468–482. DOI: 10.1056/NEJMoa2400327 PMID: 39879593

Guler, R., Ozturk, M., Sabeel, S., Motaung, B., Parihar, S. P., Thienemann, F., & Brombacher, F. (2021). Targeting molecular inflammatory pathways in granuloma as host-directed therapies for tuberculosis. *Frontiers in Immunology*, *12*, 733853. Advance online publication. DOI: 10.3389/fimmu.2021.733853 PMID: 34745105

Gulumbe, B. H., Abdulrahim, A., Ahmad, S. K., Lawan, K. A., & Danlami, M. B. (2025). WHO report signals tuberculosis resurgence: Addressing systemic failures and revamping control strategies. *Decoding Infection and Transmission*, *3*, 100044. DOI: 10.1016/j.dcit.2025.100044

Guo, J., Zhang, X., Chen, X., & Cai, Y. (2022). Proteomics in biomarker discovery for tuberculosis: Current status and future perspectives. *Frontiers in Microbiology*, *13*, 845229. DOI: 10.3389/fmicb.2022.845229 PMID: 35558124

Guo, Q., Bi, J., Lin, Q., Ye, T., Wang, Z., Wang, Z., Liu, L., & Zhang, G. (2022). Whole Genome Sequencing Identifies Novel Mutations Associated With Bedaquiline Resistance in Mycobacterium tuberculosis. *Frontiers in Cellular and Infection Microbiology*, *12*, 807095. Advance online publication. DOI: 10.3389/fcimb.2022.807095 PMID: 35694543

Guo, W., Cronk, R., Scherer, E., Oommen, R., Brogan, J., Sarr, M., & Bartram, J. (2019). A systematic scoping review of environmental health conditions in penal institutions. *International Journal of Hygiene and Environmental Health*, *222*(5), 790–803. DOI: 10.1016/j.ijheh.2019.05.001

Gupta, R. K., Lucas, S. B., Fielding, K. L., & Lawn, S. D. (2015). Prevalence of tuberculosis in post-mortem studies of HIV-infected adults and children in resource-limited settings : A systematic review and meta-analysis. *AIDS (London, England)*, *29*(15), 1987–2002. DOI: 10.1097/QAD.0000000000000802

Hanekom, S., Pharaoh, H., Irusen, E., & Daniels, K. J. (2019). Post-tuberculosis health-related quality of life, lung function and exercise capacity in a cured pulmonary tuberculosis population in the Breede Valley District, South Africa. *The South African Journal of Physiotherapy, 75*(1), 1–8. PMID: 31392293

Harada, N., Nakajima, Y., Higuchi, K., Sekiya, Y., Rothel, J., & Mori, T. (2006). Screening for tuberculosis infection using whole-blood interferon-γ and Mantoux testing among Japanese healthcare workers. *Infection Control and Hospital Epidemiology, 27*(5), 442–448. DOI: 10.1086/503346

Haribhau, B. D. (2015). Study of polysomnography in cure post-tuberculosis patients. *Journal of Evolution of Medical and Dental Sciences, 4*(67), 11616–11626. DOI: 10.14260/jemds/2015/1676

Harms, C. A., Wetter, T. J., St. Croix, C. M., Pegelow, D. F., & Dempsey, J. A. (2000). Effects of respiratory muscle work on exercise performance. *Journal of Applied Physiology, 89*(1), 131–138. DOI: 10.1152/jappl.2000.89.1.131 PMID: 10904044

Harries, A. D., Maher, D., & Nunn, P. (1997). Practical and affordable measures for the protection of health care workers from tuberculosis in low-income countries. *Bulletin of the World Health Organization, 75*(5), •••. PMID: 9447782

Hashim, Z., Tyagi, R., Singh, G. V., Nath, A., & Kant, S. (2024). Preventive treatment for latent tuberculosis from Indian perspective. In *Lung India* (Vol. 41, Issue 1). DOI: 10.4103/lungindia.lungindia_336_23

Hassan, S., Yaesoubi, R., Magnus, O. B. H., Kanthali, M., Purohit, M. R., & Mustafa, T. (2025). Factors associated with the delay in diagnosis of extrapulmonary tuberculosis at the patient and health system level: A study from a rural setting in India. *PLoS One, 20*(1), e0316273. DOI: 10.1371/journal.pone.0316273 PMID: 39775521

Haute Autorité de Santé. (2023). *Evaluation des strategies de depistage et de reperage precoce de la tuberculose pulmonaire.* https://www.has-sante.fr/upload/docs/application/pdf/2023-09/evaluation_des_strategies_de_depistage_et_de_reperage_precoce_de_la_tuberculose_pulmonaire_-_note_de_2023-09-07_09-30-39_346.pdf

Hermes, L. (2020). *Untersuchung des Risikos des Vorliegens einer Latenten Tuberkuloseinfektion in der Allgemeinbevölkerung* [Doctoral dissertation, Hamburg, Germany].

Herrero-Cortina, B., Lee, A. L., Oliveira, A., O'Neill, B., Jácome, C., Dal Corso, S., Poncin, W., Muñoz, G., Inal-Ince, D., Alcaraz-Serrano, V., Reychler, G., Bellofiore, A., Posthumus, A., Tonia, T., Chalmers, J. D., & Spinou, A. (2023). European Respiratory Society statement on airway clearance techniques in adults with bronchiectasis. *The European Respiratory Journal*, *62*(1), 2202053. DOI: 10.1183/13993003.02053-2022 PMID: 37142337

Herzmann, C., Sotgiu, G., Bellinger, O., Diel, R., Gerdes, S., Goetsch, U., Heykes-Uden, H., Schaberg, T., & Lange, C. (2017). Risk for latent and active tuberculosis in Germany. *Infection, 45*(3), 283–290. DOI: 10.1007/s15010-016-0963-2

Hibah, N. A. A., & Hasan, H.-E. A. (2015). Prevalence of latent tuberculosis infection among multinational healthcare workers in Muhayil Saudi Arabia. *Egyptian Journal of Bronchology, 9*(2), 183–187.

Hickey, M. D., Ayieko, J., Kabami, J., Owaraganise, A., Kakande, E., Ogachi, S., Aoko, C. I., Wafula, E. M., Sang, N., Sunday, H., Revill, P., Bansi-Matharu, L., Shade, S. B., Chamie, G., Balzer, L. B., Petersen, M. L., Havlir, D. V., Kamya, M. R., & Phillips, A. N. (2025). Cost-effectiveness of leveraging existing HIV primary health systems and community health workers for hypertension screening and treatment in Africa: An individual-based modeling study. *PLoS Medicine*, *22*(1), e1004531. DOI: 10.1371/journal.pmed.1004531 PMID: 39854581

Hill, N. S. (2006). Pulmonary rehabilitation. *Proceedings of the American Thoracic Society*, *3*(1), 66–74. DOI: 10.1513/pats.200511-121JH PMID: 16493153

Ho, D. E., Imai, K., King, G., & Stuart, E. A. (2011). MatchIt: Nonparametric preprocessing for parametric causal inference. *Journal of Statistical Software, 42*(8), 1–28. DOI: 10.18637/jss.v042.i08

Horton, K. C., MacPherson, P., Houben, R. M., White, R. G., & Corbett, E. L. (2016). Sex Differences in Tuberculosis Burden and Notifications in Low- and Middle-Income Countries: A Systematic Review and Meta-analysis. *PLoS Medicine*, *13*(9), e1002119. DOI: 10.1371/journal.pmed.1002119 PMID: 27598345

Houben, R. M. G. J., & Dodd, P. J. (2016). The global burden of latent tuberculosis infection: A re-estimation using mathematical modelling. *PLoS Medicine*, *13*(10), e1002152. Advance online publication. DOI: 10.1371/journal.pmed.1002152 PMID: 27780211

Huang, Y., Guo, X., Wu, Y., Chen, X., Feng, L., Xie, N., & Shen, G. (2024). Nanotechnology's frontier in combatting infectious and inflammatory diseases: Prevention and treatment. *Signal Transduction and Targeted Therapy*, *9*(1), 34. Advance online publication. DOI: 10.1038/s41392-024-01745-z PMID: 38378653

Hudson, M., Todd, H., Nalugwa, T., Schraufnagel, A., Christian, C., Boccia, D., Wingfield, T., & Shete, P. B. (2025). [Manuscript title not provided]. *medRxiv*. DOI: 10.1101/2025.03.04.25323276

Hughes, G., Bern, H., Chiang, C. Y., Goodall, R. L., Nunn, A. J., Rusen, I. D., & Meredith, S. K. (2022). QT prolongation in the STREAM Stage 1 trial. *The International Journal of Tuberculosis and Lung Disease : the Official Journal of the International Union against Tuberculosis and Lung Disease*, *26*(4), 334–340. DOI: 10.5588/ijtld.21.0403 PMID: 35351238

Husnain, A. (2025). Artificial intelligence and deep learning in healthcare, cyber security, and food systems: A comprehensive review of applications, challenges, and future directions. *Global Journal of Emerging AI and Computing*, *1*(2), 95–126. DOI: 10.70445/gjeac.1.2.2025.95-126

Hussain, A., Khurana, A. K., Goyal, A., Kothari, S., Soman, R. K., Tej, S., & Pakhare, A. (2024). Effect of pulmonary rehabilitation in patients with post-tuberculosis sequelae with functional limitation. *The Indian Journal of Tuberculosis*, *71*(2), 123–129. DOI: 10.1016/j.ijtb.2023.04.012 PMID: 38589115

Hussain, T., Tripathy, S. S., Das, S., Satapathy, P., Das, D., Thomas, B., & Pati, S. (2020). Prevalence, risk factors and health seeking behaviour of pulmonary tuberculosis in four tribal dominated districts of Odisha: Comparison with studies in other regions of India. *PLoS One*, *15*(4), e0227083. DOI: 10.1371/journal.pone.0227083 PMID: 32251467

Hu, Y. Q., Liu, K., Lai, L. Q., He, Y. R., Hong, L. P., Jiang, C. Q., Liu, S.-M., & Cao, M.-Z. (2025). Evaluation of the diagnostic efficiency of fluorescence in situ hybridization for pulmonary tuberculosis: A systematic review and meta-analysis. *Frontiers in Medicine*, *11*, 1467530. DOI: 10.3389/fmed.2024.1467530 PMID: 39835097

Huynh, J., Abo, Y. N., Triasih, R., Singh, V., Pukai, G., Masta, P., Tsogt, B., Luu, B. K., Felisia, F., Pank, N., Aung, A., Morton, A., Azzopardi, P., Koesoemadinata, R. C., Alisjahbana, B., Hill, P. C., Marais, B. J., Chiang, S. S., & Graham, S. M. (2025). Emerging evidence to reduce the burden of tuberculosis in children and young people. *International Journal of Infectious Diseases*, *107869*, 107869. Advance online publication. DOI: 10.1016/j.ijid.2025.107869 PMID: 40049398

Idrees, M., & Bilal, M. (2023). Behind Bars: A Critical Investigation of Prison's Conditions and Protection of the Prisoner's Human Rights in Pakistan. *Review of Education. Administration & Law*, *6*(2), 567–578. DOI: 10.47067/real.v6i2.332

Idris, R., Zielbauer, A. S., Koepsell, J., Kloka, J., & Wetzstein, N. (2024). Extracorporeal membrane oxygenation (ECMO) in patients with tuberculosis: Systematic review and meta-analysis of 43 cases. *BMC Pulmonary Medicine*, *24*(1), 47. Advance online publication. DOI: 10.1186/s12890-023-02715-x

Igarashi, M. (2017). Development of new antituberculosis drugs from natural products. *Bioscience, Biotechnology, and Biochemistry*, *81*(1), 32–37. DOI: 10.1080/09168451.2016.1248369 PMID: 27885931

Institute of Medicine. Indian National Science Academy, & Indian Council of Medical Research. (2012). *The global burden of drug-resistant TB*. In *Facing the reality of drug-resistant tuberculosis in India: Challenges and potential solutions: Summary of a joint workshop* (pp. 37–54). National Academies Press. https://www.ncbi.nlm.nih.gov/books/NBK100388/

International Organization for Migration. (2021). [United Nations.]. *World Migration Report*, •••, 2022.

Islam, M. S., Chughtai, A. A., Nazneen, A., Chowdhury, K. I. A., Islam, M. T., Tarannum, S., Banu, S., & Seale, H. (2020). A tuberculin skin test survey among healthcare workers in two public tertiary care hospitals in Bangladesh. *PLoS One*, *15*(12), e0243951. DOI: 10.1371/journal.pone.0243951 PMID: 33332458

Ivanova, O., Hoffmann, V. S., Lange, C., Hoelscher, M., & Rachow, A. (2023). Post-tuberculosis lung impairment: Systematic review and meta-analysis of spirometry data from 14 621 people. *European Respiratory Review : an Official Journal of the European Respiratory Society*, *32*(168), 220221. DOI: 10.1183/16000617.0221-2022 PMID: 37076175

Jackson, S., Kabir, Z., & Comiskey, C. (2024). Retrospective cohort study exploring the impact of universal Tuberculosis (TB) vaccination cessation on the epidemiology of paediatric TB in Ireland, 2011–2021. *Vaccine*, *42*(8), 2099–2105. Advance online publication. DOI: 10.1016/j.vaccine.2024.02.061

Jain, D., & Tronic, B. (2018). Tuberculosis in India: A human rights approach to healthcare. *Sw. J. Int'l L.*, *24*, 219.

Jaligidad, K. (2016). *Study of Prevalence of Cor Pulmonale in Patients with Pulmonary Tuberculosis with Reference to ECG, Echocardiographic Changes and Radiological Extent of the Disease*. Rajiv Gandhi University of Health Sciences.

Janagond, A. B., Ganesan, V., Vijay Kumar, G. S., Ramesh, A., Anand, P., & Mariappan, M. (2017). Screening of health-care workers for latent tuberculosis infection in a Tertiary Care Hospital. *International Journal of Mycobacteriology, 6*(3), 253. Advance online publication. DOI: 10.4103/ijmy.ijmy_82_17 PMID: 28776523

Jebali, R., Hedhli, A., Daoud, S., Euchi, K., Marzouki, S., Medi, W., Chikh Rouhou, S., Ouahchi, Y., Merai, S., Toujani, S., Mjid, M., & Dhahri, B. (2023). Particularité de la tuberculose pulmonaire chez les patients immunodéprimé non infecté par le VIH. *Revue des Maladies Respiratoires Actualités, 15*(1), 274. DOI: 10.1016/j.rmra.2022.11.518

Jeffries, C., Lobue, P., Chorba, T., Metchock, B., & Kashef, I. (2017). Role of the Health Department in Tuberculosis Prevention and Control—Legal and Public Health Considerations. *Tuberculosis and Nontuberculous Mycobacterial Infections*, 261-282.

Jensen, P. A., Lambert, L. A., Iademarco, M. F., & Ridzon, R. (2005). *Guidelines for preventing the transmission of Mycobacterium tuberculosis in health-care settings, 2005* (NIH Publication No. 4046398604). National Institutes of Health.

Jhaveri, T. A., Jhaveri, D., Galivanche, A., Lubeck-Schricker, M., Voehler, D., Chung, M., Thekkur, P., Chadha, V., Nathavitharana, R., Kumar, A. M. V., Shewade, H. D., Powers, K., Mayer, K. H., Haberer, J. E., Bain, P., Pai, M., Satyanarayana, S., & Subbaraman, R. (2024). Barriers to engagement in the care cascade for tuberculosis disease in India: A systematic review of quantitative studies. *PLoS Medicine, 21*(5), e1004409. DOI: 10.1371/journal.pmed.1004409 PMID: 38805509

Johnston, J. C., Cooper, R., & Menzies, D. (2022). Treatment of tuberculosis disease. *Canadian Journal of Respiratory, Critical Care, and Sleep Medicine, 6*(sup1, Suppl. 1), 66–76. DOI: 10.1080/24745332.2022.2036504

Jones, S. A., Biswas, N., & Davies, H. E. (2025). Tuberculosis Related Pleural Effusion: An Update. *Current Pulmonology Reports, 14*(1), 9. DOI: 10.1007/s13665-025-00373-4

Joshi, R., Reingold, A. L., Menzies, D., & Pai, M. (2006). Tuberculosis among health-care workers in low- and middle-income countries: A systematic review. *PLoS Medicine, 3*(10), Article e494. DOI: 10.1371/journal.pmed.0030494

Junqueira-Kipnis, A. P., Leite, L. C. D. C., Croda, J., Chimara, E., Carvalho, A. C. C., & Arcêncio, R. A. (2024). Advances in the development of new vaccines for tuberculosis and Brazil's role in the effort forward the end TB strategy. *Memorias do Instituto Oswaldo Cruz, 119*, e240093. DOI: 10.1590/0074-02760240093 PMID: 39383403

Kadam, R. A. (2017). Informed consent process: A step further towards making it meaningful! *Perspectives in Clinical Research*, *8*(3), 107–112. DOI: 10.4103/picr.PICR_147_16 PMID: 28828304

Kakande, E., Ssekyanzi, B., Abbott, R., Ariho, W., Nattabi, G., Landsiedel, K., Temple, J., Chamie, G., Havlir, D. V., Kamya, M. R., Charlebois, E. D., Balzer, L. B., & Marquez, C. (2024). Prevalence and Predictors of Tuberculosis Infection in Children and Adolescents in Rural Uganda: A Cross-sectional Study. *The Pediatric Infectious Disease Journal*, *43*(12), 1120–1127. DOI: 10.1097/INF.0000000000004475 PMID: 39018476

Kaniga, K., Hasan, R., Jou, R., Vasiliauskienė, E., Chuchottaworn, C., Ismail, N., Metchock, B., Miliauskas, S., Viet Nhung, N., Rodrigues, C., Shin, S., Simsek, H., Smithtikarn, S., Ngoc, A. L. T., Boonyasopun, J., Kazi, M., Kim, S., Kamolwat, P., Musteikiene, G., & Omar, S. V. (2022). Bedaquiline drug resistance emergence assessment in multidrug-resistant tuberculosis (MDR-TB): A 5-year prospective in vitro surveillance study of bedaquiline and other second-line drug susceptibility testing in MDR-TB isolates. *Journal of Clinical Microbiology*, *60*(1), e0291920. Advance online publication. DOI: 10.1128/JCM.02919-20 PMID: 34705538

Kanwar, S. S. (2012). Diagnostic Methods for Mycobacterium tuberculosis and Challenges in Its Detection in India. In P.-J. Cardona (Éd.), *Understanding Tuberculosis—Global Experiences and Innovative Approaches to the Diagnosis*. InTech. DOI: 10.5772/31714

Katamba, A., Mochizuki, T., Nalugwa, T., Nantale, M., Oyuku, D., Nabwire, S., Babirye, D., Musinguzi, J., Nakawesa, A., Nekesa, I., Turyahabwe, S., Joloba, M., Dowdy, D. W., Moore, D. A. J., Davis, J. L., Shete, P., Adams, K., Reza, T., Fielding, K., & Cattamanchi, A. (2024). Impact of a multicomponent strategy including decentralized molecular testing for tuberculosis on mortality: Planned analysis of a cluster-randomized trial in Uganda. *EClinicalMedicine*, *78*, 102953. Advance online publication. DOI: 10.1016/j.eclinm.2024.102953 PMID: 39659443

Katrak, S., Lowenthal, P., Shen, R., True, L., Henry, L., & Barry, P. (2021). Bedaquiline for multidrug-resistant tuberculosis and QTc prolongation in California. *Journal of Clinical Tuberculosis and Other Mycobacterial Diseases*, *23*, 100216. DOI: 10.1016/j.jctube.2021.100216 PMID: 33598568

Kaufmann, S., Dorhoi, A., Hotchkiss, R., & Bartenschlager, R. (2018). Host-directed therapies for bacterial and viral infections. *Nature Reviews. Drug Discovery*, *17*(1), 35–56. DOI: 10.1038/nrd.2017.162 PMID: 28935918

Kaur, P., Potluri, V., Ahuja, V. K., Naveenkumar, C. N., Krishnamurthy, R. V., Gangadharaiah, S. T., Shivarudraiah, P., Eswaran, S., Nirmal, C. R., Mahizhaveni, B., Dusthackeer, A., Mondal, R., Batt, S. M., Richardson, E. J., Loman, N. J., Besra, G. S., Shandil, R. K., & Narayanan, S. (2021). A multi-targeting pre-clinical candidate against drug-resistant tuberculosis. *Tuberculosis (Edinburgh, Scotland)*, *129*, 102104. DOI: 10.1016/j.tube.2021.102104 PMID: 34214859

Kazemian, S. V., Shakeri, M., Nazar, E., Nasehi, M., Sharafi, S., & Dadgarmoghaddam, M. (2024). Prevalence, treatment outcomes and determinants of TB/HIV coinfection: A 4-year retrospective review of national tuberculosis registry in a country in a MENA region. *Heliyon*, *10*(5), e26615. Advance online publication. DOI: 10.1016/j.heliyon.2024.e26615

Kengo, A., Nabeemeeah, F., Denti, P., Sabet, R., Okyere-Manu, G., Abraham, P., Weisner, L., Mosala, M. H., Tshabalala, S., Scholefield, J., Resendiz-Galvan, J. E., Martinson, N. A., & Variava, E. (2024). Assessing potential drug-drug interactions between clofazimine and other frequently used agents to treat drug-resistant tuberculosis. *Antimicrobial Agents and Chemotherapy*, *68*(5), e0158323. Advance online publication. DOI: 10.1128/aac.01583-23 PMID: 38597667

Kerkhoff, A. D., Mwamba, C., Pry, J. M., Kagujje, M., Nyangu, S., Mateyo, K., Sanjase, N., Chilukutu, L., Christopoulos, K. A., Muyoyeta, M., & Sharma, A. (2023). A mixed methods study on men's and women's tuberculosis care journeys in Lusaka, Zambia—Implications for gender-tailored tuberculosis health promotion and case finding strategies. *PLOS Global Public Health*, *3*(6), e0001372. DOI: 10.1371/journal.pgph.0001372

Khan, A., Khan, N., & Singh, R. (2024). Tuberculosis diagnosis versus GeneXpert® MTB/RIF formats. *Bioanalysis*, *16*(16), 843–848. DOI: 10.1080/17576180.2024.2349423

Khan, A., Shaikh, B. T., & Baig, M. A. (2020). Knowledge, awareness, and health-seeking behaviour regarding tuberculosis in a rural district of Khyber Pakhtunkhwa, Pakistan. *BioMed Research International*, *2020*(1), 1852015. Advance online publication. DOI: 10.1155/2020/1850541 PMID: 32382530

Khan, M. F., Ali, A., Rehman, H. M., Noor Khan, S., Hammad, H. M., Waseem, M., Wu, Y., Clark, T. G., & Jabbar, A. (2024). Exploring optimal drug targets through subtractive proteomics analysis and pangenomic insights for tailored drug design in tuberculosis. *Scientific Reports*, *14*(1), 10904. DOI: 10.1038/s41598-024-61752-6 PMID: 38740859

Kharwadkar, S., Attanayake, V., Duncan, J., Navaratne, N., & Benson, J. (2022). The impact of climate change on the risk factors for tuberculosis: A systematic review. *Environmental Research, 212*, 113436. DOI: 10.1016/j.envres.2022.113436

Khattak, M., Rehman, A., Muqaddas, T., Hussain, R., Rasool, M. F., Saleem, Z., Almalki, M. S., Alturkistani, S. A., Firash, S. Z., Alzahrani, O. M., Bahauddin, A. A., Abuhussain, S. A., Najjar, M. F., Elsabaa, H. M. A., & Haseeb, A. (2024). Tuberculosis (TB) treatment challenges in TB-diabetes comorbid patients: A systematic review and meta-analysis. *Annals of Medicine, 56*(1), 2313683. Advance online publication. DOI: 10.1080/07853890.2024.2313683

Kimbrough, W., Saliba, V., Dahab, M., Haskew, C., & Checchi, F. (2012). The burden of tuberculosis in crisis-affected populations : A systematic review. *The Lancet. Infectious Diseases, 12*(12), 950–965. DOI: 10.1016/S1473-3099(12)70225-6

Kim, H. S., Lee, S., & Kim, J. H. (2018). Real-world evidence versus randomized controlled trial: Clinical research based on electronic medical records. *Journal of Korean Medical Science, 33*(34), e213. DOI: 10.3346/jkms.2018.33.e213 PMID: 30127705

King, T. L., Kavanagh, A., Scovelle, A. J., & Milner, A. (2020). Associations between gender equality and health: A systematic review. *Health Promotion International, 35*(1), 27–41. DOI: 10.1093/heapro/day093 PMID: 31916577

Kiryukhina, L. D., Kokorina, E. V., Gavrilov, P. V., Denisova, N. V., Archakova, L. I., & Yablonskiy, P. K. (2023). Gas Exchange in Patients with Pulmonary Tuberculosis: Relationships with Pulmonary Poorly Communicating Fraction and Alveolar Volume. *Journal of Respiration, 3*(2), 107–117. DOI: 10.3390/jor3020011

Knierer, J., Gallegos Morales, E. N., Schablon, A., Nienhaus, A., & Kersten, J. F. (2017). QFT-Plus: A plus in variability?—Evaluation of new generation IGRA in serial testing of students with a migration background in Germany. *Journal of Occupational Medicine and Toxicology, 12*. *Journal of Occupational Medicine and Toxicology (London, England), 1*(1), 1. Advance online publication. DOI: 10.1186/s12995-016-0148-z PMID: 28070206

Kolamou, R., Bah, B. S. S., Kalivogui, S., Diallo, B. M., & Barry, A. A. (2023). Prévalence de la co-infection tuberculose pulmonaire/VIH entre 2018-2020 dans le Centre de Diagnostic et de Traitement de la tuberculose de Damakania, République de Guinée : Prevalence of pulmonary tuberculosis/HIV co-infection between 2018-2020 in the Tuberculosis Diagnosis and Treatment Center of Damakania, Republic of Guinea. *International Journal of Biological and Chemical Sciences, 17*(2), 683–688. DOI: 10.4314/ijbcs.v17i2.31

Ko, Y., Lee, Y., Lee, H., Lee, Y., Song, J., Hong, G., Kim, M., Lee, H., Choi, S., & Shim, E. (2015). Changes in lung function according to disease extent before and after pulmonary tuberculosis. *The International Journal of Tuberculosis and Lung Disease : the Official Journal of the International Union against Tuberculosis and Lung Disease*, *19*(5), 589–595. DOI: 10.5588/ijtld.14.0454 PMID: 25868029

Kreuter, M. W., Lukwago, S. N., Bucholtz, R. D. C., Clark, E. M., & Sanders-Thompson, V. (2003). Achieving cultural appropriateness in health promotion programs: Targeted and tailored approaches. *Health Education & Behavior*, *30*(2), 133–146. DOI: 10.1177/1090198102251021

Krippendorff, K. (2013). *Content analysis: An introduction to its methodology* (3rd ed.). SAGE.

Krishna, S., & Jacob, J. J. (2021). Diabetes mellitus and tuberculosis.

Kroesen, V. M., Gröschel, M. I., Martinson, N., Zumla, A., Maeurer, M., van der Werf, T. S., & Vilaplana, C. (2017). Non-Steroidal Anti-inflammatory Drugs As Host-Directed Therapy for Tuberculosis: A Systematic Review. *Frontiers in Immunology*, *8*, 772. DOI: 10.3389/fimmu.2017.00772 PMID: 28713389

Kumari, R. (2024). Tribal health in India: Overcoming public health challenges with a focus on tuberculosis. *Apollo Medicine*, *22*(1), 76–83. DOI: 10.1177/09760016241277333

Kunst, H., Lange, B., Hovardovska, O., Bockey, A., Zenner, D., Andersen, A. B., Hargreaves, S., Pareek, M., Friedland, J. S., Wejse, C., Bothamley, G., Guglielmetti, L., Chesov, D., Tiberi, S., Matteelli, A., Mandalakas, A. M., Heyckendorf, J., Eimer, J., Malhotra, A., & Lange, C. (2025). Tuberculosis in adult migrants in Europe: A TBnet consensus statement. *The European Respiratory Journal*, *65*(3), 2401612. DOI: 10.1183/13993003.01612-2024 PMID: 39672603

Kustanto, A., & Ul-Haq, J. (2025). Ecological factors influencing tuberculosis in Indonesia: Exploring the interplay of health resources, socioeconomic status, climatic factors, and consumption patterns. *Journal of Population and Social Studies*, *33*, 822–843. DOI: 10.25133/JPSSv332025.044

Kuupiel, D., Vezi, P., Bawontuo, V., Osei, E., & Mashamba-Thompson, T. P. (2020). Tuberculosis active case-finding interventions and approaches for prisoners in sub-Saharan Africa: A systematic scoping review. *BMC Infectious Diseases*, *20*(1), 1–14. DOI: 10.1186/s12879-020-05283-1

Lama, V. N., Flaherty, K. R., Toews, G. B., Colby, T. V., Travis, W. D., Long, Q., Murray, S., Kazerooni, E. A., Gross, B. H., Lynch, J. P.III, & Martinez, F. J. (2003). Prognostic value of desaturation during a 6-minute walk test in idiopathic interstitial pneumonia. *American Journal of Respiratory and Critical Care Medicine*, *168*(9), 1084–1090. DOI: 10.1164/rccm.200302-219OC PMID: 12917227

Lange, C., Bothamley, G., Günther, G., Guglielmetti, L., Kontsevaya, I., Kuksa, L., Lange, B., Lorent, N., Saluzzo, F., Sester, M., Tebruegge, M., Tunesi, S., & Tweed, C.Tuberculosis Network European Trials Group. (2025). A year in review on tuberculosis and non-tuberculous mycobacteria disease: A 2025 update for clinicians and scientists. *Pathogens & Immunity*, *10*(2), 1–45. DOI: 10.20411/pai.v10i2.791 PMID: 40062355

Lara-Espinosa, J. V., & Hernández-Pando, R. (2021). Psychiatric problems in pulmonary tuberculosis: Depression and anxiety. *Journal of Tuberculosis Research*, *9*(01), 31–50. DOI: 10.4236/jtr.2021.91003

Lawn, S. D., & Nicol, M. P. (2011). Xpert® MTB/RIF assay: Development, evaluation and implementation of a new rapid molecular diagnostic for tuberculosis and rifampicin resistance. *Future Microbiology*, *6*(9), 1067–1082. DOI: 10.2217/fmb.11.84 PMID: 21958145

Laycock, K. M., Eby, J., Arscott-Mills, T., Argabright, S., Caiphus, C., Kgwaadira, B., Lowenthal, E. D., Steenhoff, A. P., & Enane, L. A. (2021). Towards quality adolescent-friendly services in TB care. *The International Journal of Tuberculosis and Lung Disease : the Official Journal of the International Union against Tuberculosis and Lung Disease*, *25*(7), 579–583. DOI: 10.5588/ijtld.21.0059 PMID: 34183104

Lee, S., Lee, W., & Kang, S. K. (2021). Tuberculosis infection status and risk factors among health workers: An updated systematic review. In *Annals of Occupational and Environmental Medicine* (Vol. 33, Issue 1). DOI: 10.35371/aoem.2021.33.e17

Lee, D., Islam, M. A., Natarajan, S., Dudekula, D. B., Chung, H., Park, J., & Oh, B. (2024). Identification of Anti-Tuberculosis Drugs Targeting DNA Gyrase A and Serine/Threonine Protein Kinase PknB: A Machine Learning-Assisted Drug-Repurposing Approach. *Tropical Medicine and Infectious Disease*, *9*(12), 288. DOI: 10.3390/tropicalmed9120288 PMID: 39728815

Lee, H. K., Teo, S. S. H., Barbier, S., Tang, S. C., Yeo, G. H., & Tan, N. C. (2016). The impact of direct observed therapy on daily living activities, quality of life and socioeconomic burden on patients with tuberculosis in primary care in Singapore. *Proceedings of Singapore Healthcare*, *25*(4), 235–242. DOI: 10.1177/2010105816652148

Lee, J. Y., Kwon, N., Goo, G. Y., & Cho, S. I. (2022). Inadequate housing and pulmonary tuberculosis: A systematic review. *BMC Public Health*, *22*(1), 622. DOI: 10.1186/s12889-022-12879-6

Lee, S. W. H., Nordin, A. A., Teng, W. Y., Osman, N. N., Mohan, D. S. R., Halim, N. H. A., Rahim, F. I. A., Syafira, N., & Assri, M. (2023). *A primary health care case study in the context of the COVID-19 pandemic.*

Li, A., Yuan, S.-y., Li, Q., Li, J., Yin, X.-y., & Liu, N. (2023). Prevalence and risk factors of malnutrition in patients with pulmonary tuberculosis: A systematic review and meta-analysis. *Frontiers in Medicine*, *10*, 1173619. DOI: 10.3389/fmed.2023.1173619 PMID: 37636566

Li, H., Salinger, D. H., Everitt, D., Li, M., Del Parigi, A., Mendel, C., & Nedelman, J. R. (2019). Long-term effects on QT prolongation of pretomanid alone and in combinations in patients with tuberculosis. *Antimicrobial Agents and Chemotherapy*, *63*(10), e00445–e19. DOI: 10.1128/AAC.00445-19 PMID: 31358590

Link, B. G., & Phelan, J. C. (2001). Conceptualizing stigma. *Annual Review of Sociology*, *27*(1), 363–385. DOI: 10.1146/annurev.soc.27.1.363

Li, S., Tan, Y., Deng, Y., Bai, G., Huang, M., Shang, Y., Wang, Y., Xue, Z., Zhang, X., Wang, W., Pan, J., & Pang, Y. (2024). The emerging threat of fluroquinolone-, bedaquiline-, and linezolid-resistant Mycobacterium tuberculosis in China: Observations on surveillance data. *Journal of Infection and Public Health*, *17*(1), 137–142. Advance online publication. DOI: 10.1016/j.jiph.2023.11.018

Litvinjenko, S., Magwood, O., Wu, S., & Wei, X. (2023). Burden of tuberculosis among vulnerable populations worldwide: An overview of systematic reviews. *The Lancet. Infectious Diseases*, *23*(12), 1395–1407. DOI: 10.1016/S1473-3099(23)00372-9

Liu, J., Ren, Z.-H., Qiang, H., Wu, J., Shen, M., Zhang, L., & Lyu, J. (2020). Trends in the incidence of diabetes mellitus: Results from the Global Burden of Disease Study 2017 and implications for diabetes mellitus prevention. *BMC Public Health*, *20*(1), 1415. Advance online publication. DOI: 10.1186/s12889-020-09502-x PMID: 32943028

Liu, X., Lan, H., Bai, X., Li, Q., Wen, Y., Feng, M., & Tang, X. (2023). Sleep quality and its associated factors among patients with tuberculosis: A cross-sectional study. *Frontiers in Public Health*, *10*, 1047425. DOI: 10.3389/fpubh.2022.1047425 PMID: 36684994

Liu, Y. E., Mabene, Y., Camelo, S., Rueda, Z. V., Pelissari, D. M., Johansen, F. D. C., Huaman, M. A., Avalos-Cruz, T., Alarcon, V. A., Ladutke, L., Bergman, M., Cohen, T., Goldhaber-Fiebert, J., Croda, J., & Andrews, J. R. (2024). Mass incarceration as a driver of the tuberculosis epidemic in Latin America and projected effects of policy alternatives: A mathematical modelling study. *The Lancet. Public Health*, *9*(11), e841–e851. https://www.thelancet.com/journals/lanpub/article/PIIS2468-2667(24)00192-0/fulltext. DOI: 10.1016/S2468-2667(24)00192-0

Liu, Y., Shi, J., Li, L., Wu, T., Chu, P., Pang, Y., Guo, Y., Gao, M., & Lu, J. (2022). Spontaneous mutational patterns and novel mutations for delamanid resistance in *Mycobacterium tuberculosis. Antimicrobial Agents and Chemotherapy*, *66*(8), e0053122. Advance online publication. DOI: 10.1128/aac.00531-22 PMID: 36448833

Liu, Y., Wu, Y. H., Zhang, S. C., Liu, L., Wu, M., & Cheng, M. M. (2024). Revisiting Computer-Aided Tuberculosis Diagnosis. *IEEE Transactions on Pattern Analysis and Machine Intelligence*, *46*(4), 2316–2332. Advance online publication. DOI: 10.1109/TPAMI.2023.3330825

Lönnroth, K., Castro, K. G., Chakaya, J. M., Chauhan, L. S., Floyd, K., Glaziou, P., & Raviglione, M. C. (2010). Tuberculosis control and elimination 2010–50 : Cure, care, and social development. *Lancet*, *375*(9728), 1814–1829. DOI: 10.1016/S0140-6736(10)60483-7

Lönnroth, K., Jaramillo, E., Williams, B. G., Dye, C., & Raviglione, M. (2009). Drivers of tuberculosis epidemics: The role of risk factors and social determinants. *Social Science & Medicine*, *68*(12), 2240–2246. DOI: 10.1016/j.socscimed.2009.03.041 PMID: 19394122

Lönnroth, K., Mor, Z., Erkens, C., Bruchfeld, J., Nathavitharana, R. R., van der Werf, M. J., & Lange, C. (2017). Tuberculosis in migrants in low-incidence countries: Epidemiology and intervention entry points. *The International Journal of Tuberculosis and Lung Disease : the Official Journal of the International Union against Tuberculosis and Lung Disease*, *21*(6), 624–637. DOI: 10.5588/ijtld.16.0845 PMID: 28482956

López, M. P., Ulloa, A. P., & Escobar, F. A. (2022). Tuberculosis and prison overcrowding from the perspective of social inequities in health in Colombia, 2018. *Biomédica : Revista del Instituto Nacional de Salud*, *42*(1), 159–169. DOI: 10.7705/biomedica.5894

Lu, W., Zhu, L., Liu, Q., Chen, C., Lu, P., Ding, X., Shao, Y., & Li, Y. (2023). Progress in Epidemiology of Tuberculosis in China. In *Progress in China Epidemiology* (Vol. 1, pp. 151–186). Springer Nature Singapore., DOI: 10.1007/978-981-19-2199-5_8

Lv, X., Guo, H., Lu, X., Tang, Z., Yu, K., Xu, G., Chen, S., Zhang, R., & Guo, J. (2025). GenVS-TBDB: An open AI-generated and virtual-screened small-molecule database for tuberculosis drug discovery [Preprint]. *bioRxiv*. DOI: 10.1101/2025.04.28.650819

Lynch, J. L., Barrientos-Pérez, M., Hafez, M., Jalaludin, M. Y., Kovarenko, M., Rao, P. V., & Weghuber, D. (2020). Country-specific prevalence and incidence of youth-onset type 2 diabetes: A narrative literature review. *Annals of Nutrition & Metabolism*, *76*(5), 289–296. DOI: 10.1159/000510499 PMID: 32980841

Mabud, T. S., de Lourdes Delgado Alves, M., Ko, A. I., Basu, S., Walter, K. S., Cohen, T., Mathema, B., Colijn, C., Lemos, E., Croda, J., & Andrews, J. R. (2019). Evaluating strategies for control of tuberculosis in prisons and prevention of spill-over into communities: An observational and modeling study from Brazil. *PLoS Medicine*, *16*(1), e1002737. DOI: 10.1371/journal.pmed.1002737

Macleod, A., Nair, D., Ilbahar, E., Sellars, M., & Nolte, L. (2020). Identifying barriers and facilitators to implementing advance care planning in prisons: A rapid literature review. *Health & Justice*, *8*(1), 1–11. DOI: 10.1186/s40352-020-00123-5

MacPherson, P., Houben, R. M. G. J., Glynn, J. R., Corbett, E. L., & Kranzer, K. (2013). Pre-treatment loss to follow-up in tuberculosis patients in low- and lower-middle-income countries and high-burden countries: A systematic review and meta-analysis. *Bulletin of the World Health Organization*, *92*(2), 126–138. DOI: 10.2471/BLT.13.124800 PMID: 24623906

MacPherson, P., Shanaube, K., Phiri, M. D., Rickman, H. M., Horton, K. C., Feasey, H. R., Corbett, E. L., Burke, R. M., & Rangaka, M. X. (2024). Community-based active-case finding for tuberculosis: Navigating a complex minefield. *BMC Global and Public Health*, *2*(1), 1–14. DOI: 10.1186/s44263-024-00042-9 PMID: 39681889

Mafirakureva, N., Hunter, R., Ferraro, C. F., Willner, S., Finnie, T., & Hayward, A.. (2025). Cost-effectiveness of tuberculosis infection screening at first reception into English prisons: A model-based analysis. *medRxiv*, 2021–5. DOI: 10.1101/2025.01.11.24319317

Mahajan, R. (2013). Bedaquiline: First FDA-approved tuberculosis drug in 40 years. *International Journal of Applied & Basic Medical Research*, *3*(1), 1–2. DOI: 10.4103/2229-516X.112228 PMID: 23776831

Mahler, B., & Croitoru, A. (2019). Pulmonary rehabilitation and tuberculosis: A new approach for an old disease. *Pneumologia (Bucharest, Romania)*, *68*(3), 107–113. DOI: 10.2478/pneum-2019-0024

Mamotte, N., Wassenaar, D., Koen, J., & Essack, Z. (2010). Convergent ethical issues in HIV/AIDS, tuberculosis and malaria vaccine trials in Africa: Report from the WHO/UNAIDS African AIDS Vaccine Programme's Ethics, Law and Human Rights Collaborating Centre consultation, 10–11 February 2009, Durban, South Africa. *BMC Medical Ethics, 11*(1), 3. DOI: 10.1186/1472-6939-11-3 PMID: 20211030

Marais, B. J., Gie, R. P., Schaaf, H. S., Hesseling, A. C., Obihara, C. C., Nelson, L. J., Enarson, D. A., Donald, P. R., & Beyers, N. (2004). The clinical epidemiology of childhood pulmonary tuberculosis: A critical review of literature from the pre-chemotherapy era. *The International Journal of Tuberculosis and Lung Disease : the Official Journal of the International Union against Tuberculosis and Lung Disease*, *8*(3), 278–285. PMID: 15139465

Marks, L. R., Nolan, N. S., Liang, S. Y., Durkin, M. J., & Weimer, M. B. (2022). Infectious complications of injection drug use. *Medical Clinics, 106*(1), 187–200. https://www.medical.theclinics.com/article/S0025-7125(21)00114-0/abstract

Marme, G., Kuzma, J., Zimmerman, P. A., Harris, N., & Rutherford, S. (2024). Investigating socio-ecological factors influencing implementation of tuberculosis infection prevention and control in rural Papua New Guinea. *Journal of Public Health (Oxford, England)*, *46*(2), 267–276. DOI: 10.1093/pubmed/fdae018 PMID: 38326281

Martín, D., Barbosa, P., Ramos, J. P., Vieira, M., & Duarte, R. (2024). People first: A participatory community approach on patient-reported outcomes in tuberculosis. *Breathe (Sheffield, England)*, *20*(1), 230138. DOI: 10.1183/20734735.0138-2023 PMID: 38482186

Martinez-Garcia, M., Guan, W., De-La-Rosa, D., Athanazio, R., Oscullo, G., Shi, M., Pujal-Montaña, P., Endlich, B., Tiberi, S., Centis, R., & Migliori, G. B. (2023). Post-TB bronchiectasis: From pathogenesis to rehabilitation. *The International Journal of Tuberculosis and Lung Disease : the Official Journal of the International Union against Tuberculosis and Lung Disease*, *27*(3), 175–181. DOI: 10.5588/ijtld.22.0566 PMID: 36855043

Martinez, L., Cords, O., Horsburgh, C. R., Andrews, J. R., Acuna-Villaorduna, C., Desai Ahuja, S., Altet, N., Augusto, O., Baliashvili, D., Basu, S., Becerra, M., Bonnet, M., Henry Boom, W., Borgdorff, M., Boulahbal, F., Carvalho, A. C. C., Cayla, J. A., Chakhaia, T., Chan, P.-C., & Zhu, L. (2020). The risk of tuberculosis in children after close exposure: A systematic review and individual-participant meta-analysis. *Lancet*, *395*(10228), 973–984. DOI: 10.1016/S0140-6736(20)30166-5 PMID: 32199484

Martinez, L., Warren, J. L., Harries, A. D., Croda, J., Espinal, M. A., Olarte, R. A. L., Avedillo, P., Lienhardt, C., Bhatia, V., Liu, Q., Chakaya, J., Denholm, J. T., Lin, Y., Kawatsu, L., Zhu, L., Horsburgh, R., & Andrews, J. R. (2023). Global, regional, and national estimates of tuberculosis incidence and case detection among incarcerated individuals from 2000 to 2019: A systematic analysis. *The Lancet. Public Health, 8*(7), e511–e519. https://www.thelancet.com/journals/lanpub/article/PIIS2468-2667(23)00097-X/fulltext. DOI: 10.1016/S2468-2667(23)00097-X

Maseko, A. F., Silumbwe, A., Maritim, P., Munakampe, M. N., Chirambo, G. B., Jacobs, C., & Zulu, J. M. (2025). Factors that shape the integration of HIV and TB services in Zomba District, Malawi. *BMC Health Services Research, 25*(1), 213. DOI: 10.1186/s12913-025-12367-8 PMID: 39915793

Masini, T., Furin, J., Udwadia, Z., & Guglielmetti, L. (2023). Optimal management of drug-resistant tuberculosis: Can India lead the way? *The Indian Journal of Medical Research, 157*(2-3), 220–222. DOI: 10.4103/ijmr.ijmr_300_23 PMID: 37202941

Matteucci, K. C., Correa, A. A. S., & Costa, D. L. (2022). Recent advances in host-directed therapies for tuberculosis and malaria. *Frontiers in Cellular and Infection Microbiology, 12*, 905278. Advance online publication. DOI: 10.3389/fcimb.2022.905278 PMID: 35669122

McAdams, H. P., Erasmus, J., & Winter, J. A. (1995). Radiologic manifestations of pulmonary tuberculosis. *Radiologic Clinics of North America, 33*(4), 655–678. DOI: 10.1016/S0033-8389(22)00611-X PMID: 7610237

Mcgee, P., Jensen, P. A., Lambert, L. A., Iademarco, M. F., Ridzon, R., & Mcgee, P. (2005). Morbidity and Mortality Weekly Report Guidelines for Preventing the Transmission of Mycobacterium tuberculosis in Health-Care Settings, 2005. *MMWR. Recommendations and Reports : Morbidity and Mortality Weekly Report. Recommendations and Reports / Centers for Disease Control, 54*(RR-17).

Meca, A.-D., Mititelu-Tar ău, L., Bogdan, M., Dijmarescu, L. A., Pelin, A.-M., & Foia, L. G. (2022). Mycobacterium tuberculosis and pulmonary rehabilitation: From novel pharmacotherapeutic approaches to management of post-tuberculosis sequelae. *Journal of Personalized Medicine, 12*(4), 569. DOI: 10.3390/jpm12040569 PMID: 35455684

Meghji, J., Auld, S. C., Bisson, G. P., Khosa, C., Masekela, R., Navuluri, N., & Rachow, A. (2025). Post-tuberculosis lung disease: Towards prevention, diagnosis, and care. *The Lancet. Respiratory Medicine, 13*(5), 460–472. Advance online publication. DOI: 10.1016/S2213-2600(24)00429-6 PMID: 40127662

Mehmood, A., Abbas, R., Saeed, A., Saleem, S., Nawaz, S., & Tabassum, S. (2024). Assessment of Dyspnea in Patients with Chronic Obstructive Lung Diseases with Modified Borg Scale; Descriptive Cross-Sectional Study: Assessment of Dyspnea in Chronic Obstructive Lung Diseases. *The Healer Journal of Physiotherapy and Rehabilitation Sciences*, *4*(3), 998–1005. DOI: 10.55735/hjprs.v4i3.243

Meintjes, G., & Maartens, G. (2024). HIV-associated tuberculosis. *The New England Journal of Medicine*, *391*(4), 343–355. DOI: 10.1056/NEJMra2308181 PMID: 39047241

Melendez, J., Sánchez, C. I., Philipsen, R. H. H. M., Maduskar, P., Dawson, R., Theron, G., Dheda, K., & Van Ginneken, B. (2016). An automated tuberculosis screening strategy combining X-ray-based computer-aided detection and clinical information. *Scientific Reports*, *6*(1), 25265. DOI: 10.1038/srep25265

Menzies, D. (2022). Canadian Tuberculosis Standards 8th edition: What's new? And what's next? In (Vol. 6, pp. 333-336): Taylor & Francis.

Menzies, D., Joshi, R., & Pai, M. (2007). Risk of tuberculosis infection and disease associated with work in health care settings. *International Journal of Tuberculosis and Lung Disease, 11*(6), 593–605.

Menzies, D., Joshi, R., & Pai, M. (2007). Risk of tuberculosis infection and disease associated with work in health care settings. *The International Journal of Tuberculosis and Lung Disease : the Official Journal of the International Union against Tuberculosis and Lung Disease*, *11*(6), 593–605.

Mera, H. B., Wagnew, F., Akelew, Y., Hibstu, Z., Berihun, S., Tamir, W., Alemu, S., Lamore, Y., Mesganaw, B., Adugna, A., & Tsegaye, T. B. (2023). Prevalence and Predictors of Pulmonary Tuberculosis among Prison Inmates in Sub-Saharan Africa : A Systematic Review and Meta-Analysis. *Tuberculosis Research and Treatment*, *6226200*, 1–13. Advance online publication. DOI: 10.1155/2023/6226200

Middelkoop, K., Bekker, L.-G., Liang, H., Aquino, L. D. H., Sebastian, E., Myer, L., & Wood, R. (2011). Force of tuberculosis infection among adolescents in a high HIV and TB prevalence community: A cross-sectional observation study. *BMC Infectious Diseases*, *11*(1), 156. Advance online publication. DOI: 10.1186/1471-2334-11-156 PMID: 21631918

Migliori, G. B., Thong, P. M., Alffenaar, J. W. C., Denholm, J., Tadolini, M., Al-yaquobi, F., Blanc, F.-X., Buonsenso, D., Chesov, D., & Codecasa, L. R. (2020). Worldwide effects of coronavirus disease pandemic on tuberculosis services, January–April 2020. *Emerging Infectious Diseases*, *26*(11), 2709–2712. DOI: 10.3201/eid2611.203163 PMID: 32917293

Millington, K. A., Nightingale, R., Walker, N. F., Ringwald, B., Cantillon, D., Karmadwala, F., & Wingfield, T. (2025). Addressing the growing TB disease burden in England. *The Lancet. Respiratory Medicine*, *13*(5), 387–389. Advance online publication. DOI: 10.1016/S2213-2600(25)00088-8 PMID: 40147470

Ministry of Health and Family Welfare. (2023). *TB India 2023: Annual status report*. Directorate General of Health Services, Government of India.

Minkler, M., & Wallerstein, N. (Eds.). (2008). *Community-based participatory research for health: From process to outcomes* (2nd ed.). Jossey-Bass.

Mirzayev, F., Viney, K., Linh, N. N., Gonzalez-Angulo, L., Gegia, M., Jaramillo, E., Zignol, M., & Kasaeva, T. (2021). World Health Organization recommendations on the treatment of drug-resistant tuberculosis, 2020 update. *The European Respiratory Journal*, *57*(6), 2003300. Advance online publication. DOI: 10.1183/13993003.03300-2020 PMID: 33243847

Mishra, G., Alffenaar, J.-W., Munje, R., & Khateeb, S. (2024). Adverse drug reactions due to linezolid in the programmatic management of drug-resistant tuberculosis in India: A retrospective multicenter study. *The Indian Journal of Tuberculosis*, *71*(Suppl 1), S101–S109. DOI: 10.1016/j.ijtb.2023.04.006 PMID: 39067941

Moodley, R., & Godec, T. R. (2016). Short-course treatment for multidrug-resistant tuberculosis: The STREAM trials. *European Respiratory Review : an Official Journal of the European Respiratory Society*, *25*(139), 29–35. DOI: 10.1183/16000617.0080-2015 PMID: 26929418

Moon, H.-W., & Hur, M. (2013). Interferon-gamma release assays for the diagnosis of latent tuberculosis infection: An updated review. *Annals of Clinical and Laboratory Science, 43*(2), 221–229.

Morgan, D. L. (1997). *Focus groups as qualitative research* (2nd ed.). SAGE. DOI: 10.4135/9781412984287

Mori, T., & Leung, C. C. (2010). Tuberculosis in the Global Aging Population. *Infectious Disease Clinics of North America*, *24*(3), 751–768. DOI: 10.1016/j.idc.2010.04.011

Morley, J. E., Vellas, B., Abellan Van Kan, G., Anker, S. D., Bauer, J. M., Bernabei, R., Cesari, M., Chumlea, W. C., Doehner, W., Evans, J., Fried, L. P., Guralnik, J. M., Katz, P. R., Malmstrom, T. K., McCarter, R. J., Gutierrez Robledo, L. M., Rockwood, K., Von Haehling, S., Vandewoude, M. F., & Walston, J. (2013). Frailty Consensus : A Call to Action. *Journal of the American Medical Directors Association*, *14*(6), 392–397. DOI: 10.1016/j.jamda.2013.03.022

Mosquera-Rendón, J., Moreno-Herrera, C. X., Robledo, J., & Hurtado-Páez, U. (2023). Genome-Wide Association Studies (GWAS) Approaches for the Detection of Genetic Variants Associated with Antibiotic Resistance: A Systematic Review. *Microorganisms, 11*(12), 2866. DOI: 10.3390/microorganisms11122866 PMID: 38138010

Mostafavi, E., Nasehi, M., Shahraki, A. H., Esmaeili, S., Ghaderi, E., Sharafi, S., & Doosti-Irani, A. (2016). Comparison of the tuberculin skin test and the QuantiFERON-TB Gold test in detecting latent tuberculosis in health care workers in Iran. *Epidemiology and Health, 38*, Article e2016032. DOI: 10.4178/epih.e2016032

Mouton, J. P., Njuguna, C., Kramer, N., Stewart, A., Mehta, U., Blockman, M., De Smidt, M. F., De Waal, R. R., Parrish, A. G., Wilson, D. P. K. K., Igumbor, E. U., Aynalem, G., Dheda, M., Maartens, G., Cohen, K., Fortuin-De Smidt, M., De Waal, R. R., Parrish, A. G., Wilson, D. P. K. K., & Krebs, A. (2021). Facility and patient barriers in the implementation of isoniazid preventive therapy for people living with. *The International Journal of Tuberculosis and Lung Disease : the Official Journal of the International Union against Tuberculosis and Lung Disease, 20*(1).

Mp, W. R., & Wijiastutik, Y.MP. (2024). Ecological Analysis of Children Tuberculosis (TB) in Indonesia. [NHSJ]. *Nursing and Health Sciences Journal, 4*(1), 71–75. Advance online publication. DOI: 10.53713/nhsj.v4i1.328

Mugenyi, N., Ssewante, N., Baruch Baluku, J., Bongomin, F., Mukenya Irene, M., Andama, A., & Byakika-Kibwika, P. (2024). Innovative laboratory methods for improved tuberculosis diagnosis and drug-susceptibility testing. *Frontiers in Tuberculosis, 1*, 1295979. Advance online publication. DOI: 10.3389/ftubr.2023.1295979

Mumtaz, Z., & Salway, S. (2005). 'I never go anywhere': Extricating the links between women's mobility and uptake of reproductive health services in Pakistan. *Social Science & Medicine, 60*(8), 1751–1765. DOI: 10.1016/j.socscimed.2004.08.019 PMID: 15686807

Mumtaz, Z., & Salway, S. M. (2007). Gender, pregnancy and the uptake of antenatal care services in Pakistan. *Sociology of Health & Illness, 29*(1), 1–26. DOI: 10.1111/j.1467-9566.2007.00519.x PMID: 17286703

Munedzimwe, F., Chetty-Makkan, C. M., Mukora, R., Charalambous, S., Turner, K., & Chihota, V. (2023). "It's about time they taught us": A qualitative study evaluating the barriers to finding and screening child contacts under five at risk for TB in Gauteng Province, South Africa from the provider and caregiver perspectives. *BMC Health Services Research, 23*(1), 1415. DOI: 10.1186/s12913-023-10359-0 PMID: 38102646

Muniyandi, M., Ramesh, P. M., Wells, W. A., Alavadi, U., Sahu, S., & Padmapriyadarsini, C. (2023). The cost-effectiveness of the BEAT-TB regimen for pre-extensively drug-resistant TB. *Tropical Medicine and Infectious Disease*, *8*(8), 411. Advance online publication. DOI: 10.3390/tropicalmed8080411 PMID: 37624349

Muñoz-Torrico, M., Rendon, A., Centis, R., D'Ambrosio, L., Fuentes, Z., Torres-Duque, C., Mello, F., Dalcolmo, M., Pérez-Padilla, R., Spanevello, A., & Migliori, G. B. (2016). Is there a rationale for pulmonary rehabilitation following successful chemotherapy for tuberculosis? *Jornal Brasileiro de Pneumologia : Publicaçao Oficial da Sociedade Brasileira de Pneumologia e Tisilogia*, *42*(5), 374–385. DOI: 10.1590/S1806-37562016000000226 PMID: 27812638

Musafiri, S., Dusabejambo, V., Munganyinka, B., Manzi, O., Kalisa, L., & Rutayisire, P. (2015). The aftermath of pulmonary tuberculosis: Predictors of severe pulmonary sequelae and quality of life of patients visiting a tertiary level of care in Rwanda, East Africa. *Austin J Pulm Respir Med*, *2*(2), 1027.

Muzanyi, G., Ntale, M., Salata, R., Joloba, M., Mukonzo, J., Mafigiri, D., Mubiri, P., & Bbosa, G. (2025). Hair isoniazid levels predict TB sputum culture conversion. *The International Journal of Tuberculosis and Lung Disease : the Official Journal of the International Union against Tuberculosis and Lung Disease*, *29*(1), 1–6. DOI: 10.5588/ijtld.24.0374 PMID: 39754284

Naeije, R., & Chesler, N. (2012). Pulmonary circulation at exercise. *Comprehensive Physiology*, *2*(1), 711–741. DOI: 10.1002/j.2040-4603.2012.tb00405.x PMID: 23105961

Nafisah, S. I., & Muhammad, G. (2024). Tuberculosis detection in chest radiograph using convolutional neural network architecture and explainable artificial intelligence. *Neural Computing & Applications*, *36*(1), 111–131. Advance online publication. DOI: 10.1007/s00521-022-07258-6

Nagarajan, K., Kumarswamy, K., Begum, R., Panibatla, V., Singarajipura, A., Adepu, R., Munjattu, J. F., Sellapan, S., Arangba, S., Goswami, A., Swamickan, R., Basha, J., Dsouza, P. M., & Muniyandi, M. (2024). Self-driven solutions and resilience adapted by people with drug-resistant tuberculosis and their caregivers in Bengaluru and Hyderabad, India: A qualitative study. *The Lancet Regional Health. Southeast Asia*, *22*, 22. DOI: 10.1016/j.lansea.2024.100372 PMID: 38420270

Naidoo, K., Perumal, R., Cox, H., Mathema, B., Loveday, M., Ismail, N., Omar, S. V., Georghiou, S. B., Daftary, A., O'Donnell, M., & Ndjeka, N. (2024). The epidemiology, transmission, diagnosis, and management of drug-resistant tuberculosis—Lessons from the South African experience. *The Lancet. Infectious Diseases*, *24*(9), e559–e575. DOI: 10.1016/S1473-3099(24)00144-0 PMID: 38527475

Nardell, E. A. (2016). Transmission and institutional infection control of tuberculosis. *Cold Spring Harbor Perspectives in Medicine*, *6*(2), a018192. DOI: 10.1101/cshperspect.a018192 PMID: 26292985

Nardell, E. A., & Fennelly, K. P. (2006). Tuberculosis transmission and infection control in congregate settings. In *Reichman and Hershfield's Tuberculosis* (pp. 843–872). CRC Press.

Nasir, A., Hassan, I. I., Ma'ruf, A., Suharno, N. E., Goenharto, S., Purwanto, C. R., & Tyas, A. P. M. (2024). Coping efforts made: Psychological burden of people living with tuberculosis due to social stigma in society. A qualitative phenomenology study. *PLoS One*, *19*(7), e0303331. DOI: 10.1371/journal.pone.0303331 PMID: 39078843

Nathavitharana, R. R., Mishra, H., Sullivan, A., Hurwitz, S., Lederer, P., Meintjes, J., Nardell, E., & Theron, G. (2022). Predicting Airborne Infection Risk : Association Between Personal Ambient Carbon Dioxide Level Monitoring and Incidence of Tuberculosis Infection in South African Health Workers. *Clinical Infectious Diseases*, *75*(8), 1297–1306. DOI: 10.1093/cid/ciac183

Navarro, C. E., Benjumea-Bedoya, D., Estupiñan-Bohórquez, A. F., & Florez, I. D. (2025). Cost-effectiveness analysis comparing QuantiFERON test and tuberculin skin test for the diagnosis of latent tuberculosis infection in immunocompetent children under 15 years of age in Colombia. *BMJ Open*, *15*(3), e087333. DOI: 10.1136/bmjopen-2024-087333 PMID: 40081973

Ndjeka, N., Conradie, F., Schnippel, K., Hughes, J., Bantubani, N., Ferreira, H., Maartens, G., Mametja, D., Meintjes, G., Padanilam, X., Variava, E., Pym, A., & Pillay, Y. (2015). Treatment of drug-resistant tuberculosis with bedaquiline in a high HIV prevalence setting: An interim cohort analysis. *The International Journal of Tuberculosis and Lung Disease : the Official Journal of the International Union against Tuberculosis and Lung Disease*, *19*(8), 979–985. DOI: 10.5588/ijtld.14.0944 PMID: 26162365

Negin, J., Abimbola, S., & Marais, B. J. (2015). Tuberculosis among older adults – time to take notice. *International Journal of Infectious Diseases*, *32*, 135–137. DOI: 10.1016/j.ijid.2014.11.018

Nema, V. (2012). Tuberculosis diagnostics : Challenges and opportunities. *Lung India : Official Organ of Indian Chest Society, 29*(3), 259. DOI: 10.4103/0970-2113.99112

Nicola Martins Rodrigues, S., Henriques, H., & Henriques, M. (2021). Effectiveness of a preoperative breathing exercises intervention on patients undergoing cardiac surgery: a systematic review. *European Journal of Preventive Cardiology, 28*(Supplement_1), zwab061. 345.

Nienhaus, A., Ringshausen, F. C., Costa, J. T., Schablon, A., & Tripodi, D. (2013). IFN-gamma release assay versus tuberculin skin test for monitoring TB infection in healthcare workers. *Expert Review of Anti-Infective Therapy, 11*(1), 37–48. DOI: 10.1586/eri.12.150

Nienhaus, A., Kesavachandran, C., Wendeler, D., Haamann, F., & Dulon, M. (2012). Infectious diseases in healthcare workers—An analysis of the standardised data set of a German compensation board. *Journal of Occupational Medicine and Toxicology, 7*. *Journal of Occupational Medicine and Toxicology (London, England), 8*(1), 8. Advance online publication. DOI: 10.1186/1745-6673-7-8 PMID: 22553942

Njagi, L. N., Mecha, J. O., Mureithi, M. W., Otieno, L. E., & Nduba, V. (2024). Towards pharmacogenomics-guided tuberculosis (TB) therapy: N-acetyltransferase-2 genotypes among TB-infected Kenyans of mixed ethnicity. *BMC Medical Genomics, 17*(1), 14. Advance online publication. DOI: 10.1186/s12920-023-01788-1

Noor, L., Zutshi, K., & Aman, I. (2024). Physical Rehabilitation for Tuberculosis: A Review of Literature. *Indian Journal of Preventive and Social Medicine, 55*(4), 400–407.

Nuermberger, E. L., Martínez-Martínez, M. S., Sanz, O., Urones, B., Esquivias, J., Soni, H., Tasneen, R., Tyagi, S., Li, S. Y., Converse, P. J., Boshoff, H. I., Robertson, G. T., Besra, G. S., Abrahams, K. A., Upton, A. M., Mdluli, K., Boyle, G. W., Turner, S., Fotouhi, N., & Jiménez, E. (2022). GSK2556286 Is a Novel Antitubercular Drug Candidate Effective *In Vivo* with the Potential To Shorten Tuberculosis Treatment. *Antimicrobial Agents and Chemotherapy, 66*(6), e0013222. DOI: 10.1128/aac.00132-22 PMID: 35607978

Nyang'wa, B. T., Berry, C., Kazounis, E., Motta, I., Parpieva, N., Tigay, Z., Solodovnikova, V., Liverko, I., Moodliar, R., Dodd, M., Ngubane, N., Rassool, M., McHugh, T. D., Spigelman, M., Moore, D. A. J., Ritmeijer, K., du Cros, P., & Fielding, K.TB-PRACTECAL Study Collaborators. (2022). A 24-Week, All-Oral Regimen for Rifampin-Resistant Tuberculosis. *The New England Journal of Medicine, 387*(25), 2331–2343. DOI: 10.1056/NEJMoa2117166 PMID: 36546625

Nyang'wa, B. T., Kloprogge, F., Moore, D. A. J., Bustinduy, A., Motta, I., Berry, C., & Davies, G. R. (2021). Population pharmacokinetics and pharmacodynamics of investigational regimens' drugs in the TB-PRACTECAL clinical trial (the PRACTECAL-PKPD study): A prospective nested study protocol in a randomised controlled trial. *BMJ Open*, *11*(9), e047185. Advance online publication. DOI: 10.1136/bmjopen-2020-047185 PMID: 34489274

Nyasulu, P. S., Hui, D. S., Mwaba, P., Tamuzi, J. L., Sakala, D. Y., Ntoumi, F., Maeurer, M., Goletti, D., Petersen, E., & Zumla, A. (2025). Global perspectives on tuberculosis in prisons and incarceration centers-Risk factors, priority needs, challenges for control and the way forward. *IJID Regions*, *14*, 100621. DOI: 10.1016/j.ijregi.2025.100621

O'Grady, J., Hoelscher, M., Atun, R., Bates, M., Mwaba, P., Kapata, N., Ferrara, G., Maeurer, M., & Zumla, A. (2011). Tuberculosis in prisons in sub-Saharan Africa–the need for improved health services, surveillance and control. *Tuberculosis (Edinburgh, Scotland)*, *91*(2), 173–178. DOI: 10.1016/j.tube.2010.12.002

O'Grady, M. A., Mootz, J., Suleman, A., Sweetland, A., Teodoro, E., Anube, A., Feliciano, P., Bezuidenhout, C., Dos Santos, P. F., Fumo, W., Gouveia, L., Pinsky, I., Mello, M., Kann, B., & Wainberg, M. L. (2022). Mobile technology and task shifting to improve access to alcohol treatment services in Mozambique. *Journal of Substance Abuse Treatment*, *134*, 108549. DOI: 10.1016/j.jsat.2021.108549

Octavia, D. R., Sholikha, J., & Utami, P. R. (2024). Validity and Reliability Test of the Medication Adherence Report Scale (MARS) Questionnaire for Tuberculosis (TB) Patients. [Journal of Pharmacy and Science]. *Journal Pharmasci*, *9*(1), 7–9. Advance online publication. DOI: 10.53342/pharmasci.v9i1.362

Ogwu, M. C., & Izah, S. C. (2025). Mobile health and telemedicine for tropical diseases. In *Technological innovations for managing tropical diseases* (pp. 183–211). Springer., DOI: 10.1007/978-3-031-82622-1_8

Okeke, C. C., Ibe, C. C., Nduji, O. J., Ndulue, C. J., Ngige, O., Amuchie, C. C., Ezema, C. C., Onyeogulu, A. O., Ojo, A., Obuseh, M., Alli, O. O., Akinteye, E. I., Idion, K. N., Akpan-Udo, U. I., Okereke, I. C., & Eke, C. (2025). Pulmonary Tuberculosis-Associated Morbidity in Africa: A Systematic Review. *Cureus*, *17*(1). Advance online publication. DOI: 10.7759/cureus.77569 PMID: 39958055

Okoroafor, S. C., & Christmals, C. D. (2024). Health professions education strategies for enhancing capacity for task-shifting and task-sharing implementation in Africa: A scoping review. *The Journal of Continuing Education in the Health Professions*, *44*(3), 194–202. DOI: 10.1097/CEH.0000000000000517 PMID: 37341562

Olawade, D. B., Eberhardt, J., David-Olawade, A. C., Balogun, M. A., Bolarinwa, O. A., & Esan, D. T. (2024). Transforming multidrug-resistant tuberculosis care: The potentials of telemedicine in resource-limited settings. *Health Sciences Review (Oxford, England)*, *12*, 100185. DOI: 10.1016/j.hsr.2024.100185

Oliveira, O., Gaio, R., Correia-Neves, M., Rito, T., & Duarte, R. (2021). Evaluation of drug-resistant tuberculosis treatment outcome in Portugal, 2000–2016. *PLoS One*, *16*(4), e0250028. Advance online publication. DOI: 10.1371/journal.pone.0250028 PMID: 33878119

Olowoyo, K. S., Esan, D. T., Olowoyo, P., Oyinloye, B. E., Fawole, I. O., Aderibigbe, S., Adigun, M. O., Olawade, D. B., Esan, T. O., & Adeyanju, B. T. (2025). Treatment adherence and outcomes in patients with tuberculosis treated with telemedicine: A scoping review. *Tropical Medicine and Infectious Disease*, *10*(3), 78. DOI: 10.3390/tropicalmed10030078 PMID: 40137831

Omoteso, O. A., Fadaka, A. O., Walker, R. B., & Khamanga, S. M. (2025). Innovative strategies for combating multidrug-resistant tuberculosis: Advances in drug delivery systems and treatment. *Microorganisms*, *13*(4), 722. Advance online publication. DOI: 10.3390/microorganisms13040722 PMID: 40284559

Ong, C. W., Elkington, P. T., & Friedland, J. S. (2014). Tuberculosis, pulmonary cavitation, and matrix metalloproteinases. *American Journal of Respiratory and Critical Care Medicine*, *190*(1), 9–18. DOI: 10.1164/rccm.201311-2106PP PMID: 24713029

Ono, K., Tabusadani, M., Yamane, K., Takao, S., Mori, K., Matsumura, Y., Kuroyama, Y., Kawahara, K., Omatsu, S., Furuuchi, K., Fujiwara, K., Morimoto, K., Kimura, H., & Senjyu, H. (2022). Decreased incremental shuttle walk test distance characterized by fibrocavitary lesions in non-tuberculous mycobacterial pulmonary disease. *Expert Review of Respiratory Medicine*, *16*(4), 469–475. DOI: 10.1080/17476348.2022.2049762 PMID: 35245168

Oostvogels, S., Ley, S. D., Heupink, T. H., Dippenaar, A., Streicher, E. M., De Vos, E., Meehan, C. J., Dheda, K., Warren, R., & Van Rie, A. (2022). Transmission, distribution and drug resistance-conferring mutations of extensively drug-resistant tuberculosis in the Western Cape Province, South Africa. *Microbial Genomics*, *8*(4), 000815. Advance online publication. DOI: 10.1099/mgen.0.000815 PMID: 35471145

Osman, M., du Preez, K., Seddon, J. A., Claassens, M. M., Dunbar, R., Dlamini, S. S., Welte, A., Naidoo, P., & Hesseling, A. C. (2021). Mortality in South African children and adolescents routinely treated for tuberculosis. *Pediatrics*, *147*(4), e2020032490. Advance online publication. DOI: 10.1542/peds.2020-032490 PMID: 33692161

Oyejide, A. J., Adekunle, Y. A., Abodunrin, O. D., & Atoyebi, E. O. (2025). *Artificial intelligence, computational tools and robotics for drug discovery, development, and delivery*. Intelligent Pharmacy., DOI: 10.1016/j.ipha.2025.01.001

Padmanabhanunni, A., & Pretorius, T. B. (2025). An exploratory study of the mental health of first responders: Depression, anxiety, and post-traumatic stress disorder. *South African Journal of Psychology. Suid-Afrikaanse Tydskrif vir Sielkunde, 55*(2), 00812463251317901. DOI: 10.1177/00812463251317901

Pai, M., Nicol, M. P., & Boehme, C. C. (2016). Tuberculosis Diagnostics : State of the Art and Future Directions. *Microbiology Spectrum, 4*(5), 4.5.16. DOI: 10.1128/microbiolspec.TBTB2-0019-2016

Pai, M., Zwerling, A., & Menzies, D. (2008). Systematic review: T-cell-based assays for the diagnosis of latent tuberculosis infection: An update. *Annals of Internal Medicine, 149*(3), 177–184. https://doi.org/DOI: 10.7326/0003-4819-149-3-200808050-00268

Pai, M., Behr, M. A., Dowdy, D., Dheda, K., Divangahi, M., & Schito, M. (2023). Tuberculosis. *Nature Reviews. Disease Primers, 2*(1), 16076. DOI: 10.1038/nrdp.2016.76 PMID: 27784885

Pai, M., & Swaminathan, S. (2023). India is well placed to scale innovations in tuberculosis diagnostics. *The Indian Journal of Medical Research, 157*(2&3), 114–117. DOI: 10.4103/ijmr.ijmr_243_23 PMID: 37006022

Panezai, S., Ahmad, M. M., & Saqib, S. E. (2017). Factors affecting access to primary health care services in Pakistan: A gender-based analysis. *Development in Practice, 27*(6), 813–827. DOI: 10.1080/09614524.2017.1344188

Papathakis, P., & Piwoz, E. (2008). Nutrition and Tuberculosis: A review of the literature and considerations for TB control programs. *United States Agency for International Development, Africa's Health 2010 Project*, 1.

Pape, S., Gulma, K., Shivalli, S., & de Kiev, L. C. (2022). Diagnostic accuracy of screening algorithms to identify persons with active pulmonary tuberculosis at prison entry: Protocol of a systematic review and network meta-analysis. *Journal of Medicine and Life, 15*(12), 1464–1475. DOI: 10.25122/jml-2022-0164

Pape, S., Gulma, K., Shivalli, S., & de Kiev, L. C. (2024). Diagnostic accuracy of active pulmonary tuberculosis screening during detention admission: A systematic review. *Journal of Medicine and Life, 17*(7), 671–681. DOI: 10.25122/jml-2024-0155

Parker, W., Kaland, A., & Mlomali, M. (2013). The impact of radio dramas on tuberculosis knowledge in rural Malawi. *International Journal of Communication, 7*, 1932–1950.

Park, H.-Y., Cheon, H.-B., Choi, S. H., & Kwon, J.-W. (2021). Health-related quality of life based on EQ-5D utility score in patients with tuberculosis: A systematic review. *Frontiers in Pharmacology, 12*, 659675. DOI: 10.3389/fphar.2021.659675 PMID: 33935781

Parvez, F. M. (2021). Prevention and control of tuberculosis in correctional facilities. In *Public health behind bars: from prisons to communities* (pp. 157–193). Springer US., DOI: 10.1007/978-1-0716-1807-3_11

Pasipanodya, J. G., Miller, T. L., Vecino, M., Munguia, G., Garmon, R., Bae, S., Drewyer, G., & Weis, S. E. (2007). Pulmonary impairment after tuberculosis. *Chest, 131*(6), 1817–1824. DOI: 10.1378/chest.06-2949 PMID: 17400690

Paton, N. I., Cousins, C., Suresh, C., Burhan, E., Chew, K. L., Dalay, V. B., Lu, Q., Kusmiati, T., Balanag, V. M., Lee, S. L., Ruslami, R., Pokharkar, Y., Djaharuddin, I., Sugiri, J. J. R., Veto, R. S., Sekaggya-Wiltshire, C., Avihingsanon, A., Sarin, R., Papineni, P., & Crook, A. M. (2023). Treatment strategy for rifampin-susceptible tuberculosis. *The New England Journal of Medicine, 388*(10), 873–887. DOI: 10.1056/NEJMoa2212537 PMID: 36808186

Patton, M. Q. (2002). *Qualitative research and evaluation methods* (3rd ed.). SAGE.

Peterson, E. J. R., Ma, S., Sherman, D. R., & Baliga, N. S. (2016). Network analysis identifies Rv0324 and Rv0880 as regulators of bedaquiline tolerance in *Mycobacterium tuberculosis. Nature Microbiology, 1*(8), 16078. Advance online publication. DOI: 10.1038/nmicrobiol.2016.78 PMID: 27573104

Petil, E. D.Jr, & Caballero, N. R. (2025). Physiotherapy in community-based rehabilitation in middle and low-income countries: A scoping review. *Philippine Journal of Physical Therapy, 4*(1), 11–26. DOI: 10.46409/002.ESRL3383

Phillips, P. P. J., Mitnick, C. D., Neaton, J. D., Nahid, P., Lienhardt, C., & Nunn, A. J. (2019). Keeping phase III tuberculosis trials relevant: Adapting to a rapidly changing landscape. *PLoS Medicine, 16*(3), e1002767. Advance online publication. DOI: 10.1371/journal.pmed.1002767 PMID: 30901331

Placeres, A. F., de Almeida Soares, D., Delpino, F. M., Moura, H. S. D., Scholze, A. R., Dos Santos, M. S., Arcêncio, R. A., & Fronteira, I. (2023). Epidemiology of TB in prisoners: A metanalysis of the prevalence of active and latent TB. *BMC Infectious Diseases, 23*(1), 20. DOI: 10.1186/s12879-022-07961-8

Pontali, E., Sotgiu, G., Tiberi, S., Tadolini, M., Visca, D., D'Ambrosio, L., Centis, R., Spanevello, A., & Migliori, G. B. (2018). Combined treatment of drug-resistant tuberculosis with bedaquiline and delamanid: A systematic review. *The European Respiratory Journal, 52*(1), 1800934. Advance online publication. DOI: 10.1183/13993003.00934-2018 PMID: 29903862

Poongothai, S., Anjana, R. M., Aarthy, R., Unnikrishnan, R., Narayan, K. M. V., Ali, M. K., Karkuzhali, K., & Mohan, V. (2023). Strategies for participant retention in long term clinical trials: A participant -centric approaches. *Perspectives in Clinical Research, 14*(1), 3–9. DOI: 10.4103/picr.picr_161_21 PMID: 36909219

Potty, R. S., Kumarasamy, K., Adepu, R., Reddy, R. C., Singarajipura, A., Siddappa, P. B., Sreenivasa, P. B., Thalinja, R., Lakkappa, M. H., Swamickan, R., Shah, A., Panibatla, V., Dasari, R., & Washington, R. (2021). Community health workers augment the cascade of TB detection to care in urban slums of two metro cities in India. *Journal of Global Health, 11*, 04042. DOI: 10.7189/jogh.11.04042

Prabhune, A. G., Dadha, P., & Prabhune, A. (2025). Bridging gaps in tuberculosis control: A culturally competent approach for tribal populations in India. *Cureus, 17*(3). Advance online publication. DOI: 10.7759/cureus.80689 PMID: 40242683

Pradipta, I. S., Idrus, L. R., Probandari, A., Lestari, B. W., Diantini, A., Alffenaar, J.-W. C., & Hak, E. (2021). Barriers and strategies to successful tuberculosis treatment in a high-burden tuberculosis setting: A qualitative study from the patient's perspective. *BMC Public Health, 21*(1), 1903. DOI: 10.1186/s12889-021-12005-y PMID: 34670527

Purdey, M. (2006). Anti-lactoferrin toxicity and elevated iron: The environmental prerequisites which activate susceptibility to tuberculosis infection? *Medical Hypotheses, 66*(3), 513–517. DOI: 10.1016/j.mehy.2005.09.027

Qin, Z. Z., Ahmed, S., Sarker, M. S., Paul, K., Adel, A. S. S., Naheyan, T., Barrett, R., Banu, S., & Creswell, J. (2021). Tuberculosis detection from chest x-rays for triaging in a high tuberculosis-burden setting : An evaluation of five artificial intelligence algorithms. *The Lancet. Digital Health, 3*(9), e543–e554. DOI: 10.1016/S2589-7500(21)00116-3

Rabahi, M. F., Silva Júnior, J. L. R. D., Ferreira, A. C. G., Tannus-Silva, D. G. S., & Conde, M. B. (2017). Tuberculosis treatment. *Jornal Brasileiro de Pneumologia, 43*(6), 472–486. https://doi.org/ (Erratum published in 2018, *Jornal Brasileiro de Pneumologia, 44*(4), 340. https://doi.org/)DOI: 10.1590/S1806-37562016000000388

Rafiza, S., Rampal, K. G., & Tahir, A. (2011). Prevalence and risk factors of latent tuberculosis infection among health care workers in Malaysia. *BMC Infectious Diseases, 11*. *BMC Infectious Diseases*, *19*(1), 19. Advance online publication. DOI: 10.1186/1471-2334-11-19 PMID: 21244645

Rahman, T., Khandakar, A., Rahman, A., Zughaier, S. M., Al Maslamani, M., Chowdhury, M. H., Tahir, A. M., Hossain, M. S. A., & Chowdhury, M. E. H. (2024). TB-CXRNet: Tuberculosis and Drug-Resistant Tuberculosis Detection Technique Using Chest X-ray Images. *Cognitive Computation*, *16*(3), 1393–1412. Advance online publication. DOI: 10.1007/s12559-024-10259-3

Rahmatullah, S., Rahmawati, R., & Arifin, A. (2025). Environmental Risk Factors and Tuberculosis Transmission: A Case-Control Study in Batu Mandi District, South Kalimantan, Indonesia, 2024. *Global Health & Environmental Perspectives*, *2*(1), 12–23.

Rajagopalan, S. (2001). Tuberculosis and Aging : A Global Health Problem. *Clinical Infectious Diseases*, *33*(7), 1034–1039. DOI: 10.1086/322671

Rajoli, R. K. R., Podany, A. T., Moss, D. M., Swindells, S., Flexner, C., Owen, A., & Siccardi, M. (2018). Modelling the long-acting administration of anti-tuberculosis agents using PBPK: A proof of concept study. *The International Journal of Tuberculosis and Lung Disease : the Official Journal of the International Union against Tuberculosis and Lung Disease*, *22*(8), 937–944. DOI: 10.5588/ijtld.17.0515 PMID: 29991405

Ramey, M. E., Kaya, F., Bauman, A. A., Massoudi, L. M., Sarathy, J. P., Zimmerman, M. D., Scott, D. W. L., Job, A. M., Miller-Dawson, J. A., Podell, B. K., Lyons, M. A., Dartois, V., Lenaerts, A. J., & Robertson, G. T. (2023). Drug distribution and efficacy of the DprE1 inhibitor BTZ-043 in the C3HeB/FeJ mouse tuberculosis model. *Antimicrobial Agents and Chemotherapy*, *67*(11), e0059723. DOI: 10.1128/aac.00597-23 PMID: 37791784

Rangaka, M. X., Cavalcante, S. C., Marais, B. J., Thim, S., Martinson, N. A., Swaminathan, S., & Chaisson, R. E. (2015). Controlling the seedbeds of tuberculosis: Diagnosis and treatment of tuberculosis infection. *Lancet*, *386*(10010), 2344–2353. https://www.thelancet.com/journals/lancet/article/PIIS0140-6736(15)00323-2/fulltext. DOI: 10.1016/S0140-6736(15)00323-2

Rashid, M., & Sharma, M. (2025). AI-assisted diagnosis and treatment planning—A discussion of how AI can assist healthcare professionals in making more accurate diagnoses and treatment plans for diseases. In AI in disease detection: Advancements and applications (pp. 313–336). DOI: 10.1016/B978-0-323-95393-6.00017-5

Raviglione, M. C., & Pio, A. (2002). Evolution of WHO policies for tuberculosis control, 1948–2001. *Lancet, 359*(9308), 775–780. DOI: 10.1016/S0140-6736(02)07880-7

Ravimohan, S., Kornfeld, H., Weissman, D., & Bisson, G. P. (2018). Tuberculosis and lung damage: From epidemiology to pathophysiology. *European Respiratory Review : an Official Journal of the European Respiratory Society, 27*(147), 170077. DOI: 10.1183/16000617.0077-2017 PMID: 29491034

Reichmann, M. T., Tezera, L. B., Vallejo, A. F., Vukmirovic, M., Xiao, R., Reynolds, J., Jogai, S., Wilson, S., Marshall, B., Jones, M. G., Leslie, A., D'Armiento, J. M., Kaminski, N., Polak, M. E., & Elkington, P. (2021). Integrated transcriptomic analysis of human tuberculosis granulomas and a biomimetic model identifies therapeutic targets. *The Journal of Clinical Investigation, 131*(15), e148136. DOI: 10.1172/JCI148136 PMID: 34128839

Rentmeester, L. L., Burton, D. W., Fitzgerald, R. L., & Clark, R. F. (2014). 2014 ACMT annual scientific meeting—March 28–30, 2014 Phoenix, AZ, USA. *Journal of Medical Toxicology; Official Journal of the American College of Medical Toxicology, 10*(1), 65–99. DOI: 10.1007/s13181-013-0376-x

Ren, W., Ma, Z., Li, Q., Liu, R., Ma, L., Yao, C., Shang, Y., Zhang, X., Gao, M., Li, S., & Pang, Y. (2024). Antigen-specific chemokine profiles as biomarkers for detecting Mycobacterium tuberculosis infection. *Frontiers in Immunology, 15*, 1359555. Advance online publication. DOI: 10.3389/fimmu.2024.1359555

Resnicow, L., Baranowski, T., Ahluwalia, J. S., & Braithwaite, R. L. (1999). Cultural sensitivity in public health: Defined and demystified. *Health Education & Behavior, 26*(3), 253–267. DOI: 10.1177/109019819902600302

Reyes, H. (2007). Pitfalls of TB management in prisons, revisited. *international journal of prisoner. International Journal of Prisoner Health, 3*(1), 43–67. DOI: 10.1080/17449200601149148

Riaz, A., Zaidi, S., & Khowaja, A. R. (2015). Perceived barriers to utilizing maternal and neonatal health services in contracted-out versus government-managed health facilities in the rural districts of Pakistan. *International Journal of Health Policy and Management, 4*(5), 279–284. DOI: 10.15171/ijhpm.2015.50 PMID: 25905478

Rich, J. D., Beckwith, C. G., Macmadu, A., Marshall, B. D. L., Brinkley-Rubinstein, L., Amon, J. J., Milloy, M.-J., King, M. R. F., Sanchez, J., Atwoli, L., & Altice, F. L. (2016). Clinical care of incarcerated people with HIV, viral hepatitis, or tuberculosis. *Lancet, 388*(10049), 1103–1114. DOI: 10.1016/S0140-6736(16)30379-8

Riessman, C. K. (2008). Narrative methods for the human sciences. *Sage (Atlanta, Ga.).*

Rifat, D., Li, S.-Y., Ioerger, T., Shah, K., Lanoix, J.-P., Lee, J., Bashiri, G., Sacchettini, J., & Nuermberger, E. (2021). Mutations in fbiD (Rv2983) as a novel determinant of resistance to pretomanid and delamanid in *Mycobacterium tuberculosis. Antimicrobial Agents and Chemotherapy*, *65*(1), e01948–e20. DOI: 10.1128/AAC.01948-20 PMID: 33077652

Rimande-Joel, R., & Ekenedo, G. O. (2019). Knowledge, belief and practice of cervical cancer screening and prevention among women of Taraba, North-East Nigeria. *Asian Pacific Journal of Cancer Prevention : APJCP*, *20*(11), 3291–3298. DOI: 10.31557/APJCP.2019.20.11.3291 PMID: 31759351

Ringshausen, F. C., Schablon, A., & Nienhaus, A. (2012). Interferon-gamma release assays for the tuberculosis serial testing of health care workers: A systematic review. *Journal of Occupational Medicine and Toxicology, 7*. *Journal of Occupational Medicine and Toxicology (London, England)*, *6*(1), 6. Advance online publication. DOI: 10.1186/1745-6673-7-6 PMID: 22537915

Rizvi, N., Khan, K. S., & Shaikh, B. T. (2014). Gender: Shaping personality, lives and health of women in Pakistan. *BMC Women's Health*, *14*(1), 53. Advance online publication. DOI: 10.1186/1472-6874-14-53 PMID: 24690271

Rizvi, N., & Nishtar, S. (2008). Pakistan's health policy: Appropriateness and relevance to women's health needs. *Health Policy (Amsterdam)*, *88*(2-3), 269–281. DOI: 10.1016/j.healthpol.2008.03.011 PMID: 18479774

Roberts, C. A., Lobato, M. N., Bazerman, L. B., Kling, R., Reichard, A. A., & Hammett, T. M. (2006). Tuberculosis prevention and control in large jails: A challenge to tuberculosis elimination. *American Journal of Preventive Medicine*, *30*(2), 125–130. DOI: 10.1016/j.amepre.2005.10.018

Rodriguez, C. A., Brooks, M. B., Guglielmetti, L., Hewison, C., Jachym, M. F., Lessem, E., Varaine, F., & Mitnick, C. D. (2019). Barriers and facilitators to early access of bedaquiline and delamanid for MDR-TB: A mixed-methods study. *Public Health Action*, *9*(1), 32–41. DOI: 10.5588/pha.18.0078 PMID: 30963040

Rolland, Y., Benetos, A., Gentric, A., Ankri, J., Blanchard, F., Bonnefoy, M., De Decker, L., Ferry, M., Gonthier, R., Hanon, O., Jeandel, C., Nourhashemi, F., Perret-Guillaume, C., Retornaz, F., Bouvier, H., Ruault, G., & Berrut, G. (2011). Frailty in older population : A brief position paper from the French society of geriatrics and gerontology. *Psychologie & Neuropsychiatrie du Vieillissement*, *9*(4), 387–390. DOI: 10.1684/pnv.2011.0311

Rosenstock, I. M. (1974). Historical origins of the Health Belief Model. *Health Education Monographs*, *2*(4), 328–335. DOI: 10.1177/109019817400200403

Rust, G., Ye, J., Baltrus, P., Daniels, E., Adesunloye, B., & Fryer, G. E. (2008). Practical barriers to timely primary care access: Impact on adult use of emergency department services. *Archives of Internal Medicine, 168*(15), 1705–1710. DOI: 10.1001/archinte.168.15.1705

Saini, V., & Garg, K. (2020). Case finding strategies under national tuberculosis elimination programme (NTEP). *indian journal of tuberculosis, 67*(4), S101-S106. DOI: 10.1016/j.ijtb.2020.09.029

Sakuma, T., Tatsumi, K., Kimura, H., Honda, Y., & Kuriyama, T. (1996). Sleep oxygen desaturation in late sequelae of pulmonary tuberculosis. *Internal Medicine (Tokyo, Japan), 35*(7), 534–539. DOI: 10.2169/internalmedicine.35.534 PMID: 8842758

Saleem, J., Rahmanulla, A., Ahmed, M. G., Sultana, R., & Prashantha Kumar, B. R. (2025). *Machine learning & deep learning tools in pharmaceutical sciences: A comprehensive review.* Intelligent Pharmacy., DOI: 10.1016/j.ipha.2024.11.003

Salman Latif, M. S., Shafee, I., Ali, J., Mannan, A., Deedar, S., & Waris, S. (2022). Six Minute Walk Test in People with Tuberculosis Sequelae. *Pakistan Journal of Medical & Health Sciences, 16*(03), 935–935. DOI: 10.53350/pjmhs22163935

Sancar, B., Doğan, A., & Taş, S. (2024). Timed Up-and-Go Test and Sit-to-Stand Test in Community-Dwelling Older Person: Inter and Intraobserver Reliability Among Turkish Nurses. *International Journal of Older People Nursing, 19*(5), e12649. DOI: 10.1111/opn.12649 PMID: 39297511

Sanchez, A., Massari, V., Gerhardt, G., Espinola, A. B., Siriwardana, M., Camacho, L. A. B., & Larouzé, B. (2013). X ray screening at entry and systematic screening for the control of tuberculosis in a highly endemic prison. *BMC Public Health, 13*(1), 1–7. DOI: 10.1186/1471-2458-13-983

Sant'Anna, C. C., & de Oliveira, M. C. B. (2021). The long-running issues of tuberculosis. *The Lancet. Global Health, 9*(10), e1339–e1340. DOI: 10.1016/S2214-109X(21)00401-0 PMID: 34534470

Sant'Anna, C. C., Orfaliais, C. T., March, M. F., & Conde, M. B. (2006). Evaluation of a proposed diagnostic scoring system for pulmonary tuberculosis in Brazilian children. *The International Journal of Tuberculosis and Lung Disease : the Official Journal of the International Union against Tuberculosis and Lung Disease, 10*(4), 463–465. PMID: 16602415

Santos, M. S. D., Berra, T. Z., Scholze, A. R., Delpino, F. M., Ramos, A. C. V., Alves, Y. M., & Paulino da Costa, F. (2022). Trend and spatial distribution of drug-resistant tuberculosis in liberty-deprived populations in the State of Paraná, Brazil. *Tropical Medicine and Infectious Disease*, *7*(10), 266. DOI: 10.3390/tropicalmed7100266

Sarathy, J. P., Gruber, G., & Dick, T. (2019). Re-Understanding the Mechanisms of Action of the Anti-Mycobacterial Drug Bedaquiline. *Antibiotics (Basel, Switzerland)*, *8*(4), 261. DOI: 10.3390/antibiotics8040261 PMID: 31835707

Sarkar, M., Srinivasa, , Madabhavi, I., & Kumar, K. (2017). Tuberculosis associated chronic obstructive pulmonary disease. *The Clinical Respiratory Journal*, *11*(3), 285–295. DOI: 10.1111/crj.12621 PMID: 28268242

Satyanarayana, S., Nair, S. A., Chadha, S. S., Shivashankar, R., Sharma, G., Yadav, S., Mohanty, S., Kamineni, V., Wilson, N. C., Harries, A. D., & Dewan, P. K. (2011). From Where Are Tuberculosis Patients Accessing Treatment in India? Results from a Cross-Sectional Community Based Survey of 30 Districts. *PLoS One*, *6*(9), e24160. DOI: 10.1371/journal.pone.0024160

Sawaswong, V., Chanchaem, P., Klomkliew, P., Rotcheewaphan, S., Meesawat, S., Kemthong, T., Kaewparuehaschai, M., Noradechanon, K., Ekatat, M., Kanitpun, R., Srilohasin, P., Warit, S., Chaiprasert, A., Malaivijitnond, S., & Payungporn, S. (2024). Full-length 16S rDNA sequencing based on Oxford Nanopore Technologies revealed the association between gut-pharyngeal microbiota and tuberculosis in cynomolgus macaques. *Scientific Reports*, *14*(1), 3404. Advance online publication. DOI: 10.1038/s41598-024-53880-w

Sawyer, S. M., Afifi, R. A., Bearinger, L. H., Blakemore, S.-J., Dick, B., Ezeh, A. C., & Patton, G. C. (2012). Adolescence: A foundation for future health. *Lancet*, *379*(9826), 1630–1640. DOI: 10.1016/S0140-6736(12)60072-5 PMID: 22538178

Schablon, A., Nienhaus, A., Ringshausen, F. C., Preisser, A. M., & Peters, C. (2014). Occupational screening for tuberculosis and the use of a borderline zone for interpretation of the IGRA in German healthcare workers. *PLoS ONE, 9*(12), Article e115322. DOI: 10.1371/journal.pone.0115322

Schablon, A., Harling, M., Diel, R., Ringshausen, F. C., Torres Costa, J., & Nienhaus, A. (2010). Serial testing with an interferon-γ release assay in German healthcare workers. *GMS Krankenhaushygiene Interdisziplinär, 5*(1), Article Doc05. DOI: 10.3205/dgkh000149

Scholze, A. R., Dália Alves, J., Berra, T. Z., Santos, F. L. D., Ramos, A. C. V., Lima de Freitas, G., Galdino, M. J. Q., Pieri, F. M., & Arcoverde, M. (2022). The burden of alcohol, tobacco and others drugs among incarcerated population diagnosed with tuberculosis: Time trends and spatial determinants in Southern Brazil. *BMC Public Health, 22*(1), 999. DOI: 10.1186/s12889-022-13408-1

Schwab, T. C., Perrig, L., Göller, P. C., De la Hoz, F. F. G., Lahousse, A. P., Minder, B., & Fenner, L. (2024). Targeted next-generation sequencing to diagnose drug-resistant tuberculosis: A systematic review and meta-analysis. *The Lancet. Infectious Diseases, 24*(10), 1162–1176. DOI: 10.1016/S1473-3099(24)00263-9 PMID: 38795712

Scriba, T. J., Fiore-Gartland, A., Penn-Nicholson, A., Mulenga, H., Mbandi, S. K., Borate, B., Mendelsohn, S. C., Hadley, K., Hikuam, C., Kaskar, M., Musvosvi, M., Bilek, N., Self, S., Sumner, T., White, R. G., Erasmus, M., Jaxa, L., Raphela, R., & Innes, C.. (2021). Biomarker-guided tuberculosis preventive therapy (CORTIS): A randomised controlled trial. *The Lancet. Infectious Diseases, 21*(3), 354–365. DOI: 10.1016/S1473-3099(20)30914-2 PMID: 33508224

Seabra, B., & Duarte, R. (2024). Tuberculosis national registries and data on diagnosis delay – Is there room for improvement? *Pulmonology, 30*(2), 130–136. Advance online publication. DOI: 10.1016/j.pulmoe.2021.05.004

Segal-Maurer, S. (2017). Tuberculosis in enclosed populations. *Tuberculosis and Nontuberculous Mycobacterial Infections*, 237-259. DOI: 10.1128/9781555819866.ch14

Seidler, A., Nienhaus, A., & Diel, R. (2005). Review of epidemiological studies on the occupational risk of tuberculosis in low-incidence areas. *Respiration, 72*(4), 431–446. DOI: 10.1159/000086261

Sekandi, J. N., Buregyeya, E., Zalwango, S., Nakkonde, D., Kaggwa, P., Quach, T. H. T., Asiimwe, D., Atuyambe, L., & Dobbin, K. (2025). Effectiveness of a mobile health intervention (DOT Selfie) in increasing treatment adherence monitoring and support for patients with tuberculosis in Uganda: Randomized controlled trial. *JMIR mHealth and uHealth, 13*(1), e57991. DOI: 10.2196/57991 PMID: 39715573

Sempeera, H., Anguzu, R., & Kawooya, A. (2017). Patient attitudes towards community-based tuberculosis DOT and adherence to treatment in an urban setting; Kampala, Uganda. *The Pan African Medical Journal, 27*, 1. DOI: 10.11604/pamj.2017.27.1.11119 PMID: 28748003

Sepulveda Conwell, D., Mosher, A., Khan, A., Tapy, J., Sandman, L., Vernon, A., & Horsburgh, C. R. (2007). Factors associated with loss to follow-up in a large tuberculosis treatment trial (TBTC Study 22). *Contemporary Clinical Trials*, *28*(3), 288–294. DOI: 10.1016/j.cct.2006.09.003 PMID: 17107825

Sequera, G., Estigarribia, G., Walter, K. S., Lopez, R., Andrews, J., & Croda, J. (2023). *Tuberculosis in prisons: a growing global health concern. The Challenge of Tuberculosis in the 21st Century*. European Respiratory Society.

Shafik, W. (2024c). Generative AI for Social Good and Sustainable Development. In *Generative AI: Current Trends and Applications* (pp. 185–217). Springer. DOI: 10.1007/978-981-97-8460-8_10

Shafik, W. (2024a). Connected healthcare—the impact of Internet of Things on medical services. In *Artificial Intelligence and Internet of Things based Augmented Trends for Data Driven Systems* (pp. 181–217). CRC Press., DOI: 10.1201/9781003497318-10

Shafik, W. (2024b). Digital healthcare systems in a federated learning perspective. In *Federated Learning for Digital Healthcare Systems* (pp. 1–35). Elsevier. DOI: 10.1016/B978-0-443-13897-3.00001-1

Shafik, W. (2024d). The Future of Healthcare: AIoMT—Redefining Healthcare with Advanced Artificial Intelligence and Machine Learning Techniques. In *Artificial Intelligence and Machine Learning in Drug Design and Development* (pp. 605–634). Wiley., DOI: 10.1002/9781394234196.ch19

Shafik, W. (2024e). The Future of Healthcare: Data-Driven Trends and Innovation. In *Advancing Healthcare through Data-driven Innovations* (pp. 166–185). CRC Press. DOI: 10.1201/9781003475392-11

Shafik, W. (2025). Smart biomedical devices for smart healthcare. In *Machine Learning Models and Architectures for Biomedical Signal Processing* (pp. 421–448). Elsevier. DOI: 10.1016/B978-0-443-22158-3.00017-X

Shah, H. D., Chaudhary, S., Desai, B., Patel, J., Yasobant, S., Bhavsar, P., Saha, S., Sinha, A. K., Saxena, D., Patel, Y., & Modi, B. (2024). Exploring private sector perspectives on barriers and facilitators in availing tuberculosis care cascade services: A qualitative study from the Indian state. *BMC Primary Care*, *25*(1), 5. Advance online publication. DOI: 10.1186/s12875-023-02244-w

Shah, I., & Åhman, E. (2004). Age patterns of unsafe abortion in developing country regions. *Reproductive Health Matters*, *12*(24, Suppl.), 9–17. DOI: 10.1016/S0968-8080(04)24002-2 PMID: 15938153

Shaikh, B. T., & Hatcher, J. (2004). Health seeking behaviour and health service utilization in Pakistan: Challenging the policy makers. *Journal of Public Health (Oxford, England)*, *27*(1), 49–54. DOI: 10.1093/pubmed/fdh207 PMID: 15590705

Sharma, D., Gautam, S., Srivastava, N., & Bisht, D. (2024). In silico screening of Food and Drug Administration-approved compounds against Trehalose 2-sulfotransferase (Rv0295c) in *Mycobacterium tuberculosis*: Insights from molecular docking and dynamics simulations. *International Journal of Mycobacteriology*, *13*(1), 73–82. DOI: 10.4103/ijmy.ijmy_20_24 PMID: 38771283

Sharma, K., Ahmed, F., Sharma, T., Grover, A., Agarwal, M., & Grover, S. (2023). Potential repurposed drug candidates for tuberculosis treatment: Progress and update of drugs identified in over a decade. *ACS Omega*, *8*(20), 17362–17380. DOI: 10.1021/acsomega.2c05511 PMID: 37251185

Shaw, J. A., Irusen, E. M., Diacon, A. H., & Koegelenberg, C. F. (2018). Pleural tuberculosis: A concise clinical review. *The Clinical Respiratory Journal*, *12*(5), 1779–1786. DOI: 10.1111/crj.12900 PMID: 29660258

Shete, P. B., Kadota, J. L., Nanyunja, G., Namale, C., Nalugwa, T., Oyuku, D., Turyahabwe, S., Kiwanuka, N., Cattamanchi, A., & Katamba, A. (2023). Evaluating the impact of cash transfers on tuberculosis (ExaCT TB): A stepped wedge cluster randomised controlled trial. *ERJ Open Research*, *9*(3), 00182–02023. DOI: 10.1183/23120541.00182-2023 PMID: 37342088

Shiromwar, S. S., Khan, A. H., & Chidrawar, V. (2023). A systematic review on extensively drug-resistant tuberculosis from 2009 to 2020: Special emphases on treatment outcomes. *Revista Española de Quimioterapia*, *36*(1), 30–44. DOI: 10.37201/req/029.2022 PMID: 36503203

Shorette, K., & Phillips, N. E. (2024). (In) sufficient institutionalization? Norm articulation in the World Health Organization and infectious disease prevalence across the global South. *International Journal of Comparative Sociology*, *65*(6), 752–781. DOI: 10.1177/00207152241226449

Short, S. R. (2017). Grassroots challenges to the effects of prison sprawl on mental health services for incarcerated people. *The Fordham Urban Law Journal*, *45*, 437.

Siddiqi, K., Lambert, M.-L., & Walley, J. (2003). Clinical diagnosis of smear-negative pulmonary tuberculosis in low-income countries : The current evidence. *The Lancet. Infectious Diseases*, *3*(5), 288–296. DOI: 10.1016/S1473-3099(03)00609-1

Signorell, A., van Heerden, A., Ayakaka, I., Jacobs, B. K. M., Antillon, M., & Tediosi, F.. (2025). Effectiveness and cost-effectiveness of community-based TB screening algorithms using computer-aided detection (CAD) technology alone compared to CAD combined with point-of-care C-reactive protein testing: Protocol for a paired screen-positive trial. *medRxiv*. DOI: 10.1101/2025.01.16.25320687

Silva, D. R., Fernandes, F. F., Ferreira, J. C., Bernando, W., Dalcolmo, M. M. P., Johansen, F. D. C., & Mello, F. C. Q. (2025). Bedaquiline, pretomanid, linezolid, and moxifloxacin (BPaLM) for multidrug- or rifampin-resistant tuberculosis: A systematic review. *Jornal Brasileiro de Pneumologia : Publicaçao Oficial da Sociedade Brasileira de Pneumologia e Tisilogia*, *50*(6), e20240295. Advance online publication. DOI: 10.36416/1806-3756/e20240295 PMID: 39813501

Simpson, P. L., Simpson, M., Adily, A., Grant, L., & Butler, T. (2019). Prison cell spatial density and infectious and communicable diseases: A systematic review. *BMJ Open*, *9*(7), e026806. DOI: 10.1136/bmjopen-2018-026806

Singh, S. (2025). Public–private partnership to end tuberculosis: Challenges and opportunities. *International Journal for Equity in Health*, *24*(1), 195. DOI: 10.1186/s12939-025-02516-0 PMID: 40616075

Singh, S. J., ZuWallack, R. L., Garvey, C., & Spruit, M. A. (2013). *Learn from the past and create the future: the 2013 ATS/ERS statement on pulmonary rehabilitation* (Vol. 42). European Respiratory Society.

Singh, U. B., Rade, K., Rao, R., Kumar, N., Mattoo, S. K., & Nair, S.. (2025). Lessons and updates from India's National TB Elimination Program–Bold decisions and innovative ways of fast-tracking progress towards ending TB. *IJID Regions*. Advance online publication. DOI: 10.1016/j.ijregi.2025.100599

Slobod, D., Damia, A., Leali, M., Spinelli, E., & Mauri, T. (2022). Pathophysiology and clinical meaning of ventilation-perfusion mismatch in the acute respiratory distress syndrome. *Biology (Basel)*, *12*(1), 67. DOI: 10.3390/biology12010067 PMID: 36671759

Smyth, R., Berton, S., Rajabalee, N., Chan, T., & Sun, J. (2021). Protein Kinase R Restricts the Intracellular Survival of *Mycobacterium tuberculosis* by Promoting Selective Autophagy. *Frontiers in Microbiology*, *11*, 613963. DOI: 10.3389/fmicb.2020.613963 PMID: 33552025

Snow, K., Hesseling, A. C., Naidoo, P., Graham, S. M., Denholm, J., & du Preez, K. (2017). Tuberculosis in adolescents and young adults: Epidemiology and treatment outcomes in the Western Cape. *The International Journal of Tuberculosis and Lung Disease : the Official Journal of the International Union against Tuberculosis and Lung Disease*, *21*(6), 651–657. DOI: 10.5588/ijtld.16.0866 PMID: 28482959

Snyder, L. B. (2007). Health communication campaigns and their impact on behavior. *Journal of Nutrition Education and Behavior*, *39*(2, Suppl), S32–S40. DOI: 10.1016/j.jneb.2006.09.004

Sonone, S. V., Bhakaney, P. R., Jain, M., Yadav, V., & Vardhan, V. D. (2022). Inpatient pulmonary rehabilitation followed by Tele-Rehabilitation in a patient with Post Tubercular sequelae: A case study.

Sossen, B., Kubjane, M., & Meintjes, G. (2025). Tuberculosis and HIV coinfection: Progress and challenges towards reducing incidence and mortality. International Journal of Infectious Diseases. *International Journal of Infectious Diseases*, *107876*, 107876. Advance online publication. DOI: 10.1016/j.ijid.2025.107876 PMID: 40064284

Spruit, M. A., Singh, S. J., Garvey, C., ZuWallack, R., Nici, L., Rochester, C., Hill, K., Holland, A. E., Lareau, S. C., Man, W. D.-C., Pitta, F., Sewell, L., Raskin, J., Bourbeau, J., Crouch, R., Franssen, F. M. E., Casaburi, R., Vercoulen, J. H., Vogiatzis, I., & Wouters, E. F. M. (2013). An official American Thoracic Society/European Respiratory Society statement: Key concepts and advances in pulmonary rehabilitation. *American Journal of Respiratory and Critical Care Medicine*, *188*(8), e13–e64. DOI: 10.1164/rccm.201309-1634ST PMID: 24127811

Srinivasan, S. (2025). Patient-Centric Care in Tuberculosis Management: Addressing Challenges and Improving Health Outcomes. In *Convergence of Population Health Management, Pharmacogenomics, and Patient-Centered Care* (pp. 265-282). IGI Global. DOI: 10.4018/979-8-3693-3260-3.ch012

Srinivasan, S., & Praba Lama (2025). Patient-Centered Care for TB Patients: An Effective Approach to Corporate Social Responsibility. In Corporate Social Responsibility in Health and Social Care (pp. 183-218).IGI Global. DOI:DOI: 10.4018/979-8-3693-5991-4.ch008

Srinivasan, S., & Vallipriya, R. (2025). Bias: Understanding and Addressing Disparities in Patient Care Across Multiple Demographics. In *Cases on Physician Cultural Responsibility, Ethics, and Biases* (pp. 21-38). IGI Global Scientific Publishing. DOI: 10.4018/979-8-3693-3683-0.ch002

Srinivasan, S., & Vallipriya, R. (2025). Intercultural Communication: An Effective Strategy for the Patient Physician Relationship. In *Cases on Physician Cultural Responsibility, Ethics, and Biases* (pp. 171-192). IGI Global Scientific Publishing. DOI: 10.4018/979-8-3693-3683-0.ch008

Srinivasan, S., Rajavel, N., & Kumar, A. S. (2025). Cancer Diagnosis and Treatment Barriers Among Prisoners. In *Cancer Diagnosis, Treatment and Care: Reflections for the Education of Survivors and Healthcare Providers* (pp. 185-202). IGI Global Scientific Publishing. DOI: 10.4018/979-8-3693-5400-1.ch011

Srinivasan, S. (2021). Mental Health problems faced by Aged Inmates due to Overcrowding of Central prison in Tamil Nadu. DOI: 10.2139/ssrn.3962987

Srinivasan, S., Rajavel, N., & Mahmoudi-Dehaki, M. (2025). Elderly Inmates Living With Dementia in Central Prisons. In *Assistive Technology Solutions for Aging Adults and Individuals With Disabilities* (pp. 343–404). IGI Global Scientific Publishing., DOI: 10.4018/979-8-3693-6308-9.ch015

Srinivasan, S., Rajavel, N., & Sanchez, N. K. (2025). The Impact of AI on Elderly Inmates in Central Prison. In *Exploration of AI in Contemporary Legal Systems* (pp. 281–314). IGI Global Scientific Publishing., DOI: 10.4018/979-8-3693-7205-0.ch013

Srinivasan, S., & Tyagi, N. (2025). Respiratory Diseases Affected by Informal Workers. In *Generative AI Techniques for Sustainability in Healthcare Security* (pp. 95–124). IGI Global Scientific Publishing., DOI: 10.4018/979-8-3693-6577-9.ch006

Srinivasan, S., Vallipriya, R., & Singh, A. K. (2025). Integrated Public-Private Partnerships to Combat Tuberculosis for Improving Economic Development. In *Public Private Partnership Dynamics for Economic Development* (pp. 323–356). IGI Global Scientific Publishing., DOI: 10.4018/979-8-3693-9153-2.ch015

Srinivas, M., Jagadeesh, G. T., Kamarthi, P., Patil, N., & Venkataramanappa, J. S. (2024). Effect of Telerehabilitation in a Patient with Pulmonary Tuberculosis: A Case Study. *Indian Journal of Respiratory Care*, *13*(1), 65. DOI: 10.5005/jp-journals-11010-1088

Stancil, S. L., Mirzayev, F., & Abdel-Rahman, S. M. (2021). Profiling pretomanid as a therapeutic option for TB infection: Evidence to date. *Drug Design, Development and Therapy*, *15*, 2815–2830. DOI: 10.2147/DDDT.S281639 PMID: 34234413

Stead, D., Wasserman, S., Steenkamp, E., Parrish, A., Barr, D., & Meintjes, G. (2025). Comparative performance of urine lipoarabinomannan and urine Xpert MTB/RIF Ultra for diagnosing tuberculosis in adult inpatients with human immunodeficiency virus in East London, South Africa. *Clinical Infectious Diseases*, •••, ciaf080. Advance online publication. DOI: 10.1093/cid/ciaf080 PMID: 40172283

Stierlin, N., Risch, M., & Risch, L. (2024). Current advancements in drone technology for medical sample transportation. *Logistics (Basel)*, *8*(4), 104. DOI: 10.3390/logistics8040104

Stop, T. B. Partnership. (2020). *The Global Plan to End TB 2023–2030*. Geneva: Stop TB Partnership.

Stop, T. B. Partnership. (2025). TB REACH. https://www.stoptb.org/what-we-do/accelerate-tb-innovations/tb-reach

Storvig, E., Harstad, I., Ehrnström, B., & Iversen, V. C. (2024). Beyond the diagnosis of drug-resistant Tuberculosis in Norway: Patients' experiences before, during and after treatment. *BMC Public Health*, *24*(1), 1801. DOI: 10.1186/s12889-024-19342-8 PMID: 38971760

Story, A., Murad, S., Roberts, W., Verheyen, M., & Hayward, A. C. (2007). Tuberculosis in London : The importance of homelessness, problem drug use and prison. *Thorax*, *62*(8), 667–671. DOI: 10.1136/thx.2006.065409

Strati, A., Zavridou, M., Economopoulou, P., Gkolfinopoulos, S., Psyrri, A., & Lianidou, E. (2021). Development and analytical validation of a reverse transcription droplet digital PCR (RT-ddPCR) assay for PD-L1 transcripts in circulating tumor cells. *Clinical Chemistry*, *67*(4), 642–652. DOI: 10.1093/clinchem/hvaa321 PMID: 33421061

Subbaraman, B., Nathavitharana, R. R., Mayer, K. H., Satyanarayana, S., Chadha, V. K., Arinaminpathy, N., & Pai, M. (2019). Digital adherence technologies for the management of tuberculosis therapy: Mapping the landscape and research priorities. *BMJ Global Health*, *3*(5), e001018. DOI: 10.1136/bmjgh-2018-001018 PMID: 30364330

Subbaraman, R., Nathavitharana, R. R., Mayer, K. H., Satyanarayana, S., Chadha, V. K., Arinaminpathy, N., & Pai, M. (2019). Constructing care cascades for active tuberculosis : A strategy for program monitoring and identifying gaps in quality of care. *PLoS Medicine*, *16*(2), e1002754. DOI: 10.1371/journal.pmed.1002754

Subbaraman, R., Thomas, B. E., Kumar, S., Mishra, H., Dhir, S., & Pai, M. (2020). Evaluation of the accuracy of 99DOTS, a novel cellphone-based strategy for monitoring adherence to tuberculosis medications: Comparison of digital-adherence data with urine isoniazid testing. *Clinical Infectious Diseases, 71*(9), e513–e516. DOI: 10.1093/cid/ciaa333 PMID: 32221550

Suman, S. K., Chandrasekaran, N., & Priya Doss, C. G. (2023). Micro-nanoemulsion and nanoparticle-assisted drug delivery against drug-resistant tuberculosis: Recent developments. *Clinical Microbiology Reviews, 36*(4), e0008823. Advance online publication. DOI: 10.1128/cmr.00088-23 PMID: 38032192

Sun, Q., Li, S., Gao, M., & Pang, Y. (2024). Therapeutic Strategies for Tuberculosis: Progress and Lessons Learned. *Biomedical and Environmental Sciences, 37*(11), 1310–1323. DOI: 10.3967/bes2024.168 PMID: 39667968

Sutter, A., Landis, D., & Nugent, K. (2022). The potential role for metformin in the prevention and treatment of tuberculosis. *Journal of Thoracic Disease, 14*(6), 1758–1765. DOI: 10.21037/jtd-22-39 PMID: 35813707

Swain, S., Kumar, A., & Vishwakarma, V. K. K, A. A., Mittal, A., & Wig, N. (2024). Diagnosis and Management of Latent Tuberculosis Infection: Updates. In *Infectious Disorders - Drug Targets* (Vol. 24, Issue 4). DOI: 10.2174/0118715265 275319231124053615

Szumowski, J. D., & Lynch, J. B. (2015). Profile of delamanid for the treatment of multidrug-resistant tuberculosis. *Drug Design, Development and Therapy, 9*, 677–682. DOI: 10.2147/DDDT.S60923 PMID: 25678771

Tabachnick, B. G., & Fidell, L. S. (2013). *Using multivariate statistics* (6th ed.). Pearson.

Tahan, T. T., Gabardo, B. M., & Rossoni, A. M. (2020). Tuberculosis in childhood and adolescence: A view from different perspectives. *Jornal de Pediatria, 96*(Suppl. 1), 99–110. DOI: 10.1016/j.jped.2019.11.002 PMID: 31862302

Tait, D. R., Hatherill, M., Van Der Meeren, O., Ginsberg, A. M., Van Brakel, E., Salaun, B., Scriba, T. J., Akite, E. J., Ayles, H. M., Bollaerts, A., Demoitié, M.-A., Diacon, A., Evans, T. G., Gillard, P., Hellström, E., Innes, J. C., Lempicki, M., Malahleha, M., Martinson, N., & Roman, F. (2019). Final analysis of a trial of M72/AS01E vaccine to prevent tuberculosis. *The New England Journal of Medicine, 381*(25), 2429–2439. DOI: 10.1056/NEJMoa1909953 PMID: 31661198

Tamuzi, J. L., Muyaya, L. M., & Mbuesse, P. (2021). HIV/TB co-infection prevalence and treatment outcomes in Democratic Republic of the Congo from 2005 to 2020: Systematic review and meta-analysis. *Community Medicine and Health Education Research, 2*(1), 17–35. DOI: 10.33702/cmher.2021.2.1.4

Tanabe, M., Nakamura, A., Arai, A., Yamasaki, D., Hirano, K., Kobayashi, T., Taguchi, O., Kaneko, T., & Ito, M. (2017). The direct comparison of two interferon-gamma release assays in the tuberculosis screening of Japanese healthcare workers. *Internal Medicine, 56*(7), 773–779. https://doi.org/DOI: 10.2169/internalmedicine.56.7688

Tanimura, T., Jaramillo, E., Weil, D., Raviglione, M., & Lönnroth, K. (2014). Financial burden for tuberculosis patients in low- and middle-income countries : A systematic review. *The European Respiratory Journal, 43*(6), 1763–1775. DOI: 10.1183/09031936.00193413

Tan, Z. M., Lai, G. P., Pandey, M., Srichana, T., Pichika, M. R., Gorain, B., Bhattamishra, S. K., & Choudhury, H. (2020). Novel approaches for the treatment of pulmonary tuberculosis. *Pharmaceutics, 12*(12), 1196. Advance online publication. DOI: 10.3390/pharmaceutics12121196 PMID: 33321797

Tavoschi, L., O'Moore, É., & Hedrich, D. (2019). Challenges and opportunities for the management of infectious diseases in Europes' prisons: Evidence-based guidance. *The Lancet. Infectious Diseases, 19*(7), e253–e258. https://www.thelancet.com/journals/laninf/article/PIIS1473-3099(18)30756-4/abstract. DOI: 10.1016/S1473-3099(18)30756-4

Taylor, J., Coates, E., Brewster, L., Mountain, G., Wessels, B., & Hawley, M. S. (2015). Examining the use of telehealth in community nursing : Identifying the factors affecting frontline staff acceptance and telehealth adoption. *Journal of Advanced Nursing, 71*(2), 326–337. DOI: 10.1111/jan.12480

Teibo, T. K. A., Andrade, R. L. P., Rosa, R. J., de Abreu, P. D., Olayemi, O. A., Alves, Y. M., Vaz Tavares, R. B., da Costa, F. B. P., Dias Moura, H. S., Ferezin, L. P., Tártaro, A. F., de Campos, M. C. T., Ribeiro, N. M., Berra, T. Z., & Arcêncio, R. A. (2024). Barriers that interfere with access to tuberculosis diagnosis and treatment across countries globally: A systematic review. *ACS Infectious Diseases, 10*(8), 2600–2614. DOI: 10.1021/acsinfecdis.4c00466 PMID: 39023509

Tesfamariam, S., Ghebrenegus, A. S., Woldu, H., Fisseha, E., Belai, G., & Russom, M. (2021). Secondary erythrocytosis following drugs used in rifampicin/multidrug-resistant tuberculosis: A retrospective cohort study. *BMJ Open Respiratory Research, 8*(1), e001064. DOI: 10.1136/bmjresp-2021-001064 PMID: 34815231

Thapa, P., Narasimhan, P., Jayasuriya, R., Hall, J. J., Mukherjee, P. S., Das, D. K., & Beek, K. (2023). Barriers and facilitators to informal healthcare provider engagement in the national tuberculosis elimination program of India: An exploratory study from West Bengal. *PLOS Global Public Health, 3*(10), e0001390. DOI: 10.1371/journal.pgph.0001390

The Union. (2023). *Improving retention during TB preventive treatment through person-centred care in South-East Asia.* https://theunion.org/news/improving-retention-during-tb-preventive-treatment-through-person-centred-care-in-south-east-asia

Thee, S., Krüger, R., von Bernuth, H., Meisel, C., Kölsch, U., Kirchberger, V., & Feiterna-Sperling, C. (2019). Screening and treatment for tuberculosis in a cohort of unaccompanied minor refugees in Berlin, Germany. *PLoS One, 14*(5), e0216234. Advance online publication. DOI: 10.1371/journal.pone.0216234 PMID: 31112542

Thompson, R. R., Nalugwa, T., Oyuku, D., Tucker, A., Nantale, M., Nakaweesa, A., Musinguzi, J., Reza, T. F., Zimmer, A. J., Ferguson, O., Turyahabwe, S., Joloba, M., Cattamanchi, A., Katamba, A., Dowdy, D. W., & Sohn, H. (2023). Multicomponent strategy with decentralised molecular testing for tuberculosis in Uganda: A cost and cost-effectiveness analysis. *The Lancet. Global Health, 11*(2), e278–e286. DOI: 10.1016/S2214-109X(22)00509-5 PMID: 36669808

Tiberi, S., Du Plessis, N., Walzl, G., Vjecha, M. J., Rao, M., Ntoumi, F., Mfinanga, S., Kapata, N., Mwaba, P., McHugh, T. D., Ippolito, G., Migliori, G. B., Maeurer, M. J., & Zumla, A. (2018). Tuberculosis: Progress and advances in development of new drugs, treatment regimens, and host-directed therapies. *The Lancet. Infectious Diseases, 18*(7), e183–e198. https://www.thelancet.com/journals/laninf/article/PIIS1473-3099(18)30110-5/fulltext. DOI: 10.1016/S1473-3099(18)30110-5

Tiberi, S., Muñoz-Torrico, M., Duarte, R., Dalcolmo, M., D'Ambrosio, L., & Migliori, G. B. (2018). New drugs and perspectives for new anti-tuberculosis regimens. *Pulmonology, 24*(2), 86–98. DOI: 10.1016/j.rppnen.2017.10.009 PMID: 29487031

Timm, J., Bateson, A., Solanki, P., Paleckyte, A., Witney, A. A., Rofael, S. A. D., Fabiane, S., Olugbosi, M., McHugh, T. D., & Sun, E. (2023). Baseline and acquired resistance to bedaquiline, linezolid and pretomanid, and impact on treatment outcomes in four tuberculosis clinical trials containing pretomanid. *PLOS Global Public Health, 3*(10), e0002283. Advance online publication. DOI: 10.1371/journal.pgph.0002283 PMID: 37851685

Togun, T., Kampmann, B., Stoker, N. G., & Lipman, M. (2020). Anticipating the impact of the COVID-19 pandemic on TB patients and TB control programmes. *Annals of Clinical Microbiology and Antimicrobials*, *19*(1), 21. Advance online publication. DOI: 10.1186/s12941-020-00363-1 PMID: 32446305

Topp, S. M., Moonga, C. N., Luo, N., Kaingu, M., Chileshe, C., Magwende, G., Heymann, S. J., & Henostroza, G. (2016). Exploring the drivers of health and healthcare access in Zambian prisons: A health systems approach. *Health Policy and Planning*, *31*(9), 1250–1261. DOI: 10.1093/heapol/czw059

Torres Costa, J., Sá, R., Cardoso, M. J., Silva, R., Ferreira, J., Ribeiro, C., Miranda, M., Plácido, J. L., & Nienhaus, A. (2009). Tuberculosis screening in Portuguese healthcare workers using the tuberculin skin test and the interferon-gamma release assay. *European Respiratory Journal, 34*(6), 1423–1428. https://doi.org/DOI: 10.1183/09031936.00029909

Torres Costa, J., Silva, R., Ringshausen, F. C., & Nienhaus, A. (2011). Screening for tuberculosis and prediction of disease in Portuguese healthcare workers. *Journal of Occupational Medicine and Toxicology, 6*. *Journal of Occupational Medicine and Toxicology (London, England)*, *19*(1), 19. Advance online publication. DOI: 10.1186/1745-6673-6-19 PMID: 21658231

Trickey, A., & Trickey, A. (2017). Investigating the epidemiology of hepatitis C virus (HCV) infection in different settings. *The American Journal of Tropical Medicine and Hygiene*, *97*(6), 1920–1928. DOI: 10.4269/ajtmh.17-0019

Tsegaye Sahle, E., Blumenthal, J., Jain, S., Sun, S., Young, J., Manyazewal, T., Woldeamanuel, H., Teferra, L., Feleke, B., Vandenber, O., Rey, Z., Briggs-Hagen, M., Haubrich, R., Amogne, W., & McCutchan, J. A. (2019). Bacteriologically-confirmed pulmonary tuberculosis in an Ethiopian prison: Prevalence from screening of entrant and resident prisoners. *PLoS One*, *14*(12), e0226160. DOI: 10.1371/journal.pone.0226160

U.S. Food and Drug Administration. (2019). *Adaptive designs for clinical trials of drugs and biologics: Guidance for industry*. https://www.fda.gov/media/78495/download

U.S. Food and Drug Administration. (2022). *Submitting documents using real-world data and real-world evidence to FDA for drug and biological products: Guidance for industry*. https://www.fda.gov/media/124795/download:contentReference[oaicite:2]index=2

U.S. Food and Drug Administration. (2024). Real-world evidence in regulatory decision-making. https://www.fda.gov/science-research/science-and-research-special-topics/real-world-evidence

Uden, L., Barber, E., Ford, N., & Cooke, G. S. (2017). Risk of Tuberculosis Infection and Disease for Health Care Workers: An Updated Meta-Analysis. *Open Forum Infectious Diseases*, *4*(3), ofx137. Advance online publication. DOI: 10.1093/ofid/ofx137 PMID: 28875155

Ullah, A., Ullah, H., Lateef, M., Sultan, I. N., Tareen, A. K., & Khan, M. W. (2024). Evaluating the Diagnostic Accuracy of GeneXpert MTB/RIF Assay for the Diagnosis of Tuberculosis. *Pakistan Journal of Zoology*, *56*(2). Advance online publication. DOI: 10.17582/journal.pjz/20220527100541

Ullah, H., Ahmed, H., Salman, A., Iqbal, R., Hussaini, S. J., & Malikzai, A. (2024). The rising tide of tuberculosis in Pakistan : Factors, impact, and multi-faceted approaches for prevention and control. *Health Science Reports*, *7*(10), e70130. DOI: 10.1002/hsr2.70130

UNAIDS. (2023). UNAIDS Global Report 2023. https://thepath.unaids.org/

United Nations General Assembly. (2023). Political declaration of the high-level meeting on the fight against tuberculosis: Draft resolution submitted by the President of the General Assembly (78th session, 2023/2024). https://digitallibrary.un.org/record/4022582

Uplekar, M., Creswell, J., Ottmani, S.-E., Weil, D., Sahu, S., & Lönnroth, K. (2013). Programmatic approaches to screening for active tuberculosis [State of the art series. Active case finding/screening. Number 6 in the series]. *The International Journal of Tuberculosis and Lung Disease : the Official Journal of the International Union against Tuberculosis and Lung Disease*, *17*(10), 1248–1256. DOI: 10.5588/ijtld.13.0199

Urrego, J., Ko, A. I., Carbone, A. D. S. S., Paião, D. S. G., Sgarbi, R. V. E., Yeckel, C. W., Andrews, J. A., & Croda, J. (2015). The impact of ventilation and early diagnosis on tuberculosis transmission in Brazilian prisons. *The American Journal of Tropical Medicine and Hygiene*, *93*(4), 739–746. DOI: 10.4269/ajtmh.15-0166

Vallipriya, R., & Singh, A. K. (2025). Integrated Public-Private Partnerships to Combat Tuberculosis for Improving. *Public Private Partnership Dynamics for Economic Development*, 323.

Vaman, R. S., Valamparampil, M. J., & Nair, S. (2021). Prevalence and determinants of latent tuberculosis infection among healthcare personnel in India. *Journal of Patient Safety and Infection Control, 9*(2), 35–39. Advance online publication. DOI: 10.4103/jpsic.jpsic_19_21

van der Westhuizen, H. M., Ehrlich, R., Somdyala, N., Greenhalgh, T., Tonkin-Crine, S., & Butler, C. C. (2024). Stigma relating to tuberculosis infection prevention and control implementation in rural health facilities in South Africa—A qualitative study outlining opportunities for mitigation. *BMC Global and Public Health, 2*(1), 66. DOI: 10.1186/s44263-024-00097-8 PMID: 39681968

Van der Westhuizen, H.-M., & Dramowski, A. (2017). When students become patients: TBdisease among medical undergraduates in Cape Town, South Africa. *South African Medical Journal, 107*(6), 475–479. DOI: 10.7196/SAMJ.2017.v107i6.12260 PMID: 28604316

van Heerden, J. K., Louw, E. H., Thienemann, F., Engel, M. E., & Allwood, B. W. (2024). The prevalence of pulmonary hypertension in post-tuberculosis and active tuberculosis populations: A systematic review and meta-analysis. *European Respiratory Review : an Official Journal of the European Respiratory Society, 33*(171), 230154. DOI: 10.1183/16000617.0154-2023 PMID: 38232991

Van Rie, A., Sengupta, A., Pungrassami, P., Balthip, S., & Dawson, R. (2008). Measuring stigma associated with tuberculosis and HIV/AIDS in southern Thailand: Exploratory and confirmatory factor analysis of two new scales. *Tropical Medicine & International Health, 13*(1), 21–29. DOI: 10.1111/j.1365-3156.2007.01971.x

Vanhems, P., Barrat, A., Cattuto, C., Pinton, J.-F., Khanafer, N., Régis, C., Kim, B., Comte, B., & Voirin, N. (2013). Estimating potential infection transmission routes in hospital wards using wearable proximity sensors. *PLoS One, 8*(9), e73970. DOI: 10.1371/journal.pone.0073970 PMID: 24040129

Varma, D. M., Zahid, M. S. H., Bachelder, E. M., & Ainslie, K. M. (2020). Formulation of host-targeted therapeutics against bacterial infections. *Translational Research; the Journal of Laboratory and Clinical Medicine, 220*, 98–113. DOI: 10.1016/j.trsl.2020.03.009 PMID: 32268128

Varshney, K., Anaele, B., Molaei, M., Frasso, R., & Maio, V. (2021). Risk factors for poor outcomes among patients with extensively drug-resistant tuberculosis (XDR-TB): A scoping review. *Infection and Drug Resistance, 14*, 5429–5448. DOI: 10.2147/IDR.S339972 PMID: 34938089

Vasiliu, A., Martinez, L., Gupta, R. K., Hamada, Y., Ness, T., Kay, A., Bonnet, M., Sester, M., Kaufmann, S. H. E., Lange, C., & Mandalakas, A. M. (2024). Tuberculosis prevention: Current strategies and future directions. *Clinical Microbiology and Infection*, *30*(9), 1123–1130. DOI: 10.1016/j.cmi.2023.10.023 PMID: 37918510

Vidyasagaran, A. L., Siqueira, N. T. D., Kakchapati, S., Hall, T. F., Naznin, B., Tajree, J., . . . Elsey, H. (2024). Public–Private Mix (PPM) for Tuberculosis (TB) in Urban Health Systems in Least Developed, Low Income and Lower-Middle-Income Countries and Territories–A Systematic Review. medRxiv, 2024-05. DOI: 10.1101/2024.05.01.24306566

Villarino, M. E., Scott, N. A., Weis, S. E., Weiner, M., Conde, M. B., Jones, B., Nachman, S., Oliveira, R., Moro, R. N., Shang, N., Goldberg, S. V., & Sterling, T. R. (2015). Treatment for preventing tuberculosis in children and adolescents: A randomized clinical trial of a 3-month, 12-dose regimen of a combination of rifapentine and isoniazid. *JAMA Pediatrics*, *169*(3), 247–255. DOI: 10.1001/jamapediatrics.2014.3158 PMID: 25580725

Vinkeles Melchers, N. V., van Elsland, S. L., Lange, J. M., Borgdorff, M. W., & van den Hombergh, J. (2013). State of affairs of tuberculosis in prison facilities: A systematic review of screening practices and recommendations for best TB control. *PLoS One*, *8*(1), e53644. DOI: 10.1371/journal.pone.0053644

von Groote-Bidlingmaier, F., Patientia, R., Sanchez, E., Balanag, V.Jr, Ticona, E., Segura, P., Cadena, E., Yu, C., Cirule, A., Lizarbe, V., Davidaviciene, E., Domente, L., Variava, E., Caoili, J., Danilovits, M., Bielskiene, V., Staples, S., Hittel, N., Petersen, C., & Gupta, R. (2019). Efficacy and safety of delamanid in combination with an optimised background regimen for treatment of multidrug-resistant tuberculosis: A multicentre, randomised, double-blind, placebo-controlled, parallel group phase 3 trial. *The Lancet. Respiratory Medicine*, *7*(3), 249–259. DOI: 10.1016/S2213-2600(18)30426-0 PMID: 30630778

Vonasek, B. J., Kumwenda, T., Gumulira, J., Nyirongo, M., Heller, T., Palmer, M., McCollum, E. D., Chiunda, M., Garcia-Prats, A. J., Bélard, S., & Mvalo, T. (2024). Point-of-Care Ultrasound for Tuberculosis in Young Children with Severe Acute Malnutrition. *The Pediatric Infectious Disease Journal*, *43*(2), e65–e67. Advance online publication. DOI: 10.1097/INF.0000000000004158

Wakefield, M. A., Loken, B., & Hornik, R. C. (2010). Use of mass media campaigns to change health behavior. *Lancet*, *376*(9748), 1261–1271. DOI: 10.1016/S0140-6736(10)60809-4

Walker, T. M., Merker, M., Knoblauch, A. M., Helbling, P., Schoch, O. D., van der Werf, M. J., Kranzer, K., Fiebig, L., Kröger, S., Haas, W., Hoffmann, H., Indra, A., Egli, A., Cirillo, D. M., Robert, J., Rogers, T. R., Groenheit, R., Mengshoel, A. T., Mathys, V., & Witschi, M.MDR-TB Cluster Consortium. (2018). A cluster of multidrug-resistant *Mycobacterium tuberculosis* among patients arriving in Europe from the Horn of Africa: A molecular epidemiological study. *The Lancet. Infectious Diseases, 18*(4), 431–440. DOI: 10.1016/S1473-3099(18)30004-5 PMID: 29326013

Wallace, D., & Wallace, R. (2019). Problems with the WHO TB model. *Mathematical Biosciences, 313*, 71–80. DOI: 10.1016/j.mbs.2019.05.002

Wang, B., Wang, L., Yang, Q., Zhang, Y., Qinglai, T., Yang, X., Xiao, Z., Lei, L., & Li, S. (2024). Pulmonary inhalation for disease treatment: Basic research and clinical translations. *Materials Today. Bio, 25*, 100966. Advance online publication. DOI: 10.1016/j.mtbio.2024.100966 PMID: 38318475

Wang, H., Ji, X. B., Li, C. W., Lu, H. W., Mao, B., Liang, S., Cheng, K. B., Bai, J. W., Martinez-Garcia, M. A., & Xu, J. F. (2018). Clinical characteristics and validation of bronchiectasis severity score systems for post-tuberculosis bronchiectasis. *The Clinical Respiratory Journal, 12*(8), 2346–2353. DOI: 10.1111/crj.12911 PMID: 29790656

Wang, M. Q., Zheng, Y. F., Hu, Y. Q., Huang, J. X., Yuan, Z. X., Wu, Z. Y., Huang, L.-F., Tang, C.-T., Zhang, F.-Y., Chen, Y., He, J.-K., Guo, X.-G., & Yan, B.-M. (2025). Diagnostic accuracy of Xpert MTB/RIF Ultra for detecting pulmonary tuberculosis and rifampicin resistance: A systematic review and meta-analysis. *European Journal of Clinical Microbiology & Infectious Diseases, 44*(3), 1–22. DOI: 10.1007/s10096-024-05032-1 PMID: 39754613

Wani, R. L. S. (2013). Clinical manifestations of pulmonary and extra-pulmonary tuberculosis. *South Sudan Medical Journal, 6*(3), 52–56.

Weiner, B. (1986). *An attributional theory of motivation and emotion*. Springer-Verlag. DOI: 10.1007/978-1-4612-4948-1

WHO. (2015). *The End TB Strategy* (WHO/HTM/TB/2015.19). https://apps.who.int/iris/bitstream/handle/10665/331326/WHO-HTM-TB-2015.19-eng.pdf

WHO. (2017a). *Ethics guidance for the implementation of the End TB strategy* (WHO/HTM/TB/2017.07). Geneva: World Health Organization. https://apps.who.int/iris/bitstream/handle/10665/254820/9789241512114-eng.pdf

WHO. (2017b). *WHO issues ethics guidance to protect rights of TB patients.* https://www.who.int/news/item/22-03-2017-who-issues-ethics-guidance-to-protect-rights-of-tb-patients

WHO. (2018). *Global tuberculosis report 2018* (WHO/CDS/TB/2018.20). Geneva: World Health Organization. Retrieved from https://apps.who.int/iris/handle/10665/274453

WHO. (2022a). *Global tuberculosis report 2022.* World Health Organization. https://www.who.int/teams/global-tuberculosis-programme/tb-reports/global-tuberculosis-report-2022

WHO. (2022b). *Module 4: Drug-resistant tuberculosis treatment, 2022 update – 4. The 6-month bedaquiline, pretomanid, linezolid and moxifloxacin (BPaLM) regimen.* TB Knowledge Sharing Platform. https://tbksp.who.int/en/node/576

WHO. (2022c). *WHO operational handbook on tuberculosis: Module 4: Treatment – drug-susceptible tuberculosis treatment.* World Health Organization. https://www.who.int/publications/i/item/9789240050761

Widiastuti, E., Cahyati, W. H., & Rahayu, S. R. (2024). Analysis of Voluntary Counseling and Testing (VCT) Service Utilization Factors in Tuberculosis (TB) Patients in Semarang City. *PROMOTOR, 7*(1), 42–45. Advance online publication. DOI: 10.32832/pro.v7i1.511

Wild, V., Jaff, D., Shah, N. S., & Frick, M. (2017). Tuberculosis, human rights and ethics considerations along the route of a highly vulnerable migrant from sub-Saharan Africa to Europe. *The International Journal of Tuberculosis and Lung Disease : the Official Journal of the International Union against Tuberculosis and Lung Disease, 21*(11), 1075–1085. DOI: 10.5588/ijtld.17.0324 PMID: 28911349

Willis, G. B. (2005). Cognitive interviewing: A tool for improving questionnaire design. *Sage (Atlanta, Ga.).*

Witte, K. (1992). Putting the fear back into fear appeals: The extended parallel process model. *Communication Monographs, 59*(4), 329–349. DOI: 10.1080/03637759209376276

Wondmeneh, T. G., & Mekonnen, A. T. (2023). The incidence rate of tuberculosis and its associated factors among HIV-positive persons in Sub-Saharan Africa: A systematic review and meta-analysis. *BMC Infectious Diseases, 23*(1), 613. DOI: 10.1186/s12879-023-08533-0

Wong, Y. J., Noordin, N. M., Keshavjee, S., & Lee, S. W. H. (2021). Impact of latent tuberculosis infection on health and wellbeing: A systematic review and meta-analysis. *European Respiratory Review : an Official Journal of the European Respiratory Society, 30*(159), 200260. DOI: 10.1183/16000617.0260-2020 PMID: 33408089

Woodman, M., Haeusler, I. L., & Grandjean, L. (2019). Tuberculosis genetic epidemiology: A Latin American perspective. *Genes, 10*(1), 53. DOI: 10.3390/genes10010053

World Health Organization. (2014). *The End TB Strategy*. https://www.who.int/publications/i/item/9789241506838

World Health Organization. (2014). *The End TB Strategy*. World Health Organization.

World Health Organization. (2018). *Compendium of WHO guidelines and associated standards : Ensuring optimum delivery of the cascade of care for patients with tuberculosis* (2nd ed). World Health Organization. https://iris.who.int/handle/10665/272644

World Health Organization. (2019). *WHO consolidated guidelines on tuberculosis: Module 1: Prevention - infection prevention and control*. Geneva: World Health Organization. Retrieved from https://www.who.int/publications/i/item/9789241550512

World Health Organization. (2020). *Global Tuberculosis Report 2020* (1st ed.). World Health Organization.

World Health Organization. (2021). *WHO Consolidated Guidelines on Tuberculosis. Module 2 : Screening - Systematic Screening for Tuberculosis Disease* (1st ed.). World Health Organization.

World Health Organization. (2021). *WHO consolidated guidelines on tuberculosis. Module 2: screening-systematic screening for tuberculosis disease*. World Health Organization.

World Health Organization. (2021). *WHO consolidated guidelines on tuberculosis: Module 3 – Diagnosis: Rapid diagnostics for tuberculosis detection, 2021 update*. Geneva: World Health Organization. https://www.who.int/publications/i/item/9789240029415

World Health Organization. (2023). *Global Tuberculosis Report 2023*. World Health Organization.

World Health Organization. (2023, November 7).. . *Global Tuberculosis Report, 2023*, https://www.who.int/teams/global-tuberculosis-programme/tb-reports/global-tuberculosis-report-2023

World Health Organization. (2024). 1.3 Drug-resistant TB. *Global Tuberculosis Report, 2024,* •••. https://www.who.int/teams/global-tuberculosis-programme/tb-reports/global-tuberculosis-report-2024/tb-disease-burden/1-3-drug-resistant-tb

World Health Organization. (2025). Global programme on tuberculosis & lung health. https://www.who.int/teams/global-tuberculosis-programme/the-end-tb-strategy

World Health Organization. (s. d.). *Global Programme on Tuberculosis & Lung Health.* Consulté 27 avril 2025, à l'adresse https://www.who.int/teams/global-tuberculosis-programme/populations-comorbidities

Wozniak, J. M., Li, W., & Parker, C. G. (2024). Chemical proteomic mapping of reversible small molecule binding sites in native systems. *Trends in Pharmacological Sciences, 45*(11), 969–981. DOI: 10.1016/j.tips.2024.09.001 PMID: 39406592

Wu, D., Wang, L., & Zhang, L. (2024). Efficacy and safety of step-by-step Baduanjin exercise based on doctor-nurse-patient integration mode for pulmonary rehabilitation in patients after lobectomy due to pulmonary tuberculosis: A randomized controlled clinical trial. *Journal of Cardiothoracic Surgery, 19*(1), 520. DOI: 10.1186/s13019-024-03042-w PMID: 39252121

Wu, S., Litvinjenko, S., Magwood, O., & Wei, X. (2023). Defining tuberculosis vulnerability based on an adapted social determinants of health framework : A narrative review. *Global Public Health: An International Journal for Research, Policy and Practice, 18*(1), 2221729. DOI: 10.1080/17441692.2023.2221729

Wytrychowski, K., Hans-Wytrychowska, A., Piesiak, P., Majewska-Pulsakowska, M., & Rożek-Piechura, K. (2020). Pulmonary rehabilitation in interstitial lung diseases: A review of the literature. *Advances in Clinical and Experimental Medicine, 29*(2), 257–264. DOI: 10.17219/acem/115238 PMID: 32101645

Xu, Z., Chen, W., & Li, X. (2021). Effects of comprehensive nursing intervention combined with respiratory functional exercises on pulmonary function and self-care ability in patients with pulmonary tuberculosis: Results of a randomized trial. *Annals of Palliative Medicine, 10*(7), 7543–7550. DOI: 10.21037/apm-21-1178 PMID: 34353042

Yadav, S. (2024). BPaLM regimen against drug-resistant tuberculosis in India: A need of the hour. *Cureus, 16*(9), e68421. Advance online publication. DOI: 10.7759/cureus.68421 PMID: 39360094

Yadav, S. (2024). Stigma in Tuberculosis: Time to Act on an Important and Largely Unaddressed Issue. *Cureus, 16*(6), e61964. DOI: 10.7759/cureus.61964 PMID: 38978939

Yang, H., Liu, Q., Wu, Y., He, K., Zeng, Q., & Liu, M. (2024). Paradoxical tuberculosis-associated immune reconstitution inflammatory syndrome in initiating ART among HIV-Infected patients in China-risk factors and management. *BMC Infectious Diseases*, *24*(1), 272. Advance online publication. DOI: 10.1186/s12879-024-09080-y

Yang, Y., Wei, L., Wang, S., Ke, L., Zhao, H., Mao, J., Li, J., & Mao, Z. (2022). The effects of pursed lip breathing combined with diaphragmatic breathing on pulmonary function and exercise capacity in patients with COPD: A systematic review and meta-analysis. *Physiotherapy Theory and Practice*, *38*(7), 847–857. DOI: 10.1080/09593985.2020.1805834 PMID: 32808571

Yanifitri, D. B., Arliny, Y., Utami, W. A., & Winardi, W. (2024). Cycloserine- and Fluoroquinolone-Induced Seizure in Multidrug-Resistance Tuberculosis (MDR-TB) Patient: A Case Report. *Jurnal Respirasi*, *10*(1), 61–68. Advance online publication. DOI: 10.20473/jr.v10-I.1.2024.61-68

Yap, P., Tan, K. H. X., Lim, W. Y., Barkham, T., Tan, L. W. L., Chen, M. I.-C., Wang, Y. T., & Chee, C. B. E. (2018). Prevalence of and risk factors associated with latent tuberculosis in Singapore: A cross-sectional survey. *International Journal of Infectious Diseases, 72*, 55–62. DOI: 10.1016/j.ijid.2018.05.004

Yerezhepov, D., Gabdulkayum, A., Akhmetova, A., Kozhamkulov, U. A., Rakhimova, S. E., Kairov, U. Y., Zhunussova, G., Kalendar, R. N., & Akilzhanova, A. (2024). Vitamin D status, VDR, and TLR polymorphisms and pulmonary tuberculosis epidemiology in Kazakhstan. *Nutrients*, *16*(4), 558. DOI: 10.3390/nu16040558 PMID: 38398882

Ye, Z., Li, L., Yang, L., Zhuang, L., Aspatwar, A., Wang, L., & Gong, W. (2024, October). Impact of diabetes mellitus on tuberculosis prevention, diagnosis, and treatment from an immunologic perspective. *Exploration*, *4*(5), 20230138. DOI: 10.1002/EXP.20230138 PMID: 39439490

Yimer, S. A., Kalayou, S., Homberset, H., Birhanu, A. G., Riaz, T., Zegeye, E. D., Lutter, T., Abebe, M., Holm-Hansen, C., Aseffa, A., & Tønjum, T. (2020). Lineage-specific proteomic signatures in the *Mycobacterium tuberculosis* complex reveal differential abundance of proteins involved in virulence, DNA repair, CRISPR-Cas, bioenergetics and lipid metabolism. *Frontiers in Microbiology*, *11*, 550760. DOI: 10.3389/fmicb.2020.550760 PMID: 33072011

Yin, Z., Yang, Y., Hu, C., Li, J., Qin, B., Yang, X., & Zhang, L. (2024). Wearable respiratory sensors for health monitoring. *NPG Asia Materials*, *16*(1), 8. DOI: 10.1038/s41427-023-00513-9

Yoshikawa, A., Araki, K., & Matsumoto, T. (2025). Simulation-based infection prevention and control training for medical and healthcare students: A systematic review. *Frontiers in Medicine, 12*, 1529557. DOI: 10.3389/fmed.2025.1529557 PMID: 40438369

Young, C., Walzl, G., & Du Plessis, N. (2020). Therapeutic host-directed strategies to improve outcome in tuberculosis. *Mucosal Immunology, 13*(2), 190–204. DOI: 10.1038/s41385-019-0226-5 PMID: 31772320

Yuen, C. M., Puma, D., Millones, A. K., Galea, J. T., Tzelios, C., Calderon, R. I., Brooks, M. B., Jimenez, J., Contreras, C., Nichols, T. C., Nicholson, T., Lecca, L., Becerra, M. C., & Keshavjee, S. (2021). Identifying barriers and facilitators to implementation of community-based tuberculosis active case finding with mobile X-ray units in Lima, Peru : A RE-AIM evaluation. *BMJ Open, 11*(7), e050314. DOI: 10.1136/bmjopen-2021-050314

Zary, M., Mohamed, M. S., Kafie, C., Chilala, C. I., Bahukudumbi, S., Foster, N., Gore, G., Fielding, K. L., Subbaraman, R., & Schwartzman, K. (2024). The performance of digital technologies for measuring tuberculosis medication adherence: A systematic review. *BMJ Global Health, 9*(1), e015633. Advance online publication. DOI: 10.1136/bmjgh-2024-015633 PMID: 39013639

Zein-Eddine, R., Le Meur, A., Skouloubris, S., Jelsbak, L., Refrégier, G., & Myllykallio, H. (2025). Genome wide analyses reveal the role of mutator phenotypes in the emergence of drug resistance inMycobacterium tuberculosis. DOI: 10.1101/2025.01.17.633521

Zenner, D., Southern, J., Van Hest, R., DeVries, G., Stagg, H. R., Antoine, D., & Abubakar, I. (2013). Active case finding for tuberculosis among high-risk groups in low-incidence countries [State of the art series. Case finding/screening. Number 3 in the series]. *The International Journal of Tuberculosis and Lung Disease : the Official Journal of the International Union against Tuberculosis and Lung Disease, 17*(5), 573–582. DOI: 10.5588/ijtld.12.0920

Zhang, L., Yang, Z., Wu, F., Ge, Q., Zhang, Y., Li, D., Gao, M., & Liu, X. (2024). Multiple cytokine analysis based on QuantiFERON-TB gold plus in different tuberculosis infection status: An exploratory study. *BMC Infectious Diseases, 24*(1), 28. Advance online publication. DOI: 10.1186/s12879-023-08943-0

Zhang, S., Huang, X., Zhao, X., Li, B., Cai, Y., Liang, X., & Wan, Q. (2022). Effect of exercise on bone mineral density among patients with osteoporosis and osteopenia: A systematic review and network meta-analysis. *Journal of Clinical Nursing, 31*(15-16), 2100–2111. DOI: 10.1111/jocn.16101 PMID: 34725872

Zhang, Y., Zhou, L., Liu, Z.-W., Chai, C.-L., Wang, X.-M., Jiang, J.-M., & Chen, S.-H. (2020). Multidrug-resistant tuberculosis transmission among middle school students in Zhejiang Province, China. *Infectious Diseases of Poverty*, *9*(1), 57. Advance online publication. DOI: 10.1186/s40249-020-00670-x PMID: 32460836

Zhao, B., Zheng, H., Timm, J., Song, Z., Pei, S., Xing, R., Guo, Y., Ma, L., Li, F., Li, Q., Li, Y., Huang, L., Teng, C., Wang, N., Gupta, A., Juneja, S., Huang, F., Zhao, Y., & Ou, X. (2024). Prevalence and genetic basis of *Mycobacterium tuberculosis* resistance to pretomanid in China. *Annals of Clinical Microbiology and Antimicrobials*, *23*(1), 40. DOI: 10.1186/s12941-024-00697-0 PMID: 38702782

Zhao, Q., Wang, L., Tao, T., & Xu, B. (2013). Impacts of the "transport subsidy initiative on poor TB patients" in Rural China: A patient-cohort based longitudinal study in rural China. *PLoS One*, *8*(11), e82503. DOI: 10.1371/journal.pone.0082503 PMID: 24282623

Zheng, S., Gu, Y., Gu, Y., Zhao, Y., Li, L., Wang, M., Jiang, R., Yu, X., Chen, T., & Li, J. (2025). Machine learning–enabled virtual screening indicates the anti-tuberculosis activity of aldoxorubicin and quarfloxin with verification by molecular docking, molecular dynamics simulations, and biological evaluations. *Briefings in Bioinformatics*, *26*(1), bbae696. Advance online publication. DOI: 10.1093/bib/bbae696 PMID: 39737570

Zhou, F., Zhang, L., Gao, L., Hao, Y., Zhao, X., Liu, J., Lu, J., Li, X., Yang, Y., Chen, J., & Deng, Y. (2014). Latent tuberculosis infection and occupational protection among health care workers in two types of public hospitals in China. *PLoS One*, *9*(8), e104673. Advance online publication. DOI: 10.1371/journal.pone.0104673 PMID: 25157814

Zhuang, L., Ali, A., Yang, L., Ye, Z., Li, L., Ni, R., An, Y., Ali, S. L., & Gong, W. (2024). Leveraging computer-aided design and artificial intelligence to develop a next-generation multi-epitope tuberculosis vaccine candidate. *Infectious Medicine*, *3*(4), 100148. DOI: 10.1016/j.imj.2024.100148 PMID: 39687693

Zhu, H., Zhou, X., Zhuang, Z., Li, L., Bi, J., & Mi, K. (2023). Advances of new drugs bedaquiline and delamanid in the treatment of multi-drug resistant tuberculosis in children. *Frontiers in Cellular and Infection Microbiology*, *13*, 1183597. Advance online publication. DOI: 10.3389/fcimb.2023.1183597 PMID: 37384221

Zimenkov, D., Ushtanit, A., Gordeeva, E., Guselnikova, E., Schwartz, Y., & Stavitskaya, N. (2025). High prevalence of atpE mutations in bedaquiline-resistant *Mycobacterium tuberculosis* isolates, Russia. *Emerging Infectious Diseases*, *31*(3), 525–536. DOI: 10.3201/eid3103.241488 PMID: 40023803

Zong, Z., Huo, F., Shi, J., Jing, W., Ma, Y., Liang, Q., Jiang, G., Dai, G., Huang, H., & Pang, Y. (2018). Relapse Versus Reinfection of Recurrent Tuberculosis Patients in a National Tuberculosis Specialized Hospital in Beijing, China. *Frontiers in Microbiology, 9*. Advance online publication. DOI: 10.3389/fmicb.2018.01858 PMID: 30154770

Zulu, J. M., Maritim, P., Halwiindi, H., Chavula, M. P., Munakampe, M., Matenga, T. F. L., Mweemba, C., Sinyangwe, N. N., Habib, B., Musukuma, M., Silumbwe, A., Wang, B., Kaonga, P., Chewe, M., Fisa, R., Banda, J., Mubanga, A., & Phiri, H. (2024). Implementation strategies for decentralized management of multidrug-resistant tuberculosis: Insights from community health systems in Zambia. *Archives of Public Health = Archives Belges de Santé Publique, 82*(1), 157. DOI: 10.1186/s13690-024-01384-4 PMID: 39277746

Zuo, X., Dong, Z., Zhang, P., Zhu, X., Qiao, C., Yang, Y., & Lou, P. (2022). Cognitive-behavioral therapy on psychological stress and quality of life in subjects with pulmonary tuberculosis: A community-based cluster randomized controlled trial. *BMC Public Health, 22*(1), 2160. DOI: 10.1186/s12889-022-14631-6 PMID: 36419020

Zwerling, A., van den Hof, S., Scholten, J., Cobelens, F., Menzies, D., & Pai, M. (2012). Interferon-gamma release assays for tuberculosis screening of healthcare workers: A systematic review. *Thorax, 67*(1), 62–70. DOI: 10.1136/thx.2010.143180

About the Contributors

Sheehama J – Brief biography Qualifications: 1.Graduated with the Philosophy Doctor (PhD) in Biomedical Sciences at Kazan State University in Russia, 2008 2.High Education Pedagogy Post Graduate Diploma – Kazan State University, 2008 3.Graduated with the Master of Sciences in Medical Microbiology at Kazan State University in Rissia, 2005 4.Pre-University Certificate in Natural Sciences and Voronezh state University, Russia, 2000 Post Doctorate Training and Qualifications: 1.Commonwealth Professional Scholarship Award at Cardiff University, UK, 2019 – strengthening Health systems through training and research 2.UNESCO- Merck at Geneva, Switzerland, 2015 – Africa research capacity empowerment. 3.Postdoctoral Executive professional at Harvard School of Public Health, Boston, USA 2013- Building Design and Engineering Approaches to Airborne Infection Control 4.Management and Leadership Certificate at GiZ and HTV University, Saarland, Germany, 2011 - Health Project Management and Leadership 5.Postdoctoral Certificate; Health Management and Leadership in public health, University of Washington, USA, 2011 - Health Management and Leadership in public health: Work and Professional Experience: 1.Director University of Namibia HP & Oshakati Campuses 2021 – to date 2.President of Russian Alumni Association of Namibia 2018 – to date 3.Deputy Director Academic Affairs and Research; January 2016 – to Date, University of Namibia 4.Consultant – WHO: Namibia National TB Infection Prevention and Control Guidelines Review; August – September 2020 5.Honorary Senior Lecturer, Cardiff University, UK; June 2020 – to date 6.Consultant – WHO: AFRO II Integrated Vector borne diseases Management Project; October 2017 – February 2019 7.Coordinator School of Medicine and UNAM Health Sciences Northern Namibia Teaching Hospitals; January 2016 – to Date 8.Deputy Associate Dean, University of Namibia; June 2012 - December 2015 9.Senior Lecturer Biomedical Sciences, UNAM School of Medicine; August 2013 - to date 10.Head of Department Medical Microbiology UNAM School of Medicine; January 2012 – September 2012 11.Lecturer Biomedical Sciences (Medical Biochemistry,

Microbiology, Infection Control) UNAM School of Medicine; September 2009 – August 2013

***

Tarun Kumar Bhatt is an Associate Professor at the Central University of Rajasthan, India. His research focuses on clinical biotechnology, parasitology, in-silico and in-vitro drug screening, vaccine development, and parasite diagnostics. He has published widely in the field of malaria biology and molecular parasitology.

Samia Boussaa is currently Professor in ISPITS (Institut Supérieur des Professions Infirmières et des Techniques de Santé) of Rabat (Morocco). She obtained her PhD, in Ecology and Epidemiology, at Cadi Ayyad University (Morocco) and at Strasbourg University (France) in 2008. Her research is focused on Medical Entomology, Vector Borne Disease and especially on Epidemiology of leishmaniasis in Morocco.

Chakrapani Chaturvedi has a doctorate in community health nursing and is an accomplished professor of community health at the Faculty of Nursing, Banasthali Vidyapith, India. He had more than 15 years of expertise in primary healthcare services and participation in National Health programs He is highly regarded as an influential educator and community leader, actively contributing to grassroots health advancements. He is dedicated to improving the standard of nursing education and public health training. He is dedicated to enhancing community health results via education, service, research, and leadership.

Sakshi Chaturvedi is a distinguished associate professor in the nursing department at Banasthali Vidyapith, India. With more than 15 years of pedagogical experience, she has significantly contributed to nursing education and research while committing to the enhancement of primary care health services.

Shailendra Choudhary holds an Diploma in community medicine. He has vast experience in primary health care, district health administration, and the implementation of health care programs. He is a distinguished healthcare leader and administrator.

Ida Evangeline, presently working as an Assistant Professor in the Department of Electrical and Electronics Engineering at the Government College of Engineering, Tirunelveli, Tamilnadu, India. She obtained her Bachelor's in Electrical and Electronics Engineering from Manonmaniam Sundaranar University in 2003, and Master's in Power Systems Engineering from Anna University, Chennai, Tamilnadu,

India in 2005. She completed her PhD degree in 2023 at Anna University, Chennai, Tamilnadu, India. She has published six research papers in international journals. Her current research interests include optimal power flow, renewable energy, soft computing, machine learning, and deep learning.

Attuluri Vamsi Kumar is a faculty member in the Department of Medical Laboratory Sciences at the Regional Institute of Paramedical and Nursing Sciences (RIPANS), under the Ministry of Health & Family Welfare, Government of India. Based in Zemabawk, Mizoram, his work focuses on advancing diagnostic methodologies and strengthening laboratory education in resource-limited settings.

Ravinesh Mishra is currently working as Dean, School of Pharmacy and Emerging Sciences at Baddi University of Emerging Sciences and Technology, Baddi, Himachal Pradesh. He holds a B. Pharm. from CCS University (2003), M. Pharm. from Rajiv Gandhi University of Health Sciences, Bengaluru (2007), and Ph.D. in Pharmaceutical Sciences from Jamia Hamdard University, New Delhi (2011). With over 18 years of professional experience, Dr. Mishra has qualified GATE twice and was awarded the UGC and CSIR fellowships during his doctoral studies. He received the prestigious DST Young Scientist Award in 2010 and has also undergone short-term toxicological trainings. Dr. Mishra has made significant contributions to pharmaceutical research with over 80 publications, 14 patents, 3 books, and 10 book chapters to his credit. He has guided several M. Pharm students and Ph.D. scholars. His achievements have been recognized with awards from the Society of Toxicology and Therapeutic Drug Monitoring & Clinical Toxicology.

Archan Mitra is a dedicated and accomplished media and communication specialist with over 12 years of experience in academia, research, and industry. Expertise in teaching, research, and curriculum development, with significant contributions to the fields of journalism, mass communication, and environmental sustainability. Proven ability to lead interdisciplinary 4+ projects, such as the development of the GREEN MBA initiative for IIM Kashipur and World Bank and other digital education programs, showcasing a commitment to innovative pedagogy and sustainable practices. Published extensively, including 35+ Scopus-indexed articles and 10+ authored books on emerging topics such as artificial intelligence and media, New Media and digital transformation, Science Communication, and Environmental communication. Recognized for peer-review excellence with over 80+ journal reviews. Adept at leveraging advanced tools and technologies, including Adobe Creative Suite, SPSS, and multimedia platforms, to deliver impactful research and teaching outcomes. With specializing in NVIVO analysis. Strong academic leadership skills demonstrated through roles such as Research Coordinator and

Media Centre In-Charge, enhancing institutional outreach, accreditation, and student success. Passionate about bridging traditional and digital media paradigms, fostering inclusive learning environments, and contributing to sustainable development through scholarly work.

Debasis Mitra is a faculty member in the Department of Microbiology at Graphic Era (Deemed to be University), Dehradun, Uttarakhand, India. His research interests include medical microbiology, host–pathogen interactions, and microbial biotechnology. He has contributed to teaching and guiding students in microbiology and allied health sciences, and actively engages in academic and research activities aimed at advancing microbial sciences.

Dhruvi Patel is an Assistant Professor in Medical Laboratory Technology at Parul University, Vadodara. She specializes in clinical diagnostics and is committed to quality education in paramedical sciences.

Nivedita Priya is an Assistant Professor of Medical Biochemistry at the Parul Institute of Paramedical and Health Sciences, Faculty of Medicine, Parul University, Vadodara. Her research focuses on clinical biochemistry, with published studies on thyroid autoimmunity and iron-deficiency anemia.

Ruma Roy is a dynamic media professional with a strong academic foundation in Mass Communication and Journalism, having earned her postgraduate degree from Visva Bharati University and a gold medal in her undergraduate studies. She brings a diverse portfolio of experiences, including roles as a content moderator at ByteDance and a social media expert at Immigration Ultimate. With hands-on expertise in SEO, content moderation, social media management, and customer service, she is also proficient in tools like Adobe Premiere Pro, Photoshop, Canva, and MS Office Suite. Ruma is a dedicated team player, known for her discipline, adaptability, and relentless drive to acquire new skills across domains. Outside her professional pursuits, she is an accomplished classical dancer and award-winning painter with accolades from institutions like Pracheen Kala Kendra. Ruma blends creativity with strategic communication, making her a valuable asset in any multidisciplinary team.

Wasswa Shafik (Member, IEEE) received a Bachelor of Science degree in information technology from Ndejje University, Uganda, a Master of Engineering degree in Information Technology (Computer and Communication Networks) from Yazd University, Iran, and a PhD in Computer Science with the School of Digital Science, Universiti Brunei Darussalam, Brunei Darussalam. He is also the Founder and Research Director of the Dig Connectivity Research Laboratory (DCRLab) after serving as a Research Associate at the Network Interconnectivity Research Laboratory at Yazd University. Prior to this, he worked as a Community Data Analyst at Population Services International (PSI-Uganda), a Community Data Officer at the Programme for Accessible Health Communication (PACE-Uganda), a Research Assistant at the Socio-Economic Data Centre (SEDC-Uganda), Uganda, an Assistant Data Officer at TechnoServe, Kampala, Uganda, and Asmaah Charity Organization as Cheif Executive Officer. He has hundreds of publications with renowned publishers. His research interests include Artificial Intelligence, Neural Networks, Computer Vision, Smart Agriculture, Digital Health, and Green Computing.

Bhartendu Sharma is currently working as an Associate Professor, Head of Department, School of Pharmacy and Emerging Sciences at Baddi University of Emerging Sciences and Technology, Baddi, Himachal Pradesh. He holds M. Pharm in Pharmaceutical Chemistry and earned his Ph.D. in Pharmaceutical Sciences, bringing with him over 13 years of academic and research experience. Dr. Sharma has been actively involved in both teaching and research, contributing to the development of future pharmaceutical professionals. His areas of interest include drug design and synthesis, medicinal chemistry, and pharmaceutical analysis. He has guided numerous undergraduate, postgraduate and PhD scholars and is committed to fostering research-oriented learning. Over the years, he has contributed to several research publications in reputed journals and has participated in various national and international conferences. Dr. Sharma is dedicated to academic excellence, innovation in pharmaceutical education, and continuous professional development.

Priya Sharma is currently working as an Assistant Professor, School of Pharmacy and Emerging Sciences at Baddi University of Emerging Sciences and Technology, Baddi, Himachal Pradesh. She holds M. Pharm in Pharmaceutics and earned her Ph.D. in Pharmaceutical Sciences. With over 5 years of academic and research experience, she is actively involved in both teaching and guiding students in the field of pharmaceutical sciences. Her core areas of interest include novel drug delivery systems, formulation and development, and pharmaceutical technology. She has participated in several national/ international conferences and workshops, and is committed to continuous learning and innovation in pharmaceutical education. Dr. Sharma has also contributed to research publications and is keen on expanding her research profile through interdisciplinary collaborations.

Ajay K. Singh is working as an Associate Professor (Research) in the Department of Humanities and Social Science, Graphic Era (Deemed to be University) Dehradun. He has worked as Assistant Professor (Economics) in the School of Liberal Arts & Management, DIT University Dehradun for 6 years. He did Post-Doctorate Research with EDI of India, Ahmedabad, Gujarat (India). He received MPhil (Economics) from DAVV Indore (India), and PhD (Economics) from IIT Indore (India. He has published several research papers in the diversified area such as climate change, agricultural productivity, assessment of food security; estimation of GFSI, development of environmental sustainability index (ESI) and its association with socio-economic indicators; measurement and determinants of entrepreneurship ecosystem, and dimension of sustainable development and its interlinkages with economic development.

Ukbe Sirayder is an Assistant Professor in the Department of Physiotherapy and Rehabilitation at Nuh Naci Yazgan University, Kayseri, Türkiye, where he also serves as the Head of Department. He completed his master's and doctoral studies in Cardiopulmonary Rehabilitation at Hacettepe University. His academic and research interests include cardiopulmonary rehabilitation, exercise physiology, and clinical applications in physical therapy. Dr. Sirayder is actively involved in teaching, research, and professional development activities aimed at advancing evidence-based rehabilitation practices.

Arti Thakur is an Associate Professor at the Institute of Allied Health Sciences, Desh Bhagat University, Mandi Gobindgarh. She specialises in clinical diagnostics and is dedicated to advancing education and research in paramedical sciences.

R. Vallipriya has been working in the Department of Physical Sciences at the Institute of Education (Affiliated to Tamilnadu Teacher Education University) as an Assistant Professor. With a wealth of experience, Mrs. R.Vallipriya has accumulated 12 years of extensive teaching. Her scholarly contributions include publishing 7 papers, with 1 peer review in various UGC-CARE, SCOPUS, and peer-reviewed journals.

Srinivasan Vasan is an Assistant Professor in the Department of Humanities and Social Sciences at Graphic Era (Deemed to be University), with 14 years of teaching and field expertise. He has served in the Ministry of Health and Family Welfare, as a Guest Faculty, and as a Mobilization Training Specialist with the State Government. Recently, he contributed to a tuberculosis project funded by GFATM and USAID. He has published 60 papers, with 20 more under peer review in UGC-CARE and SCOPUS journals.

Index

A

B

C

D

E

G

H

I

L

M

N

O

P

R

S

T

V

X

www.ingramcontent.com/pod-product-compliance
Lightning Source LLC
LaVergne TN
LVHW062335300926
849161LV00007B/1703